ATLAS OF
PEDIATRIC
ORTHOPEDIC
SURGERY

ATLAS OF
PEDIATRIC
ORTHOPEDIC
SURGERY

Volume II

MIHRAN O. TACHDJIAN, M.D.

Professor of Orthopedic Surgery
Northwestern University Medical School
Attending Orthopedic Surgeon
The Children's Memorial Hospital
Chicago, Illinois

W.B. SAUNDERS COMPANY
A Division of Harcourt Brace & Company

Philadelphia   London   Montreal   Toronto   Sydney   Tokyo

W.B. SAUNDERS COMPANY
A Division of
Harcourt Brace & Company

The Curtis Center
Independence Square West
Philadelphia, Pennsylvania 19106

Library of Congress Cataloging-in-Publication Data

Tachdjian, Mihran O.
Atlas of pediatric orthopedic surgery/Mihran O. Tachdjian.—1st ed.

p. cm.

ISBN 0–7216–3733–7

1. Pediatric orthopedics—Atlases.   I. Title.
[DNLM: 1. Orthopedics—in infancy & childhood—atlases.
WS 17 T117a 1994]

RD732.3.C48T328 1994

617.3′0083—dc20

DNLM/DLC   93–31640

Volume One   ISBN 0–7216–5448–7
Volume Two   ISBN 0–7216–5449–5
Two Volume Set   ISBN 0–7216–3733–7

ATLAS OF PEDIATRIC ORTHOPEDIC SURGERY

Printed in the United States of America

Last digit is the print number: 9   8   7   6   5   4   3   2   1

Dedicated to Dr. Paul P. Griffin

. . . my close friend,
who has devoted his life to teaching
and the care of the disabled child
and who is a master of the art of
the practice of pediatric orthopedic surgery.

Preface

This atlas describes and illustrates the standard and attested operative procedures performed in pediatric orthopedics. Of the surgical techniques described, 124 are taken from the second edition of *Pediatric Orthopedics;* these have been revised. One hundred thirty-two new surgical procedures have been added.

The resident and fellow in training will learn details of surgical technique by first observing, next assisting, and then operating under the supervision of an experienced surgeon and teacher. This atlas is intended to serve as a guide; modifications can be made, depending on the individual deformity, findings at surgery, and complexity of the problem. Each operative case is different. One should follow the principles that are based on biologic facts and past experience of successful surgery. It is vital to pay meticulous attention to detail—preoperatively, at surgery, and postoperatively.

On the page opposite each plate, indications, requisites, and requirements for blood for transfusion, image intensifier radiographic control, or special instrumentation are listed for each procedure. Preoperative planning is crucial!

In the beginning of the atlas I have given an overview of the total care of the child and some practical points of basic surgical technique. The practice of orthopedic surgery is an art. The operative procedure is only a portion of what is involved in the management of the whole child.

Preparation of this atlas has been a challenging task. I have tried to describe and illustrate my preferred methods of operative procedures learned from personal experience for the past four decades. I hope that the reader will find it useful as a guide to the surgical care of children with neuromusculoskeletal disorders.

MIHRAN O. TACHDJIAN

Acknowledgments

I wish to thank the three new illustrators of this atlas, Ms. Marguerite Aitken, Ms. Cynthia Eller, and Ms. Janice Ruvido, with whom I have greatly enjoyed working. I am also greatly indebted to the late Mr. Ernie Beck, whose superb artistry has been a landmark for medical illustrators.

I also thank the staff at W. B. Saunders for their efforts.

Special thanks to Dr. Robert Winter for his assistance in preparing the chapter on the spine.

Finally, I would like to express my deep gratitude to Mrs. Lynn Ridings, without whose editorial assistance and collaboration this difficult task would not have come to fruition.

Principles of the Practice of Pediatric Orthopedic Surgery

The practice of surgery is an art as well as a science. The following practical points and general principles of surgery are presented for the sake of thoroughness in provision of total care to the child.

INDICATIONS AND OBJECTIVES OF SURGERY

Objectives and indications for surgery should be clearly defined, discussed with the parents and patient, and recorded. Explain clearly what you propose to do, the reasons for performing the operation, and the results to be expected. Be realistic in your goals. Alternate methods of management should be discussed and reasons given why you propose to perform the operative procedure for that particular problem. Often the parents and patient want to know the natural history of the deformity if left untreated. Is open surgery absolutely necessary? Can the deformity be corrected by intensive physical therapy, casts, or orthotic devices? Prolonged immobilization in cast causes muscle atrophy and joint contracture, whereas early open surgery will rapidly correct deformity and restore function. The effectiveness and safety of surgery and its advantages and disadvantages should be compared with that of nonoperative methods of management. The philosophy and practice among most physicians is that nonsurgical methods of treatment should always be tried initially and only after they fail should operative procedures be employed. In certain deformities, however, such as rigid intrinsic talipes equinovarus, surgery is more conservative and simpler than nonoperative methods of management.

Parents often like to know the worst outcome that can occur following surgery. *Non nocere*—Do no harm!—is one of the basic requisites of surgery. The problems, complications, and dangers of the operation should be clearly explained to the parents and to the adolescent patient.

TIMING OF THE OPERATION

Timing is important. What is the best age? Should a clubfoot be corrected surgically at three months, six months, or one year of age? Should a congenital high scapula be transferred distally at one year or at three years of age? What are the risks of early surgery versus the drawbacks of postponing it to a later date? For example, a septic hip should be drained immediately because it is an emergency procedure; a heel cord lengthening to correct equinus deformity in spastic cerebral palsy should be delayed until the child is three to four years of age, when adequate postoperative care can be provided.

SEQUENCE OF OPERATIVE PROCEDURES

When involvement is bilateral, should you operate on both sides during the same procedure or should you stage them? What should be the interval between the two operations? A child may need two, three, or more surgical procedures for treatment of a complex problem. For example, with a high dislocation of a hip (antenatal or teratologic), open reduction with femoral shortening and possibly innominate osteotomy are needed; should you operate on both hips on the same day or stagger them two or three weeks apart? Most surgeons prefer to stage such extensive operative procedures, whereas a patient with spastic cerebral palsy can readily tolerate multilevel surgery, such as bilateral hip adductor myotomy, iliopsoas tenotomy and hamstring and heel cord lengthening. Some surgeons prefer to operate on both feet for correction of talipes equinovarus at the same sitting; others prefer to stage the procedures because of the potential for excessive blood loss and the necessity for blood transfusion with its inherent risks.

BLOOD LOSS

Blood loss may be significant during a major orthopedic operation. An estimate of the probable amount of blood loss should be forecast and arrangements made for obtaining adequate blood and cross-matching. In the modern era of autoimmune deficiency (human immunodeficiency virus, or HIV) syndrome and hepatitis B, the family should be given the option to donate blood by a designated donor or, in the older patient, to have autologous blood available. As a general policy, a patient who is donating autologous blood should weigh at least 110 pounds and be 17 years of age. He may be younger with parental consent. A red blood cell saver may be used, especially in spine surgery. Arrangements should be made in advance for the blood saver and its possible problems, and complications should be discussed with the family and patient. Certain religious groups, such as Jehovah's Witnesses, will refuse blood transfusion. This can create special problems, which should be handled individually.

PREOPERATIVE LABORATORY STUDIES

Preoperative studies should consist of a complete blood count and urinalysis.

Sickle Cell Disease

For African American children, a sickle cell preparation should be arranged when scheduling the operation. Order it far ahead of the day of surgery. If findings are positive, a hemoglobin electrophoresis should be done to determine the exact hemoglobinopathy. It behooves the surgeon to remember that a sickle cell test may be negative in an infant under four months of age but can subsequently change to positive; therefore, a negative sickle cell preparation in a young infant needs to be performed again when he or she is older.

Pregnancy Test

A pregnancy test in teenagers who have reached menarche is appropriate, provided that first a recent menstrual history is taken and the patient and parents are informed. A routine chest radiogram should not be made unless there is cardiopulmonary pathology. HIV and hepatitis B screenings are still a controversial issue.

Contagious Diseases

It is vital to inquire whether the child has been recently exposed to a contagious disease, such as chickenpox or measles. A child would be extremely uncomfortable in a cast with the skin lesions caused by these diseases.

Allergies and Medications

The surgeon should know whether the child has any allergies, whether he or she has been or is presently taking medication, and whether there have been any adverse reactions to the drugs. Most importantly, ask whether there has been any unusual bruising or bleeding; it is best to detect a bleeding disorder *before* surgery. Ask about previous surgical procedures and how they were tolerated. A family history of difficulty with surgery or anesthesia should be investigated.

Latex gloves and other products, such as Penrose drains, should not be used for patients with myelomeningocele during surgery because of the great probability of allergy and anaphylactic shock. It is best to use non-latex gloves, such as those made of neoprene. Other patients who may have similar allergies to latex products include those who have experienced multiple catheterizations and latex exposure.

Chronic Illness

Chronically ill patients who have been taking long-term medication require special preoperative assessment and laboratory studies. For patients with cerebral palsy and other central nervous system disorders who are taking seizure medications, a recent neurologic assessment and blood level determinations of anticonvulsant medications are indicated. After neurologic clearance—and if the blood levels of the medications are within normal, not toxic ranges—the child should take seizure medication on the morning of surgery with a small sip of water. It is my policy that children who are receiving anti-seizure medication see the anesthesiologist preoperatively because many of these medications can affect cardiopulmonary, liver, and kidney function and blood coagulation. The anesthesiologist should be familiar with the patient's history long before the day of surgery. Children with shunts should be provided with appropriate neurosurgical consultation.

Asthma

Asthmatic children require special preoperative assessment by an allergist to determine whether their medications are adequate. In the past, it was a common practice to start an aminophylline infusion; however, this rarely is needed now because beta$_2$ agonists, like nebulized albuterol, are very effective and less cardiotoxic. Nebulized albuterol is often provided just before surgery.

Occasionally, children with asthma may require prednisone treatment several days prior to surgery. Patients who have received steroid therapy treatment for rheumatoid arthritis, asthma, or organ transplantation during the past year require administration of steroids perioperatively.

Diabetes

The diabetic patient who is insulin-dependent will require glucose infusion and insulin injection in divided doses administered the day before surgery, during surgery, and postoperatively. The primary physician in charge of medication management should be the endocrinologist or pediatrician, who, in conjunction with the anesthesiologist, will plan the perioperative management.

Patients who have received *salicylates* or *nonsteroidal anti-inflammatory agents,* such as tolmetin sodium (tolectin), naprosyn, or ibuprofen, may experience bleeding problems on the operating table. It is best to stop such medications three to four weeks before surgery.

Prematurity

Premature infants up to six months of age are at high risk for apnea spells during recovery and postoperatively. They should be admitted and observed with an apnea monitor for at least 12 hours. Do not schedule the premature baby for outpatient surgery; however, a morning admission on the day of surgery can be arranged.

Upper Respiratory Disease

The most common problem associated with an anesthetic concerns patients with upper respiratory infection, including coughing, rhinorrhea, and pulmonary congestion. These children are at high risk for airway obstruction, laryngospasm, and a stormy anesthetic course. They should not be anesthetized until after the symptoms have disappeared unless it is an emergency.

Malignant Hyperthermia

Because malignant hyperthermia is a very serious complication of some anesthetics, it is crucial to interrogate the family about any temperature control problems, any difficulties with previous operations or anesthesia, or symptoms compatible with the syndrome in the patient, the parents, and immediate family. The surgeon must remember that patients with malignant hyperthermia syndrome show a greater incidence of kyphoscoliosis, clubfoot, winged scapula, hyperlaxity of joints, and repeated dislocations than do healthy children. As a rule, I recommend that children with myopathies, arthrogryposis, and central core disease also be managed as if they are in the high-risk group.

Atlantoaxial Instability

Atlantoaxial instability can be a serious problem, such as in Down syndrome, skeletal dysplasias (such as Morquio's disease), and rheumatoid arthritis. It is vital to assess stability of the cervical spine by flexion-extension views and magnetic resonance imaging (MRI) studies.

Physical Health

When elective surgical procedures are to be performed, it is prudent to have the patient in the best physical condition possible. If in doubt, obtain preoperative pediatric and anesthesia consultations. The anesthesiologist should discuss risks of anesthesia with the family.

PREOPERATIVE ORTHOPEDIC CONSULTATION

When a surgical procedure is being discussed with the family and patient, the approximate site and length of incisions should be mentioned. Often an adolescent is more concerned with the cosmesis of the scar than the surgery itself. The possibility of a drain and the type and extent of cast immobilization—below-knee, above-knee, or hip spica—should be discussed: I also give my patients a choice of color of cast. Other details of interest are whether the child will be able to bear full weight or whether crutches with partial or non-weight bearing will be used. Instructing the child in how to walk with crutches before surgery is much simpler than teaching the patient who is in discomfort in the cast after surgery. The expected total length of time in the cast should be estimated and the physical therapy program after cast removal outlined. If internal fixation devices are to be used, explain when removal will be necessary, what is involved, whether a general or local anesthetic with sedation will be used, and whether or not another cast will be applied. Mention the possibility that you may not be able to remove the fixation device or that it may break.

When special physical or occupational therapy is required, especially after surgery for neuromuscular disorders such as cerebral palsy or myelomeningocele, it is best that the postoperative therapy program be outlined and discussed by the physical therapist and occupational therapist and the appropriate arrangements made. A patient-therapist and surgeon-therapist rapport should be established to ensure optimal results.

Discuss the length of the hospital stay, and indicate whether the parents can stay with the child. The child should be allowed to bring an object of comfort, such as a favorite teddy bear or blanket. Address the transport of the child from the hospital to the home and any special equipment required in the home, such as a sitting or reclining wheelchair or hospital bed with a trapeze, or whether the child will be in home traction. The discharge nurse from the hospital should be involved preoperatively to assist in solving difficult problems of home management.

Because the nursing staff interacts with the patients and families more than any other members of the health care team, they are in the best position to provide the physician with information regarding obvious or subtle changes in a patient's condition or response to treatment. It is therefore essential that the nurses and physicians maintain an environment that is conducive to collaboration in an effort to best meet the physical as well as psychosocial needs of the patients and their families.

PAIN CONTROL

A great concern for children and their families is postoperative pain. Assure these patients that they will be made as comfortable as possible but that a slight degree of discomfort is desirable to prevent total inactivity, atelectasis, and pulmonary complications. At present, patient-controlled analgesia in the older child and adolescent is used. The anesthesiologist may perform one caudal anesthetic injection at the end of surgery to provide significant analgesia for lower extremity procedures that lasts for several hours postoperatively. Epidural anesthesia has its drawbacks, especially because there is a potential for compartment syndrome following procedures such as osteotomy of the tibia. It is best that the anesthesiologist be involved in the discussion of postoperative pain control with the family, patient, and surgeon.

If possible, arrangements should be made for the parents to bring the child to the operating room and recovery area preoperatively so that the child is familiarized with the area.

PSYCHOLOGIC STATE OF THE PATIENT

The patient's psychologic state is not always easy to assess, but it is important, particularly when the child's cooperation is required after surgery. The adequacy of postoperative care often dictates the difference between success or failure of a surgical procedure, especially one affecting the muscular system.

HOME AND FAMILY SITUATION

The family should be well informed and prepared for provision of an intensive postoperative care and therapy training program. These questions should be addressed: Who will take care of the child after discharge? Are both parents working, or is there a single parent? How interested are they in the child?

OUTPATIENT PROCEDURES

Outpatient surgery has become very popular because of the demands of insurance companies to curtail health care costs. There are advantages and disadvantages. It minimizes the disturbances of life for the patient and family. However, there is increased risk of postoperative complications from early discharge. *The surgeon should demand and dictate what is best for the child.*

The prerequisites for outpatient surgery are as follows:

1. The child should be in good general health, with only a minimal possibility of surgical and anesthesia problems and complications arising.

2. The procedure should not be very painful; only minimal medication for pain control, such as simple acetaminophen (Tylenol) or Tylenol with codeine, is anticipated.

3. The patient should not be sent home with a drain.

Before discharge, it is vital that the patient be fully awake and responsive, is not vomiting, and can tolerate oral fluids. Neurovascular function should be normal. If in doubt, the cast must be bivalved. Clear instructions should be given, preferably in writing as to cast or wound care and when to return for follow-up. The patient and family should understand the potential complications that can develop and they should be reported.

PATIENT TRANSFER

During transfer of the patient from the waiting-holding area to the operating room, it is reassuring and comforting to the patient and the parents if the surgeon accompanies and assists in this move. The surgeon should again confirm with the parents and patient that the correct limb is being operated on. The surgeon should reiterate the expected length of time during which the patient will be in the operating room and that the parents will be able to speak with the surgeon after the procedure. A few words of assurance, such as, "I'll take good care of Billy—don't worry," will relax the nervous parents and patient.

THE OPERATING ROOM

When the child is wheeled to the operating room, there should be a professional demeanor, an atmosphere of tranquility, and a minimum level of noise. Demand that the assisting staff turn off loud music. Assist in transferring the patient to the operating table. Provide for the privacy of the patient by appropriate cover by sheets or clothing. If radiograms are to be made during surgery, be sure that the table is radiolucent. The radiopaque strips of the heating pad will obscure the operative site; pull them out of the field proximally—this is a problem, particularly with hip surgery.

Before anesthetizing the patient, be sure the image intensifier machine is functioning and a competent x-ray technician is available. When scheduling, specify image intensifier radiographic control. If only one or two machines are available, the orchestration of cases is important.

Do not anesthetize the child unless recent radiograms are on the x-ray viewing box and you personally verify and check the correct limb and site of surgery. Bring the pertinent office or outpatient preoperative notes to the operating room. It is the personal responsibility of the surgeon to see that the correct limb is operated on. Do not depend on the operating room schedule, the nursing staff, or resident staff.

After the proper level of anesthesia is achieved, if tourniquet ischemia is to be used, the surgeon should personally supervise or apply the tourniquet and the level of tourniquet pressure.

PATIENT POSITION

The surgeon directs the proper positioning of the patient on the operating table. Secure the proper posture by sandbags or adhesive strapping. Bony prominences are adequately padded to prevent pressure sores. Nerves, such as the ulnar nerve at the elbow or the common peroneal nerve at the fibular head-neck, must be relieved of all pressure. When the patient is placed on a fracture table, the greater sciatic notch and perineum should be well padded. Discuss any special positions, such as prone or lateral, with the anesthesiologist before the anesthetic is administered.

SPECIAL INSTRUMENTATION

When an operative procedure is expected to take more than two hours, insert a Foley catheter into the bladder for urine drainage. Catheterization is carried out under sterile conditions.

The surgeon should consult with the operating room nurse well in advance of the surgery time so that the proper instruments can be obtained and sterilized. This is particularly true when special instruments are required for a particular operation. Such planning ahead will prevent unnecessary delay during surgery.

THE INCISION

In planning the site and extent of the incision, the surgeon should obtain adequate exposure but should not ignore cosmesis. The appearance of the scar should be pleasing, not unsightly. Draw the proposed incision with a sterile pencil. As a rule, straight incisions look less conspicuous than S-shaped or curved ones. When making an ilioinguinal approach to the hip, use Salter's "bikini" incision, not that described for a Smith-Peterson approach. Also, a transverse adductor incision is preferable to that of a longitudinal one in adductor myotomy of the hip. When performing a procedure around the upper arm, employ an axillary medial incision if possible. For wound closure, use the subcuticular technique; an absorbable suture may be used in the fearful child. I prefer 00 subcuticular nylon; it is very easy to remove, causes little pain, and avoids problems of foreign body reaction, allergy, and rejection and discharge of absorbable suture material.

OPERATIVE TECHNIQUE

Gentle handling of tissues is vital. Rough and forceful retraction of skin and muscles causes tissue necrosis and increases the chance of infection. Atraumatic technique is the hallmark of a good surgeon. The growth plate and articular cartilage are sacred; they should not be injured.

Repeat irrigation of the wound during surgery removes all debris and dead tissue. Blood vessels should be clamped and coagulated before division; such a technique controls bleeding and conserves blood. Venous drainage of the limb should be preserved as much as possible. Do not divide sensory nerves. After completion of the operation prior to wound closure, the wound is thoroughly irrigated and Ace bandage compression is applied and the tourniquet released. The wound should be completely dry before closure. Insert closed suction drainage in all cases, particularly when bone work has been performed. Blood oozing from the divided surfaces of cancellous bone will cause hematoma and infection.

A fast surgeon who is fighting the clock is not necessarily technically superb. Manual dexterity and eye-hand coordination are important. Plan and think ahead. A surgeon and the assistants should know the steps of the procedure. The competent surgeon knows what to do and how to do it. The scrub nurse should anticipate the needs of the surgeon and should be prepared to hand over the next instrument before being asked for it. Such teamwork can decrease the actual operating time.

IMMOBILIZATION IN A CAST

Operations on bones and joints often necessitate immobilization in a cast. Children ordinarily do not respect Ace or other bandages; they take them off. Therefore, the surgeon may prefer to use a cast as a method of postoperative dressing and support. The trauma of repeated dressing care and bandage changes is more disturbing to a child than cast care. Frequently I recommend the use of a posterior cast mold and Ace bandage support if postoperative swelling is anticipated; this is particularly important when there is a possibility of compartment syndrome, such as following osteotomy of the tibia or both bones of the forearm. The splint is applied in the operating room, and before the child goes home, a plaster of Paris or plastic cast is applied. All bony prominences and nerves should be adequately padded, and the cast should be well molded.

The parents and patients are indoctrinated on cast care; written instructions are provided. I insist that parents sign a statement that written instructions on cast care and details of postoperative care, such as when to be seen again, have been provided. There should be no diversity of opinion between the surgeon, resident, nurse, or therapist. Instructions given should be uniform.

THE OPERATIVE RECORD

The operation should be dictated in detail. The operative record includes the following: (1) name of the patient, (2) medical record number, (3) name of attending physician, (4) name of assisting physician, (5) preoperative diagnosis, (6) postoperative diagnosis, (7) indications for surgery, (8) surgical procedures performed, (9) alternate methods of management, (10) possible problems and complications, (11) type of anesthesia, (12) position of the patient, (13) technique of preparing the operative site, (14) surgical exposure, (15) findings at surgery, (16) operative procedure, (17) total tourniquet time and pressure, (18) blood loss, (19) wound closure, (20) sponge count, (21) cast application and dressings, (22) return visit or readmission, and (23) weight-bearing status.

PHYSIOTHERAPY AND OCCUPATIONAL THERAPY

The therapist is a vital member of the team who provides care of the patient's neuromusculoskeletal system. It is beyond the scope of this volume to cover details of therapy. The therapist should be involved preoperatively and should develop a working relationship and communication between the child and parent. It is unfortunate that most orthopedic residents have a limited knowledge of the usefulness of physiotherapy and occupational therapy; such modalities of therapy in the child are different from those of the adult.

The surgeon and therapist should work together. For neuromuscular disorders and complex problems of the upper and lower limbs, I strongly recommend that the therapist assess the child preoperatively and be involved in the decision-making process. In certain cases, I invite the therapist to come to the operating room and observe surgery. Such a professional working relationship between the therapist and surgeon should improve the overall care of the child.

When making a request for physical or occupational therapy, include the following: diagnosis, aim of treatment, previous treatment (especially surgery), and special precautions. Attach a copy of the office notes and operative report for the therapist's information.

Always remember to show warmth, gentleness, and consideration of the child as a whole person. An orthopedic surgeon must remember that there is a fourth dimension to pediatric orthopedic surgery—growth. Treatment is not concluded until the child becomes an adult.

Contents

Volume II

10   Spine

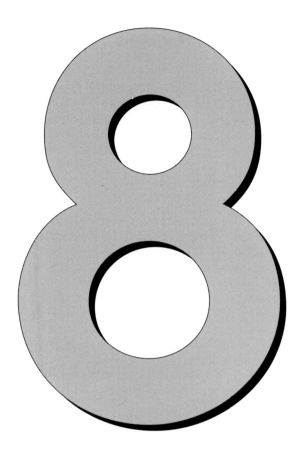

Leg

PLATE 150 **Brown's Femorofibular Arthroplasty with Shortening of the Upper Fibular Shaft**

Indications. Bilateral complete absence or longitudinal deficiency with a functional foot and adequate motor strength in the quadriceps femoris and hamstrings. Determine the pathologic anatomic dysfunction by magnetic resonance imaging. Brown's procedure is controversial; some surgeons prefer bilateral knee disarticulation.

Patient Position. Supine.

Operative Technique

A. A lazy S–shaped incision is made. It begins laterally and distally at the junction of the upper one fourth and lower three fourths of the fibula and extends proximally to the knee joint level, where it curves medially and then upward to the lower fourth of the thigh. Subcutaneous tissue is divided in line with the skin incision. The skin flaps are developed and retracted. (*Note*: In Brown's original description, a U-shaped incision was made on the anterior aspect of the knee joint; this makes exposure of the upper part of the fibula and fibular shortening very difficult.)

B. Next, the patella and patellar tendon are identified, and a longitudinal incision is made through the capsular structures lateral to the patella.

C. The patellar tendon is traced as far distally as possible, sectioned at its lowest point, and reflected proximally. The knee joint capsule is incised, and the lower end of the femur is exposed.

D. By blunt and sharp dissection, the upper fibular shaft is exposed. Stay anterior to avoid injury to the common peroneal nerve. About 0.5 to 1 cm. of the tip of the epiphysis is resected to create a flat surface at the upper end of the fibula.

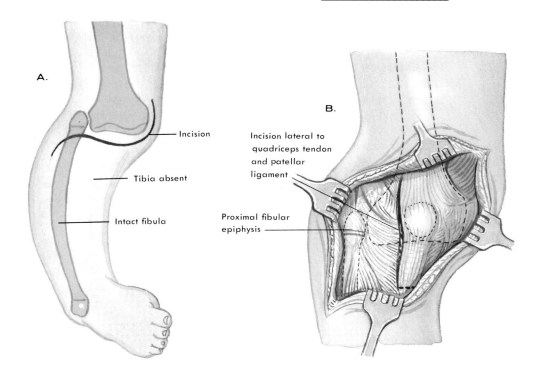

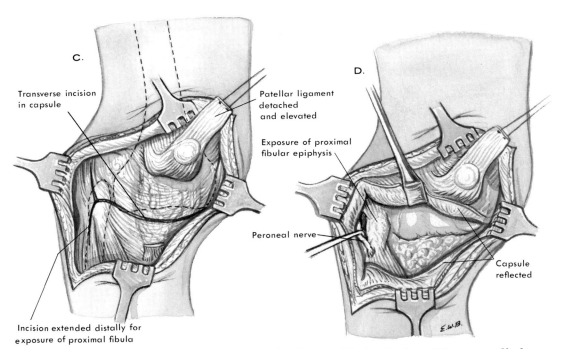

Plate 150. A.–H., Brown's femorofibular arthroplasty with shortening of the upper fibular shaft.

E. One to 2 cm. of the upper diaphysis of the fibula is resected at its metaphyseal junction, and all soft-tissue attachments between the upper end of the fibula and the distal femur are released. The upper segment of the fibula is placed in weight-bearing alignment below the femoral condyles.

F. An intramedullary Steinmann pin is inserted into the fibular segments and driven into the femoral condyle in the intercondylar notch.

G. and **H.** The patellar tendon is reattached, and the quadriceps mechanism is repaired. The wound is closed in the usual manner, and a hip spica cast is applied for immobilization.

Postoperative Care. In about four to six weeks the intramedullary pin is removed, and an above-knee cast is applied for an additional two to four weeks until the fibular osteotomy is healed. After removal of the cast, passive and active exercises are gradually instituted to restore range of motion of the knee and to develop motor strength of the quadriceps muscle.

Initially, the limb is supported in an above-knee orthosis with a drop lock knee and a plastic ankle-foot component to maintain alignment of the foot and knee. Splinting at night is continued for a prolonged period; this prevents the development of a flexion contracture of the knee and varus deviation of the foot and ankle.

REFERENCES

Brown, F. W.: Construction of a knee joint in congenital total absence of the tibia. A preliminary report. J. Bone Joint Surg., 47-A:695, 1965.

Brown, F. W.: The Brown operation for total hemimelia tibia. *In*: Aitken, G. T. (ed.): Selected Lower Limb Anomalies. National Academy of Sciences, 1971, pp. 20–28.

Brown, F. W., and Pohnert, W. H.: Construction of a knee joint in meromelia tibia (congenital absence of the tibia). A 15-year follow-up study. J. Bone Joint Surg., 54-A:1333, 1972.

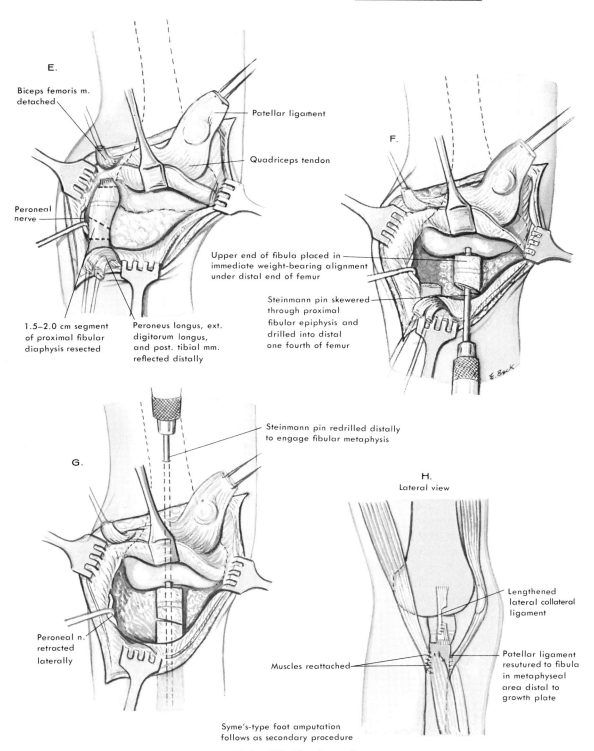

E.

Biceps femoris m. detached

Patellar ligament

Quadriceps tendon

Peroneal nerve

Upper end of fibula placed in immediate weight-bearing alignment under distal end of femur

Steinmann pin skewered through proximal fibular epiphysis and drilled into distal one fourth of femur

1.5–2.0 cm segment of proximal fibular diaphysis resected

Peroneus longus, ext. digitorum longus, and post. tibial mm. reflected distally

F.

G.

Steinmann pin redrilled distally to engage fibular metaphysis

H.
Lateral view

Peroneal n. retracted laterally

Lengthened lateral collateral ligament

Muscles reattached

Patellar ligament resutured to fibula in metaphyseal area distal to growth plate

Syme's-type foot amputation follows as secondary procedure

Plate 150. (Continued)

PLATE 151   Valgization Osteotomy of the Proximal Tibia to Correct Tibia Vara Using Plate and Screws

Indications

1. A child four years of age or older with stage II or III Langenskiöld tibia vara deformity with a tibiofemoral angle greater than 15 degrees, a metaphyseal-diaphyseal angle of 14 degrees or greater, and an epiphyseal-metaphyseal angle of 40 degrees or more.

2. Stage IV Langenskiöld tibia vara deformity with impending closure of a medial physis of the upper tibia. Operate before the age of eight years. In a child nine years and older, there is considerable recurrence of deformity with a guarded prognosis.

Radiographic Control. Image intensifier.

Patient Position. The patient is placed in the supine position, and the entire lower limb is prepared and draped. A sterile pneumatic tourniquet is used for proper visualization and determination of the biomechanical axis of the hip, thigh, knee, and ankle.

Operative Technique

A. and **B.** First, an oblique osteotomy of the fibula is performed through a separate 3- to 4-cm. lateral incision at the juncture of its proximal and distal thirds. Avoid injury to the peroneal nerve.

Then, through an anterolateral incision, the proximal metaphysis and upper portion of the tibial diaphysis are subperiosteally exposed. It is crucial to stay in a subperiosteal plane to avoid vascular injury. The level of osteotomy is below the insertion of the patellar tendon. Do not damage the proximal tibial physis and the anterior apophyseal extension of the proximal tibial tuberosity. If in doubt, it is best to confirm the level of osteotomy by radiograms. Next, a threaded Steinmann pin of appropriate diameter is inserted through the midshaft of the tibia, parallel to the ankle joint, and another threaded Steinmann pin is inserted through the proximal tibial metaphysis parallel to the knee joint. With a "starter" and drill holes, the line of a cuneiform osteotomy is outlined; the medial limb of the buttress is in the proximal fragment to ensure locking of the fragments.

C. and **D.** The osteotomy is completed with sharp chisels. The distal fragment is angulated laterally and rotated outward, correcting both the varus and the medial rotation deformity. With medial sliding of the upper end of the shaft in the concave surface of the metaphyseal fragment, stable contact of the osteotomized fragments is obtained. It is important to obtain mild valgus angulation of 5 to 10 degrees. Do not place the tibia in marked valgus. Next, the osteotomized tibial fragments are transfixed with criss-cross threaded Steinmann pins, and anteroposterior and lateral radiograms are made with the knee in full extension (including the knee and ankle) to document the degree of correction into physiologic valgus. Obtain long films to assess alignment of the mechanical axis of the lower limb. In unilateral tibia vara, the two limbs should be carefully compared to see that they are symmetrical. In bilateral involvement, each knee and tibia should be placed in physiologic genu valgum. It is important to provide symmetry to the limbs.

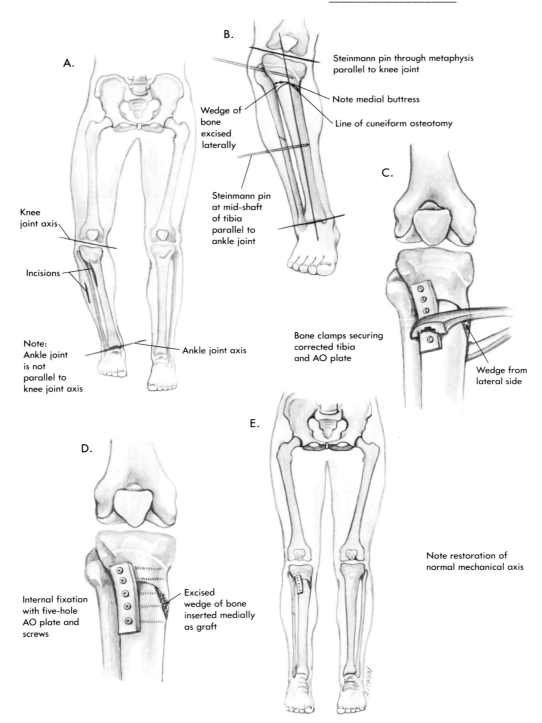

A. Knee joint axis

Incisions

Note: Ankle joint is not parallel to knee joint axis

Ankle joint axis

B. Steinmann pin through metaphysis parallel to knee joint

Note medial buttress

Line of cuneiform osteotomy

Wedge of bone excised laterally

Steinmann pin at mid-shaft of tibia parallel to ankle joint

C. Bone clamps securing corrected tibia and AO plate

Wedge from lateral side

D. Internal fixation with five-hole AO plate and screws

Excised wedge of bone inserted medially as graft

E. Note restoration of normal mechanical axis

Plate 151. A.–E., Valgization osteotomy of the proximal tibia to correct tibia vara using plate and screws.

This author recommends internal fixation with an AO five-hole compression plate that is placed laterally. Some surgeons may prefer to place the plate medially because of the simplicity of its application; this author has found subcutaneous position of the plate bothersome to some patients.

Prior to internal fixation the tourniquet should be released and the circulatory status of the limb is carefully ascertained; entrapment of the anterior tibial artery where it passes through the interosseous membrane should be ruled out. Determine anterior and lateral compartment pressure if vascular status is in question. If there is circulatory compromise, the limb should be returned immediately to the uncorrected position. Peroneal nerve injury is ordinarily not a problem following proximal tibial osteotomy to correct varus.

If the circulation of the limb is normal, the tibial fragments are fixed with the AO compression plate. The excised wedge is used as bone graft to fill in the defect created medially.

Some surgeons prefer internal fixation with criss-cross threaded Steinmann pins. They find this method of fixation adequate; however, it is important that the knee in the cast be in full extension to immobilize the proximal fragment.

E. Next, an anterior fasciotomy is performed to prevent compartment syndrome. After complete hemostasis, a Hemovac drain is inserted and the wound is closed in routine manner. An above-knee posterior splint is applied, incorporating the foot-ankle in neutral position with the knee flexed 30 to 45 degrees. The region of the fibular head-neck should be well padded to relieve pressure on the common peroneal nerve.

Postoperative Care. In the postoperative period the neurovascular status is carefully observed for compromise. This is definitely a potential hazard. Two to three days postoperatively a solid above-knee cast is applied with the ankle and knee in the same position as above.

Ordinarily, the osteotomy heals in six weeks. Four weeks after operation, if there is enough callus to prevent change or loss of position, the cast is removed and an above-knee cast is applied with the knee in full extension and the ankle-foot free, allowing partial to gradual full weight-bearing. If criss-cross pins are used, the percutaneous Steinmann pins are removed four weeks after radiograms disclose enough callus to prevent change or loss of position. Another above-knee cast is applied for an additional three or four weeks, at which time the osteotomy usually will have healed. The plate and screws are removed six to nine months after surgery. After plate and screw removal, the limb is protected by an above-knee walking cast. These are the principal drawbacks of internal fixation with plate and screws.

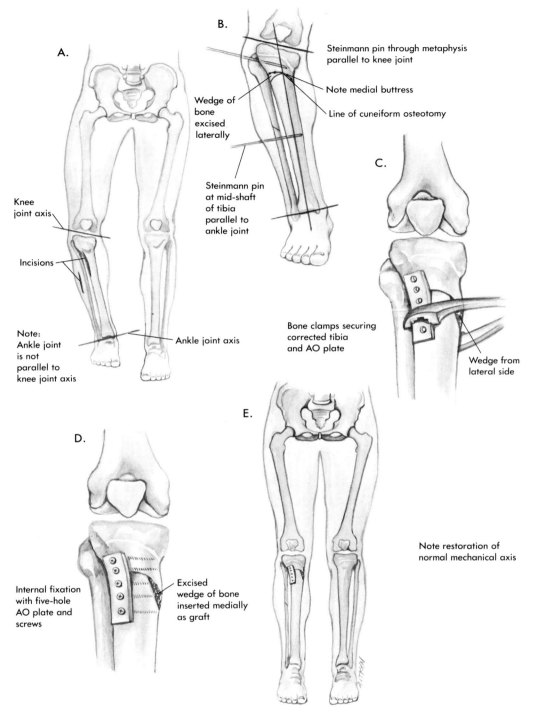

A.

Knee
joint axis

Incisions

Note:
Ankle joint
is not
parallel to
knee joint axis

Ankle joint axis

B.

Steinmann pin through metaphysis
parallel to knee joint

Note medial buttress

Line of cuneiform osteotomy

Wedge of
bone
excised
laterally

Steinmann pin
at mid-shaft
of tibia
parallel to
ankle joint

C.

Bone clamps securing
corrected tibia
and AO plate

Wedge from
lateral side

D.

Internal fixation
with five-hole
AO plate and
screws

Excised
wedge of bone
inserted medially
as graft

E.

Note restoration of
normal mechanical axis

Plate 151. (Continued)

PLATE 152

Oblique Wedge Osteotomy of the Proximal Tibia at the Metaphyseal-Diaphyseal Juncture to Correct Tibia Vara and Excessive Medial Tibial Torsion (Wagner Technique)

Indications. Tibia vara in the older child and adolescent. The oblique wedge resection technique achieves angular and rotational realignment of the proximal tibia. As compared with the transverse wedge osteotomy, it has the following advantages:

1. Axial displacement is minimal.
2. It provides a large cancellous surface, and therefore the osteotomy heals more rapidly.
3. It is more stable.

Radiographic Control. Image intensifier.

Patient Position. The procedure is performed with the patient supine on a radiolucent operating table. A bag under the ipsilateral hip-pelvis prevents lateral rotation of the hip and maintains the lower limb in neutral rotation. In the short, fat lower limb, prepare the whole lower limb and hip, and drape sterile to clinically assess adequate correction of the deformity. A sterile tourniquet is applied on the proximal thigh.

Operative Technique. First, through a separate longitudinal 5-cm. incision in the middle third of the leg, the fibula is subperiosteally exposed, and a short oblique osteotomy is performed with a power saw (see Plate 151).

Caution! Close the fibular incision after release of the tourniquet when the tibial osteotomy has been performed and internally fixed. Drain the fibular wound. Complete hemostasis should be achieved. Lateral compartment syndrome may occur!

The proximal one third of the diaphysis of the tibia and metaphysis is exposed through an 8- to 10-cm. longitudinal incision described and illustrated in Plate 151. In the oblique wedge osteotomy for correction of proximal tibia vara, the osteotomy will hinge medially; therefore, the periosteum is not elevated on its upper medial metaphyseal corner. Also, the subperiosteal exposure of the lateral aspect of the tibial shaft should be distal enough to excise an adequately long oblique wedge—this is critical.

A.–D. The first step is to outline the long oblique wedge based laterally and distally to be excised. If only angular deformity (varus) is to be corrected, the width of the wedge of bone is the same both anteriorly and posteriorly; however, when excessive medial torsion is to be corrected also, along with varus, the wedge of bone to be resected is wider anteriorly than posteriorly. The inferior tibial fragment will rotate laterally when the osteotomized surfaces are apposed.

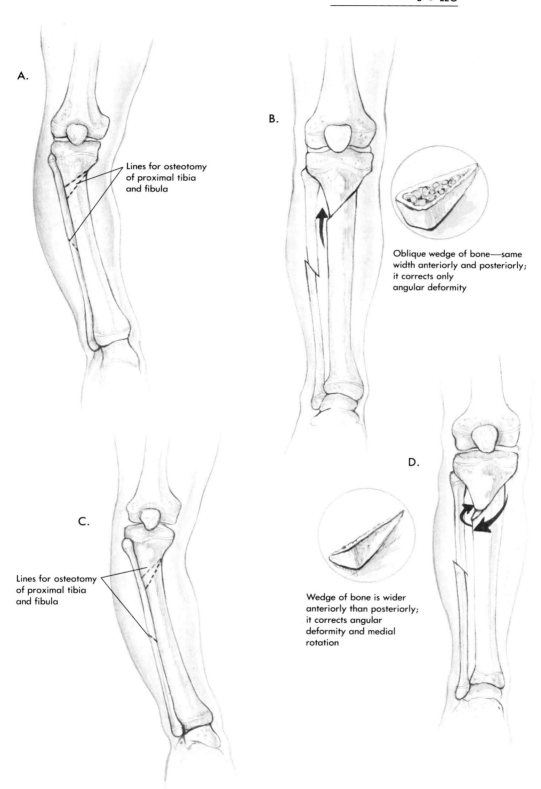

A.

Lines for osteotomy
of proximal tibia
and fibula

B.

Oblique wedge of bone—same
width anteriorly and posteriorly;
it corrects only
angular deformity

C.

Lines for osteotomy
of proximal tibia
and fibula

D.

Wedge of bone is wider
anteriorly than posteriorly;
it corrects angular
deformity and medial
rotation

Plate 152. A.–H., Oblique wedge osteotomy of the proximal tibia at the metaphyseal-diaphyseal juncture to correct tibia vara and excessive medial tibial torsion (Wagner technique).

E. Under image-intensifier radiographic control, determine the exact site of the upper tibial physis. Mark it with a stout Keith needle. Growth should not be disturbed.

With a power drill, two guide wires are directed distal-lateral to proximal-medial; superomedially, the two pins meet 0.5 to 1.0 cm. distal to the medial tibial physis. The width of the wedge inferolaterally is estimated clinically or calculated following Williams' guidelines.

F. Insert a Chandler retractor under the periosteum, posterolaterally protecting the soft tissue and neurovascular structures. The periosteum and a thin shell of cortex are left intact superomedially. The oblique wedge of bone is resected with a power saw and AO sharp osteotomes.

G. The tibial fragments are manipulated and the bone surfaces are apposed. The adequacy of correction obtained is assessed clinically and by anteroposterior and lateral radiograms of the entire tibia, including the knee and ankles. The osteotomy can be temporarily fixed with two threaded Steinmann pins. If more correction is desired, more bone can be resected; if overcorrected, bone graft fragments taken from the wedge of bone are reinserted at the osteotomy site.

H. The threaded Steinmann pins (if used for temporary fixation) are removed. Internal fixation is carried out by two cortical screws inserted through separate stab wounds from the medial side of the subcutaneous surface of the tibia. The screws are directed perpendicular to the plane of osteotomy. Their ends should engage the opposite cortex and not injure the lateral part of the upper tibial physis. Final radiograms of the leg are made in the anteroposterior and lateral projections.

The tourniquet is released and complete hemostasis is achieved. *A fasciotomy of the anterior compartment is performed.* Do not commit the mistake of deleting this vital step of surgery despite the completely dry operative field—*Volkmann's ischemia can develop.*

The periosteum is closed with 00 Tycron interrupted sutures. Both wounds—tibial and fibular—are drained with medium-sized Hemovac suction tubes. The subcutaneous tissue is closed with 00 Vicryl interrupted sutures and the skin with 00 subcuticular nylon. An above-knee cast is applied with the knee flexed 30 degrees and the ankle and foot in neutral position.

Postoperative Care. If necessary, the cast is bivalved (not split) and the sheath wadding is cut to the skin with sterile scissors. Assess and record neurovascular function every four hours. The suction tubes are removed on the first or second postoperative day, depending on the amount of drainage.

Ambulation with toe-touch gait, with crutch support (three-point), is allowed by the second or third postoperative day. The cast is changed in three weeks and is removed six weeks after surgery when there is adequate healing.

REFERENCES

Wagner, H.: Orthopaedic corrections in children with vitamin D-resistant rickets. *In*: Weil, U. H. (ed.): Acetabular Dysplasia. Skeletal Dysplasia in Childhood. Berlin: Springer-Verlag, 1978, pp. 183–197.

Williams, A. T.: Tibial realignment by oblique wedge osteotomy. Int. Orthop., 10:171, 1986.

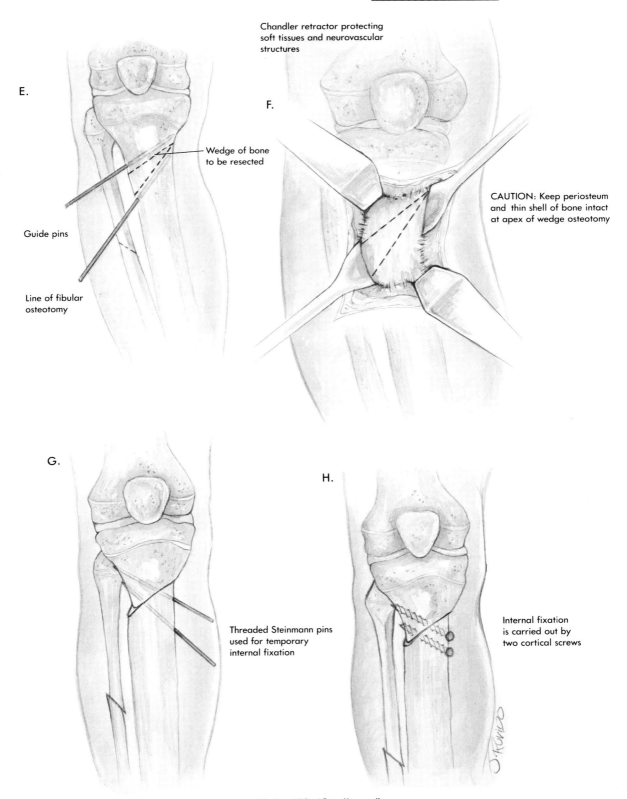

E.

Wedge of bone
to be resected

Guide pins

Line of fibular
osteotomy

F.

Chandler retractor protecting
soft tissues and neurovascular
structures

CAUTION: Keep periosteum
and thin shell of bone intact
at apex of wedge osteotomy

G.

Threaded Steinmann pins
used for temporary
internal fixation

H.

Internal fixation
is carried out by
two cortical screws

Plate 152. (Continued)

PLATE 153   Oblique Coronal Osteotomy of the Proximal Tibia at the Metaphyseal-Diaphyseal Juncture to Correct Tibia Vara

Indications. Correction of angular and rotational deformity of the proximal tibia in Blount's disease (tibia vara).

Principle. A pure rotational deformity requires an osteotomy in the transverse plane. Varus or valgus deformities are corrected by an osteotomy in the frontal (coronal) plane. Flexion-extension deformity requires an osteotomy in the sagittal plane. In Blount's disease there is both varus and medial rotation deformity, and following the principle proposed by MacEwen and Shands for correction of rotational angular deformity of the proximal femur, Rab introduced a technique of an oblique proximal tibial osteotomy. The line of osteotomy is directed from anterior-distal to posterior-proximal. The greater the vertical (frontal) direction, the greater the correction of varus deformity.

Radiographic Control. Image intensifier.

Patient Position. The operative procedure is performed with the patient supine with the entire lower limb including the hip prepared and draped sterile. Adequate visualization of the lower limb is vital. A sterile pneumatic tourniquet is used for tourniquet ischemia.

Operative Technique

A. Rab has presented a nomogram to calculate the angle of oblique osteotomy. The degree of valgization is found on the vertical axis, and the desired degree of rotational correction is found on the horizontal axis. The dark line at their intersection describes the osteotomy angle down from the horizontal axis.

B. First, an osteotomy of the fibula is performed in its middle one third or at the juncture of the proximal and middle thirds through a 4-cm. longitudinal incision (see Plate 152). Then the anteromedial and anterolateral surfaces of the proximal diaphysis and metaphysis are subperiosteally exposed through a 6- to 8-cm. longitudinal incision. The incision in the periosteum is Y-shaped. Chandler retractors are introduced subperiosteally with the knee in flexion to protect neurovascular structures posteriorly.

C. Under image-intensifier radiographic control, a smooth Steinmann pin is drilled into the tibia at the desired angle for the osteotomy. The pin is inserted 1 cm. distal to the proximal tibial tubercle and directed toward the posterior cortex to terminate at a safe distance from the growth plate. Under image-intensifier radiographic control, the angle and depth of the pin are determined.

D. With a power saw the tibia is osteotomized distal to the pin. As the saw penetrates deep into bone, frequent image-intensifier radiograms are made to visualize its depth and direction. The greater part of the cut in the tibia is made from its anteromedial side because this approach is easier. When the osteotomy is completed, do not manipulate and tear the periosteum on the posterior surface of the tibia.

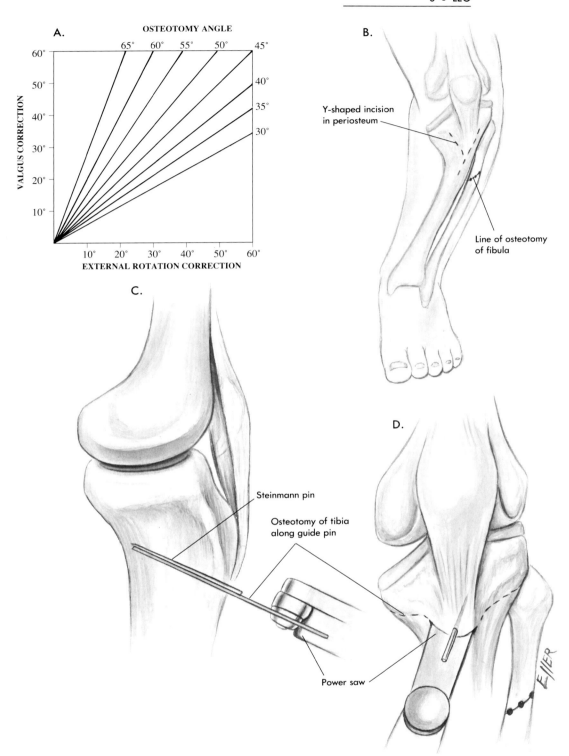

Plate 153. A.–F., Oblique coronal osteotomy of the proximal tibia at the metaphyseal-diaphyseal juncture to correct tibia vara.

E. Next, a 3.5-mm. cortical screw is used to transfix the osteotomized fragments. The screw hole is started lateral to the tibial tubercle. The screw should engage both tibial fragments and penetrate the posterior cortex of the distal fragment. It is best to overdrill in the proximal fragment to allow some mobility.

F. The assistant holds the leg, the tourniquet is released, and complete hemostasis is achieved. Be sure to perform a fasciotomy of the anterior compartment to prevent compartment syndrome. A medium-sized Hemovac suction tube is inserted for drainage, and the wound is closed in the routine fashion.

The osteotomized tibia is manipulated, correcting both varus and medial rotation. The position of the osteotomy is verified by image intensifier, and a final large radiogram in the anteroposterior and lateral projections is made. An above-knee cast is applied. It is important that the knee is in complete extension.

Postoperative Care. Toe-touch is allowed with a three-point crutch gait. Radiograms are made at ten days and 21 days to check maintenance of alignment and healing. The cast is changed, and another cast is applied. Depending on the degree of healing and the stability of the osteotomized fragments, greater weight-bearing is allowed. The osteotomy usually heals in six to eight weeks.

REFERENCES

MacEwen, G. D., and Shands, A. R., Jr.: Oblique trochanteric osteotomy. J. Bone Joint Surg., 49-A:345, 1967.

Rab, G. T.: Oblique tibial osteotomy for Blount's disease (tibia vara). J. Pediatr. Orthop., 8:715, 1988.

E.

F.

Correction of
varus deformity
and medial rotation

Cortical screw
transfixing osteotomy

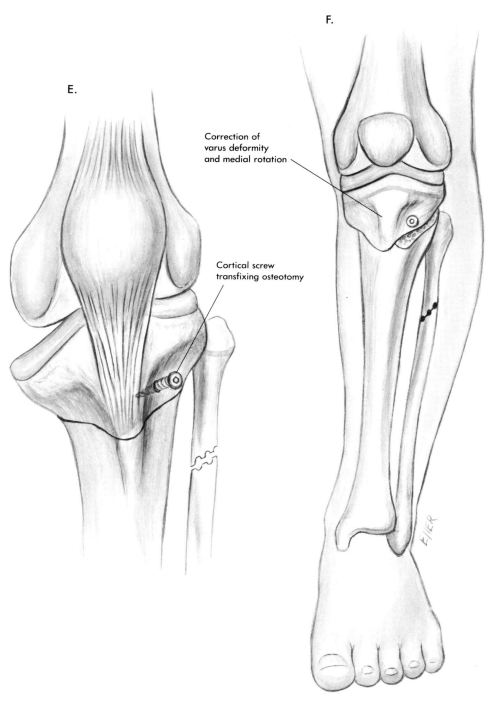

Plate 153. (Continued)

PLATE 154 Valgization Osteotomy of the Proximal Tibia to Correct Tibia Vara with Tibial Lengthening with the Use of the OF-Garches Limb Lengthener

Indications. Tibia vara in the adolescent or in the older child.

Radiographic Control. Image intensifier.

Special Instrumentation

1. Orthofix (OF)-Garches tibial lengthener (with a T-clamp capable of moving only in one plane and swiveling screw seats to allow convergent siting of the outer screws).

2. Kirschner wires, 2 mm. in diameter.

3. Use 6/5-mm. cancellous screws and 6/5-mm. cortical screws. Measure the length and thread length for the cancellous and cortical screws ahead of time on a lateral radiogram using the transparent template provided by Orthofix.

4. Standard Orthofix application equipment with assembly templates.

Operative Technique

A1. and **A2.** The Orthofix-Garches limb lengthener is designed to allow lengthening of the tibia in the upper metaphyseal region with simultaneous ability to control valgus or varus deviation. The angular correction may be gradual or immediate; the latter is recommended only for varus. When valgus deformity is corrected immediately, there is a definite risk of stretching and injury to the common peroneal nerve. When the plan is to correct angular deformity, the locking pin of the compression-distraction unit is placed anteriorly, as shown in A1. When simple lengthening is to be carried out after correction of the angular deformity, the locking pin of the compression-distraction unit is inserted on the medial side, as shown in A2.

B. If a tibial lengthening is to be performed with correction of tibia vara, first transfix the distal diaphysis of the fibula to the tibia with an oblique screw inserted inferosuperiorly at an angle of about 30 degrees. This maneuver prevents any proximal displacement of the lateral malleolus during the tibial lengthening. This is combined with resection of 0.5 cm. of the shaft of the fibula.

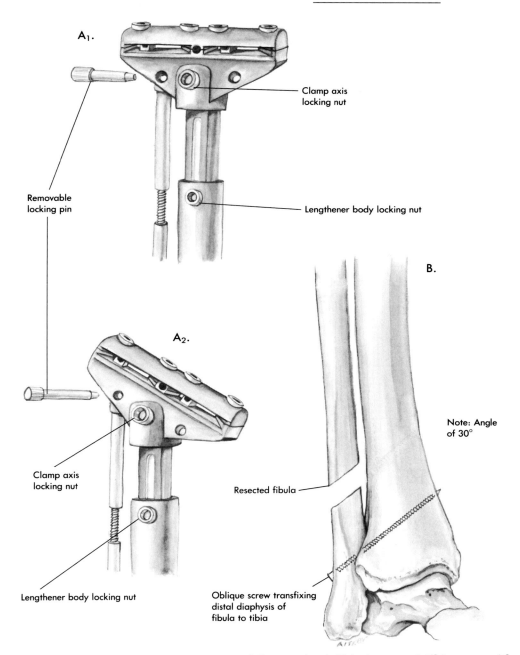

A₁.

Removable
locking pin

Clamp axis
locking nut

Lengthener body locking nut

A₂.

Clamp axis
locking nut

Lengthener body locking nut

B.

Note: Angle
of 30°

Resected fibula

Oblique screw transfixing
distal diaphysis of
fibula to tibia

Plate 154. A.–O., Valgization osteotomy of the proximal tibia to correct tibia vara with tibial lengthening with the use of the OF-Garches limb lengthener.

C1.–C4. Determine the knee joint line and mark the proximal tibial tubercle with indelible ink. Under image-intensifier radiographic control, position a T-clamp template on the upper tibia. Be sure there is adequate space from the skin by means of a guard. It is vital that the T-clamp be parallel to the superior surface of the tibia and in the frontal plane. C1 and C3 show the correct position of the template T-clamp, whereas the position in C2 and C4 is incorrect.

Correct
position

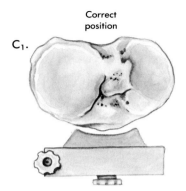

C₁.

Incorrect
position

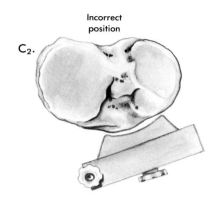

C₂.

T-CLAMP TEMPLATE

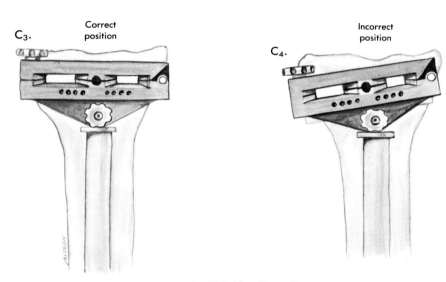

C₃.

Correct
position

C₄.

Incorrect
position

Plate 154. (Continued)

D1. and **D3.** When the upper tibial growth plate is open, the level of the T-clamp template is inferior to the proximal tibial physis.

D2. and **D4.** In the skeletally mature patient, the T-clamp template is immediately below the subarticular bony plate of the articular surface of the tibia.

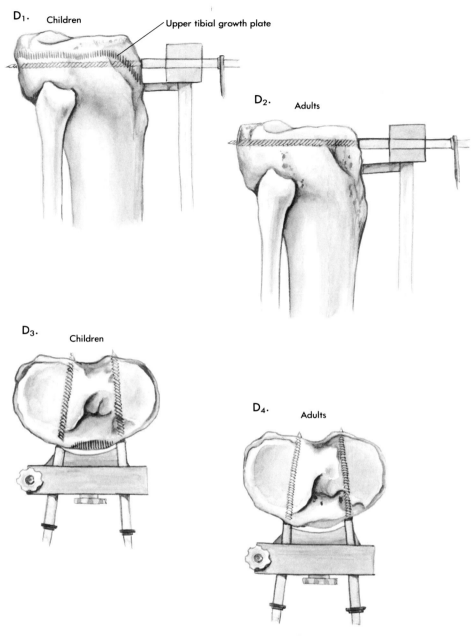

D₁. Children

Upper tibial growth plate

D₂. Adults

D₃. Children

D₄. Adults

Plate 154. (Continued)

D5. If the T-clamp is placed too high, the screws may penetrate the joint. If it is placed too distal, the level of the osteotomy may be low in the diaphysis rather than at the metaphysis. The clamp axis locking nut should be placed at the same level as the osteotomy is planned.

E. After the T-clamp template is properly positioned it is anchored temporarily to the tibia by means of Kirschner wires through holes in the template. Verify the proper positioning of the T-clamp template by regular anteroposterior and lateral radiograms.

F. Adjust the body of the template so that it is parallel to the tibial diaphysis. It should be the same distance from the tibia as the T-clamp. Tighten the clamp axis locking nut of the template. Insert Kirschner wires through holes in the body template, transfixing it to the tibia.

D₅.

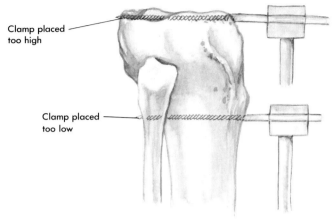

Clamp placed too high

Clamp placed too low

E. Kirschner wires

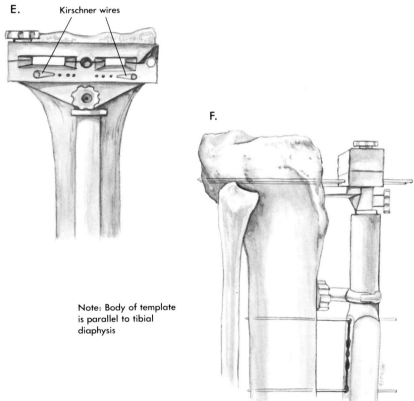

Note: Body of template is parallel to tibial diaphysis

F.

Plate 154. (Continued)

G. Insert the proximal cancellous screws first, following the steps and technique described in Plate 156.

H. The screws should be inserted obliquely so that they converge posteriorly. The tips of the screws converge but do not touch each other. They should not converge too much in order to avoid loss of stability or bending while angular correction is performed. There should be adequate penetration of the posterior cortex, but it should be no more than one thread. In the growing skeleton, the middle screw is not inserted because it will disturb growth. In the adult, however, a third middle screw is inserted.

I1. and **I2.** Insert the diaphyseal screws, and remove the Kirschner wires, template, and screw guides.

G.

H.

Obliquely inserted
cancellous screws

Note: Screws converge
posteriorly

I_2.

I_1.

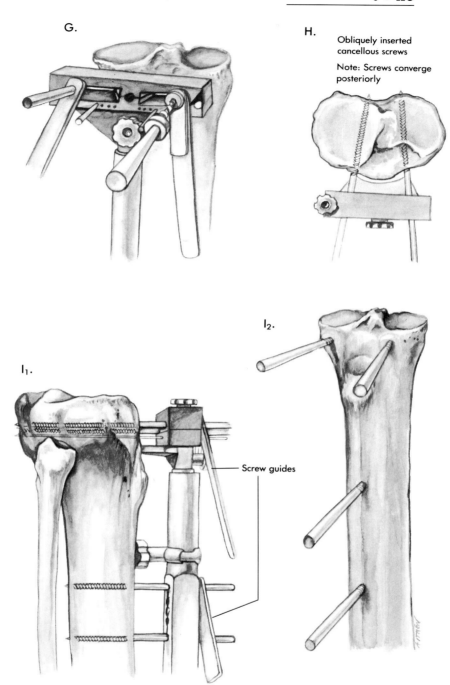

Screw guides

Plate 154. (Continued)

J1. and **J2.** Through an anteromedial or anterolateral approach, expose the upper tibial metaphyseal-diaphyseal region in the routine fashion through a 4-cm. longitudinal incision. Divide the periosteum, and subperiosteally expose the osteotomy site, which in children is immediately distal to the proximal tibial tubercle. Perform an osteotomy first by drilling holes and then by using a sharp osteotome, as described in Plate 156. The level of tibial osteotomy varies according to whether there is ligamentous laxity of the knee joint. If the knee is stable, the osteotomy level is distal to the insertion of the patellar tendon. If the knee joint is lax, the osteotomy should be proximal to the insertion of the patellar tendon. The osteotomy site should be at the same level as the clamp axis locking nut.

K. The body of the OF-Garches limb lengthener is then positioned, leaving the upper clamp open. When the body has been fitted into position, the clamp cover is secured tightly into place.

L. The locking pin is inserted as shown in A2 (medially), and the completeness of the osteotomy is double-checked by distracting the two bone fragments several millimeters using the compression-distraction unit.

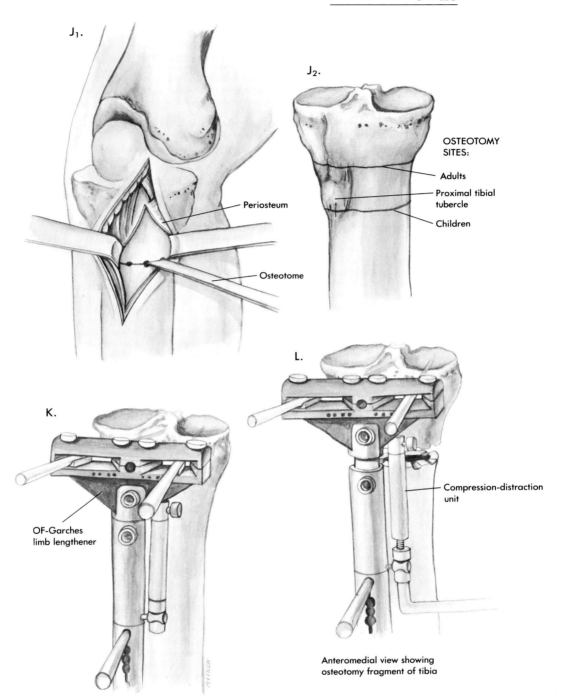

J₁.

Periosteum

Osteotome

J₂.

OSTEOTOMY
SITES:

Adults

Proximal tibial
tubercle

Children

K.

OF-Garches
limb lengthener

L.

Compression-distraction
unit

Anteromedial view showing
osteotomy fragment of tibia

Plate 154. (Continued)

M. The clamp axis and lengthener body locking nuts are tightened. The periosteum is sutured meticulously, a Hemovac suction tube is inserted, and the wound is closed in the usual fashion.

N1. and **N2.** Next, a decision is made as to whether instantaneous correction of the angular deformity should be performed, or varus or valgus deformity should be corrected gradually with distraction.

Even for angular correction only, I suggest performing 0.5 to 1.0 cm. lengthening first and then correction—this will prevent possible stress on the screws due to compression of the cortices. When gradual lengthening is desired, it is performed ten days after surgery. The compression-distraction unit is placed on the medial side with a removable locking pin inserted anteriorly. The clamp axis locking nuts are loosened, and distraction is carried out at a rate of a quarter-turn four times per day. When correction is achieved, the clamp axis locking nut and the lengthener body locking nut are both tightened.

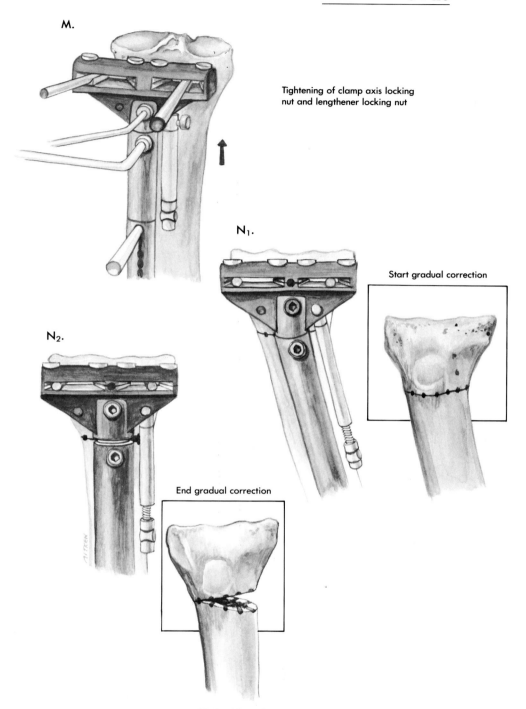

M.

Tightening of clamp axis locking
nut and lengthener locking nut

N₁.

Start gradual correction

N₂.

End gradual correction

Plate 154. (Continued)

O1.–O3. If immediate correction is desired, the T-clamp is placed parallel to the upper surface of the tibia and the body, 1 to 2 cm. anterior and parallel to the diaphysis. Tibial osteotomy is performed, using a subtraction or dome technique, 1 cm. below the proximal tibial tubercle. Fibular osteotomy is always performed. For varus correction, the compression-distraction unit is placed laterally, and for valgus correction it is placed medially with the removable locking pin positioned as in A2. The clamp axis locking nut and the lengthener body locking nut are both loosened. Correction is then carried out by manipulation until the desired alignment is achieved. Then the clamp axis locking nut is tightened and compression is exerted along the axis of the bone, if needed, with the removable locking pin positioned as in A1.

Postoperative Care. Toe-touch is allowed with a three-point crutch gait. Radiograms are made at ten days and 21 days to check maintenance of alignment and healing. The cast is changed, and another cast is applied. Depending on the degree of healing and the stability of the osteotomized fragments, greater weight-bearing is allowed. The osteotomy usually heals in six to eight weeks.

REFERENCES

DeBastiani, G.: Lengthening of the lower limbs in achondroplasts. First International Conference on Human Achondroplasia, Rome, November 19–21, 1986.

DeBastiani, G., Aldegheri, R., and Renzi-Brivio, L.: Indicazioni particolari dei fisatori esterni. G. Ital. Fissatore Esterno, 504:31, 1979.

DeBastiani, G., Aldegheri, R., and Renzi-Brivio, L.: Fissatore esterno assiale. Chir. Organi Mov., 65:287, 1979.

DeBastiani, G., Aldegheri, R., and Renzi-Brivio, L.: The treatment of fractures with a dynamic axial fixator. J. Bone Joint Surg., 66-B:538, 1984.

DeBastiani, G., Aldegheri, R., Renzi-Brivio, L., and Trivella, G.: Limb lengthening by distraction of the epiphyseal plate. A comparison of two techniques in the rabbit. J. Bone Joint Surg., 68-B:545, 1986.

DeBastiani, G., Aldegheri, R., Renzi-Brivio, L., and Trivella, G.: Chondrodiastasis-controlled symmetrical distraction of the epiphyseal plate. Limb lengthening in children. J. Bone Joint Surg., 68-B:550, 1986.

DeBastiani, G., Aldegheri, R., Renzi-Brivio, L., and Trivella, G.: Limb lengthening by callus distraction (callotasis). J. Pediatr. Orthop., 7:129, 1987.

O₁.

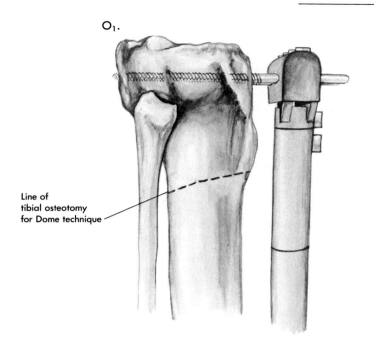

Line of
tibial osteotomy
for Dome technique

O₂.

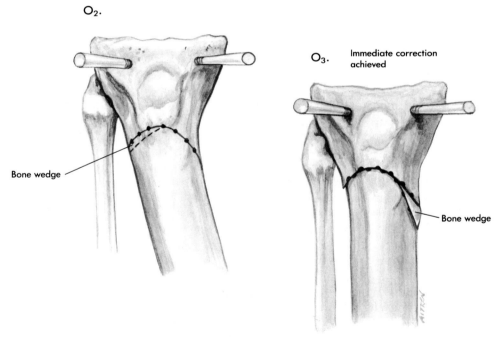

Bone wedge

O₃.   Immediate correction
achieved

Bone wedge

Plate 154. (Continued)

PLATE 155   Wagner's Tibial Diaphyseal Lengthening

Indications. Lower limb length disparity of 5 cm. or more in a patient of normal stature.

Requisites

1. Joints should be stable proximal and distal to the elongated bone. In tibial lengthening, the knee and ankle should be stable. The absence of cruciate ligaments is a relative contraindication.
2. Neuromuscular function should be normal.
3. Circulation should be normal.
4. Skin and soft tissues should be relatively normal.
5. Bone structure should be normal and strong.
6. The patient should be mentally stable with no psychological dysfunction.
7. The patient should be at an age to be cognizant of the complications of limb lengthening and to be cooperative in the postoperative regimen.

Patient Position. Supine.

Operative Technique. Tibial lengthening differs from femoral lengthening in a few respects.

A.–C. In tibial lengthening, the apparatus is applied on the anteromedial aspect of the leg, where skin is less sensitive and the tibia is subcutaneous. Because of the thinness of the soft-tissue coverage, pin tract problems are minimized. The tibia is not, of course, the only bone affected by tibial lengthening. Because the traction forces of the bars of the apparatus pull on the soft tissues, the distal physis and proximal physis of the fibula must be protected. Bony fusion of the distal tibia and fibula is not recommended, because the resultant rigidity of the ankle mortise will cause degenerative arthritis of the ankle later in life. Therefore, the fibula is transfixed to the tibia by two cortical screws immediately above and below the osteotomy site; these are positional screws with threads penetrating all four cortices, preventing approximation of osteotomized fibular segments to the tibia. The positional screws are removed after bone healing occurs.

The tibial lengthening apparatus is *not* put on distraction prior to division of the fibula. Rather, the fibula is first divided and then tension force is applied on the apparatus (after which the tibia is osteotomized). As the apparatus is on the medial aspect of the leg, tethering forces of the intact fibula will cause valgus deviation of the osteotomized tibial segments.

Anterior angulation and pressure on the skin are problems created by the strong pull of the triceps surae muscle; therefore, it is best to fix the tibial segments in slight posterior angulation after the initial osteotomy. It is vital to check alignment very closely; frequent adjustments may be required to prevent anterior bowing and valgus deformity.

The first phase of Wagner's tibial diaphyseal lengthening procedure entails insertion of Schanz screws (D–M); application of the apparatus (N and O); osteotomy (P–W); and lengthening (Z and AA).

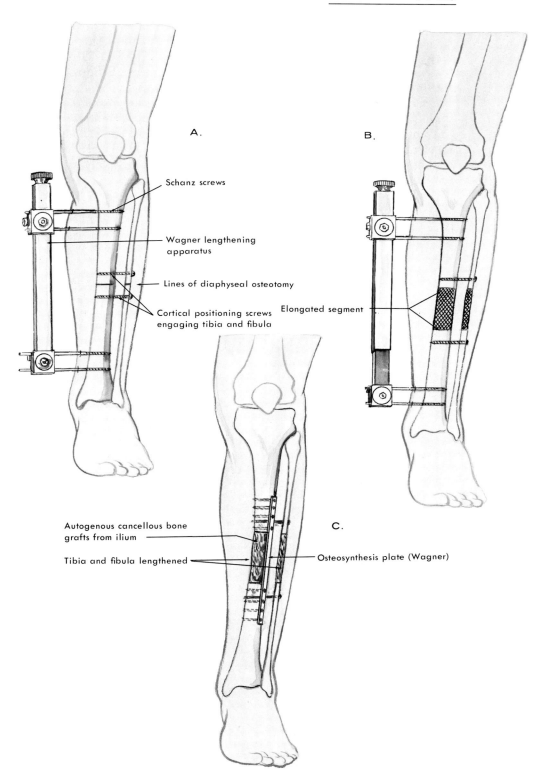

A.

B.

Schanz screws

Wagner lengthening
apparatus

Lines of diaphyseal osteotomy

Elongated segment

Cortical positioning screws
engaging tibia and fibula

Autogenous cancellous bone
grafts from ilium

C.

Tibia and fibula lengthened

Osteosynthesis plate (Wagner)

Plate 155. A.–FF., Wagner's tibial diaphyseal lengthening.

D.–O. Under image-intensifier radiographic control, two pairs of Schanz screws are inserted parallel to the knee and ankle joint axes through medial incisions into the proximal and distal ends of the tibial metaphysis. The technique is similar to that described for femoral lengthening. The upper Schanz screws are distal to the proximal tibial tubercle. The proximal physis and distal physis of the tibia must not be injured. Additionally, staying a distance of 2 cm. from the growth plate provides safety from pin tract infection. The position and depth of the screws are checked on anteroposterior and lateral radiograms. The tibial lengthening apparatus is applied posteriorly to provide space anteriorly for surgical exposure of the tibial shaft. Tension forces are not applied on the apparatus at this stage.

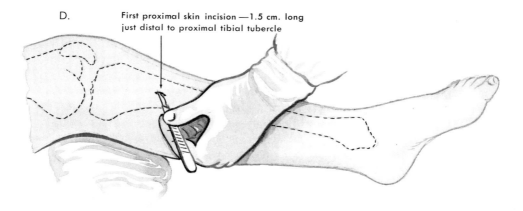

D.

First proximal skin incision —1.5 cm. long
just distal to proximal tibial tubercle

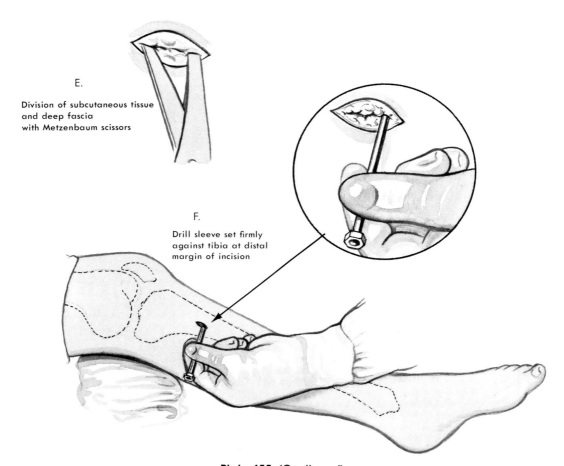

E.

Division of subcutaneous tissue
and deep fascia
with Metzenbaum scissors

F.

Drill sleeve set firmly
against tibia at distal
margin of incision

Plate 155. (Continued)

D.–O. Under image-intensifier radiographic control, two pairs of Schanz screws are inserted parallel to the knee and ankle joint axes through medial incisions into the proximal and distal ends of the tibial metaphysis. The technique is similar to that described for femoral lengthening. The upper Schanz screws are distal to the proximal tibial tubercle. The proximal physis and distal physis of the tibia must not be injured. Additionally, staying a distance of 2 cm. from the growth plate provides safety from pin tract infection. The position and depth of the screws are checked on anteroposterior and lateral radiograms. The tibial lengthening apparatus is applied posteriorly to provide space anteriorly for surgical exposure of the tibial shaft. Tension forces are not applied on the apparatus at this stage.

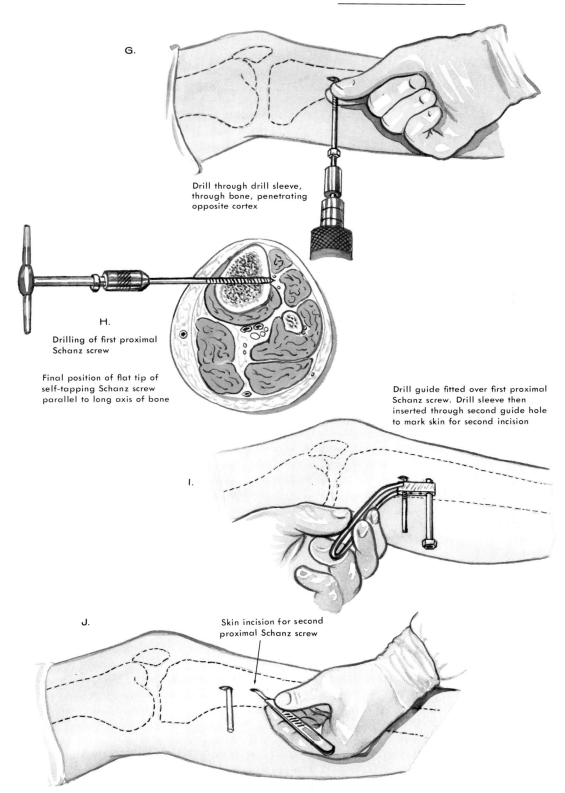

G.

Drill through drill sleeve, through bone, penetrating opposite cortex

H.

Drilling of first proximal Schanz screw

Final position of flat tip of self-tapping Schanz screw parallel to long axis of bone

Drill guide fitted over first proximal Schanz screw. Drill sleeve then inserted through second guide hole to mark skin for second incision

I.

J.

Skin incision for second proximal Schanz screw

Plate 155. (Continued)

D.–O. Under image-intensifier radiographic control, two pairs of Schanz screws are inserted parallel to the knee and ankle joint axes through medial incisions into the proximal and distal ends of the tibial metaphysis. The technique is similar to that described for femoral lengthening. The upper Schanz screws are distal to the proximal tibial tubercle. The proximal physis and distal physis of the tibia must not be injured. Additionally, staying a distance of 2 cm. from the growth plate provides safety from pin tract infection. The position and depth of the screws are checked on anteroposterior and lateral radiograms. The tibial lengthening apparatus is applied posteriorly to provide space anteriorly for surgical exposure of the tibial shaft. Tension forces are not applied on the apparatus at this stage.

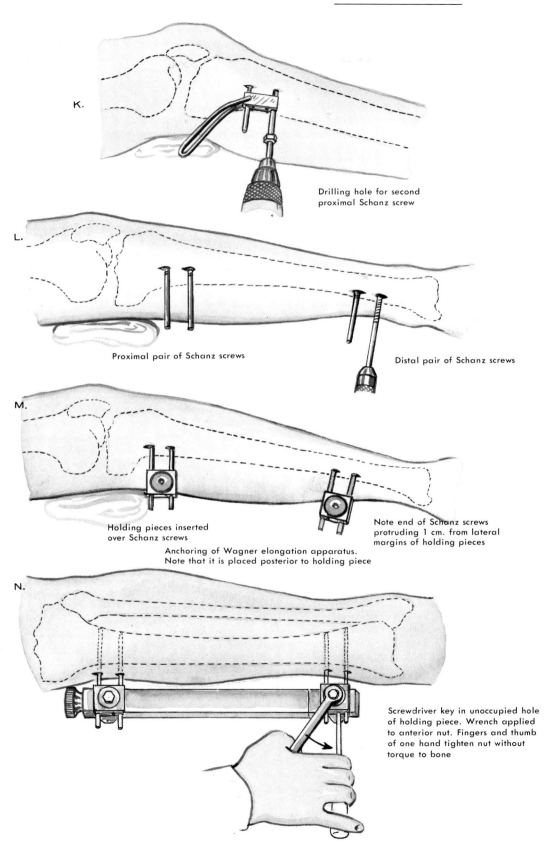

K. Drilling hole for second proximal Schanz screw

L. Proximal pair of Schanz screws

Distal pair of Schanz screws

M. Holding pieces inserted over Schanz screws

Note end of Schanz screws protruding 1 cm. from lateral margins of holding pieces

Anchoring of Wagner elongation apparatus. Note that it is placed posterior to holding piece

N. Screwdriver key in unoccupied hole of holding piece. Wrench applied to anterior nut. Fingers and thumb of one hand tighten nut without torque to bone

Plate 155. (Continued)

D.–O. Under image-intensifier radiographic control, two pairs of Schanz screws are inserted parallel to the knee and ankle joint axes through medial incisions into the proximal and distal ends of the tibial metaphysis. The technique is similar to that described for femoral lengthening. The upper Schanz screws are distal to the proximal tibial tubercle. The proximal physis and distal physis of the tibia must not be injured. Additionally, staying a distance of 2 cm. from the growth plate provides safety from pin tract infection. The position and depth of the screws are checked on anteroposterior and lateral radiograms. The tibial lengthening apparatus is applied posteriorly to provide space anteriorly for surgical exposure of the tibial shaft. Tension forces are not applied on the apparatus at this stage.

P. A 7- to 10-cm. longitudinal incision is made in the middle third of the fibula. The subcutaneous tissue and fascia are divided in line with the skin incision.

Q. The peroneal muscles are gently elevated from the posterior intermuscular septum and retracted anteriorly.

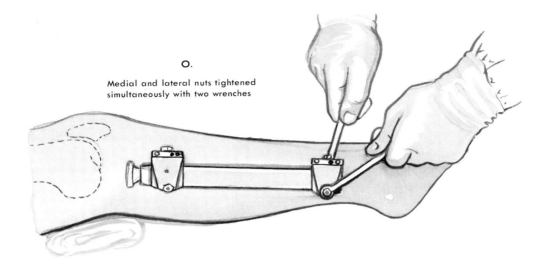

O.

Medial and lateral nuts tightened
simultaneously with two wrenches

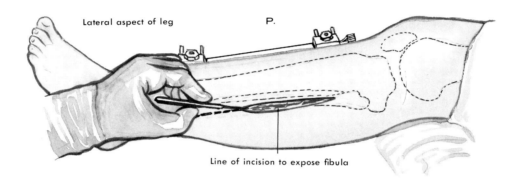

Lateral aspect of leg   P.

Line of incision to expose fibula

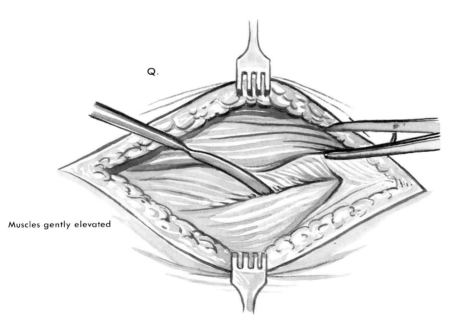

Q.

Muscles gently elevated

Plate 155. (Continued)

R. The anterior intermuscular septum is sectioned and, with a periosteal elevator, is released from the interosseous border of the fibula.

S. The interosseous membrane is sectioned from the lateral (or interosseous) border of the tibia. Injury to the interosseous vessels and nerves should be avoided. On the posterior surface of the interosseous membrane, there are numerous vessels that may cause troublesome bleeding.

At this time the site of the osteotomy of the fibula should be determined. Measured with a ruler, the site should be exactly midway between the upper and lower pairs of the Schanz screws. A smooth Kirschner wire is inserted into the fibula to mark the site of the osteotomy. Leverage is applied to the fibula to elevate it anteriorly, and the fibula is transfixed to the tibia. Next, a flat lever retractor is introduced on the posterior surface of the fibula, the anterior surface of the interosseous membrane, and the posterior surface of the tibia. Posterior depression of the interosseous membrane keeps vessels and nerves out of harm's way and provides space for screw fixation and osteotomy.

T. The sites for the positioning screws are marked. One site should be 11 mm. to one side of the Kirschner wire; the other site should be 11 mm. to the other side of the wire. The Kirschner wire marks the site of the osteotomy of the tibia and fibula. The locations of the transfixing screws do not interfere with the screws of the Wagner osteosynthesis plate on the tibia during the second phase of the operation.

A 3.2-mm. drill is used to drill holes across both bones; the holes are tapped. To prevent splitting of the fibula, the edges of its drill holes are flattened by countersinking.

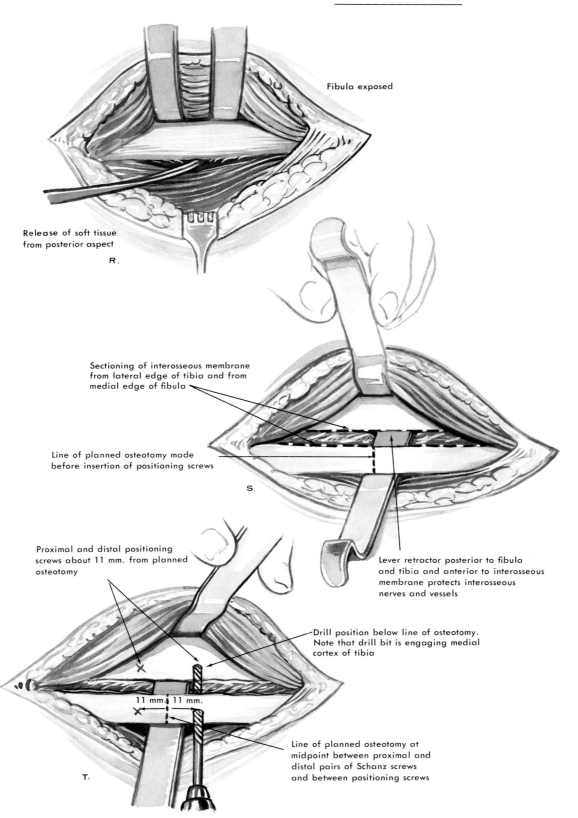

Fibula exposed

Release of soft tissue
from posterior aspect

R.

Sectioning of interosseous membrane
from lateral edge of tibia and from
medial edge of fibula

Line of planned osteotomy made
before insertion of positioning screws

S.

Lever retractor posterior to fibula
and tibia and anterior to interosseous
membrane protects interosseous
nerves and vessels

Proximal and distal positioning
screws about 11 mm. from planned
osteotomy

Drill position below line of osteotomy.
Note that drill bit is engaging medial
cortex of tibia

11 mm. 11 mm.

Line of planned osteotomy at
midpoint between proximal and
distal pairs of Schanz screws
and between positioning screws

T.

Plate 155. (Continued)

U. The positioning screws are inserted, and their site and length are double-checked on anteroposterior and lateral radiograms.

The Kirschner wire marking the site of the osteotomy of the fibula is removed, and the fibula is divided transversely with a reciprocating saw under normal saline irrigation. Biologically it is preferable to perform corticotomy of the fibula with sharp osteotomes, thereby preserving its endosteal blood supply.

Distraction force is applied on the lengthening apparatus by turning its handle counterclockwise three, four, or five turns.

V. An incision is made 1 cm. from the lateral edge of the anterior border on the crest of the tibia. The subcutaneous tissue and deep fascia are divided longitudinally in line with the skin incision. The antecrural muscles are elevated from the lateral surface of the tibia. The lateral surface of the tibia is exposed. A Chandler elevator is placed on the anterior aspect of the tibia.

W. Through the anterior wound, the positioning fibulotibial screws are visualized; a transverse osteotomy of the tibia is then carried out midway between the two positioning screws with a reciprocating saw under irrigation. Upon completion of the osteotomy, the gap between the two tibial segments springs open. It is this author's current preference to perform corticotomy of the tibia with sharp osteotomes and not to disturb the endosteal blood supply.

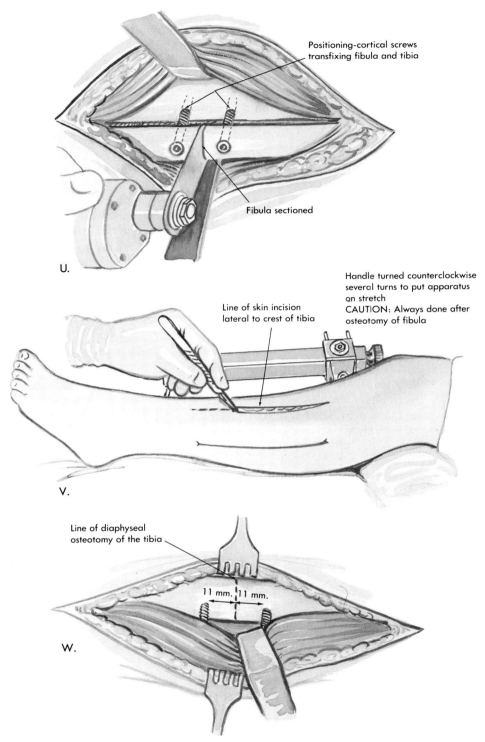

U.

Positioning-cortical screws transfixing fibula and tibia

Fibula sectioned

V.

Line of skin incision lateral to crest of tibia

Handle turned counterclockwise several turns to put apparatus on stretch
CAUTION: Always done after osteotomy of fibula

W.

Line of diaphyseal osteotomy of the tibia

11 mm. 11 mm.

Plate 155. (Continued)

X. and **Y.** To avoid anterior compartment syndrome, the deep fascia is left open or elongated in alternating oblique cuts. Sometimes, if the fascia is taut, it is best to extend the skin incision proximally and excise the fascia, thereby preventing possible compression of the superficial peroneal nerve. Suction drainage tubes are inserted. Only the subcutaneous tissues and skin are closed. Povidone-iodine (Betadine) treated dressings are applied over the sites of the Schanz screws. A posterior below-knee cast and compression dressing are applied.

Lengthening of the tibia is commenced on the third to fifth day after surgery. The rate of lengthening recommended by this author is a quarter-turn eight times a day: six turns counterclockwise (distracting) and two turns clockwise (compressing). Biologically it is preferable to employ dynamized distraction and compression. That is, three successive lengthening (counterclockwise) quarter-turns are followed by a compressive (clockwise) quarter-turn and then by three successive counterclockwise turns (distraction) followed by one quarter-turn clockwise (compression). The time schedule is set so that lengthening is performed during waking hours.

Screw tract care is similar to that required with femoral lengthening. Starting on the third day after surgery, the screw sites are cleaned three times a day with sponges dipped in alcohol. The dressings that are applied are disinfected with alcohol (continued use of Betadine corrodes the apparatus). Tenting of the skin edges is relieved by incisions when indicated. Radiograms obtained once a week allow one to check alignment; a radiopaque Bell Thompson ruler placed next to the tibia aids in determining the amount of lengthening that has been achieved.

Z. and **AA.** The patient is allowed to ambulate, and physical therapy is performed to maintain the range of motion in the knee and ankle joints. During the process of tibial lengthening, the triceps surae will shorten, and significant equinus deformity may develop. As a rule, preoperatively, if the ankle cannot be dorsiflexed to neutral position, lengthening of the heel cord is performed (usually three to six months prior to tibial lengthening). Lengthening of the Achilles tendon during the process of tibial lengthening is indicated when there is progressive equinus and restriction of ankle motion. *If the range of ankle motion is less than 20 degrees,* elongation of the heel cord should be performed immediately. Range of motion is more important than the degree of equinus. Rigidity of the ankle joint must be avoided; ankle motion and function must be preserved. If equinus develops but the range of motion in the ankle is greater than 20 degrees, lengthening of the heel cord is performed at the time of internal fixation. Professor Wagner recommends the following technique for lengthening of the heel cord.

With the apparatus in place, the patient in a prone position, and a pneumatic tourniquet on the proximal thigh, the lower limb is carefully prepared and draped. A longitudinal incision is made on the medial border of the tendo Achillis. The incision should be long, extending from the junction of the upper and middle thirds of the leg to the insertion of the Achilles tendon at the os calcis. The subcutaneous tissue and the paratenon are divided in line with the skin incision. Injury to the veins should be avoided. The Achilles tendon is divided by a very long incision in the coronal plane. It begins anteriorly in the distal part and ends posteriorly in the proximal part, so that the muscle fibers stay with the upper part. A capsulotomy of the ankle or subtalar joints is unnecessary if dorsiflexion of the ankle to the neutral position was possible preoperatively.

The position for suturing of the tricep surae's split tendons is one in which the ankle is dorsiflexed 15 to 20 degrees beyond neutral. The wound is closed in the usual fashion. No cast is applied. Ambulation is allowed with partial weight-bearing of 10 to 15 pounds on the lower limb the day after surgery. There is usually no pain and no swelling.

Percutaneous lengthening of the heel cord is not recommended.

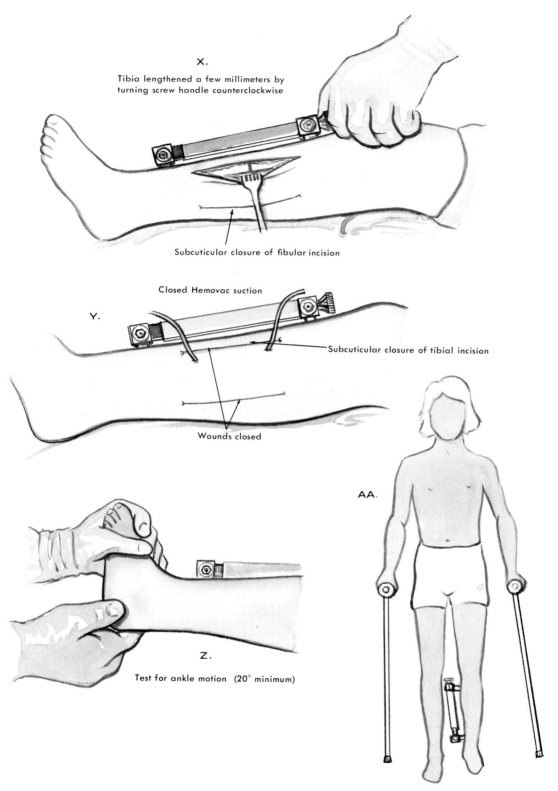

X.
Tibia lengthened a few millimeters by
turning screw handle counterclockwise

Subcuticular closure of fibular incision

Closed Hemovac suction

Y.

Subcuticular closure of tibial incision

Wounds closed

Z.
Test for ankle motion (20° minimum)

AA.

Plate 155. (Continued)

The second phase of the Wagner procedure involves plating the elongated tibial segment with the Wagner osteosynthesis plate (BB–DD) and bone grafting (EE).

BB. The anterolateral surface of the tibia is exposed through the incision used for the tibial osteotomy.

CC. When the elongated segment is identified, two Chandler retractors are placed over the proximal tibial segment; two Chandler retractors are placed over the distal tibial segment as well. It is imperative not to enter the channel of the screw tracts because of possible contamination.

DD. The distracted area is plated with an eight-hole Wagner osteosynthesis plate; four cortical screws are inserted above, and three or four cortical screws are inserted below. The plate is straight (not bent), and it is anchored on the lateral surface of the tibia.

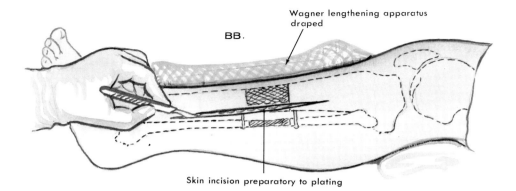

Wagner lengthening apparatus draped

BB.

Skin incision preparatory to plating

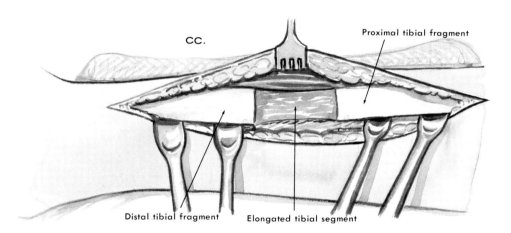

CC.

Proximal tibial fragment

Distal tibial fragment   Elongated tibial segment

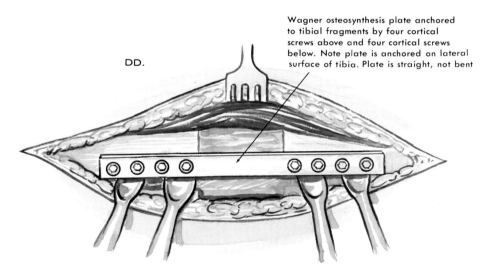

Wagner osteosynthesis plate anchored to tibial fragments by four cortical screws above and four cortical screws below. Note plate is anchored on lateral surface of tibia. Plate is straight, not bent

DD.

Plate 155. (Continued)

EE. The elongated segment is packed with autogenous cancellous bone grafts harvested from the ilium. The skin and subcutaneous tissue are closed over closed-suction drains. The positional screws fixing the tibia to the fibula are not removed. If there is delayed healing of the fibula, it may be grafted at this time.

FF. The Schanz screws and the Wagner external fixation apparatus are removed. Immobilization in a cast is not required.

Postoperative Care. As soon as the patient is comfortable, he or she is permitted to be up and around—using a three-point crutch gait and toe-touch on the lengthened limb—until there is progressive consolidation.

The third phase of the Wagner tibial lengthening procedure—the exchange of the rigid plate for a flexible semitubular plate—is the same as that described for Wagner's femoral lengthening procedure (see Plate 137).

EE.

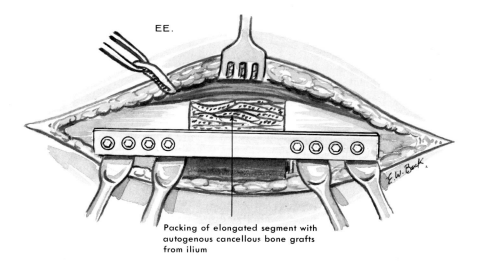

Packing of elongated segment with
autogenous cancellous bone grafts
from ilium

FF.

(Wagner lengthening apparatus
removed)

Tibia and fibula
lengthened 5–6 cm.

Autogenous cancellous bone
grafts from ilium

Osteosynthesis plate

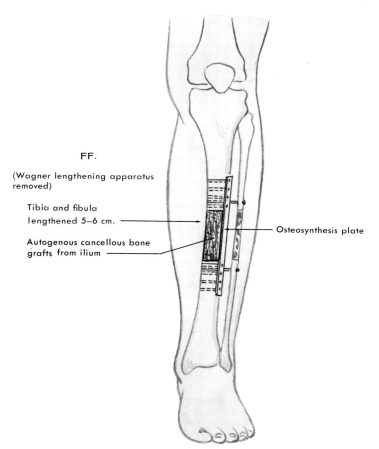

Plate 155. (Continued)

PLATE 156 · Tibial Lengthening by Callotasis (Callus Distraction)

Indications. Lower limb length disparity of 5 cm. or more in a patient of normal stature.

The choice of Orthofix limb-lengthener for tibial elongation depends on the length of the diaphysis and the amount of distraction planned. The 5-cm. lengthener is used when the minimum tibial length is 12 cm.; it allows maximum lengthening of 5 cm. The 5.5-cm. lengthener allows maximum lengthening of 5.5 cm. and is used when the minimum tibial length is 19.5 cm. The 10-cm. leg lengthener allows 10 cm. of maximum lengthening and is used when the minimum tibial length is 24 cm. It is feasible to begin with a small device and later substitute a larger lengthener if extra distraction is necessary.

Preparatory to the steps detailed in the following section, a 2-cm. segment of the diaphysis in the lower third of the fibula is excised through a separate incision in the usual fashion.

Patient Position. Supine.

Radiographic Control. Image intensifier.

Operative Technique

A. and **B.** The screws and lengthening device are placed anteriorly, just medial to the crest of the tibia. The technique for insertion of the individual screws is described in Plate 138; the only difference is that the most superior screw in the proximal tibia is cancellous. The other three screws are cortical. The cortical screws are 6 mm. in diameter; the cancellous screw is 5 mm. in diameter. When the diameter of the tibia is less than 15 mm. and the 5-cm. leg-lengthener is utilized, the cortical screws that are to be used should be 4.5 mm. in diameter; the cancellous screw should have a diameter of 3.5 mm. Screw length and thread length are estimated by assessing the radiograms and subtracting the 15 per cent magnification factor in the radiograms.

The first screw (which is cancellous) is inserted anteriorly and perpendicular to the longitudinal axis and 2 cm. inferior to the tibial plateau; it should be extracapsular. In the growing skeleton, the most proximal tibial screw is 1 cm. distal to the proximal tibial physis.

Next, the rigid template is placed in line with and parallel to the anteromedial aspect of the leg. It is vital to be as anterior as possible, immediately medial to the crest of the tibia. The first screw belongs in the most proximal hole of the template, the second (a cortical screw) in the most distal hole.

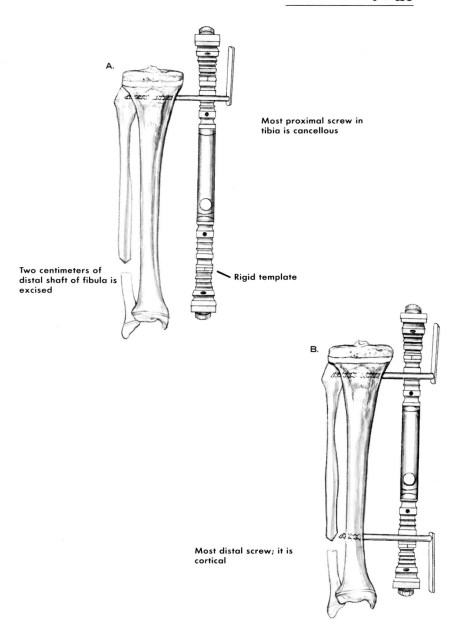

A.

Most proximal screw in
tibia is cancellous

Two centimeters of
distal shaft of fibula is
excised

Rigid template

B.

Most distal screw; it is
cortical

Plate 156. A.–M., Tibial lengthening by callotasis (callus distraction).

C. The third screw (also a cortical screw) is inserted into the fourth hole distal to the first screw.

D. The fourth screw (the final cortical screw) is placed in the superior hole of the distal set of screws. If the leg is large or the tibia fairly skeletally mature, it is advisable to insert three screws in the proximal set and sometimes three screws in the distal set. (See Steps **H.** and **I.** on page 851 and Steps **L.** and **M.** on p. 855.)

C.

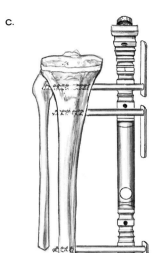

Third screw is placed in
the fifth groove of
the most proximal set
of grooves of the
template

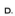

D.

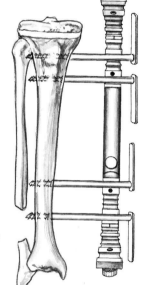

The fourth screw is
placed in the most
proximal groove of the
distal set of grooves of
the template

Plate 156. (Continued)

E. The rigid template is removed. An Orthofix leg-lengthener of appropriate size is then applied.

F. *Corticotomy* is performed 1 cm. inferior to the most distal of the proximal set of screws. A longitudinal incision is made on the anterolateral aspect of the leg. The periosteum is exposed, longitudinally incised, and elevated.

E.

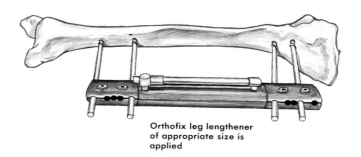

Orthofix leg lengthener
of appropriate size is
applied

F.

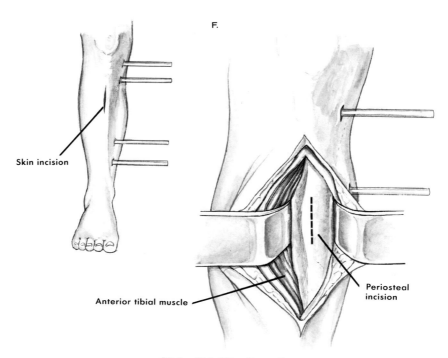

Skin incision

Anterior tibial muscle

Periosteal
incision

Plate 156. (Continued)

G. A 4.8-mm. drill is inserted into a short Orthofix screw guide. The drill stop is adjusted so that the tip of the drill guide protrudes 5 mm. beyond the end of the screw guide. A drill bit of the appropriate size is inserted into the drill guide.

H. Holes are drilled into the medial, lateral, and anterior cortices, with damage to the bone marrow being prevented by the drill stop. The stop is removed for drilling through the cortices medially and laterally.

I. Next, the holes are joined by chiseling the bone *without* penetrating the marrow. Be sure that the medial and lateral cortices of the tibia are completely osteotomized. The posterior cortex is broken by flexing the leg.

Caution! Do not use the screws as a lever to achieve acute flexion at the corticotomy site, because loosening of the screws may occur.

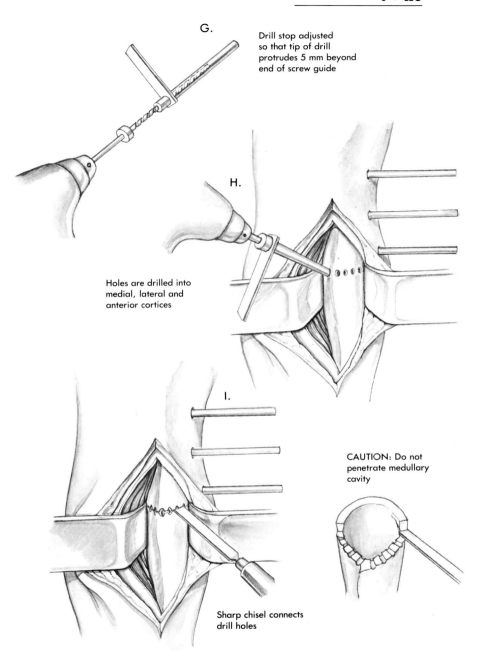

G.

Drill stop adjusted so that tip of drill protrudes 5 mm beyond end of screw guide

H.

Holes are drilled into medial, lateral and anterior cortices

I.

Sharp chisel connects drill holes

CAUTION: Do not penetrate medullary cavity

Plate 156. (Continued)

J. The periosteum is closed meticulously with interrupted sutures.

K. The Orthofix leg-lengthener is placed on the previously inserted screws. The body of the device should be parallel with the tibial shaft.

J.

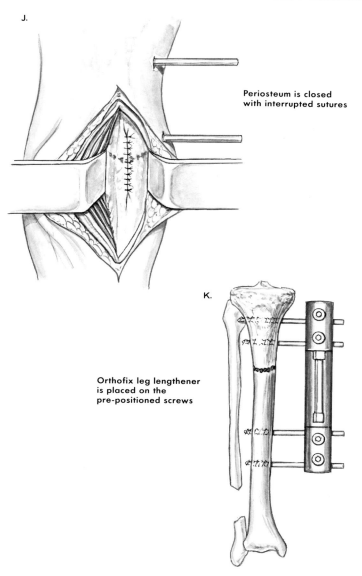

Periosteum is closed
with interrupted sutures

K.

Orthofix leg lengthener
is placed on the
pre-positioned screws

Plate 156. (Continued)

L. and **M.** Any slack in the system is tightened, and the separation of the corticotomy is double-checked by distracting the bony fragments. (If the corticotomy is proved complete this way, the osteotomized fragments are then returned to their original positions.)

Postoperative Care. The wound is drained for 24 to 48 hours after operation, and routine screw tract care is provided as outlined in the femoral lengthening section.

Distraction is begun 10 to 14 days after the corticotomy if by this time radiograms show evidence of early callus formation. The rate of distraction is the same as that outlined for femoral lengthening. Seven days after the start of distraction, radiograms are obtained to confirm separation of the corticotomy with callus continuity. Radiographic follow-up is scheduled for every 14 to 21 days thereafter. If the response of the callus in the elongated segment is poor, distraction is stopped for seven days and then recommenced. If a gap develops in the callus, compression should be applied—at the rate used for distraction—until the gap is eliminated. A wait of seven days should precede resumption of distraction.

During the lengthening process, any axial displacement that may take place is corrected by adjusting the axial position of the lengthener.

When the desired length is obtained, the body-locking screw is tightened and the distraction attachment removed. Full weight-bearing is allowed. When radiograms show good consolidation of the callus, the body-locking screw is loosened; dynamic axial loading is started and continued until adequate cortex is formed all around the elongated segment. At this time the stability of the elongated segment is tested clinically with the fixator removed and the body-locking screw tightened.

If the elongated segment is stable, the screws are left in place for four to six days and then removed. Removal will require appropriate sedation or, in the case of the apprehensive child or adolescent, general anesthesia.

If the elongated segment is mechanically unstable, the fixator is reapplied and dynamic axial loading restarted.

All during this period, physical therapy is performed daily to maintain function of the elongated limb. Again, function is never sacrificed for length.

Healing index is an expression of the number of days required to achieve 1 cm. of lengthening; the figure is obtained by dividing the overall treatment time in days by the total amount of lengthening achieved in centimeters. The healing index, in the experience of Professor DeBastiani, is 36 days for the femur, 41 days for the tibia, and 24 days for the humerus.

REFERENCES

DeBastiani, G.: Lengthening of the lower limbs in achondroplasts. First International Conference on Human Achondroplasia, Rome, November 19–21, 1986.

DeBastiani, G., Aldegheri, R., and Renzi-Brivio, L.: Indicazioni particolari dei fisatori esterni. G. Ital. Fissatore Esterno, 504:31, 1979.

DeBastiani, G., Aldegheri, R., and Renzi-Brivio, L.: Fissatore esterno assiale. Chir. Organi Mov., 65:287, 1979.

DeBastiani, G., Aldegheri, R., and Renzi-Brivio, L.: The treatment of fractures with a dynamic axial fixator. J. Bone Joint Surg., 66-B:538, 1984.

DeBastiani, G., Aldegheri, R., Renzi-Brivio, L., and Trivella, G.: Limb lengthening by distraction of the epiphyseal plate. A comparison of two techniques in the rabbit. J. Bone Joint Surg., 68-B:545, 1986.

DeBastiani, G., Aldegheri, R., Renzi-Brivio, L., and Trivella, G.: Chondrodiastasis-controlled symmetrical distraction of the epiphyseal plate. Limb lengthening in children. J. Bone Joint Surg., 68-B:550, 1986.

DeBastiani, G., Aldegheri, R., Renzi-Brivio, L., and Trivella, G.: Limb lengthening by callus distraction (callotasis). J. Pediatr. Orthop., 7:129, 1987.

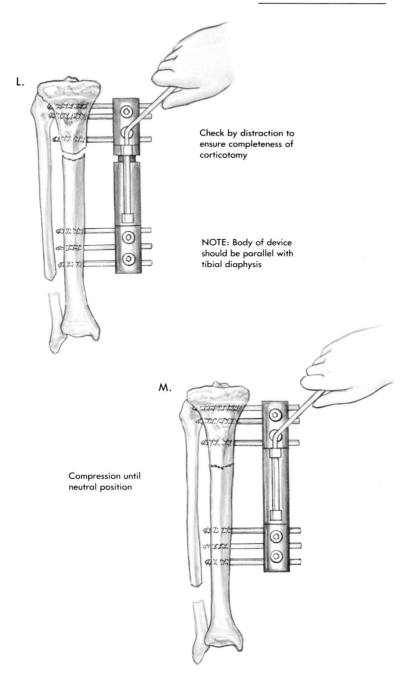

L.

Check by distraction to
ensure completeness of
corticotomy

NOTE: Body of device
should be parallel with
tibial diaphysis

M.

Compression until
neutral position

Plate 156. (Continued)

PLATE 157 | Tibial Segmental Bone Transport by Compression-Distraction

This technique is based on the biologic principle of distraction osteogenesis. The new bone formed by callus distraction fills the bony gap.

Indications

1. Reconstruction of non-unions such as in congenital pseudarthrosis of the tibia.
2. Major post-traumatic defects in long bones as a complication of severe limb injuries in which contaminated, devascularized segments of cortical bone have been excised or lost.
3. In chronic osteomyelitis in which infected necrotic bone is removed to enhance healing. Ordinarily, defects greater than 2.5 to 3 cm. require bone transport.
4. In tumor resection.

Contraindications and Requisites. Those listed in limb lengthening (Plate 137) apply to segmental long bone transport. The treatment course is prolonged, requiring strict compliance by the patient and family during the postoperative period. In tumor resection the contraindications to limb salvage apply to segmental bone transport. In traumatic injuries with neurovascular compromise, segmental bone transport should not be performed.

Prior to segmental bone transport, the surgeon should carry out the following steps.

1. Excise all devitalized or infected segments of bone.
2. Obtain a culture; initially give broad-spectrum antibiotics and then change to an antibiotic to which the organism is sensitive.
3. Debride thoroughly until soft tissues and bone bleed. The wound should be thoroughly irrigated; it should be clean.
4. Square off the bone ends.
5. Excise all interposed fragments that might interfere with transport.
6. In non-union, remove the old hardware.
7. Individualize the soft-tissue cover; it may be obtained by split-thickness skin graft, rotational flaps, or muscle pedicle free vascularized graft. Obtain appropriate plastic surgical consultation in difficult problems. In some cases the wound is allowed to granulate initially and is closed during the distraction period.
8. Often in acute trauma, initially the limb is provisionally stabilized by standard fixation to maintain length and alignment. Avoid overdistraction.

Radiographic Control. Image intensifier.

Blood for Transfusion. No.

Transport Systems. Two types of transport systems are available—the Orthofix and the Ilizarov. When the distal or proximal fragments are too small and osteoporotic, satisfactory screw fixation is not feasible and the use of the Orthofix system is contraindicated; the Ilizarov fixator can often be used in such a case. Otherwise, it is a matter of experience and personal choice of the surgeon. Both systems are technically demanding, the Ilizarov more so than the Orthofix. On the thigh the external rings of the Ilizarov fixator are cumbersome, making it difficult for the patient to sit or lie down.

In this plate the Orthofix system is described and illustrated.

SEGMENTAL BONE TRANSPORT BY THE ORTHOFIX SYSTEM

Special Equipment

1. Assembly kit for standard Orthofix fixator: drill bits, screw sleeves, drill sleeves, trocar, Allen wrench, and T-wrench.

2. Screws: conventional screws for the standard fixator can be used. Choose long screws; 4 to 5 cm. of the screw shank should protrude beyond the skin. The longer length screws allow translational adjustments.

This author recommends the use of cutting edge screws that cut through skin and soft tissues sharply, reducing the degree of discomfort and scarring usually associated with the pressure of conventional screws on soft tissues. The screw tracts heal more readily.

3. Segmental lengthener bodies: the choice of the frame depends on the length of the affected bone.

   a. 400-mm. segmental lengthener body (catalog No. 50510*), used in adults or adolescents or when a joint is crossed.

   b. 300-mm. segmental lengthener body (catalog No. 50500).

   c. Pediatric long segmental slide lengthener kit with three clamps (catalog No. 50.020).

   d. Straight clamp templates (catalog No. 14.107) used for diaphyseal defects. Three templates should be available.

   e. Two T-clamps (catalog No. 50.520) and two T-clamp templates (catalog No. 14.108) used for metadiaphyseal or metaphyseal defects. The use of a T-clamp is crucial for stable fixation on the articular end of the defect.

Preoperative Planning. Determine the proposed sites of corticotomy and insertion of three pairs of screws.

The first step is to make full-length anteroposterior and lateral radiograms of the tibia and femur. Second, determine lower limb lengths, preferably by computed tomography (CT) scan, if not feasible by Bell Thompson ruler. Third, assess mechanical axis deviation.

---

*The numbers refer to the catalog number of Orthofix equipment.

Operative Technique

A. and **B.** In the *tibia,* the level of corticotomy should be below the insertion of the patellar tendon, 2 cm. below the most distal screw of the proximal group or 2 cm. proximal to the most proximal screw of the distal clamp. The corticotomy level is proximal when the defect-gap is distal or central and distal for a proximal gap.

A.   B.

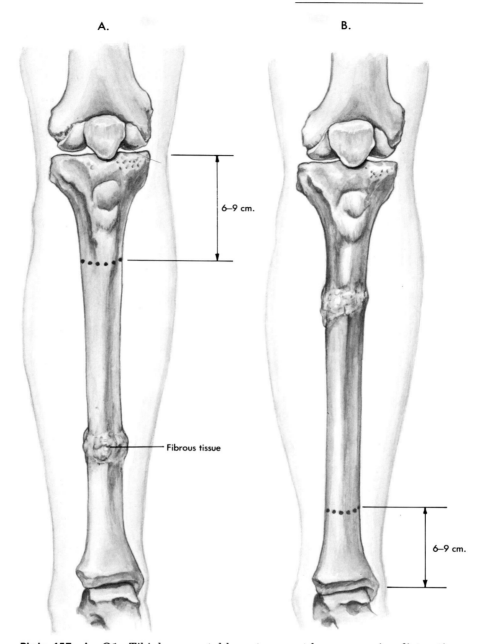

6–9 cm.

Fibrous tissue

6–9 cm.

Plate 157. A.–Q1., Tibial segmental bone transport by compression-distraction.

C. and **D.** In the *femur,* for distal gaps the level of corticotomy is 2 cm. below the most distal screw of the proximal clamp; for proximal gaps, the level of corticotomy is 2 cm. above the most proximal screw of the distal clamp.

C.   D.

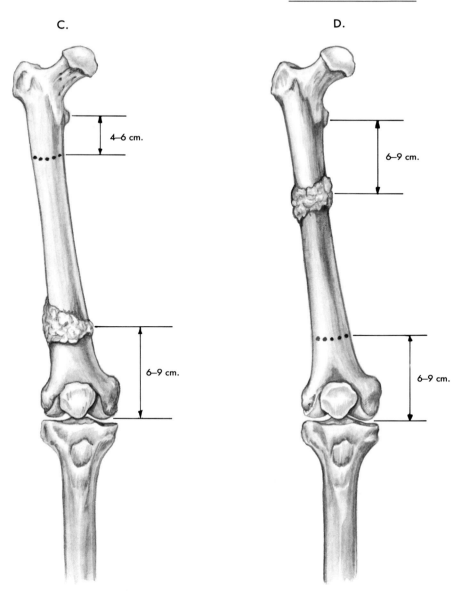

4–6 cm.

6–9 cm.

6–9 cm.

6–9 cm.

Plate 157. (Continued)

Determination of Level of Screw Sites

E. In the *tibia,* three sets of two screws are inserted: *in the long segment,* (1) three screws are proximal (in the growing skeleton and open proximal tibial physis only two screws) and (2) two screws are distal to the proposed site of corticotomy; however, in the short segment, (3) two screws are inserted on the other side of the gap. The screws should not be closer than 2 cm. to the corticotomy site or the gap. This measure provides adequate purchase and stability of fixation; also, when screw tract inflammation develops, it is not close to the gap or corticotomy site.

F. Straight clamps are preferred when the bone length in the short segment between the gap and adjacent joint (in the drawing, the ankle) is at least 7 cm.

E.
Medial application

F.
Anterior application

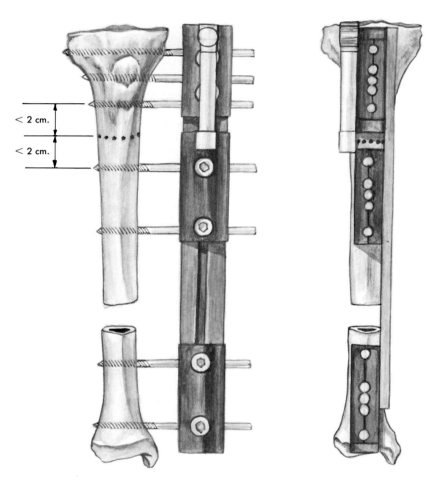

< 2 cm.

< 2 cm.

Pseudarthrosis fibrous tissue
excised and bone surfaces squared

Plate 157. (Continued)

G. A T-clamp is used when the gap is metadiaphyseal or metaphyseal or when less than 7 cm. of bone is present between the gap and the joint in the short segment.

In the tibia the screws and Orthofix transport system can be applied anteriorly, medially, or anteromedially, depending on local soft-tissue conditions. If feasible, anterior application is preferred.

H. In the *femur,* when the gap is distal, three screws are inserted in the *proximal femur*; two screws are positioned in the intertrochanteric region to allow the level of corticotomy to be high—4 to 6 cm. below the lesser trochanter. The distal set of screws is inserted next—one screw is metaphyseal and the other two screws are diaphyseal-metaphyseal. The two screws in the central segment (the one to be transported) should be located superoinferiorly in the middle of the segment.

In the *femur,* the screws and the bone segmental transport system are applied laterally.

Patient Position. The affected lower limb is prepared and draped sterile in the usual orthopedic fashion. A sterile pneumatic tourniquet for tourniquet ischemia is used as necessary and desired, especially during debridement and corticotomy. Preoperatively, depending on the site of the gap and proposed site of corticotomy, the exact level and position of screws are determined; under image-intensifier radiographic control, these sites are located and marked on the skin with indelible sterile ink.

Screw insertion. Correct insertion of screws is crucial. First, the most proximal and the most distal screws are inserted.

In the diaphysis, cortical screws are used; they are predrilled with a 4.8-mm drill bit. In the metaphysis, cancellous screws are used; they are predrilled with a 3.2-mm. drill bit. The screws should be longer than usual to accommodate the natural taper of the lower limb; the shank of the proximal screws should protrude at least 4 cm. beyond the skin, and the distal screws should protrude 8 cm. Two threads protrude through the far cortex, and four or five threads should remain outside the adjacent cortex. The screw lengths are chosen by using the x-ray screw selector transparency provided by Orthofix. Both the template and definitive screw clamps fit the body of the transport system; therefore, a separate template body is not required.

G.

H.

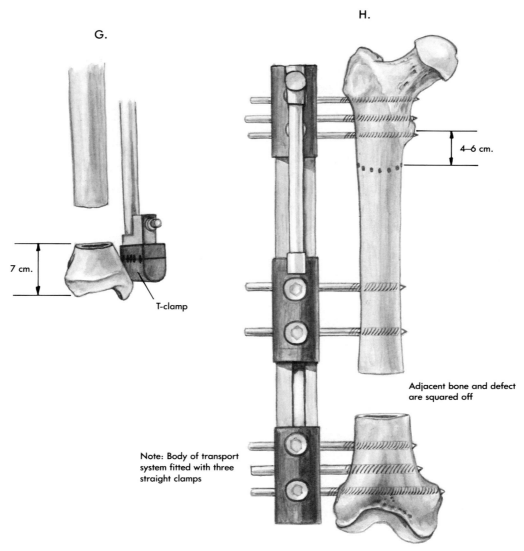

7 cm.

T-clamp

4–6 cm.

Adjacent bone and defect
are squared off

Note: Body of transport
system fitted with three
straight clamps

Plate 157. (Continued)

I. These straight clamps are mounted onto the transport body when the gap is diaphyseal and the shorter segment is more than 7 cm. in length. In the *tibia,* the 300-mm. segmental body lengthener (catalog No. 50500) is usually used.

J. When the gap is metaphyseal or diaphyseal-metaphyseal or when the gap is diaphyseal but too close to the joint (the short segment is 7 cm. or less), a T-clamp is used for fixation. Mount the T-clamp template to the transport system.

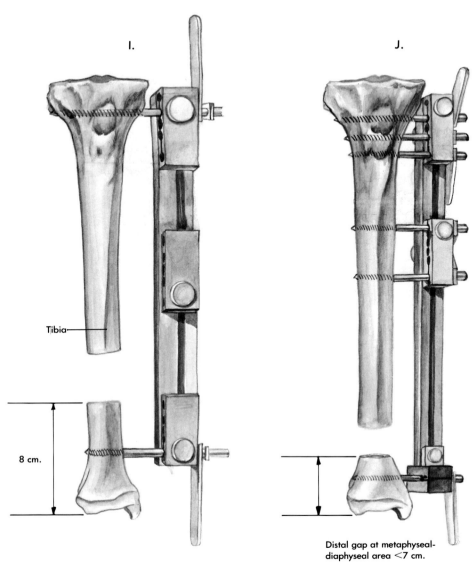

I.   J.

Tibia

8 cm.

Distal gap at metaphyseal-
diaphyseal area <7 cm.

Plate 157. (Continued)

K. and **L.** First, insert the screw in the shortest bone segment most adjacent to the joint—in this instance, the ankle joint. In anterior applications of the segmental bone transport system, this screw is inserted perpendicular to the shaft of the bone; it is crucial that the first screw be aligned properly in the sagittal plane in anterior applications; in medial applications the first screw must be aligned properly in the coronal plane.

In choosing the site of the first screw, consideration should be given to the location of the second screw in the same clamp adjacent to the gap; there should be 2 cm. of good bone between the screw and the gap.

The technique of drilling and screw insertion is performed through sleeves as described and illustrated in Plates 138 and 156.

K.

Anterior application

L.

Medial application

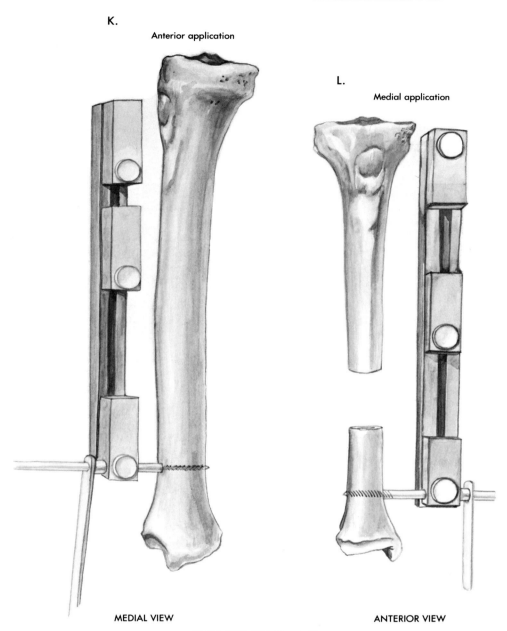

MEDIAL VIEW

ANTERIOR VIEW

Plate 157. (Continued)

M. and **N.** Insert the second screw opposite the first screw at the proximal end of the segmental lengthener. Use the template clamp on the transport body as a guide. Be sure the proximal and distal segments are aligned anatomically. There should be no rotational or angular malalignment.

A vital consideration in the placement of the second screw is the position of the template for the middle (central) segment. Determine this by image-intensifier radiography. The holes of the template should be visualized as perfect circles overlying the central segment. Make the necessary adjustments for the site of the second (i.e., the most proximal) screw so that the clamp template for the middle segment is directly over the middle segment of bone.

It is best to support the position of the middle screw template by drilling one or two 0.062-mm. Kirschner wires through the holes of the middle template into the central bone segment. The Kirschner wires also serve as guides for eventual screw insertion into the central segment.

O. Insert the second screw, and axially align the bone transport system. Inspect the position of the screws in the middle segment and that of the additional screws in the proximal and distal segments.

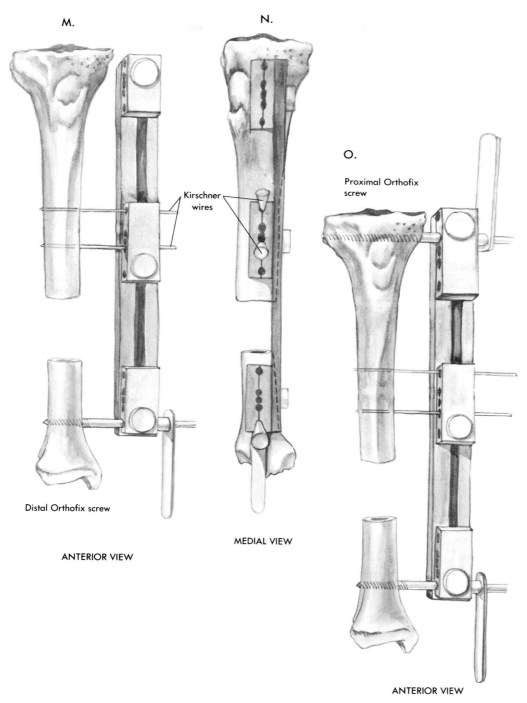

M.

N.

O.

Proximal Orthofix
screw

Kirschner
wires

Distal Orthofix screw

ANTERIOR VIEW

MEDIAL VIEW

ANTERIOR VIEW

Plate 157. (Continued)

P. Any malalignment in the plate at right angles to the fixator is corrected, and the two additional screws in the proximal and the second screw in the distal segments are inserted.

Q. Finally, insert the two screws in the central segment. Be sure the proximal and distal screws in the middle segment are as near to the center of the transport segment as possible.

P.

Q.

Temporary
Kirschner
wires

Central segment
Orthofix screws

Orthofix template

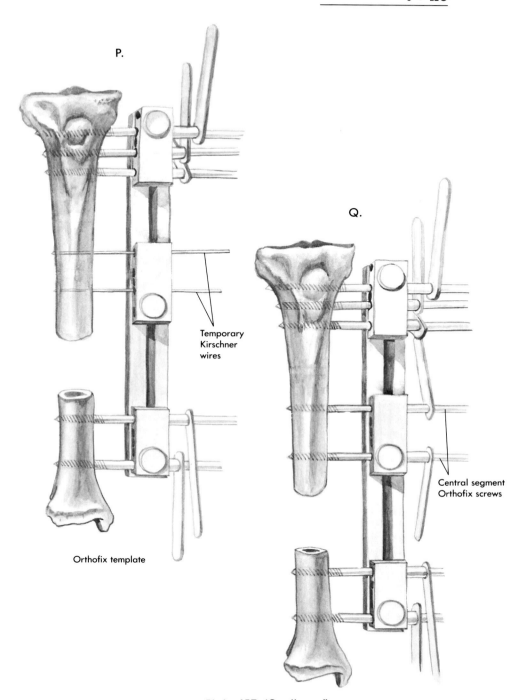

Plate 157. (Continued)

R. Remove the screw clamp templates and the body of the segmental lengthener. By image-intensifier radiography, check the position of the screws; they should purchase both cortices.

S. Remove the template clamps from the body of the segmental lengthener, and mount the definitive clamps onto the frame. Place the lengthener onto the screws with the body of the frame parallel to the long axis of the tibia. To allow dressings and pin site care, there should be 2 to 2.5 cm. of space between the skin of the leg and the body of the lengthener. Tauten the clamps onto the screws and onto the transport body.

R. ANTEROMEDIAL VIEW

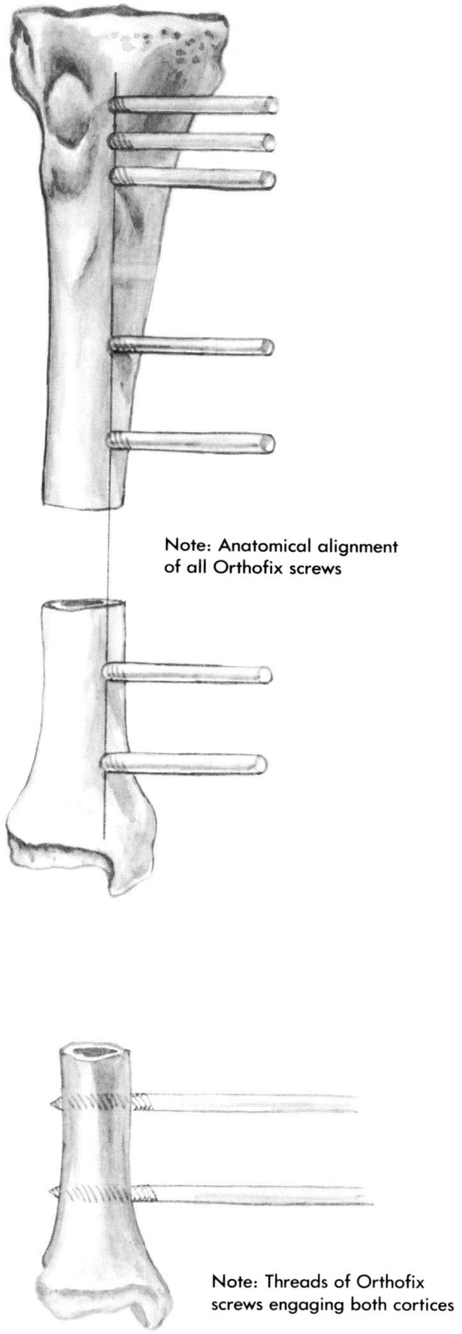

S.

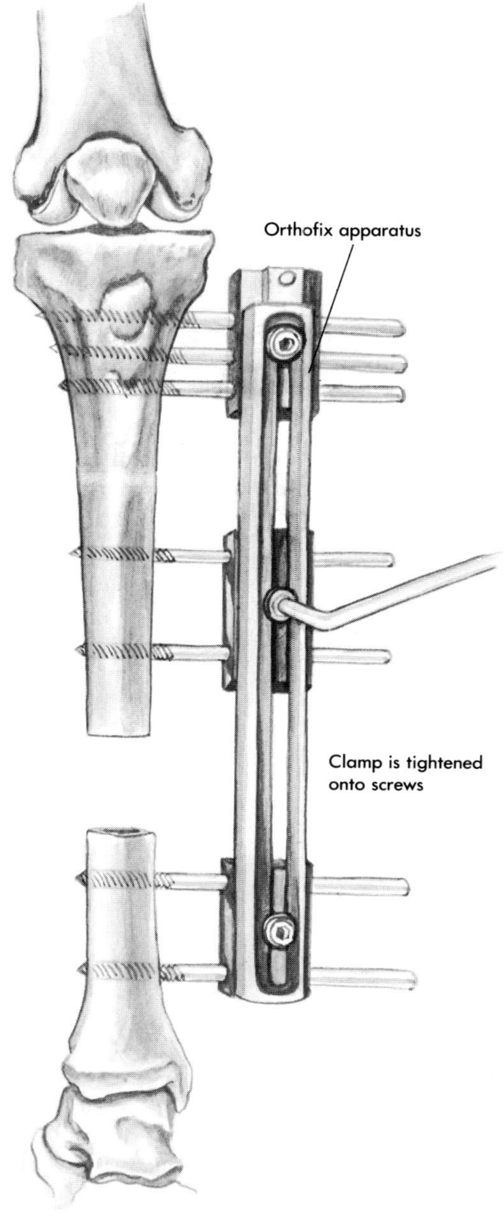

Orthofix apparatus

Note: Anatomical alignment
of all Orthofix screws

Clamp is tightened
onto screws

Note: Threads of Orthofix
screws engaging both cortices

Plate 157. (Continued)

T1. and **T2.** Any medial or lateral translation of the segments is corrected at this time. Loosen the distal screw clamp, and by changing the distance between the skin of the leg at the distal screws and the fixator body, displace the distal segment medially or laterally. A decrease in the gap translates the distal fragment toward the fixator body and vice versa; an increase in the gap translates the distal fragment away from the fixator body. When the ankle and distal tibia are translated medially, pull and move the distal tibia–ankle toward the fixator body (T1); when they are translated laterally, displace the distal tibia–ankle away from the fixator body (T2). Secure the new correct position of the segments by retightening the clamp or the screws.

T₁.

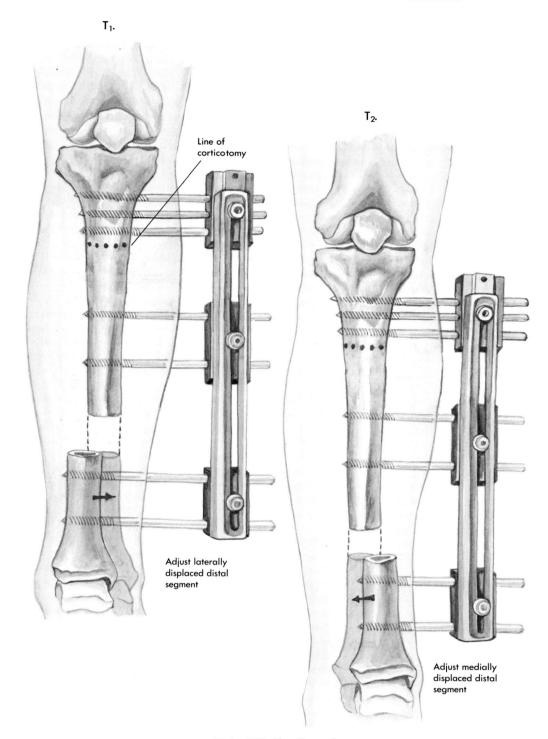

T₂.

Line of
corticotomy

Adjust laterally
displaced distal
segment

Adjust medially
displaced distal
segment

Plate 157. (Continued)

U. Apply a compression-distraction apparatus between the middle and proximal clamps.

V. A corticotomy of the proximal tibia is performed through a 5-cm longitudinal incision as described in Plate 156. There should be at least 2 cm. of space between the corticotomy site and the immediately adjacent screws. Meticulous longitudinal incision and stripping of the periosteum are important. Chandler retractors are placed subperiosteally. A series of holes is made through the anterior and posterior cortices with a 4.8-mm. drill bit inserted through a drill guide. AO sharp osteotomes are used to complete the osteotomy. Do not use a power saw!

W. Distract the compression-distraction unit, and verify that the osteotomy is complete by the gap between the proximal and middle segments.

U.

V.

W.

Testing completeness
of corticotomy

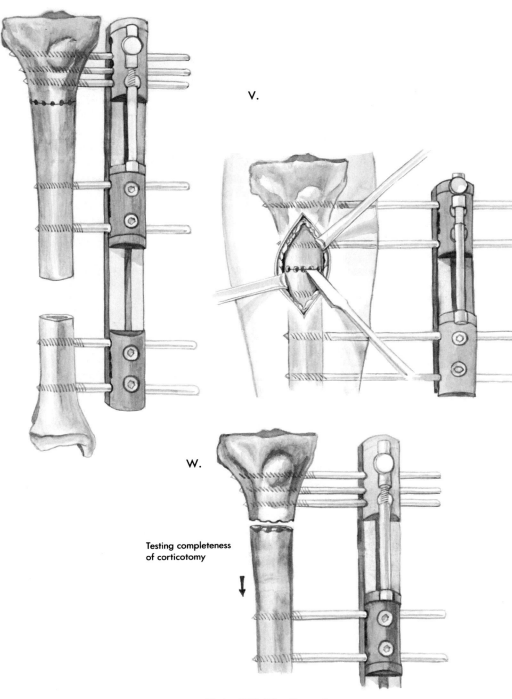

Plate 157. (Continued)

X. The corticotomy is closed, and the bolts connecting the screw clamps to the body of the segmental lengthener are tautened.

The tourniquet is released. Complete hemostasis is achieved, and the periosteum is meticulously closed with 00 Vicryl or other absorbable sutures.

A medium-sized Hemovac is inserted into the wound. Fasciotomy of the anterior compartment is performed, and the wound is closed in the usual fashion.

The corticotomy wound and screw-skin interfaces are covered with sterile dressings. The leg and foot are supported in a posterior splint with the foot-ankle in neutral position.

Postoperative Care. The lower limb is elevated for a few days until postoperative swelling subsides. The Hemovac suction tubes are removed one to three days after surgery, depending on local wound conditions and the amount of drainage. The patient is allowed to be ambulatory as soon as he or she is comfortable with partial weight-bearing in a three-point crutch gait.

Passive and active range of motion exercises of the ankle and knee are performed several times a day to prevent contractural deformity and to restore normal motor strength of muscles controlling the knee and ankle. Physiotherapy is continued during the entire course of bone transport.

Pin site care is provided daily. Sterile water is used to clean the skin around the screws. Excessive activity of the patient and mobility of the limb may cause irritation of the soft tissues by the pins and result in serous drainage. *Do not mistake the serous drainage for infection.* Continue simple pin site care with sterile water, and restrain the patient from strenuous activity. An adagio performance is appropriate.

If screw tract infection develops with increased warmth and redness of soft tissues around the pins and purulent drainage, cultures are taken and appropriate antibiotic therapy is administered. Radiograms are made to rule out osteolysis. Pin site release may be indicated if there is excessive pressure and bunching of soft tissues ahead of the advancing pin. The use of cutting screws has minimized the problem. Occasionally, a screw may become loose; in such an instance, the loose screw is removed and replaced.

Y. *Transport.* On the seventh to tenth day, the locking bolt on the central (i.e., middle) clamp is released and the middle bone segment is advanced distally by turning the compression-distraction apparatus (C-D unit connecting the proximal and distal bone segments) counterclockwise one-quarter turn four times a day; i.e., 0.25 mm. distraction is carried out for each one-quarter turn, or 1 mm. distraction per day. Anteroposterior and lateral radiograms of the tibia are made on the fourth day (to check if a gap is opening) and once a week thereafter. The rate of transport is adjusted according to local wound conditions, age of the patient (the younger the patient, the more rapid the osteogenesis), and the radiographic appearance. In the younger child distraction may be more rapid, 1.5 mm. per day, and in the adolescent or adult it may be 0.75 or 0.50 mm. per day. In performing a diaphyseal corticotomy, proceed at a slow rate.

Transport (i.e., distraction) is continued until the central segment docks with the end segment. Soft-tissue and pin site problems are managed as outlined earlier. Alignment between the bone segments may require adjustment. This is performed in the operating room under strict sterile conditions under appropriate sedation or general anesthesia. Medial or lateral translation is rectified by loosening the middle clamp screws and moving the screw shanks further out from, or further into, the clamp.

X.

Y.

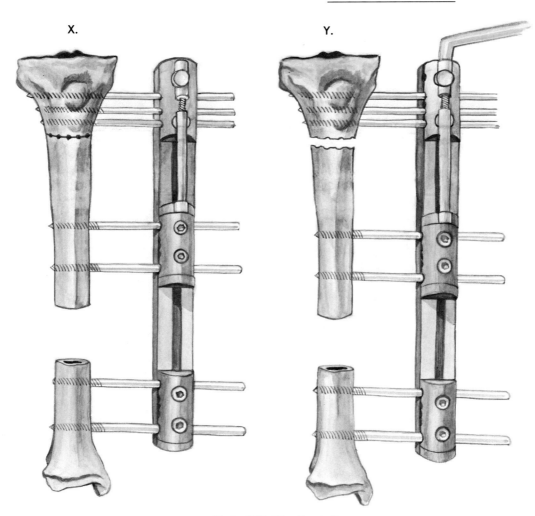

Plate 157. (Continued)

The Docking Procedure

A1. At the end of the transport, the middle and end bone segments should be apposed and anatomically aligned.

Remove the locks of the central clamp on the rail.

B1. Attach a compression-distraction unit between the middle and distal segments, and remove the distal locking screw and washer. Turn the screw of the compression-distraction unit clockwise for compression, then lock the distal clamp to the rail. Assess consolidation and maintenance of alignment at the docking site and also at the elongated segment by periodic anteroposterior and lateral radiograms.

A₁.   B₁.

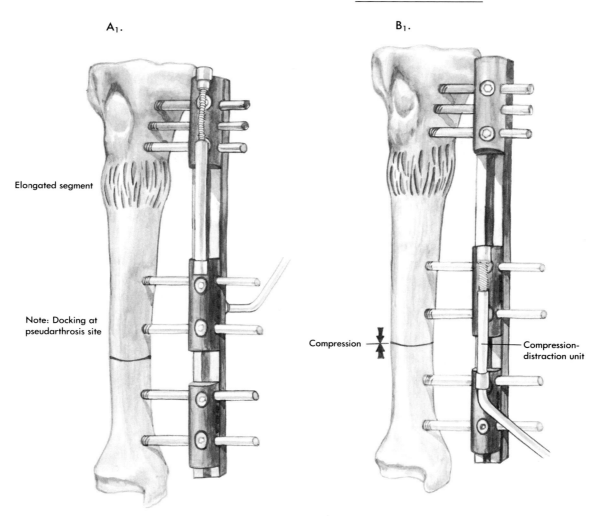

Elongated segment

Note: Docking at
pseudarthrosis site

Compression

Compression-
distraction unit

Plate 157. (Continued)

Dynamization of the Docking Site

C1. When adequate union is achieved between the transported segment and the end distal tibial segments, the docking site is dynamized by loosening the distal clamp and attaching the dyna-ring above the loosened distal clamp.

The docking site and the segment of newly formed distracted callus bone often heal at different rates. The unilateral three-clamp bone transport system allows individual dynamization and removal of clamp and screws between the docking site and distraction callus. When there is solid consolidation at the docking site but inadequate healing of distraction callus, only the distal clamp and screw are removed; the middle and proximal clamps are left intact until consolidation of the distraction callus takes place.

Management of the Distraction Callus

The beginning of the neutralization period of the distraction osteogenesis site depends on whether the lower limbs are even or there is limb length disparity and limb lengthening is planned.

D1. When tibial lengthening is indicated and planned, the middle clamp is locked on the rail, the locking screw on the proximal clamp is removed, and tibial lengthening is performed as outlined in Plate 156. On equalization of limb lengths, lock the proximal clamp on the rail, remove the compression-distraction unit, and begin the neutralization period.

C₁.

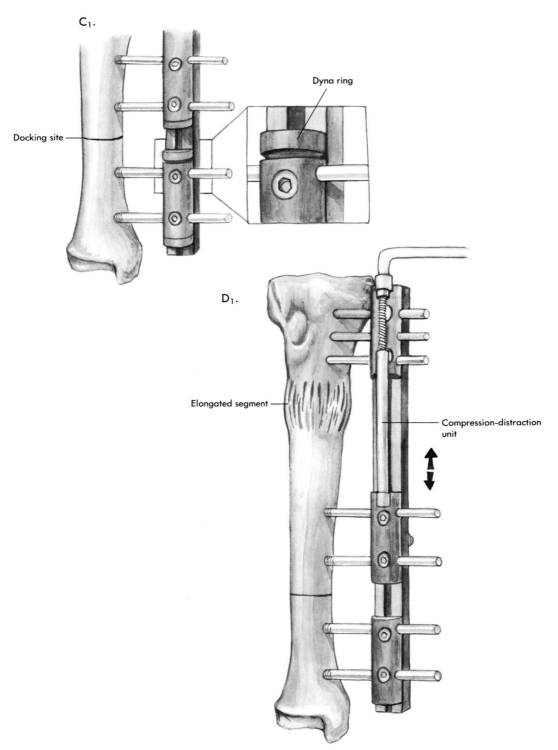

Docking site

Dyna ring

D₁.

Elongated segment

Compression-distraction unit

Plate 157. (Continued)

E1. When limb lengths are even to begin with, and limb lengthening is not indicated, lock the proximal and middle clamps to the rail, remove the compression-distraction unit, and commence the neutralization period.

E₁.

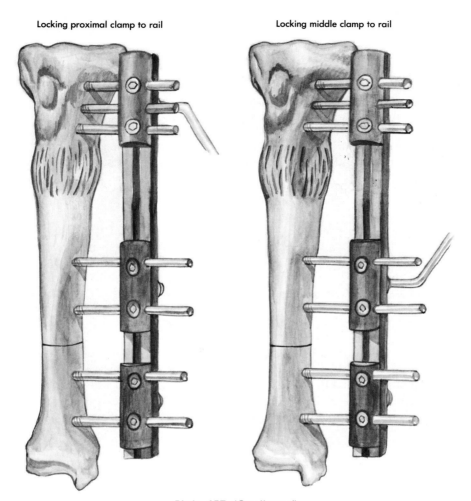

Locking proximal clamp to rail   Locking middle clamp to rail

Plate 157. (Continued)

F1. *Dynamization of the distraction-osteogenesis segment.* During the neutralization period, anteroposterior, lateral, and oblique radiograms of the tibia are made periodically, and healing of the elongated segment is assessed. There should be continuity of the cortices in at least three of four surfaces, that is, medial, lateral, anterior, and posterior.

To dynamize, lock the middle and distal clamps to the rail, remove the proximal clamp locking screw, and attach the dyna-ring below the proximal clamp.

Removal of the Clamps and Screw. When there is adequate cortex formation in all four planes and canalization of the medullary cavity, all the screws and clamps are removed.

The limb is protected in an above-knee orthosis with an anterior shell on the leg for an additional three to six months to prevent stress fracture.

Delayed Healing. Delayed healing may occur at the docking site or at the distraction osteogenesis segment, requiring various modalities of treatment to stimulate healing, such as autogenous bone graft or allograft, bone marrow injection, or the use of the bone growth stimulator.

G1. In the femur when the defect is distal, proximal corticotomy and proximal to distal transport are performed. For secure and stable fixation, three screws are inserted in the proximal femur. As stated earlier, the corticotomy site is 4 to 6 cm. distal to the lesser trochanter. Surgical approach is through an anterior incision, dividing the deep fascia and developing the space between rectus femoris medially and sartorius laterally. The fibers of vastus intermedius are divided, and the periosteum is opened.

H1. The distal screws in the femur should be perpendicular to the femoral shaft and not to the axis of the knee joint. There is a normal valgus of the knee. When the distal screw is inserted parallel to the knee joint surface, it will cause either varus malpositioning between the proximal and distal segments or lateral tracking of the transported segment.

F₁.

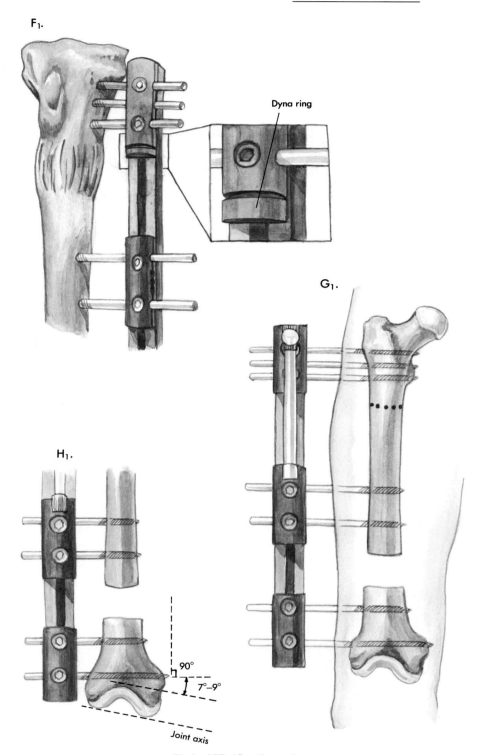

Dyna ring

G₁.

H₁.

90°

7°–9°

Joint axis

Plate 157. (Continued)

I1. and **J1.** First, the proximal screw is inserted. Next, the most distal screw is inserted; it is crucial that the position of the screw in the distal segment be correct. If malpositioned, the screws in the middle clamp will miss the bone in the transport segment—they should engage the bone.

K1. and **L1.** A T-clamp is used when the end fragment is small. Use of image-intensifier radiographic control and appropriate planning of the site of screw insertion are crucial. The posterior and anterior screws should be equidistant from the respective posterior and anterior cortices of the femoral condyles (K1). If the posterior screw is placed too far anteriorly, the anterior screw will miss the bone (L1).

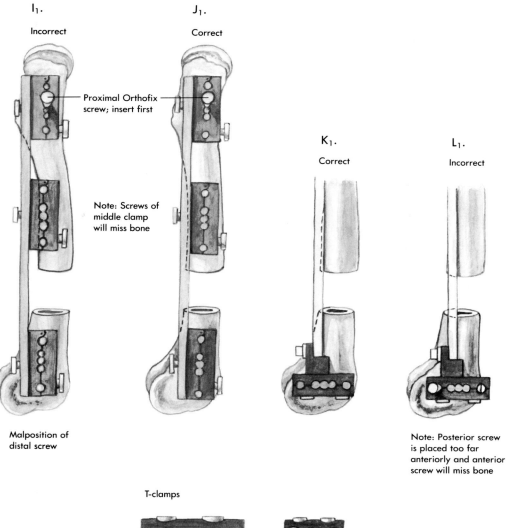

I₁.

Incorrect

J₁.

Correct

Proximal Orthofix
screw; insert first

Note: Screws of
middle clamp
will miss bone

Malposition of
distal screw

K₁.

Correct

L₁.

Incorrect

Note: Posterior screw
is placed too far
anteriorly and anterior
screw will miss bone

T-clamps

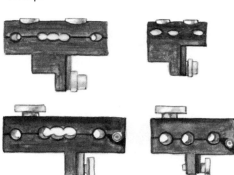

Plate 157. (Continued)

M1. and **N1.** The swiveling clamp is used for immediate or late correction of angular deformity by manipulation of the bone segments at the callus site.

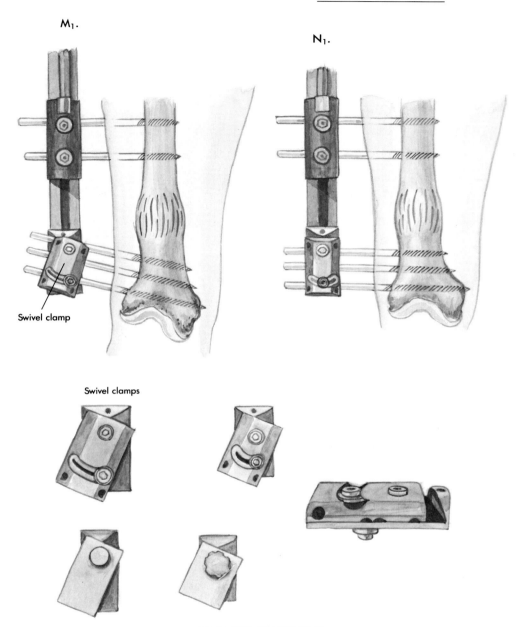

Plate 157. (Continued)

O1.–Q1. *Ball-joint coupling.* When unlocked, ball-joint coupling allows free rotation and 36 degrees of angular derotation in any plane.

O₁.

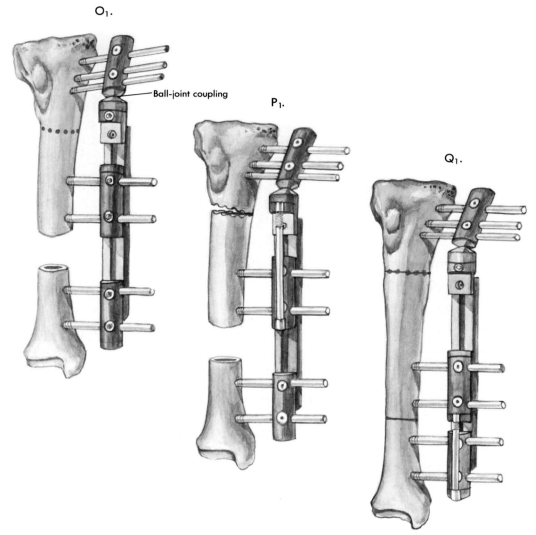

Ball-joint coupling

P₁.

Q₁.

Plate 157. (Continued)

PLATE 158   **Single-Level Tibial Lengthening (Ilizarov Method)**

Indications. Limb length disparity in the tibia greater than 5 cm. in a patient of normal stature.

Requisites

1. The knee and ankle joint should be stable.
2. Circulation should be normal.
3. There should be no skin or soft tissue problems.
4. Bone structures should be normal.
5. Psychosocially, the patient should be stable.
6. The patient should be cooperative and cognizant of the postoperative program.

Never sacrifice function for length!

Radiographic Control. Image intensifier.

Blood for Transfusion. No.

Patient Position. Supine.

Stages. Lengthening of the tibia or any long bone consists of the following stages:

1. Preoperative planning and assembly of the apparatus.
2. Application of the Ilizarov fixator.
3. A three- to ten-day period of latency prior to distraction.
4. A period of distraction, with the time dependent on the total length desired (approximately 1.0 mm. per day).
5. A period of complete immobilization and fixation of the elongated segment.
6. A period of two to three weeks of dynamization of the immobilized bone fragments and regenerated bone between them with cessation of distraction-compression.
7. Removal of the Ilizarov fixator and support of the elongated bone in a cast or brace, depending on the individual case.

Operative Technique

Preassembly

A. Assemble the frame prior to surgery under nonsterile conditions according to clinical measurements of the circumference and length of the patient's leg and radiographic mensuration of the distance between the proximal and distal tibial physes. This preassembly of the apparatus will save considerable time in the operating room. A preassembled frame will necessitate adjustments during surgery.

When lengthening with simultaneous correction of deformity of the tibia is planned, it is desirable to make a plastic model of the limb. Draw the mechanical axis deviation and apex of deformity from tracings of standing anteroposterior (AP) and lateral radiograms of the entire lower limb. The apex and plane of deformity are determined. Preoperative planning is crucial.

The Ilizarov Frame. The most proximal ring, a "five-eighths" ring, is open posteriorly so that it does not restrict knee flexion.

Note: A five-eighths ring is not strong by itself; it must be used in combination with a full ring.

Additional strength can be provided by the use of a half-pin inserted antero-posteriorly, perpendicular to the longitudinal axis of the tibia and attached to the proximal full ring by the Rancho mounting technique. The half-pin is secured to the ring by a two-hole or three-hole pin-gripping clamp. The second proximal and the two distal rings are full rings that consist of two half-rings of the same size, joined by two bolts and nuts.

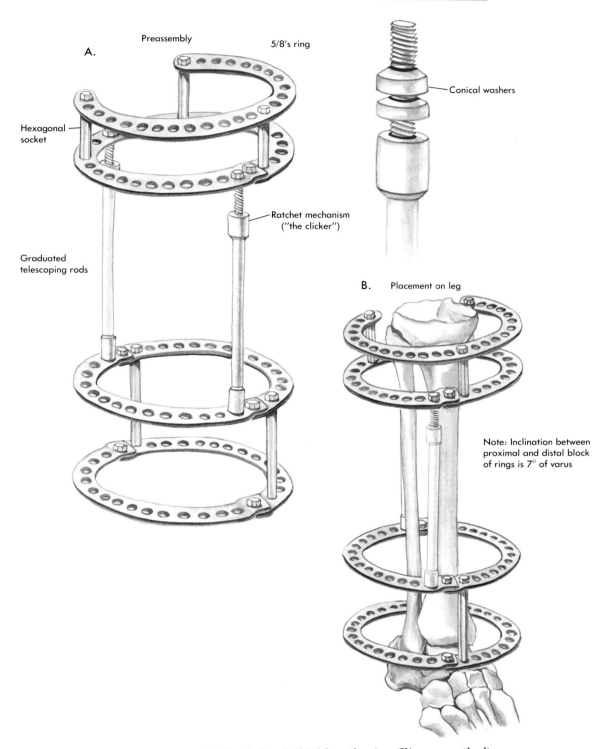

A.

Preassembly

5/8's ring

Hexagonal socket

Graduated telescoping rods

Conical washers

Ratchet mechanism ("the clicker")

B.   Placement on leg

Note: Inclination between proximal and distal block of rings is 7° of varus

Plate 158. A.–Q., Single-level tibial lengthening (Ilizarov method).

Selection of Proper Ring Size. The internal diameter of the ring should be large enough to allow clearance of two fingerbreadths (about 3 cm.) from the skin at the widest part of the leg. A simple method is to measure the diameter of the widest part of the leg. This is done in both the frontal and sagittal planes by choosing the largest diameter and then adding 6 cm. to this measurement. A final check should be made by actual fitting of the ring around the patient's leg.

Level of Rings. Ring level is obtained by measuring the distance between the proximal tibial physis and distal tibial physis on the radiograms, with the 15 per cent x-ray magnification taken into account. Also, the frame is fitted on the patient's leg before surgery and checked by AP and lateral radiograms. The proximal ring should be just distal to the proximal tibial physis, and the distal ring should be just proximal to the distal tibial physis.

Connection of Rings with Telescoping and Threaded Rods. The proximal block consists of a five-eighths ring and a full ring. The distal block consists of two full rings. The rings are connected with 40-mm. sockets, short bolts, and one hexagonal socket at each end of the five-eighths ring.

Proximal and Distal Blocks

The proximal block is connected by hexagonal sockets. The sockets are placed at each end of the five-eighths ring. The central socket is placed on the medial side of the central connecting bolt.

The distal block is connected with two 40-mm. hexagonal sockets placed on the medial sides of the central bolts both anteriorly and posteriorly.

The distal block and proximal block are connected with telescoping graduated connecting rods, one each on the lateral side of the central bolts anteriorly and posteriorly. Conical washers must be used to connect the two blocks. They consist of a convex and concave component with a spherical surface. The washers are placed on the threaded rod. The convex surface is applied against the ring. Connect the threaded rod to the equivalent side of the proximal block at the first hole lateral to the central bolt. Add a conical washer and nut to each. This allows tilting of the ring up to 7½ degrees in each direction. Measure the length of the threaded rod protruding from the telescoping rod on the front and the back. The front should be 1 to 1½ cm. longer than the back. Lock the frame tilted 7 degrees higher on the medial side and 7 degrees higher anteriorly. The medial side is the side with the socket.

Placement of Frame on Leg

B. Make sure that all connections are tight. The frame should be firm. Insert the foot-ankle through the rings and position the frame on the leg.

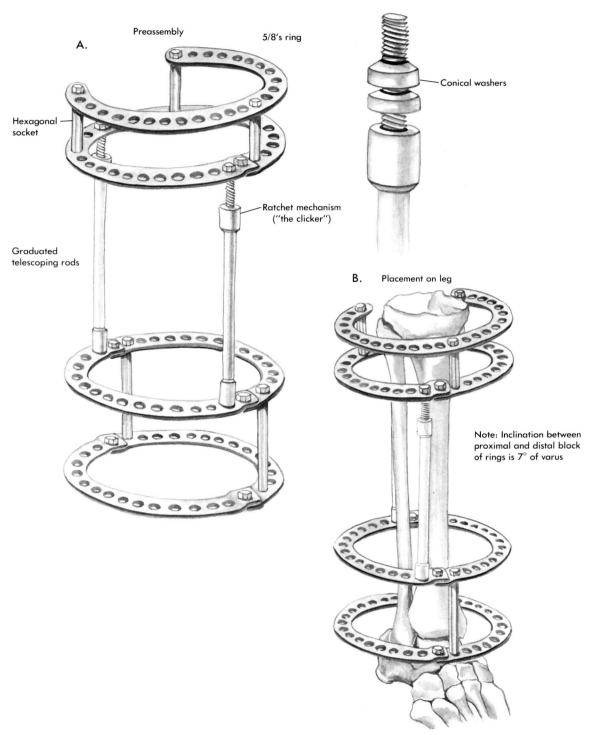

A. Preassembly
5/8's ring

Hexagonal socket

Conical washers

Ratchet mechanism ("the clicker")

Graduated telescoping rods

B. Placement on leg

Note: Inclination between proximal and distal block of rings is 7° of varus

Plate 158. (Continued)

Reference Wires

C. The first wire is inserted in the frontal plane. The wire should be at an inclination of 7 degrees to the knee joint. It is inserted from the lateral side. A 1.8-mm. olive wire should exit more proximally on the medial than on the lateral side. Its plane is similar to the inclination of the proximal block of rings.

The second wire, a 1.8-mm. smooth wire, is inserted from the lateral side in the frontal plane just proximal to the ankle joint and parallel to the tibial plafond. Extend the frame so that it fills the space between the two wires. The proximal block should be flush with the proximal reference wire, and the distal block should be flush with the distal reference wire.

Centering

D. *Lateral.* Center and fix the apparatus to the two frontal reference wires. One person holds the frame with one to two fingerbreadths of space between the rings anteriorly and the crest of the tibia. There should be two fingerbreadths of space left in circumference around the soft tissues of the leg. Check that the anterior rod is parallel with the crest of the tibia from the lateral view.

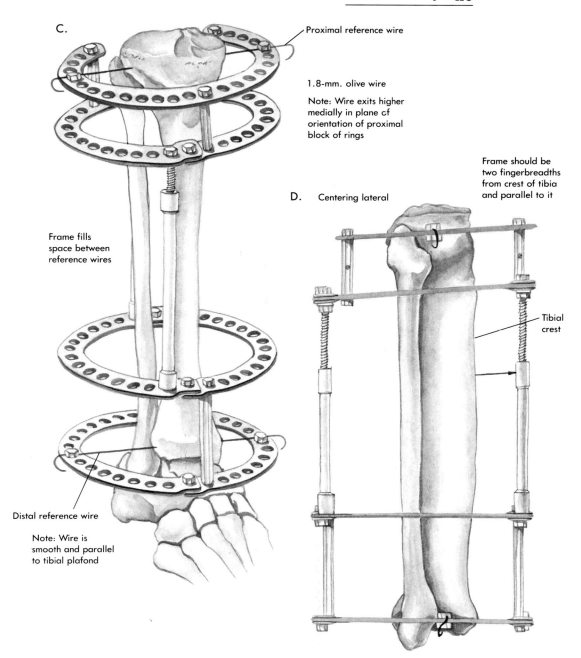

C.

Proximal reference wire

1.8-mm. olive wire

Note: Wire exits higher medially in plane cf orientation of proximal block of rings

Frame fills space between reference wires

Distal reference wire

Note: Wire is smooth and parallel to tibial plafond

Frame should be two fingerbreadths from crest of tibia and parallel to it

D.   Centering lateral

Tibial crest

Plate 158. (Continued)

E. *Anteroposterior.* Center the central fixation bolts so that they are over the crest of the tibia proximally and distally. In case the distal block is not centered correctly, it can be shifted medially or laterally because the distal reference wire is smooth. After centering, the rest of the wires can be inserted.

Following lateral and anteroposterior centering, I recommend secure fixation of the Ilizarov apparatus to the tibia by two Ilizarov half-pins inserted anteroposteriorly at right angles to the longitudinal axis of the tibia, immediately medial to the crest of the tibia. The proximal half-pin is attached to the full ring of the proximal block of rings by a two- or three-hole pin-gripping clamp, whereas the distal half-pin is similarly secured to the superior full ring of the distal block of rings.

Fibular Wires

F. Insert a fibular wire in each block next. The proximal block should be on the most proximal ring and inserted through the head of the fibula. The second wire is inserted on the second most distal ring through the fibula. The two wires are in the same direction. Tension the wires as described in Plate 250 (Appendix).

E.   Centering AP

Insertion of fibular wires

Fibular wire
through proximal
ring block

F.

Proximal transverse
reference wire

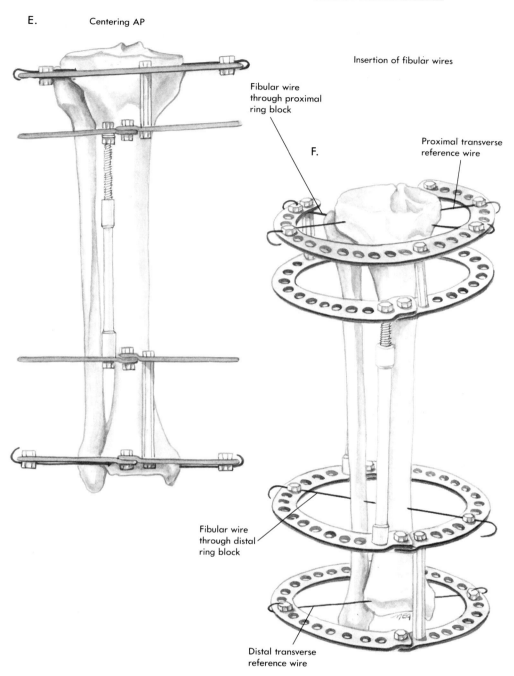

Fibular wire
through distal
ring block

Distal transverse
reference wire

Plate 158. (Continued)

Medial Face Wires

G. Insert two more wires, one in the proximal block and one in the distal block, parallel to the medial surface of the tibia. The proximal wire runs through the second ring from the top. It enters anterolaterally at the tibial crest and exits posteromedially. The distal wire enters between the tendons of tibialis anterior and extensor hallucis longus; it is an olive wire. It exits at the posteromedial corner.

The fibular wires are perpendicular to the medial face wires. This configuration provides maximal biomechanical strength with the wires at 90-degree angles to each other.

Transverse Wires

H. The last two olive wires are transverse in the frontal plane, inserted from the medial side on the second ring in the proximal block and the second to last in the distal block. All the wires are tensioned (see Plate 250).

G.

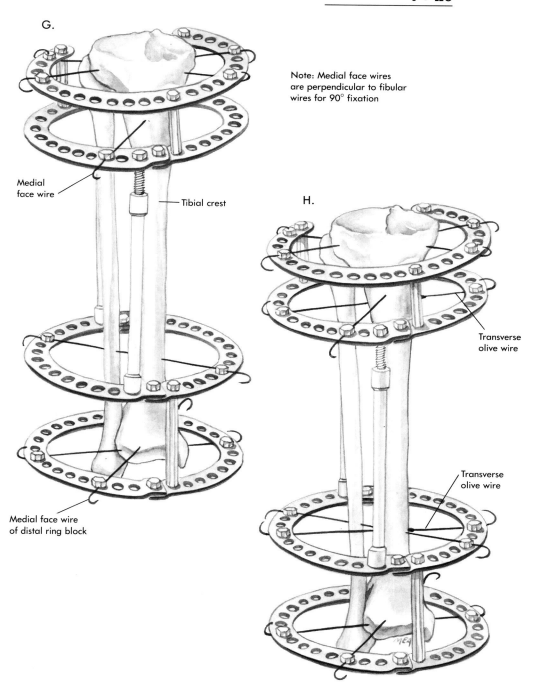

Note: Medial face wires
are perpendicular to fibular
wires for 90° fixation

Medial
face wire

Tibial crest

H.

Transverse
olive wire

Transverse
olive wire

Medial face wire
of distal ring block

Plate 158. (Continued)

Fibular Osteotomy

I. Divide the fibula at the juncture of the medial and distal thirds through a 2-cm. longitudinal incision. Expose it subperiosteally, and divide it with an electric saw.

Tibial Corticotomy

J. *Preparation.* First, remove the connecting rods between the proximal and distal blocks of rings. Check the stability, and perform the toggle test for motion. There should not be any movement either in flexion-extension or varus-valgus angulation.

I. Fibular osteotomy

J. Preparation for corticotomy

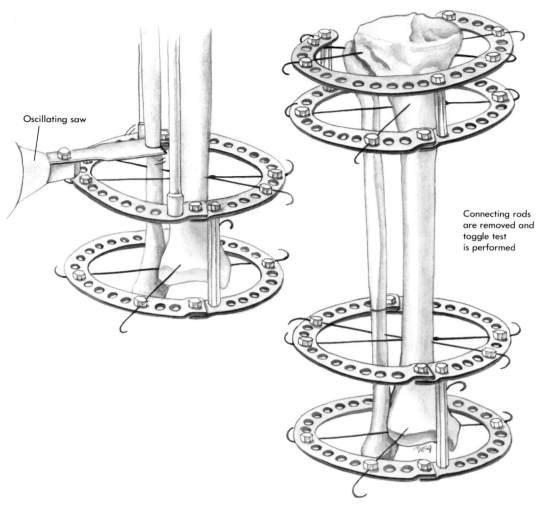

Oscillating saw

Connecting rods
are removed and
toggle test
is performed

Plate 158. (Continued)

K.–M. *Procedure.* Make a 1- to 2-cm. anterior incision over the anterior crest of the tibia just distal to the second proximal ring. The direction of the osteotomy is posterodistal. First, elevate the periosteum and insert two Chandler retractors to protect the soft tissues. Second, cut the anterior cortex of the tibia with a sharp osteotome. Change to a 5-mm. sharp osteotome, and cut the medial and lateral cortices. Once you have gone through the posteromedial corner, cut down the lateral side reaching the posterolateral corner. Leave the posterior cortex intact. Twist the osteotome laterally to break the posterior cortex.

K.

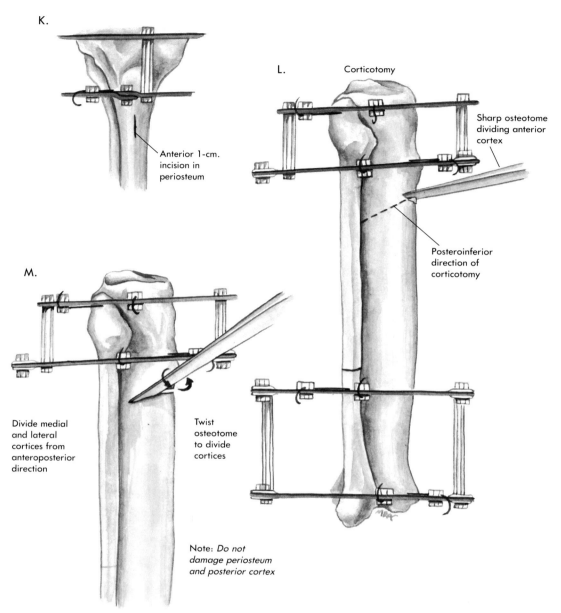

Anterior 1-cm. incision in periosteum

L.   Corticotomy

Sharp osteotome dividing anterior cortex

Posteroinferior direction of corticotomy

M.

Divide medial and lateral cortices from anteroposterior direction

Twist osteotome to divide cortices

Note: *Do not damage periosteum and posterior cortex*

Plate 158. (Continued)

External Rotation Osteoclasis

N. and **O.** Rotate the distal block of rings laterally in relation to the proximal block. Do not rotate it medially because of the potential for stretching and damage to the peroneal nerve. An alternate method for breaking the posterior cortex is with a Gigli saw. Confirm the completeness of the corticotomy with image-intensifier radiographic control.

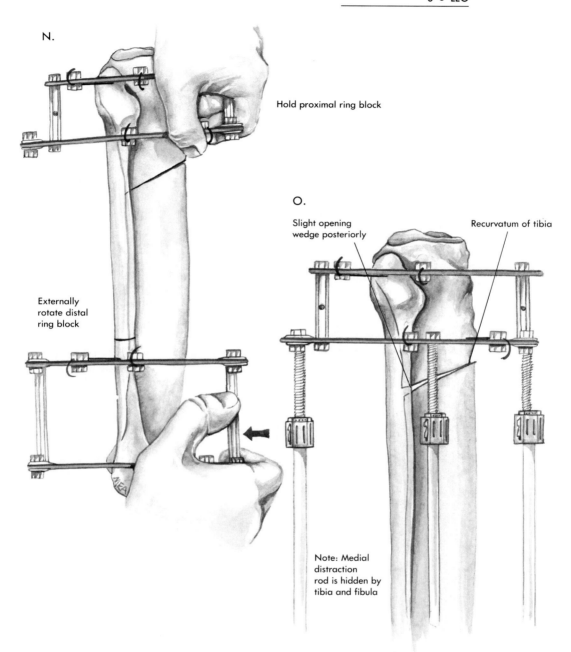

N.

Hold proximal ring block

Externally
rotate distal
ring block

O.

Slight opening
wedge posteriorly

Recurvatum of tibia

Note: Medial
distraction
rod is hidden by
tibia and fibula

Plate 158. (Continued)

P. Reattach the connected graduated telescoping rods as they were before. There should be a "clicker" placed on the rods for distraction-compression (see Lengthening by Distraction).

Final adjustments are made to ensure that there are 7 degrees of varus and 7 degrees of recurvatum between the proximal and distal blocks of rings.

Postoperative Care

Latency Period. Distraction is not carried out for three to ten days postoperatively, depending on the patient's age and extent of vascular and soft-tissue disruption at corticotomy. In children and adolescents, a three- to five-day wait is adequate; in the older patient, a seven- to ten-day wait is preferable. The start of distraction is delayed when there has been disruption of the medullary circulation and of the endosteal and periosteal soft tissues, as manifested by displacement of the bone ends.

Lengthening by Distraction

Q. Distraction totaling 1.0 mm. per day is achieved in incremental gains, e.g., four advances of 0.25 mm. each day. The lengthening is performed by turning the "clicker" one-quarter turn. One full turn is equivalent to 1.0 mm.

The most simple and reliable method of distraction is by the use of graduated telescoping rods (GTRs). The square head is easy to turn with the fingers. The ratchet mechanism is released by depressing the lever (the bar). After one-quarter of a turn, the lever pops into locking position by itself with a clicking sound (the "clicker"). This is click number 1. The square head on each side has indented dots numbered 1, 2, 3, and 4. Each number is calibrated to equal one-quarter of a turn, or 0.25 mm. of distraction. To distract further, depress the safety lever and turn the square head clockwise toward the increasing number. To compress, turn the clicker counterclockwise toward the decreasing number.

It may be necessary to change the rate of distraction, depending on the radiographic findings. The rate is slowed to 0.75 mm. or 0.50 mm. per day when consolidation of new bone is delayed. The rate may need to be increased to 1.25 mm. or 1.50 mm. per day if consolidation takes place prematurely.

An autodistractor that produces a 1-mm. revolution of the threaded rod in 64 micromotions per day has become available. The mechanism is powered by a battery carried on the patient's clothing or belt. Preliminary, limited experience indicates that the healing index is decreased by the smooth quasi-continuous distraction of the autodistractor. Additionally, the patient is freed of the responsibility for distraction. The main disadvantage is cost.

Pin Site Care. It is crucial to provide meticulous pin site care in order to prevent infection. The pin sites should be free of crust and drainage. There should be as little motion as possible of the skin and soft tissues at the pin sites.

The patient and parents are instructed as to pin site care. It is best for pediatric patients to provide their own pin care with the assistance or supervision of the parents whenever possible. Pin care is performed twice a day, once in the morning and once in the evening.

Supplies required include 2 x 2-inch Sof-Wick IV sponges (supplied by Johnson & Johnson), Ilizarov sponges, plastic clips for each pin site, normal saline, hydrogen peroxide, and cotton swabs if drainage or a crust is present.

To perform pin care:

1. The parents and patient should thoroughly wash their hands.
2. All clips are removed.
3. All Ilizarov sponges are removed, checked for drainage, and discarded if soiled.
4. Sof-Wick sponges are removed and checked for drainage.
5. Saline is used to loosen any Sof-Wick sponge that sticks to the skin.
6. The sponges are discarded.

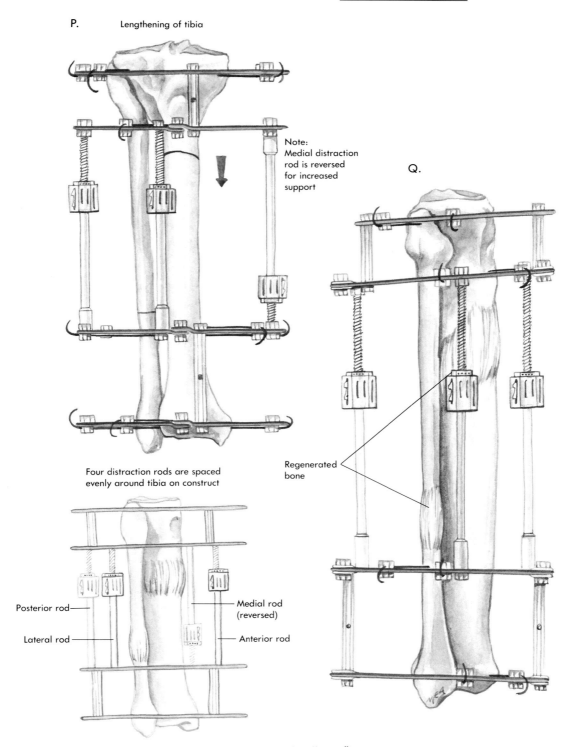

P.   Lengthening of tibia

Note:
Medial distraction
rod is reversed
for increased
support

Q.

Four distraction rods are spaced
evenly around tibia on construct

Regenerated
bone

Posterior rod

Lateral rod

Medial rod
(reversed)

Anterior rod

Plate 158. (Continued)

7. Pin sites are checked for drainage.

8. Pin sites are cleansed free of drainage or crust with saline solution and a cotton swab. A new cotton swab is used for each pin site.

9. If the drainage or crust is too hard to clean with saline, hydrogen peroxide is used for cleansing.

10. The pin sites are checked for swelling or increasing redness.

11. Sof-Wick IV sponge is placed.

12. Ilizarov sponges are placed.

13. The clip is placed firmly so that the sponges are tight against the skin.

Patients are discharged after learning pin site care, turning of the graduated telescoping rods, and completing the physical therapy program. They are allowed to bear weight partially on the affected limb with the support of three-point crutch gait. The patient is allowed to take a shower three weeks postoperatively if the wound condition permits.

The patient should return to the surgeon's office or clinic once a week during the period of elongation. Radiograms are made as necessary. The family is instructed to report any of the following problems to the surgeon or the nurse clinician:

1. Oral temperature higher than 101.5°F.
2. Increasing redness and/or swelling at the pin site.
3. Change in color of drainage at the pin site.
4. Change in the intensity and type of pain.
5. Inability to turn the clicker.
6. Bending of the clicker rod.
7. Change in sensitivity or ability to move any part of the limb being corrected.
8. Swelling of the limb.

Physical Therapy. It is vital for the child to participate in physical therapy several times a day to maintain and increase range of adjacent joints and to increase muscle strength. Early weight-bearing, as tolerated, is essential for stimulation of new bone formation. Fixation by the Ilizarov method is stable. Radiograms obtained once or twice a month are checked for signs of translational and rotational malalignments; hinges are used to correct such problems if necessary. The distraction is stopped when the desired length is achieved. When complications develop during elongation, they are managed appropriately (Table 8–1).

Complete Immobilization and Fixation. This is the period during which the regenerated bone calcifies and ossifies. The healing index (time of beginning of distraction to removal of the apparatus) varies and usually takes 30 to 45 days for each centimeter of lengthening.

Removal of the apparatus ensues when three standards are met:

1. Radiographically, the regenerated bone should be normotrophic, exhibiting normal cortex formation and medullary cavitation along the elongated segment. Computed tomography (CT) is the best way to determine the maturation and canalization of the regenerated bone. The metallic connecting rods are temporarily removed when the CT scan is performed.

2. With the connecting rods of the apparatus removed, the regenerated bone should be stable when tested clinically.

3. With the connecting rods removed, the patient should subjectively feel that the limb is firm under the stress of loading; there should be no pain on weight-bearing or walking.

Dynamization. During the dynamization period, the nuts at the sides of the connecting rod attachments are loosened and axial loading is applied by the patient bearing weight. Duration of this stage is ordinarily two to three weeks. Radiograms are repeated, and the maturity and stability of the regenerated bone is assessed.

Table 8-1. Problems and Complications of Limb Lengthening

I. **Intraoperative**
   A. *Pin insertion*—Injury to nerves and vessels by penetration of the pins or screws
   B. *Corticotomy*
      1. Disturbance of endosteal and medullary blood supply
      2. Oblique or comminuted fracture at site of osteotomy
      3. Stretching and paresis of common peroneal nerve

II. **Immediate Postoperative Period**
   A. Compartment syndrome
   B. Skin necrosis and slough
   C. Wound infection

III. **During Distraction Period**
   A. *Screw or pin tract problems*
      1. Soft-tissue necrosis
      2. Soft-tissue infection
      3. Osteomyelitis
   B. *Contracture of muscles*
   C. *Muscle weakness*
   D. *Neurologic compromise*
      1. Common peroneal nerve—due to compression by taut fascial band
      2. Lateral popliteal nerve—due to physeal separation of proximal fibular epiphysis
      3. Femoral or sciatic nerve—extremely rare, usually not encountered when distraction is gradual—less than 2 mm./day
   E. *Vascular problems*
      1. Hypertension
      2. Late erosion of the vessels by the pins
      3. Deep vein thrombosis
      4. Sudeck's atrophy
      5. Edema and hypertrophic swelling of the soft tissues of the limb
   F. *Joint subluxation-dislocation*
   G. *Joint stiffness*
   H. *Axial deviations*
      1. Tibia
         a. Valgus and anterior angulation (procurvatum) when elongated segment is proximal metaphysis or midshaft
         b. Varus and procurvatum—when elongated segment is proximal metaphysis and midshaft
      2. Femur
         a. Varus or procurvatum—when elongated segment is proximal metaphysis and midshaft
         b. Valgus and procurvatum when elongated segment is distal metaphysis
      3. Humerus
         a. Varus and flexion—when elongated segment is proximal metaphysis
         b. Flexion—when elongated segment is midshaft or distal metaphysis
      4. Forearm—flexion in both radius and ulna

IV. **Delayed Consolidation**

V. **Stress Fracture and Plastic Bowing of the Elongated Segment**

VI. **Mental Disturbance—Psychosis**

Removal of the Ilizarov Apparatus. This is usually performed in the operating room; children and apprehensive adolescents usually require general anesthesia.

When removing the Ilizarov fixator, follow this sequence:

1. Release the tension on all wires; failure to do so will cause severe pain when the wires under tension are cut.
2. Cut the wires.
3. With image intensifier or regular radiography, determine the position of the olive wires. Always extract the wires toward the olive.
4. Use large pliers or a power drill to extract the wires.
5. The direction of pull of the wires should be parallel to the direction of the wire position and orientation to bone.
6. Be cautious with half-pins; they may break.
7. Remove the connectors of the rings one by one.

After removal of the fixator, there is a definite risk of stress fracture of the newly generated bone, even after minor trauma. I recommend protecting the limb in a plastic knee-ankle-foot orthosis with an anterior plastic shell. (This orthosis is appropriate after tibial lengthening, but a hip-knee-ankle-foot orthosis is called for after femoral lengthening. The hip and knee joints are freed with a drop-lock, allowing motion, and the ankle joint is also allowed motion.)

The patient is weaned from the orthosis gradually. If the regenerated bone fractures, the limb should be immobilized in a cast. The fracture will heal rapidly, and the new bone stimulated by the fracture is better than the previous regenerated bone.

REFERENCES

Bianchi-Maiocchi, A., and Aronson, J. (Eds.): Operative Principles of Ilizarov: Fracture Treatment, Non-union Osteomyelitis, Lengthening, Deformity Correction. Baltimore, Williams & Wilkins, 1991.

Fauré, C., and Merloz, P.: Transfixation: Atlas of Anatomical Sections for the External Fixation of Limbs. New York, Springer-Verlag, 1987.

Golyakhovsky, V., and Frankel, V.: Operative Manual of Ilizarov Techniques. St. Louis, Mosby-Year Book Inc., 1993.

Green, S. A.: Complications of External Skeletal Fixation. Springfield, Ill., Charles C Thomas, 1981.

Green, S. A. (Ed.): Basic Ilizarov techniques. Tech. Orthop., 5:4, 1990.

Ilizarov, G. A.: Transosseous Osteosynthesis: Theoretical and Clinical Aspects of the Regeneration and Growth of Tissue. New York, Springer-Verlag, 1991.

Ilizarov, G. A.: The tension-stress effect on the genesis and growth of tissues. I: The influence of stability of fixation and soft-tissue preservation. Clin. Orthop., 238:249, 1989.

Ilizarov, G. A.: The tension-stress effect on the genesis and growth of tissues. II. The influence of rate and frequency of distraction. Clin. Orthop., 239:263, 1990.

Lehman, W. (Ed.): Operation Room Guide to Cross Sectional Anatomy of the Extremities and Pelvis. New York, Raven Press, 1989.

Paley, D.: Current techniques of limb lengthening. J. Pediatr. Orthop., 8:73, 1988.

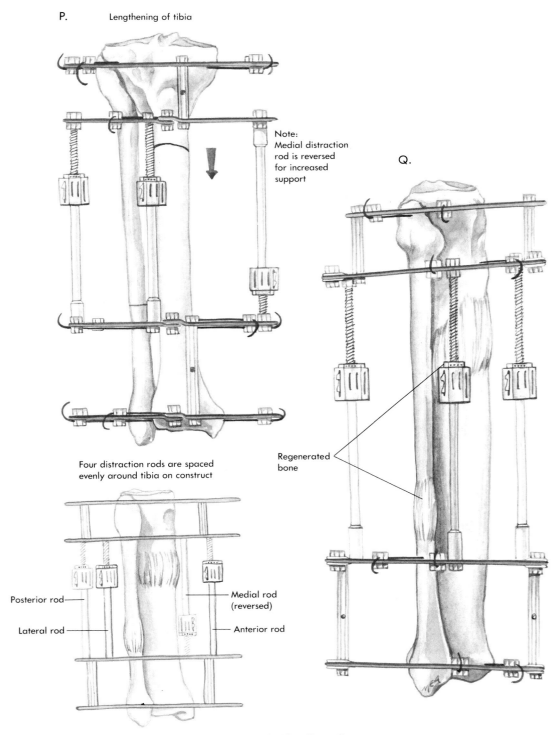

P.   Lengthening of tibia

Note:
Medial distraction
rod is reversed
for increased
support

Q.

Four distraction rods are spaced
evenly around tibia on construct

Regenerated
bone

Posterior rod

Lateral rod

Medial rod
(reversed)

Anterior rod

Plate 158. (Continued)

PLATE 159 — Epiphyseodesis of the Proximal Tibia and Fibula (Green Modification of the Phemister Technique)

Indications. Leg length inequality of less than 5 cm. When shortening of the tibia is greater than 5 cm., lengthening of the tibia should be considered.

Growth arrest of the proximal fibula is performed first, because this provides more adequate exposure and facilitates proper identification of the common peroneal nerve. Ask the anesthesiologist not to paralyze the patient. After 20 to 30 minutes of tourniquet ischemia, stimulation of the common peroneal nerve will fail to produce contraction of the innervated muscles. If the lateral side of the proximal tibial physis is arrested first, normal details of anatomy will be obscured by blood and distorted by the dissection.

Patient Position. The patient is placed in the semilateral position with the lateral side of the surgically prepped leg facing upward and the knee flexed 30 degrees. A sterile sandbag or a sterile folded sheet is placed under the knee for support.

Operative Technique

A. The knee joint line, the head of the fibula, and the proximal tibial tubercle are identified. A 30-degree slanted oblique incision is made midway between the proximal tibial tubercle and the fibular head; it begins proximally 1 cm. inferior to the joint line and 1 cm. anterior to the fibular head and extends distally and forward for a distance of 5 cm. The subcutaneous tissue is divided, and the wound flaps are widely undermined and retracted.

B. and **C.** The head of the fibula is in line with the proximal growth plate of the tibia. (In the illustration, the head of the fibula is abnormally high.) The capsule of the knee joint, the insertion of the biceps tendon, and the fibular collateral ligament of the knee are identified.

The common peroneal nerve lies close to the medial border of the biceps femoris muscle in the popliteal fossa; then it passes distally and laterally between the lateral head of the gastrocnemius and the biceps tendon. Behind the fibular head it is subcutaneous. At the site of origin of the peroneus longus muscle at the head and neck of the fibula, the common peroneal nerve winds anteriorly around the fibular neck and then passes deep to the peroneus longus muscle and branches into the superficial and deep peroneal nerves.

D. The origins of the toe extensors, extensor hallucis longus, and anterior tibial muscles, along with a cuff of periosteal flap, are elevated from the arcuate line. With a periosteal elevator, the origin of the peroneus longus muscle is detached from the head of the fibula; keeping the dissection anterior to the fibular head prevents injury to the nerve.

EPIPHYSIODESIS OF PROXIMAL TIBIA AND FIBULA

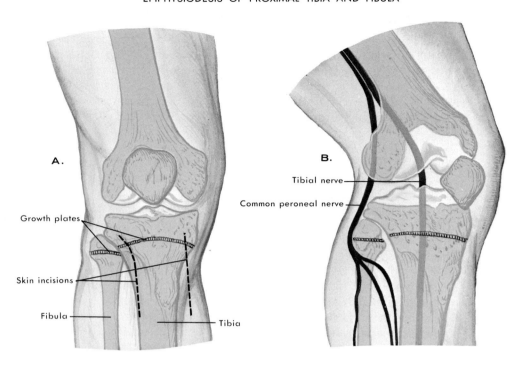

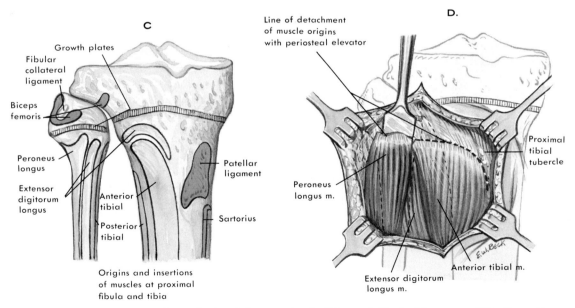

Plate 159. A.–H., Epiphyseodesis of the proximal tibia and fibula (Green modification of the Phemister technique).

E. and **F.** With a straight needle, the site of the growth plate of the proximal fibula is identified. Next, a longitudinal incision is made on the anterior aspect of the fibular head and is extended distally to include the growth plate. A rectangular piece of bone (¼ inch wide and ½ inch long) is removed from the proximal fibula, straddling the physis. Three fourths of the length of the bone graft includes the fibular head, so that only one fourth of the graft length includes the metaphysis. The growth plate is thoroughly curetted, the ends of the bone graft are reversed (180 degrees), and the piece of bone is placed securely back in the graft bed. At times, this author simply curets the growth plate and dispenses with the latter steps.

Note: A nerve stimulator should always be available in the operating room; if it is not clear whether a strand of tissue is fibrous or neural, its nature should be positively determined by stimulation. Of course, the patient should not be paralyzed by the anesthetic agent.

The lateral aspect of the proximal tibial physis is already exposed for the fibular epiphyseodesis. A longitudinal incision is made midway between the anterior and posterior borders of the lateral tibia. The periosteum is elevated, and a rectangular piece of bone (ordinarily ½ inch wide and ¾ inch long or at times ⅜ inch wide and ⅝ inch long) is resected in a manner similar to that described for the bone graft technique with the distal femur. The growth plate is drilled with diamond-shaped drill bits of increasing size in the anterior, posterior, and *proximal* directions. A hand drill is used. Some surgeons prefer to use a power drill. The steps of the epiphyseodesis are the same as those outlined in Plate 133 (G–K) for epiphyseodesis of the distal femur.

G. and **H.** The medial side of the proximal tibial physis is exposed by a longitudinal incision about 5 cm. long, beginning 1 cm. distal to the joint line and continuing distally midway between the proximal tibial tubercle and the postero-medial margin of the tibia. The subcutaneous tissue and deep fascia are divided in line with the skin incision.

Caution! Do not damage the infrapatellar branch of the saphenous nerve. The anterior margins of the sartorius tendon and tibial collateral ligament are partially elevated and retracted posteriorly.

The steps for growth arrest of the proximal tibial physis follow the steps described for distal femoral epiphyseodesis. The rectangular piece of bone graft removed from the tibia, usually ½ inch wide and ¾ inch long (or ⅜ inch wide and ⅝ inch long), is smaller than that removed from the femur. Prior to closure of the wound, the tourniquet is released and complete hemostasis is secured (otherwise, bleeding in the anterior tibial compartment will cause compartment syndrome, muscle ischemia, and paralysis).

Postoperative Care. Following closure of the wound, the region of the fibular head is well padded and the limb is immobilized in an above-knee cast that includes the foot and ankle. The knee is in 30 degrees of flexion, and the foot and ankle are in neutral position. The postoperative care is the same as that following distal femoral epiphyseodesis.

REFERENCES

Green, W. T., and Anderson, M.: Experiences with epiphyseal arrest in correcting discrepancies in length of the lower extremities in infantile paralysis. J. Bone Joint Surg., 29:659, 1947.

Green, W. T., and Anderson, M.: Discrepancy in length of the lower extremities. A.A.O.S. Instructional Course Lectures, 8:294, 1951.

Green, W. T., and Anderson, M.: Epiphyseal arrest for the correction of discrepancies in length of the lower extremities. J. Bone Joint Surg., 39-A:353, 1957.

Phemister, D. B.: Operative arrestment of longitudinal growth of bones in the treatment of deformities. J. Bone Joint Surg., 15:1, 1933.

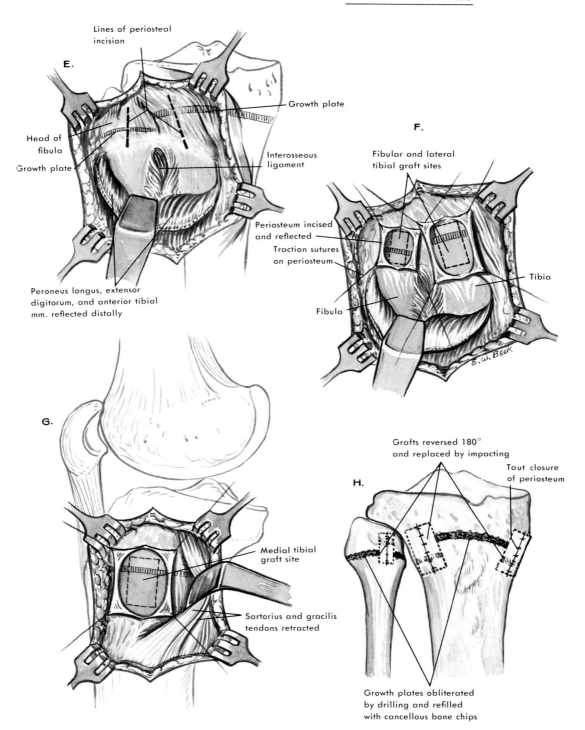

E.

Lines of periosteal
incision

Growth plate

Head of
fibula

Growth plate

Interosseous
ligament

Peroneus longus, extensor
digitorum, and anterior tibial
mm. reflected distally

F.

Fibular and lateral
tibial graft sites

Periosteum incised
and reflected

Traction sutures
on periosteum

Tibia

Fibula

G.

Medial tibial
graft site

Sartorius and gracilis
tendons retracted

H.

Grafts reversed 180°
and replaced by impacting

Taut closure
of periosteum

Growth plates obliterated
by drilling and refilled
with cancellous bone chips

Plate 159. (Continued)

PLATE 160 ## McFarland's Posterior Bypass for Congenital Pre-pseudarthrosis of the Tibia

Indications. Incipient phase of congenital pseudarthrosis of tibia in infants six to nine months of age before they pull themselves up to a standing position, take their initial steps, and fall. It may be used in the older child.

Objective. To reduce the risk of fracture by placing a graft posteriorly, spanning the pre-pseudarthrosis site.

Radiographic Control. Image intensifier.

Blood for Transfusion. Yes, especially if iliac bone graft is used. Other sources of autogenous bone graft are the opposite tibia and rib.

Patient Position. The patient is placed supine, and the operative procedure is performed under tourniquet ischemia.

Operative Technique

A. The posterior surface of the tibia is exposed through a posteromedial longitudinal incision, extending from the proximal to the distal metaphyses of the tibia. The subcutaneous tissue is divided in line with the skin incision.

B. The skin flaps are retracted, and the fascia is incised. Avoid injury to the saphenous vein. The tibia is exposed extraperiosteally to prevent a devitalizing effect on the bone ends from extensive stripping of the periosteum. The flexor digitorum longus, soleus, and posterior tibial muscles are extraperiosteally elevated and retracted posterolaterally.

Dissect and meticulously excise the cuff of proliferated fibrous ("hamartomatous") tissue surrounding the tibia at the site of the impending "pseudarthrosis" site.

Next, the thickened periosteum on the posterior concave surface of the tibia at the potential pseudarthrosis site is resected. Thoroughly release any tethering soft-tissue contractures posteriorly on the concave posterior surface of the anteriorly angulated tibia. If the triceps surae is taut, it is lengthened at its musculotendinous junction by the Vulpius technique.

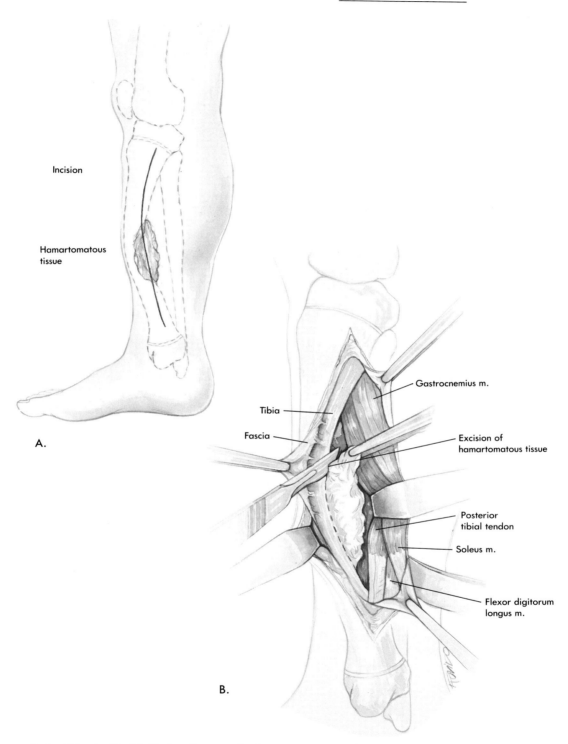

Incision

Hamartomatous
tissue

A.

Gastrocnemius m.

Tibia

Fascia

Excision of
hamartomatous tissue

Posterior
tibial tendon

Soleus m.

Flexor digitorum
longus m.

B.

Plate 160. A.–D., McFarland's posterior bypass operation for congenital pre-pseudarthrosis of the tibia.

C. and **D.** Under radiographic control, the distal and proximal tibial metaphyses are identified. A unicortical slot of appropriate size is made in the center of the posterior surface of the distal tibial metaphysis into which the autogenous bone graft from the opposite tibia is inserted. Proximally, the bone graft is inserted into a similar slot in the center of the posterior surface of the upper tibial metaphysis.

It is vital that the graft be placed on the posterior surface of the tibia (not posteromedial); it should lie straight, vertical with its upper end as far above the apex of the pre-pseudarthrosis site as possible.

Proximally, the graft is transfixed to the tibia with one unicortical, cancellous screw. Distally, the graft is sutured to the tibia with 00 Tycron or similar sutures passed through power-drilled holes in the lower end of the graft and the distal tibial metaphysis. This measure ensures secure anchorage of the graft in the desired position.

The graft should be stable, lying vertically, under compression between the knee and ankle; its ends should be embedded in healthy cancellous bone proximally and distally, well away from the lesion. The space between the longitudinal strut graft and the impending pseudarthrosis site is packed with long corticocancellous graft slivers and cancellous bone chips. It is also best to place some cancellous bone grafts at each end of the bypass graft to ensure incorporation and enhance its rate of healing. The tourniquet is released and, after complete hemostasis and insertion of a Hemovac drainage tube, the wound is closed in the usual fashion. The involved lower limb is immobilized in an above-knee cast with the knee flexed 45 degrees. If bone graft is harvested from the opposite tibia, the graft donor leg is also immobilized in a below-knee cast with the ankle and foot in neutral position.

Postoperative Care. In four to six weeks the normal leg from which the graft was harvested can be out of the cast, but the leg with the incipient pseudarthrosis is immobilized in a non–weight-bearing above-knee cast for four weeks. Then the patient is allowed to bear weight in an above-knee cast for an additional four weeks. Usually by then the graft is incorporated. The cast is removed, sutures are taken out, and another above-knee cast with the knee in 10 degrees of flexion is applied. As the child gets older and more stable in gait, and the graft incorporation becomes more solid, the cast is changed to a high AFO (ankle-foot orthosis) with an anterior shell. For the initial 6 to 12 months the leg is protected in a night orthosis, but later it may be free at night.

REFERENCES

Eyre-Brook, A. L., Baily, RA. J., and Price, C. H. G.: Infantile pseudarthrosis of the tibia: Three cases treated successfully by delayed autogenous by-pass graft, with some comments on the causative lesion. J. Bone Joint Surg., 51-B:604, 1969.
McFarland, B.: Pseudarthrosis of the tibia in childhood. J. Bone Joint Surg., 33-B:36, 1951.

POSTERIOR VIEW

MEDIAL VIEW

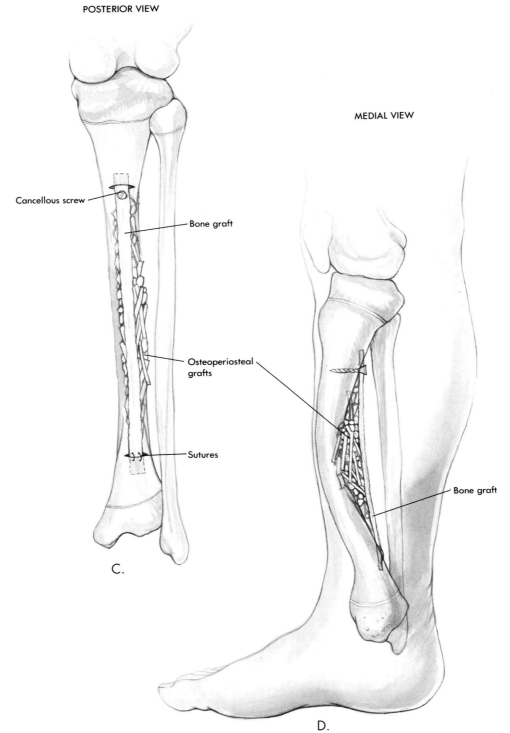

Cancellous screw

Bone graft

Osteoperiosteal
grafts

Sutures

Bone graft

C.

D.

Plate 160. (Continued)

PLATE 161 **Treatment of Congenital Pseudarthrosis of the Tibia by Dual Graft and Intramedullary Pin Fixation**

Indications. Established pseudarthrosis of the tibia. Some surgeons may prefer primary use of the Ilizarov fixator or free vascularized bone graft.

Blood for Transfusion. Yes.

Radiographic Control. Image intensifier.

Special Instrumentation. Intramedullary pin of surgeon's choice.

Patient Position. Supine.

Operative Technique

A. Over the anteromedial aspect of the tibia, a gentle, curved incision is made, starting just distal to the proximal tibial tubercle; then it curves posteriorly and extends distally parallel with the posteromedial margin of the tibia. At the distal end of the tibia the incision swings forward to end at the anterior border of the tibia.

B. The subcutaneous tissue and the fascia are incised in line with the skin incision. The wound flaps are mobilized and retracted to their respective sides. The saphenous vein and nerve are identified and protected from injury. The veins that cross the field are clamped, divided, and coagulated. The site of pseudarthrosis is exposed.

C. The heavy cuff of proliferated fibrous tissue and thickened periosteum surrounding the bone at the pseudarthrosis site is meticulously dissected. This dissection should be very thorough posteriorly. To expose the posterior surface of the tibia, the periosteum is dissected longitudinally and immediately in front of the anterior margin of the flexor digitorum longus and soleus muscles, which are extraperiosteally elevated and retracted posteriorly. The thickened periosteum and dense fibrous tissue are completely excised down to healthy muscle and bone.

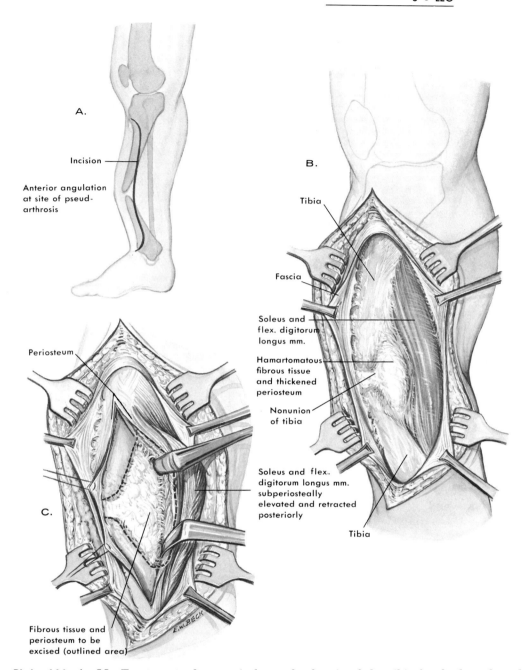

Plate 161. A.–M., Treatment of congenital pseudarthrosis of the tibia by dual graft and intramedullary pin fixation.

D. The sclerotic bone from the ends of the proximal and distal fragments is resected with a rongeur, preserving as much length of the bone as possible.

E. Next, the medullary canal of the ends of each fragment is drilled in both directions with progressively larger sizes of diamond-head hand drills.

F. Then, by manipulation, the anterior bowing of the tibia is corrected completely, and the viable ends of the bone fragments are impacted and telescoped together. At times, the Achilles tendon may have to be lengthened through a separate incision to correct the anterior bowing. If the fibula is intact and is holding the tibial bone fragments apart, it is essential to resect an adequate segment through a lateral incision.

G. An intramedullary Steinmann pin of appropriate size is used to impact and hold the fibular fragments firmly together. It is best to insert the Steinmann pin retrograde, that is, first from the proximal end of the distal fragment of the fibula, drilling out through the lateral malleolus, and then holding the fibular fragments together and drilling the pin into the proximal fragment. The Steinmann pin through the fibula also provides better fixation and more secure alignment of the tibial fragments.

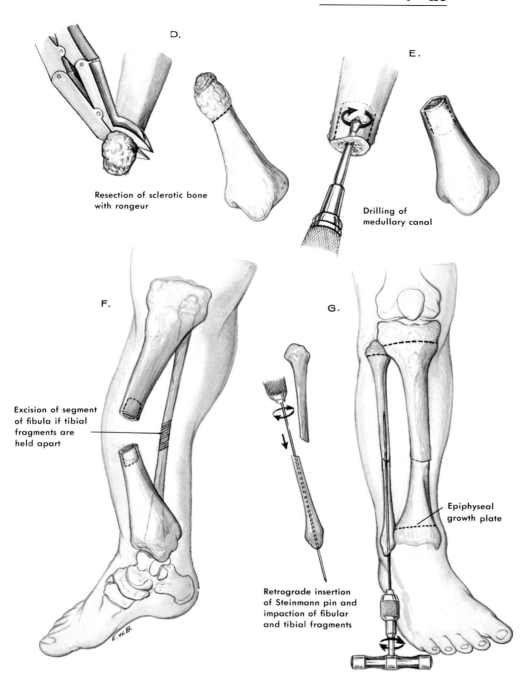

D. Resection of sclerotic bone with rongeur

E. Drilling of medullary canal

F. Excision of segment of fibula if tibial fragments are held apart

G. Epiphyseal growth plate

Retrograde insertion of Steinmann pin and impaction of fibular and tibial fragments

E.W.B.

Plate 161. (Continued)

H. During the manipulative reduction it is best to convert the anterior bowing of the tibia to 15 to 20 degrees of posterior angulation.

I. and **J.** Next, the beds for the grafts on the lateral and posterior surfaces of the tibia are prepared by removing a shaving of bone with an osteotome or gouge. The bone grafts should extend at least 2 to 3 inches on the proximal fragment and as far distally as possible on the distal fragment, but without injuring the distal tibial epiphyseal plate.

An osteoperiosteal bone graft is removed from the patient's normal tibia and is divided transversely in half. At each end of the graft a hole is made with a sharp towel clip or drill, and 0 or 00 Tycron sutures are inserted through the holes. One half of the graft is placed on the posterior surface and the second half on the lateral surface of the tibia, and they are sutured to the proximal and distal tibial fragments. The space between the grafts and the site of pseudarthrosis is packed with long bone graft slivers and cancellous bone chips.

K. At this stage, an external fixator may be applied instead of intramedullary pin fixation. In this drawing, a Wagner lengthening apparatus with two Schanz screws proximally and two Schanz screws distally is illustrated. At present this author recommends the use of the Ilizarov wires and apparatus—fixation is more secure and allows compression-distraction osteogenesis.

With a few interrupted sutures, the flexor digitorum longus, gastrocnemius soleus, and anterior tibial muscles are reattached to the tibia. Skin and subcutaneous tissue are closed in the usual manner. Abundant sterile sheath wadding is applied.

L. and **M.** When the distal fragment is short, instead of using the Wagner, De Bastiani Orthofix, or Ilizarov lengthening apparatus, the tibial fragments are fixed with a large intramedullary Steinmann pin. The Steinmann pin is drilled distally from the proximal end of the distal fragment across the center of the distal tibial epiphysis, across the ankle and subtalar joints, and out of the skin through the plantar aspect of the heel. Then the tibial fragments are aligned and held together, and the Steinmann pin is drilled into the proximal tibial fragment. The pin is directed in such a way that its proximal end will engage the posterior cortex of the tibia 1 to 2 inches distal to the proximal tibial epiphyseal plate. The distal end of the pin is cut just under the skin, and the heel is well padded while the cast is applied.

Postoperative Management. Cast immobilization is continued until there is radiologic evidence of definite bony union. This may take as long as six months or more. The cast is changed every six to eight weeks, as necessary. If an intramedullary tarsotibial nail is used, it is left in place when cast immobilization is discontinued.

Following removal of the cast, the child should use an above-knee orthosis with an anterior shell on the leg, and ankle and knee joints that are free to allow normal weight-bearing stresses for stimulation of bone formation. The brace protection is continued until skeletal maturity or until the medullary canal of the tibia has normal diameter and there are no areas of sclerosis. The intramedullary pin is not removed; it is left in place as an internal splint until the patient is skeletally mature. It is changed to a longer intramedullary pin if necessary.

If the hamartomatous fibrous tissue regenerates, it should be excised before bony changes are produced.

REFERENCES

Boyd, H. B.: Congenital pseudarthrosis. Treatment by dual bone grafts. J. Bone Joint Surg., 23:497, 1941.

Boyd, H. B., and Sage, F. P.: Congenital pseudarthrosis of the tibia. J. Bone Joint Surg., 40-A:1245, 1958.

Guilleminet, M.: Pseudarthrose congénitale du tibia. Rev. Chir. Orthop., 39:690, 1953.

Guilleminet, M., and Ricard, R.: Sur le traitement de la pseudarthrose congénitale du tibia. Valeur de la double greffe visée. Rev. Chir. Orthop., 39:3, 1953.

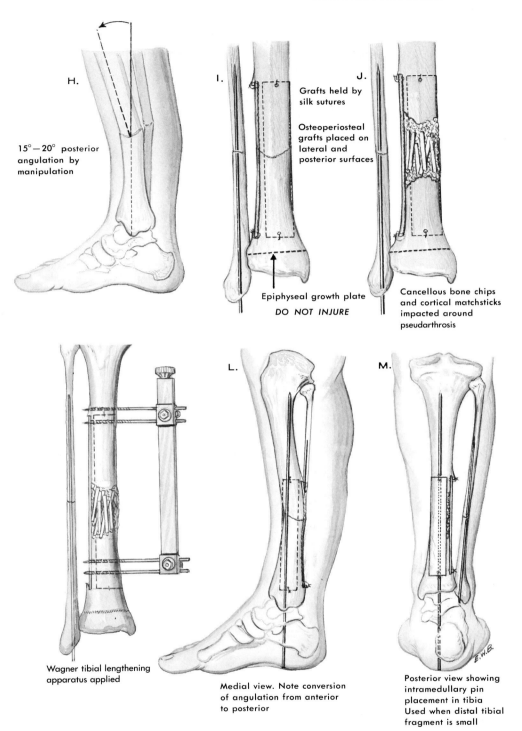

H.

15° — 20° posterior angulation by manipulation

I.

Grafts held by silk sutures

Osteoperiosteal grafts placed on lateral and posterior surfaces

Epiphyseal growth plate
DO NOT INJURE

J.

Cancellous bone chips and cortical matchsticks impacted around pseudarthrosis

Wagner tibial lengthening apparatus applied

L.

Medial view. Note conversion of angulation from anterior to posterior

M.

Posterior view showing intramedullary pin placement in tibia Used when distal tibial fragment is small

E.W.B.

Plate 161. (Continued)

Guilleminet, M., and Ricard, R.: Pseudarthrose congénitale du tibia et son traitement. Paris: Masson, 1958.

Makin, A. S.: Congenital pseudarthrosis of tibia treated by twin grafts. Proc. R. Soc. Med., 38:71, 1944.

McElvenny, R. T.: Congenital pseudo-arthrosis of the tibia. Findings in one case and a suggestion as to possible etiology and treatment. Q. Bull. Northwest. Univ. Med. Sch., 23:413, 1949.

Purvis, G. D., and Holder, J. E.: Dual bone graft for congenital pseudarthrosis of the tibia: Variations of technic. South. Med. J., 53:926, 1960.

Scott, C. R.: Congenital pseudarthrosis of the tibia. A.J.R.: 42:104, 1939.

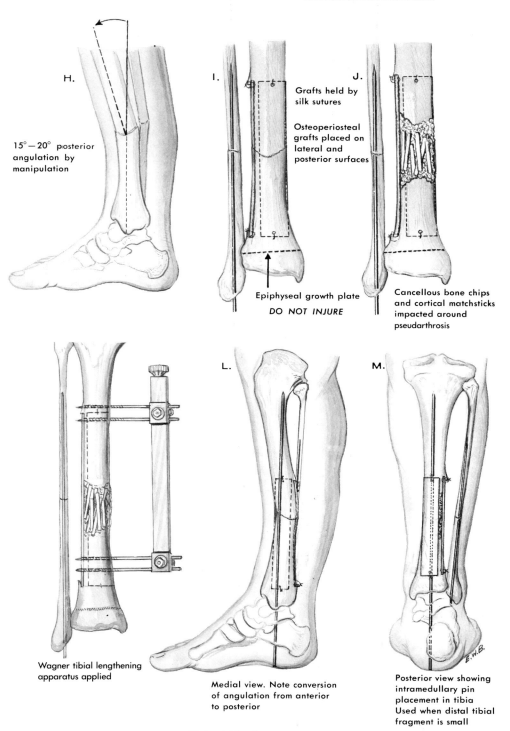

H.

15°—20° posterior angulation by manipulation

I.

Grafts held by silk sutures

Osteoperiosteal grafts placed on lateral and posterior surfaces

Epiphyseal growth plate
DO NOT INJURE

J.

Cancellous bone chips and cortical matchsticks impacted around pseudarthrosis

Wagner tibial lengthening apparatus applied

L.

Medial view. Note conversion of angulation from anterior to posterior

M.

Posterior view showing intramedullary pin placement in tibia Used when distal tibial fragment is small

Plate 161. (Continued)

PLATE 162   **Surgical Decompression of the Leg in Compartment Syndrome by a Single- or Double-Incision Open Fasciotomy**

Indications. Compartment syndrome and impending Volkmann's ischemia in any or all of the compartments of the leg.

Related Anatomic Principles

A.–G. A thorough knowledge of the detailed anatomy of the leg is vital to avoid injury to neurovascular structures during fasciotomy. There are four osteofascial compartments in the leg: (1) anterior, (2) lateral, (3) superficial posterior, and (4) deep posterior. Each compartment contains important nerves and vessels.

The deep fascia of the leg envelops the crural muscles. Anterolaterally, it blends with the periosteum or the subcutaneous surface of the tibia and the head and malleolus of the fibula. Distally, it is continuous with the extensor and flexor retinacula. On the anterior and proximal parts of the leg, the deep fascia is thick and dense, whereas posteriorly and laterally, where it covers the gastrocnemius and soleus, it is thin.

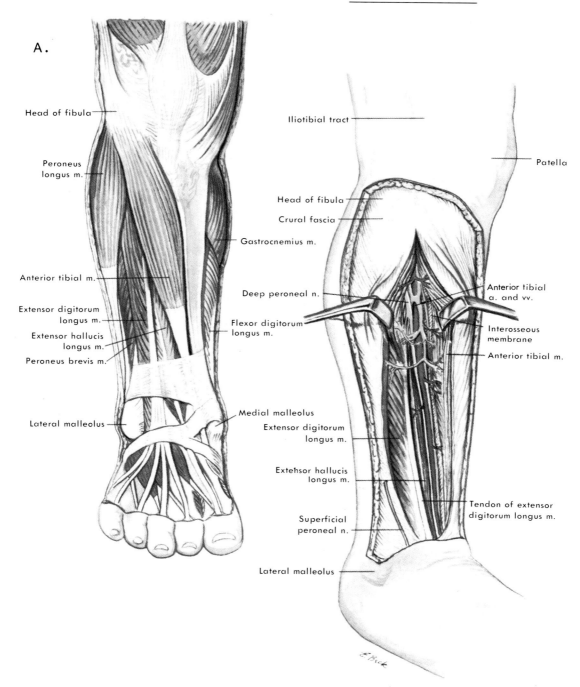

A.

Head of fibula

Peroneus longus m.

Anterior tibial m.

Extensor digitorum longus m.

Extensor hallucis longus m.

Peroneus brevis m.

Lateral malleolus

Gastrocnemius m.

Medial malleolus

Iliotibial tract

Patella

Head of fibula

Crural fascia

Deep peroneal n.

Flexor digitorum longus m.

Anterior tibial a. and vv.

Interosseous membrane

Anterior tibial m.

Extensor digitorum longus m.

Extensor hallucis longus m.

Superficial peroneal n.

Lateral malleolus

Tendon of extensor digitorum longus m.

Plate 162. A.–S., Surgical decompression of the leg in compartment syndrome by a single- or double-incision open fasciotomy. **A.–G.,** Related anatomic principles.

A., Muscles and tendons on anterior aspect of right leg and foot. Dissection of the lateral aspect of the right leg shows the relations of anterior tibial vessels and deep peroneal nerve.

The *anterior compartment* is bounded medially by the periosteum of the tibia, posteriorly by the interosseous membrane, laterally by the anterior intermuscular septum of the leg, and anteriorly by the deep fascia of the leg. The anterior compartment contains the tibialis anterior, extensor hallucis longus, extensor digitorum longus, and peroneus tertius (if present) muscles; the deep peroneal nerve; and the anterior tibial artery and vein.

The *deep peroneal nerve* originates at the bifurcation of the common peroneal nerve between the metaphysis of the fibula and peroneus longus muscle. In the proximal third of the leg the nerve traverses anteriorly deep to the extensor digitorum longus in an oblique course to the front of the interosseous membrane. In the proximal third of the leg the deep peroneal nerve lies lateral to the anterior tibial artery. In the middle third of the leg the deep peroneal nerve descends in front of the artery, and in the lower third it is often on the lateral side of the artery. The deep peroneal nerve supplies motor branches to the tibialis anterior, extensor hallucis longus, extensor digitorum longus, and peroneus tertius. It is crucial that during epimysiotomy the muscular branches of the deep and superficial peroneal nerve not be injured.

The surgeon should be knowledgeable as to the anatomic course and relations of the *anterior tibial artery,* which originates as a terminal branch of the popliteal artery at the distal border of the popliteus. It traverses from the posterior to the anterior aspect of the leg between the two heads of the posterior tibial muscle and enters at the front of the leg through to the upper border of the interosseous membrane.

In the upper two thirds of the leg the anterior tibial artery lies in front of the interosseous membrane, whereas in the lower third of the tibia it lies in front of the tibia and ankle joint midway between the malleoli. On the dorsum of the foot the anterior tibial artery becomes the dorsalis pedis artery.

In the upper third of the leg the anterior tibial artery lies between the tibialis anterior and extensor digitorum longus with the deep peroneal nerve on the lateral side. In the middle third of the leg the anterior tibial artery is between the extensor hallucis longus and the tibialis anterior, with the deep peroneal nerve in front of the artery. In the upper two thirds of the leg the anterior tibial artery is covered and escorted by the extensor hallucis longus and anterior tibial muscles and by the deep fascia. In the lower third of the leg and in the ankle the anterior tibial artery is covered by the deep fascia, extensor retinacula, and skin. At the ankle the extensor hallucis longus tendon traverses anterior to the anterior tibial artery from the lateral to the medial side.

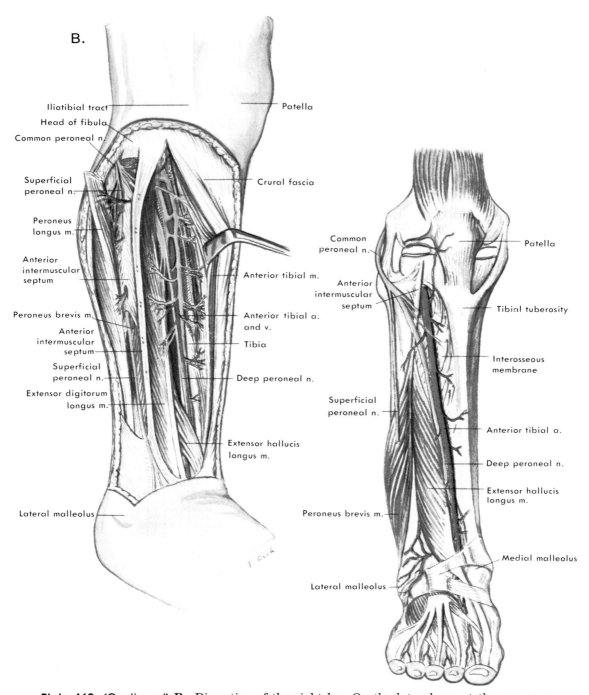

B.

Iliotibial tract
Head of fibula
Common peroneal n.
Superficial peroneal n.
Peroneus longus m.
Anterior intermuscular septum
Peroneus brevis m.
Anterior intermuscular septum
Superficial peroneal n.
Extensor digitorum longus m.
Lateral malleolus

Patella
Crural fascia
Anterior tibial m.
Anterior tibial a. and v.
Tibia
Deep peroneal n.
Extensor hallucis longus m.

Common peroneal n.
Anterior intermuscular septum
Superficial peroneal n.
Peroneus brevis m.
Lateral malleolus

Patella
Tibial tuberosity
Interosseous membrane
Anterior tibial a.
Deep peroneal n.
Extensor hallucis longus m.
Medial malleolus

Plate 162. (Continued) **B.,** Dissection of the right leg. On the lateral aspect the peroneus longus muscle is divided at its origin and retracted posteriorly to show the common peroneal nerve and its subdivision into the superficial and deep peroneal branches; the tibialis anterior is retracted medially to expose the relations of the deep peroneal nerve and the anterior tibial vessels. On the anterior view of the leg, the peroneus longus, anterior tibial, and extensor digitorum longus muscles are excised to demonstrate the course and anatomic relations of the anterior tibial vessels and peroneal nerves.

The *lateral compartment* is bounded medially by the lateral surface of the shaft of the fibula, anteriorly by the anterior intermuscular septum, posteriorly by the posterior retinacular septum, and laterally by the deep fascia of the leg. It contains the peroneus longus, the peroneus brevis, and the superficial peroneal nerve.

Proximally, after its bifurcation from the common peroneal nerve, the *superficial peroneal nerve* lies deep to the peroneus longus; then it passes distally and anteriorly between the peronei and the extensor digitorum longus. At the distal third of the leg the superficial peroneal nerve divides into a *medial branch,* which passes in front of the ankle joint, and a *lateral branch,* which passes along the lateral part of the dorsum of the foot. The superficial peroneal nerve gives its vascular branches to peroneus longus and brevis proximally in its course between the muscles.

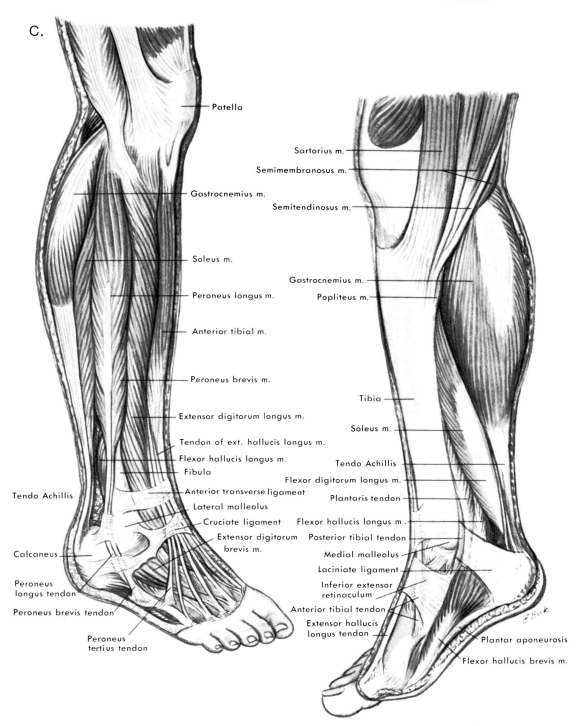

C.

Patella

Sartorius m.

Semimembranosus m.

Semitendinosus m.

Gastrocnemius m.

Gastrocnemius m.

Popliteus m.

Soleus m.

Peroneus longus m.

Anterior tibial m.

Tibia

Peroneus brevis m.

Soleus m.

Extensor digitorum longus m.

Tendo Achillis

Tendon of ext. hallucis longus m.

Flexor digitorum longus m.

Flexor hallucis longus m.

Plantaris tendon

Fibula

Flexor hallucis longus m .

Anterior transverse ligament

Posterior tibial tendon

Lateral malleolus

Medial malleolus

Tendo Achillis

Cruciate ligament

Laciniate ligament

Extensor digitorum
brevis m.

Inferior extensor
retinaculum

Calcaneus

Anterior tibial tendon

Peroneus
longus tendon

Extensor hallucis
longus tendon

Peroneus brevis tendon

Plantar aponeurosis

Peroneus
tertius tendon

Flexor hallucis brevis m.

Plate 162. (Continued) C., Muscles of the right leg—lateral and medial aspects.

The *superficial posterior compartment* is bounded medially, posteriorly, and laterally by the deep fascia of the leg and anteriorly by the deep transverse fascia of the leg. It contains the sural nerve, the gastrocnemius, the soleus, and the plantaris. Proximally, the sural nerve is deep to the deep fascia and descends between the medial and lateral heads of gastrocnemius. In the middle of the leg it pierces the deep fascia, and soon after it receives a sensory communicating branch of the common peroneal nerve. Distally, it traverses on the lateral margin of the Achilles tendon midway between the lateral malleolus and calcaneus.

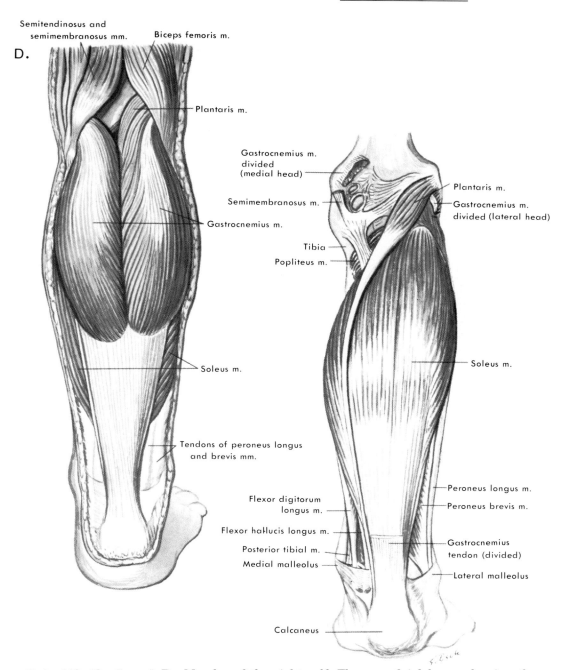

Semitendinosus and
semimembranosus mm.

Biceps femoris m.

D.

Plantaris m.

Gastrocnemius m.
divided
(medial head)

Semimembranosus m.

Gastrocnemius m.

Tibia

Popliteus m.

Plantaris m.

Gastrocnemius m.
divided (lateral head)

Soleus m.

Soleus m.

Tendons of peroneus longus
and brevis mm.

Peroneus longus m.

Peroneus brevis m.

Flexor digitorum
longus m.

Flexor hallucis longus m.

Posterior tibial m.

Medial malleolus

Gastrocnemius
tendon (divided)

Lateral malleolus

Calcaneus

Plate 162. (Continued) D., Muscles of the right calf. The superficial layer, showing the
gastrocnemius muscle and, deep to it, the soleus and plantaris muscles.

The *deep posterior compartment* is bounded posteriorly by the deep transverse fascia of the leg, laterally by the shaft of the fibula, medially by the deep fascia of the leg, and anteriorly by the tibial shaft and the interosseous membrane. It contains the popliteus, the flexor hallucis longus, the flexor digitorum longus, the tibialis posterior, the tibial nerve, and the posterior tibial vessels.

E.

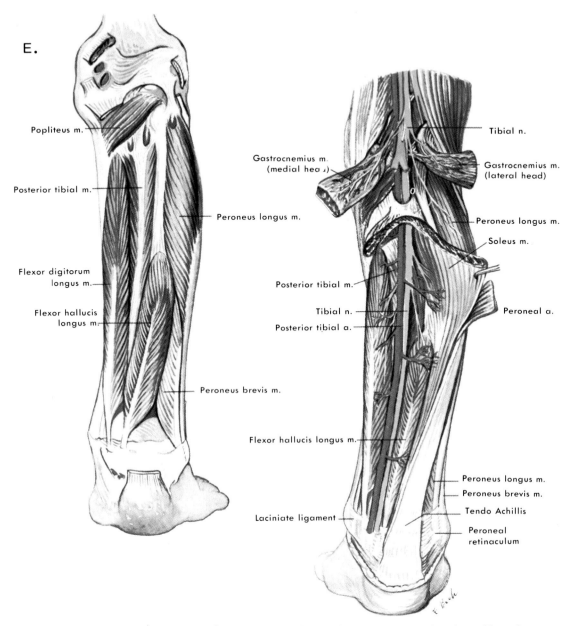

Popliteus m.

Posterior tibial m.

Flexor digitorum longus m.

Flexor hallucis longus m.

Peroneus longus m.

Peroneus brevis m.

Gastrocnemius m. (medial head)

Posterior tibial m.

Tibial n.

Posterior tibial a.

Flexor hallucis longus m.

Laciniate ligament

Tibial n.

Gastrocnemius m. (lateral head)

Peroneus longus m.

Soleus m.

Peroneal a.

Peroneus longus m.

Peroneus brevis m.

Tendo Achillis

Peroneal retinaculum

Plate 162. (Continued) **E.,** Deep posterior crural muscles. Dissection of right calf to show tibial nerve and posterior tibial artery.

F. Cross-sectional anatomy of the leg at its proximal and distal thirds.

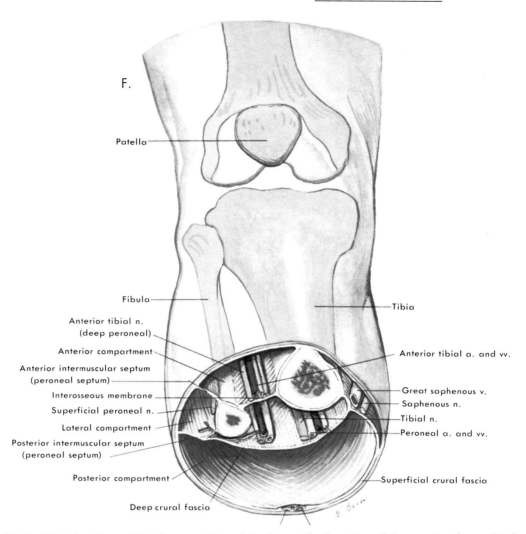

F.

Patella

Fibula

Tibia

Anterior tibial n.
(deep peroneal)

Anterior compartment

Anterior intermuscular septum
(peroneal septum)

Interosseous membrane

Superficial peroneal n.

Lateral compartment

Posterior intermuscular septum
(peroneal septum)

Posterior compartment

Deep crural fascia

Anterior tibial a. and vv.

Great saphenous v.

Saphenous n.

Tibial n.

Peroneal a. and vv.

Superficial crural fascia

Plate 162. (Continued) F., Cross section of the leg at the junction of the proximal one third and distal two thirds. The anterior, lateral, and posterior compartments are shown. Note the relationship of the vessels and nerves.

G. Cross-sectional anatomy of the leg at its proximal, middle, and distal thirds.

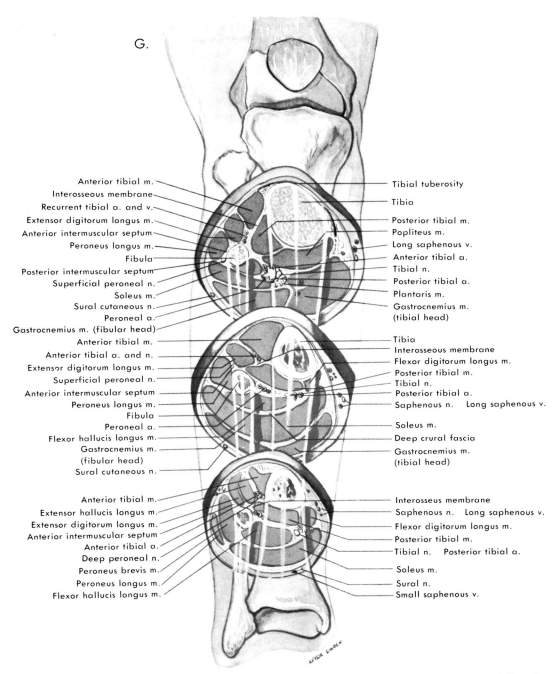

G.

Anterior tibial m.
Interosseous membrane
Recurrent tibial a. and v.
Extensor digitorum longus m.
Anterior intermuscular septum
Peroneus longus m.
Fibula
Posterior intermuscular septum
Superficial peroneal n.
Soleus m.
Sural cutaneous n.
Peroneal a.
Gastrocnemius m. (fibular head)

Tibial tuberosity
Tibia
Posterior tibial m.
Popliteus m.
Long saphenous v.
Anterior tibial a.
Tibial n.
Posterior tibial a.
Plantaris m.
Gastrocnemius m.
(tibial head)

Anterior tibial m.
Anterior tibial a. and n.
Extensor digitorum longus m.
Superficial peroneal n.
Anterior intermuscular septum
Peroneus longus m.
Fibula
Peroneal a.
Flexor hallucis longus m.
Gastrocnemius m.
(fibular head)
Sural cutaneous n.

Tibia
Interosseous membrane
Flexor digitorum longus m.
Posterior tibial m.
Tibial n.
Posterior tibial a.
Saphenous n.   Long saphenous v.
Soleus m.
Deep crural fascia
Gastrocnemius m.
(tibial head)

Anterior tibial m.
Extensor hallucis longus m.
Extensor digitorum longus m.
Anterior intermuscular septum
Anterior tibial a.
Deep peroneal n.
Peroneus brevis m.
Peroneus longus m.
Flexor hallucis longus m.

Interosseus membrane
Saphenous n.   Long saphenous v.
Flexor digitorum longus m.
Posterior tibial m.
Tibial n.   Posterior tibial a.
Soleus m.
Sural n.
Small saphenous v.

Plate 162. (Continued) G., Cross sections of the right leg at the proximal, middle, and distal thirds.

Patient Position. Supine.

Operative Technique

   H. *Anterolateral approach.* The anterior and lateral compartments are decompressed through a 10- to 15-cm. longitudinal *anterolateral incision* placed midway between the fibular shaft and the tibial crest. This site of the incision is over the anterior intermuscular septum, which separates the anterior and lateral compartments, thereby permitting access to both compartments. Initially the incision can be smaller and extended proximally and distally as necessary.

   The subcutaneous tissue is divided in line with the skin incision. The wound flaps are undermined, and the deep fascia is widely exposed.

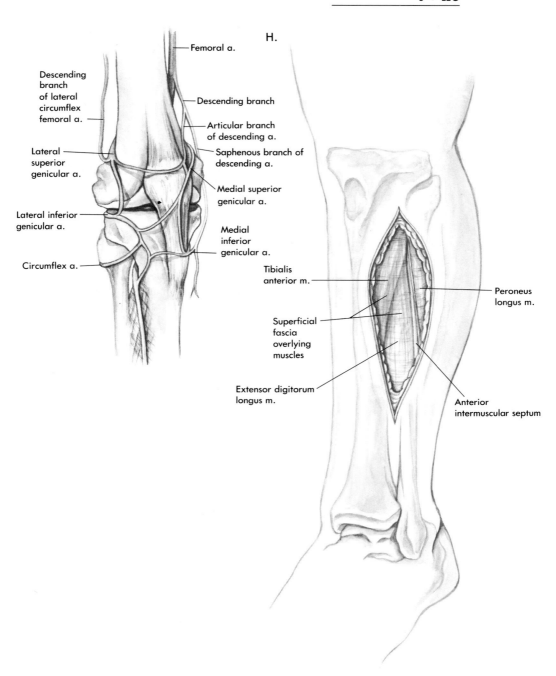

H.

Femoral a.

Descending branch of lateral circumflex femoral a.

Descending branch

Articular branch of descending a.

Saphenous branch of descending a.

Lateral superior genicular a.

Medial superior genicular a.

Lateral inferior genicular a.

Medial inferior genicular a.

Circumflex a.

Tibialis anterior m.

Peroneus longus m.

Superficial fascia overlying muscles

Extensor digitorum longus m.

Anterior intermuscular septum

Plate 162. (Continued) **H.–R.,** Operative technique. **S.,** Postoperative care.

I. Make small stab wounds with a scalpel in the deep fascia over the anterior compartment in the center of the wound, and then divide the deep fascia with Metzenbaum scissors transversely to extend to the lateral compartment. Identify the anterior intermuscular septum, which is an extension of the deep fascia cf the leg to the fibula. Locate and do not injure the superficial peroneal nerve, which lies immediately posterior to the anterior intermuscular septum in the lateral compartment.

J. Using Metzenbaum scissors with their tips slightly open, divide the deep fascia of the anterior compartment; distally, the tips of the scissors are directed slightly toward the great toe and, proximally, toward the patella.

Accessory incisions are made proximally and distally if there is any question of the thoroughness of the fasciotomy. Leave the scissors in place and make a 2-cm. longitudinal incision over its tip; perform further sectioning of the fascia through the accessory incisions.

K. The *lateral compartment* is decompressed by incising the deep fascia of the leg throughout its entire length parallel to the shaft of the fibula.

Caution! Keep the fascial incision posterolaterally, and do not injure the superficial proximal nerve, which is anterior and immediately posterior to the anterior intermuscular septum of the leg. The Metzenbaum scissors are directed proximally toward the head of the fibula and distally toward the lateral malleolus.

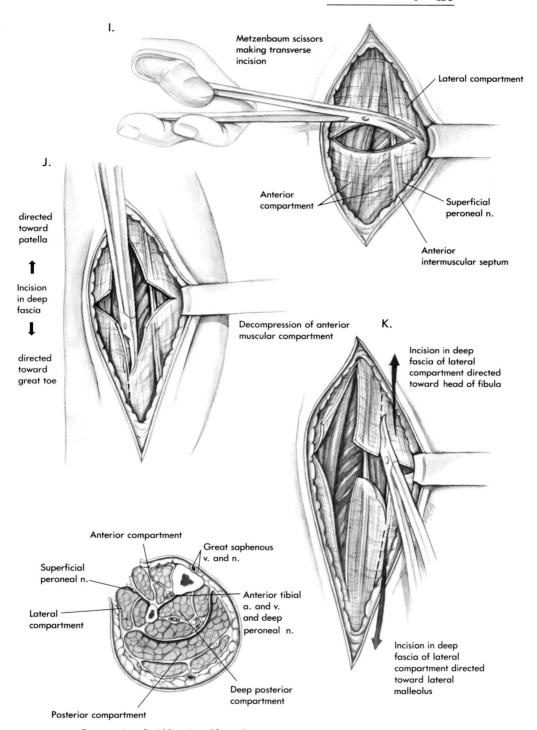

I.

Metzenbaum scissors making transverse incision

Lateral compartment

Anterior compartment

Superficial peroneal n.

Anterior intermuscular septum

J.

directed toward patella

↑

Incision in deep fascia

↓

directed toward great toe

Decompression of anterior muscular compartment

K.

Incision in deep fascia of lateral compartment directed toward head of fibula

Incision in deep fascia of lateral compartment directed toward lateral malleolus

Anterior compartment

Great saphenous v. and n.

Superficial peroneal n.

Lateral compartment

Anterior tibial a. and v. and deep peroneal n.

Posterior compartment

Deep posterior compartment

Cross-section of mid-leg viewed from above

Plate 162. (Continued)

L. The superficial and deep posterior compartments of the leg are decompressed through the posteromedial approach.

Make a 10- to 15-cm. longitudinal incision 2 cm. posterior to the medial border of the tibia.

Caution! Avoid injury to the saphenous nerve and vein, which descend on the medial side of the leg immediately posterior to the medial border of the leg. Posterior placement of the incision avoids injury to these structures. The subcutaneous tissue is divided in line with the skin incision. The wound flaps are undermined and retracted, expanding the posterior aspect of the deep fascia of the leg.

M. Identify the saphenous nerve and vein, and retract them anteriorly.

N. Make a 3- to 4-cm. transverse incision and identify the intermuscular septum between the deep and superficial posterior compartments of the leg. Identify the Achilles tendon distally and posteriorly in the superficial posterior compartment and the tendon of the flexor digitorum longus in the deep posterior compartment.

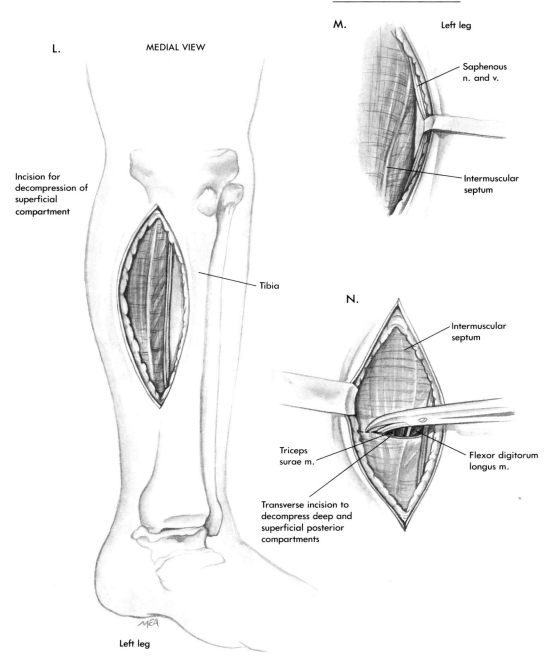

L.

MEDIAL VIEW

Incision for
decompression of
superficial
compartment

Tibia

Left leg

M.   Left leg

Saphenous
n. and v.

Intermuscular
septum

N.

Intermuscular
septum

Triceps
surae m.

Flexor digitorum
longus m.

Transverse incision to
decompress deep and
superficial posterior
compartments

Plate 162. (Continued)

O. Decompress the superficial posterior compartment first. With Metzenbaum scissors divide the deep fascia of the leg as far proximally as possible and then distally posterior to the medial malleolus.

P. Finally the deep posterior compartment is decompressed by incising the fascia under the soleus bridge, first proximally and then distally toward the medial malleolus. It is crucial to release the soleus all the way distal to its attachments to the tibia.

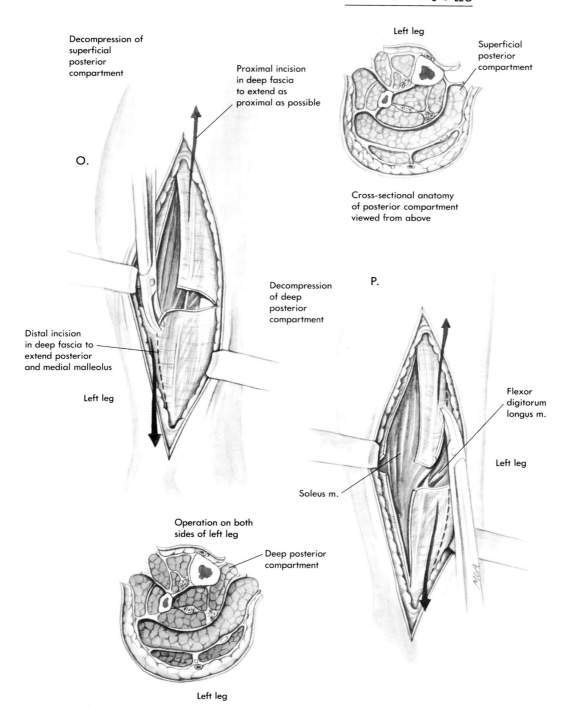

Decompression of superficial posterior compartment

Proximal incision in deep fascia to extend as proximal as possible

O.

Distal incision in deep fascia to extend posterior and medial malleolus

Left leg

Left leg

Superficial posterior compartment

Cross-sectional anatomy of posterior compartment viewed from above

Decompression of deep posterior compartment

P.

Flexor digitorum longus m.

Left leg

Soleus m.

Operation on both sides of left leg

Deep posterior compartment

Left leg

Plate 162. (Continued)

Q. and **R.** When there is impending Volkmann's ischemia to the muscles, simple release of the deep fascia is not adequate. It is vital to divide the fascial sheath of each muscle (the epimysium or perimysium) from its lower to upper margins.

Caution! Avoid inadvertent injury to any nerve branches that penetrate the epimysium.

Do not section or debride muscle! Initially it is very difficult to distinguish between a necrotic muscle and an ischemic muscle, which has the potential of recovery.

Perform a final check of pressure in each compartment. The wounds are irrigated and left open. Sterile dressings are applied. The skin and subcutaneous tissue are usually not closed. The lower limb is supported in a posterior splint with the foot-ankle in neutral position.

Q.   MEDIAL VIEW

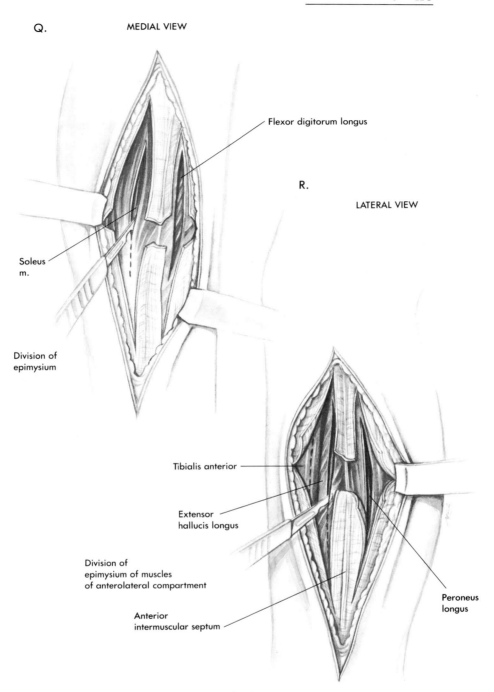

Flexor digitorum longus

R.

LATERAL VIEW

Soleus
m.

Division of
epimysium

Tibialis anterior

Extensor
hallucis longus

Division of
epimysium of muscles
of anterolateral compartment

Anterior
intermuscular septum

Peroneus
longus

Plate 162. (Continued)

Postoperative Care

S. Dressings are changed daily, as necessary, using strict sterile technique. Depending on the wound condition in five to seven days after fasciotomy, the wound is closed using the vertical mattress near-far, far-near suturing technique.

In cases of marked swelling the wounds are debrided every few days until a healthy granulation tissue bed is present, and then they are covered with split-thickness graft. This author recommends the consultation and help of a competent plastic surgeon in such an instance.

Passive and active exercises are performed several times a day to maintain range of motion of the ankle and foot. Appropriate splinting is carried out to prevent development of contracture.

REFERENCES

Allen, M. J., Stirling, A. J., Crawshaw, C. V., and Barnes, M. R.: Intracompartmental pressure monitoring of leg injuries: An aid to management. J. Bone Joint Surg., 67-B:53, 1985.

Arciero, R. A., Shishido, N. S., and Pau, T. J.: Acute anterolateral compartment syndrome secondary to rupture of the peroneus longus muscle. Am. J. Sports Med., 12:366, 1984.

Bass, R. R., Allison, E. J., Jr., Reines, H. D., Yeager, J. C., and Pryor, W. H., Jr.: Thigh compartment syndrome without lower extremity trauma following application of pneumatic antishock trousers. Ann. Emerg. Med., 12:382, 1983.

Christenson, J. T., and Wulff, K.: Compartment pressure following leg injury: The effects of diuretic treatment. Injury, 16:591, 1985.

Clancey, G. J.: Acute posterior compartment syndrome in the thigh. A case report. J. Bone Joint Surg., 67-A:1278, 1985.

Matsen, F. A. III, and Clawson, D. K.: The deep posterior compartmental syndrome of the leg. J. Bone Joint Surg., 57-A:34, 1975.

Mubarak, S. J., and Hargens, A. R.: Compartment syndromes and Volkmann's contracture. Philadelphia: W. B. Saunders Co., 1981, pp. 147–165.

S.

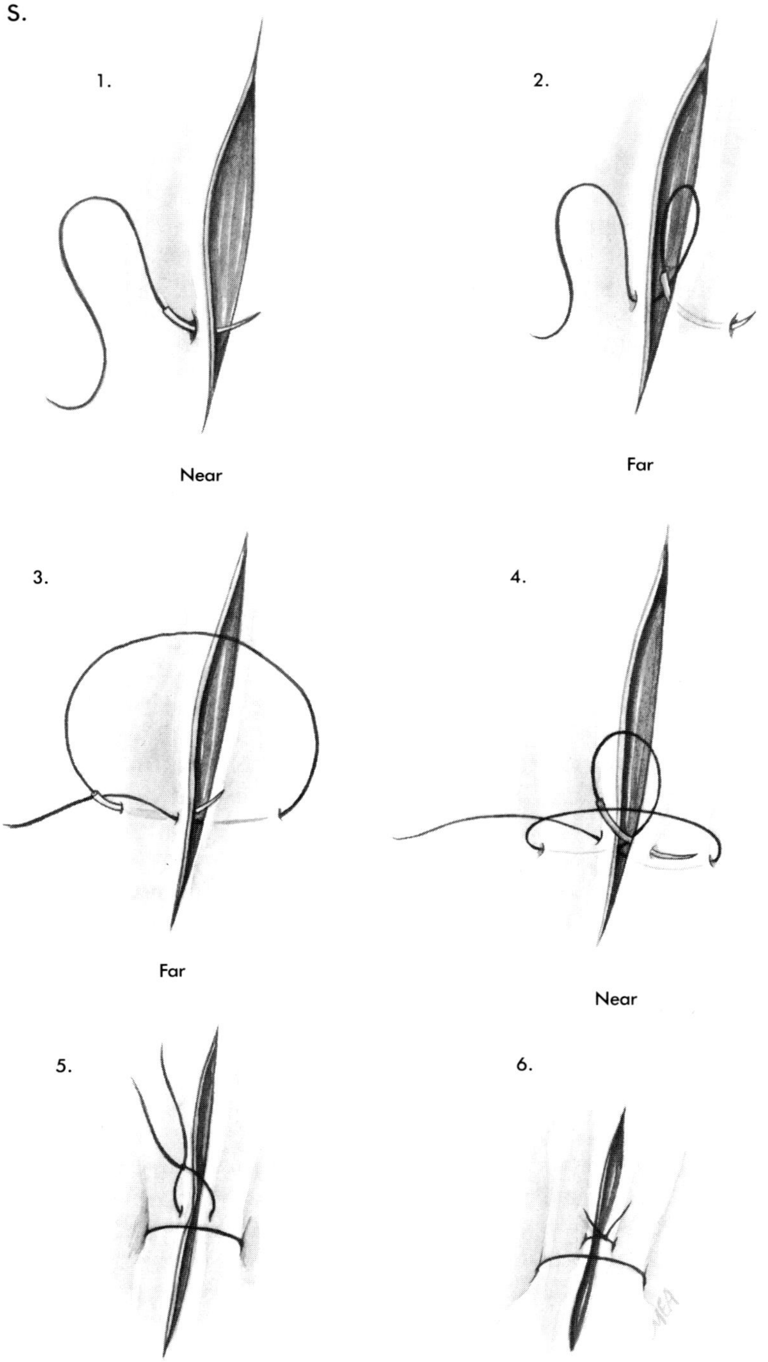

1.

Near

2.

Far

3.

Far

4.

Near

5.

6.

Plate 162. (Continued)

PLATE   163 ## Treatment of Congenital Pseudarthrosis of the Fibula (Langenskiöld Technique)

Indications. Congenital pseudarthrosis of the fibula with minimal valgus deformity of the ankle.

Caution! If the valgus deformity of the ankle is moderate (15 to 20 degrees) or severe (greater than 20 degrees), supramalleolar osteotomy of the tibia is required to correct it. When there is associated pseudarthrosis of the tibia, do not perform supramalleolar osteotomy of the tibia, because consequent development of pseudarthrosis will become a severe problem. It is safer to perform an asymmetrical medial stapling of the tibia at the appropriate skeletal age.

Radiographic Control. Image intensifier.

Blood for Transfusion. Yes.

Patient Position. Supine.

Operative Technique

A. The distal part of the fibular shaft and anterolateral tibial metaphysis are exposed through a longitudinal incision that begins at the anterolateral part of the lateral malleolus and extends proximally for a distance of 7 to 10 cm. The subcutaneous tissue is incised in line with the skin incision. The skin margins are undercut, elevated, and retracted.

B. The veins crossing the field are coagulated and divided. The superficial peroneal nerves are carefully identified and protected out of harm's way by retraction. Next, the deep fascia and lateral part of the transverse crural ligament are incised in line with the skin incision; the fascial flaps are developed and retracted. The cruciate ligament in the distal extremity of the wound is identified and left intact.

C. The peroneal tendons and muscles are identified posterolateral to the fibula and are retracted posteriorly. The peroneus tertius muscle (located in the anterior aspect of the fibula) is mobilized and retracted medially with extensor digitorum longus muscle and tendons and the extensor hallucis longus and anterior tibial muscles. The lateral part of the distal tibial shaft and the metaphysis are exposed extraperiosteally.

Next, with Keith needles and under image-intensifier radiographic control, the levels of the distal fibular and tibial physes are identified. The growth plates should not be disturbed. The site of pseudarthrosis of the fibula is exposed.

Make a vertical incision through the periosteum of the distal fibular shaft and metaphysis, stopping 1 cm. short of the distal fibular physis. Distally, a horizontal cut is made in the periosteum of the fibula to prevent inadvertent stripping of the periosteum-perichondrium from the growth plates. The periosteum is elevated, and the distal fibular shaft and metaphysis are exposed.

Next, the distal part of the anterolateral tibial diaphysis and metaphysis is subperiosteally exposed through an "inverted T" incision in the periosteum. The horizontal limb of the T is 1 cm. superior to the distal tibial physis.

Caution! Do not injure the anterior tibial vessels and the deep branch of the peroneal nerve; they are located between the anterior tibial and extensor hallucis muscles and tendon, passing directly anterior to the distal tibial metaphysis-epiphysis. If in doubt, identify the deep branch of the peroneal nerve and anterior tibial artery prior to incising the periosteum.

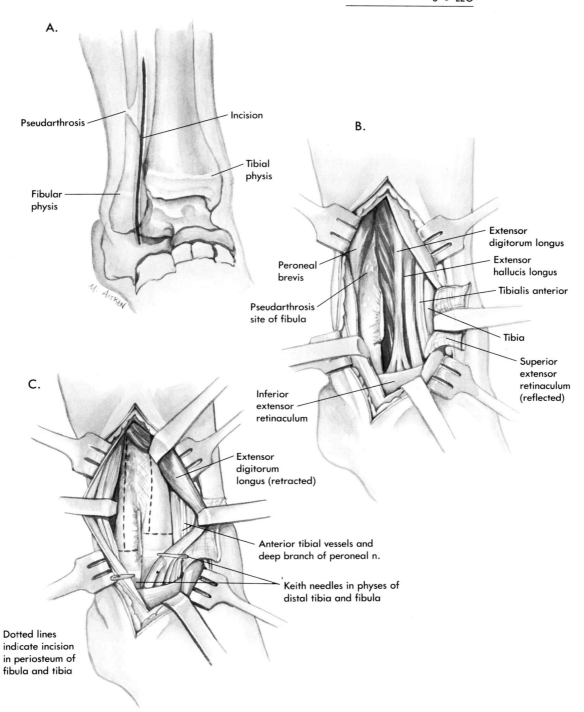

A.

Pseudarthrosis

Incision

Tibial physis

Fibular physis

M. AITKEN

B.

Peroneal brevis

Pseudarthrosis site of fibula

Extensor digitorum longus

Extensor hallucis longus

Tibialis anterior

Tibia

Superior extensor retinaculum (reflected)

Inferior extensor retinaculum

C.

Extensor digitorum longus (retracted)

Anterior tibial vessels and deep branch of peroneal n.

Keith needles in physes of distal tibia and fibula

Dotted lines indicate incision in periosteum of fibula and tibia

Plate 163. A.–F., Treatment of congenital pseudarthrosis of the fibula (Langenskiöld technique).

D. Next, the level of tibiofibular synostosis is determined. It should be at the upper part of the distal tibial metaphysis. With an electric saw or AO sharp osteotome, the distal segment of the fibula is osteotomized at the intended level of the synostosis. With an electric drill, a hole is made on the lateral aspect of the tibia at the site of the attachment of the interosseous membrane. The size of the tibial hole should correspond to the diameter of the fibula, it should be at a level parallel with the upper cut surface of the fibular metaphysis, and in depth it should extend well into cancellous bone of the tibia. Next, a 1- to 2-cm. square of the periosteum above the hole in the tibia is excised.

E. This author transfixes the fibula to the tibia with one cancellous positioning screw from the lateral aspect of the fibula into the metaphysis of the tibia, 1 to 1.5 cm. distal to the hole in the tibia and away from the distal tibial physis.

F. Autogenous bone is then taken from the ilium for the graft; it should be long enough to extend from the lateral surface of the fibula into the cancellous bone of the tibial metaphysis, and its width should correspond to the diameter of the cut surface of the fibula. The iliac bone graft is inserted into the hole in the tibia perpendicular to the long axis of the tibia and extending laterally in close approximation to the upper cut surface of the fibula. The space between the lateral surface of the tibia and the graft is packed with strips of cancellous bone from the ilium.

The pneumatic tourniquet is released, complete hemostasis is achieved, and the wound is closed in the usual fashion.

Postoperative Care. A below-knee cast is applied with the ankle and foot in neutral position. Partial weight-bearing is allowed as soon as the patient is comfortable. Full weight-bearing is allowed in three weeks. The cast is removed in six weeks. Range of ankle motion exercises and muscle strengthening exercises are performed several times a day.

Internal fixation with a cancellous screw allows early weight-bearing and a shorter period of immobilization in the cast.

If the surgeon prefers to follow the original Langenskiöld technique and not internally fix with a screw, the foot-ankle-leg are immobilized in a below-knee cast for a period of three or four months. Full weight-bearing is not permitted for the first two months.

REFERENCES

Langenskiöld, A.: Pseudarthrosis of the fibula and progressive valgus deformity of the ankle in children. Treatment by fusion of the distal and fibular metaphyses: a review of three cases. J. Bone Joint Surg., 49-A:463, 1967.

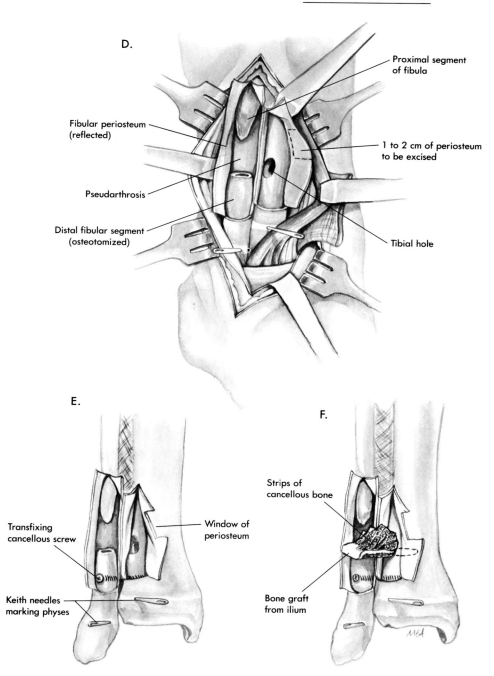

D.

Proximal segment
of fibula

Fibular periosteum
(reflected)

1 to 2 cm of periosteum
to be excised

Pseudarthrosis

Distal fibular segment
(osteotomized)

Tibial hole

E.

Transfixing
cancellous screw

Window of
periosteum

Keith needles
marking physes

F.

Strips of
cancellous bone

Bone graft
from ilium

Plate 163. (Continued)

PLATE   164 **Excision of the Proximal Fibula with Multiple Hereditary Exostoses**

Indications

1. Sarcomatous change.
2. Large exostosis causing pressure on common peroneal nerve and disturbing the proximal tibiofibular articulation and knee joint function.
3. Grotesque deformity.

Special Instrumentation. Nerve stimulator. Ask the anesthesiologist not to paralyze the patient.

Caution! After 20–30 minutes of tourniquet ischemia, the peroneal nerve will not respond to stimulation.

Radiographic Control. Image intensifier.

Patient Position. The patient is placed in semilateral decubitus position. With a pneumatic tourniquet on the proximal thigh, the lower limb is prepared and draped in the usual fashion.

Operative Technique

A. The incision begins 5 to 7 cm. above the knee joint line, in line with the biceps femoris tendon, and extends distally and laterally to the head of the fibula, where it curves forward for a distance of 5 to 7 cm. The subcutaneous tissue is divided in line with the skin incision, and the deep fascia is sectioned.

B. The iliotibial band is retracted anteriorly, and the long head of the biceps femoris is carefully exposed by blunt dissection. The common peroneal nerve is identified along its medial border and is retracted distally. Great care is exercised not to injure the common peroneal nerve by vigorous retraction.

C. The fibular collateral ligament is sectioned near its insertion and tagged with 00 nonabsorbable sutures. The upper end and proximal shaft of the fibula with the multiple exostoses are exposed. The biceps femoris tendon is sectioned at its insertion to the head of the fibula and reflected proximally. The peroneus longus and brevis muscles are elevated subperiosteally and deviated distally; stay anterior and do not damage the nerve supply to the peroneal muscles. The gastrocnemius and soleus muscles are retracted posteriorly. The level of section of the fibular shaft is determined.

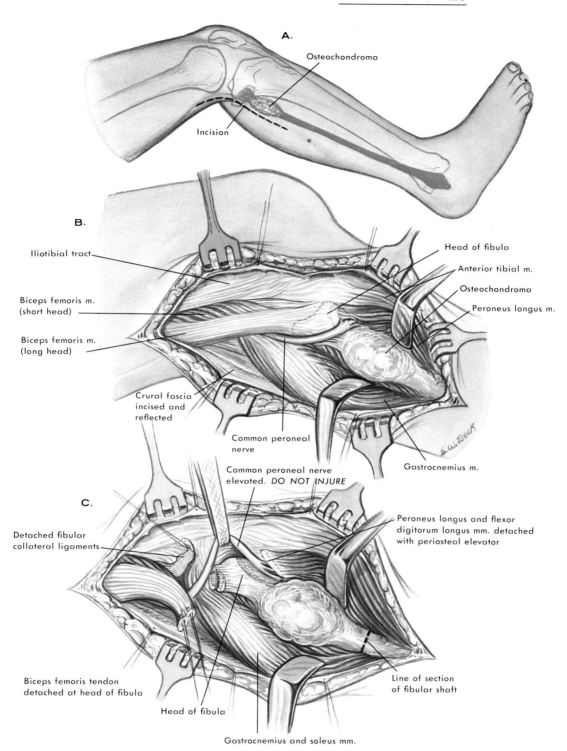

A.

Osteochondroma

Incision

B.

Iliotibial tract

Biceps femoris m.
(short head)

Biceps femoris m.
(long head)

Crural fascia
incised and
reflected

Common peroneal
nerve

Head of fibula

Anterior tibial m.

Osteochondroma

Peroneus longus m.

E.W.BECK

Gastrocnemius m.

Common peroneal nerve
elevated. *DO NOT INJURE*

C.

Detached fibular
collateral ligaments

Peroneus longus and flexor
digitorum longus mm. detached
with periosteal elevator

Biceps femoris tendon
detached at head of fibula

Head of fibula

Line of section
of fibular shaft

Gastrocnemius and soleus mm.

Plate 164. **A.–E.,** Excision of the proximal fibula with multiple hereditary exostoses.

D. The shaft of the fibula is sectioned with an electric saw, and the proximal fibular segment is pulled laterally and proximally. By extraperichondrial and extraperiosteal dissection it is completely excised. The tourniquet is released, and complete hemostasis is achieved.

E. The biceps femoris tendon and the fibular collateral ligament are firmly reattached to the lateral condyle of the tibia; drill holes in the tibia and anchor the tendon and ligament securely to bone with nonabsorbable sutures. The extensor digitorum longus and peroneus longus muscles are sutured to overlying soleus and gastrocnemius muscles. The wound is closed in layers in the usual fashion. An above-knee cast is applied with the knee in about 30 degrees of flexion and the foot and knee in neutral position.

Postoperative Care. The cast is removed six weeks after operation, and graduated active and passive exercises are performed to obtain full extension and flexion of the knee and to restore normal motor strength of the muscles controlling the knee.

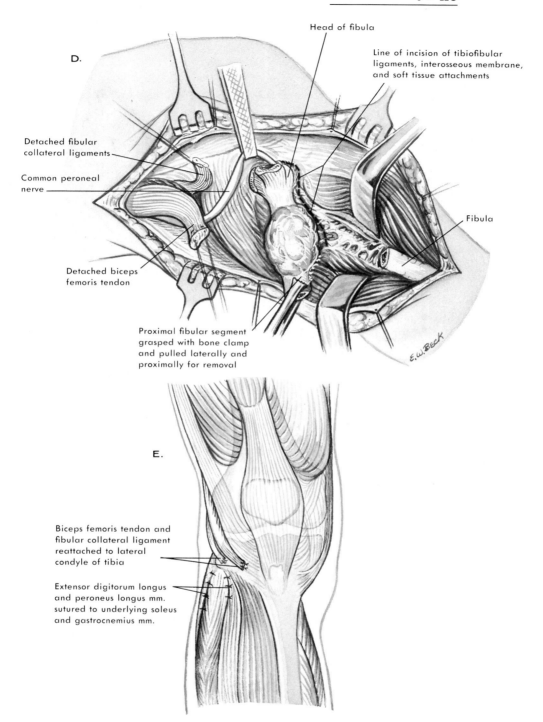

D.

Head of fibula

Line of incision of tibiofibular ligaments, interosseous membrane, and soft tissue attachments

Detached fibular collateral ligaments

Common peroneal nerve

Fibula

Detached biceps femoris tendon

Proximal fibular segment grasped with bone clamp and pulled laterally and proximally for removal

E.W.BECK

E.

Biceps femoris tendon and fibular collateral ligament reattached to lateral condyle of tibia

Extensor digitorum longus and peroneus longus mm. sutured to underlying soleus and gastrocnemius mm.

Plate 164. (Continued)

PLATE   165
Below-Knee Amputation

Indications

1. Malignant tumor of the lower leg or foot in which limb salvage is not feasible.

2. Severe congenital malformation with a functionless foot and ankle when Syme amputation is not appropriate.

Patient Position. The level of amputation is determined preoperatively. With the patient in supine position, a pneumatic tourniquet is applied on the proximal thigh.

Operative Technique

A. and **B.** The line of incision for the anterior and posterior flaps is marked on the skin, and the anteroposterior diameter of the leg at the level of bone section is measured. The anterior flap can be fashioned slightly longer than the posterior flap, or they may be made of equal length, as the position of the scar is not especially important in prosthetic fitting. The length of each flap is half the anteroposterior diameter of the leg.

C. and **D.** The incisions are deepened to the deep fascia, which is divided in line with the skin incision. The anterior and posterior flaps are raised proximally in one layer, including skin, subcutaneous tissue, and deep fascia. Over the anteromedial surface of the tibia, the periosteum is incised with the deep fascia, and both are elevated as a continuous layer to the intended level of amputation.

In the interval between the extensor digitorum longus and peroneus brevis muscles, the superficial peroneal nerve is identified; the nerve is pulled distally, is sharply divided, and is allowed to retract proximally well above the end of the stump.

The anterior tibial vessels and deep peroneal nerve are identified, doubly ligated, and divided.

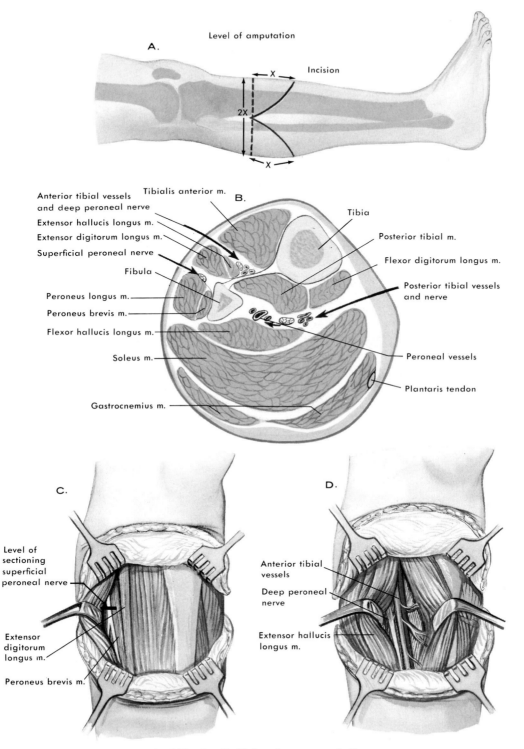

Plate 165. A.–J., Below-knee amputation.

E. and **F.** The muscles in the anterior tibial compartment are sectioned about 0.75 cm. distal to the level of bone section. The tibial crest is beveled as follows: Beginning 2 cm. proximal to the level of amputation, a 45-degree distal oblique cut is made, ending 0.5 cm. anterior to the medullary cavity.

G. Then the tibia is transversely sectioned. The angle of division should be at right angles to the axis of the bone.

H. The fibula is cleared of surrounding muscle and, with a Gigli saw, it is sectioned 2 to 3 cm. proximal to the distal end of the tibia. The bone ends are smoothed and rounded with a rasp. All periosteal fringes are excised, and the wound is irrigated with normal saline to remove bone dust.

Next the posterior muscles in the leg are sectioned. The posterior tibial and peroneal vessels are carefully identified, doubly ligated, and then divided. The tibial nerve is pulled distally and divided with a sharp knife. A fascial flap is developed from the gastrocnemius aponeurosis so that it can be brought forward to cover the end of the stump.

I. and **J.** The tourniquet is released following application of hot laparotomy pads and pressure over the cut surfaces of the muscles and bones. After five minutes the pads are removed and complete hemostasis is secured. The wound should be completely dry. The fascia of the gastrocnemius muscle is brought anteriorly and sutured to the fascia. Muscles may be partially excised if they are bulky at the side of the stump. Hemovac suction drainage catheters are placed deep to the triceps surae fascia. The subcutaneous tissue and skin are closed with interrupted sutures. A nonadherent dressing and a cylinder cast are applied for immediate prosthetic fitting.

Postoperative Care. The patient is fitted with a prosthesis as soon as he or she is comfortable and is instructed in gait training.

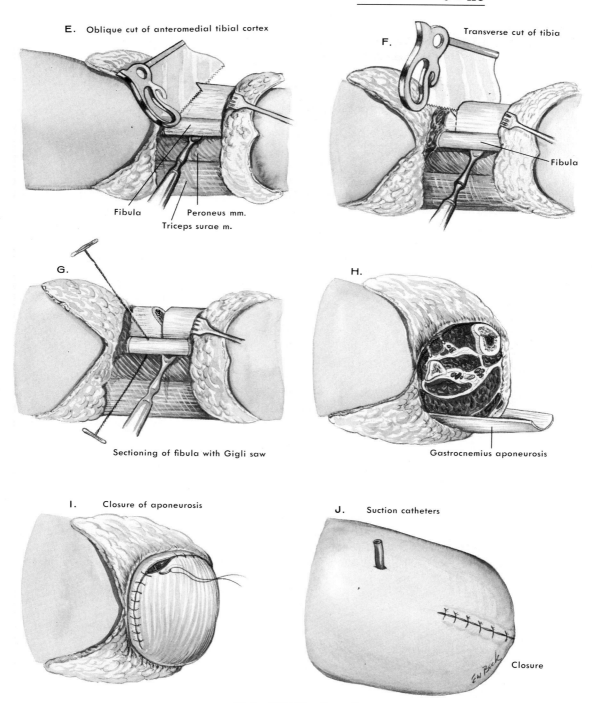

E. Oblique cut of anteromedial tibial cortex

Fibula

Peroneus mm.

Triceps surae m.

F. Transverse cut of tibia

Fibula

G.

Sectioning of fibula with Gigli saw

H.

Gastrocnemius aponeurosis

I. Closure of aponeurosis

J. Suction catheters

Closure

Plate 165. (Continued)

PLATE 166 **Medial Rotation Osteotomy of the Tibia and Fibula to Correct Lateral Tibiofibular Torsion**

Indications. Severe lateral tibiofibular torsion.

Radiographic Control. Image intensifier.

Patient Position. With the patient in supine position, the operated lower limb is rotated medially.

Operative Technique

A. First, an osteotomy of the fibula is performed at the juncture of its middle and distal thirds. A 5-cm. longitudinal incision is centered over the fibula at the intended level of osteotomy. The subcutaneous tissue is divided in line with the skin incision. The skin flaps are developed and retracted. The deep fascia is divided and retracted.

B. and **C.** The peroneal muscles and tendons are identified and retracted posteriorly. The periosteum of the fibula is exposed and incised longitudinally. The fibula is exposed subperiosteally, and Chandler elevator-retractors are inserted subperiosteally, protecting underlying soft tissues. With an electric oscillating saw, a transverse osteotomy of the fibula is performed from an anterior to a posterior direction. Do not divide the fibula lateromedially, as an overzealous, aggressive novice surgeon may inadvertently extend the osteotomy to the tibia.

The completion of the osteotomy of the fibula is double-checked with an ordinary osteotome. The wound is irrigated and packed with gauze for hemostasis.

D. Next, proceed to expose the tibia through an anterolateral approach. This author prefers to perform osteotomy of the tibia in its middle third and fix it internally with a six-hole AO compression plate. The incision begins 1 cm. lateral and 3 cm. distal to the proximal tibial tubercle and extends distally and laterally to the juncture of the middle and distal thirds of the tibia, midway between the tibial crest and fibula. Upon medial rotation of the distal segment of the leg, the obliquely directed skin incision will become vertical and cosmetically more pleasing.

Caution! Distally do not extend the incision too far laterally; you will end up with an oblique instead of vertical longitudinal scar.

Adequate skin should be left superiorly between the fibular and tibial skin incisions. The skin flaps are elevated and retracted.

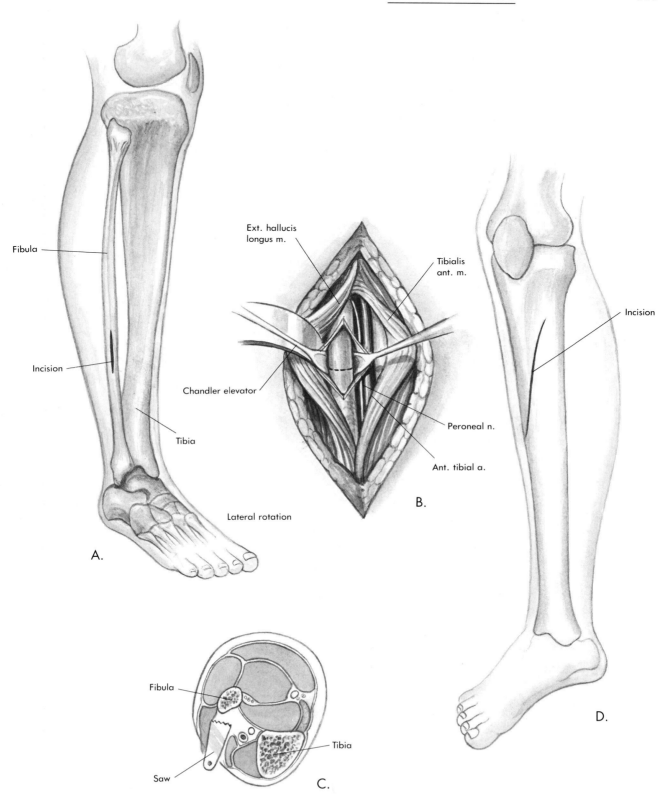

Fibula

Incision

Tibia

Lateral rotation

A.

Ext. hallucis
longus m.

Tibialis
ant. m.

Chandler elevator

Peroneal n.

Ant. tibial a.

B.

Incision

Fibula

Tibia

Saw

C.

D.

Plate 166. A.–H., Medial rotation osteotomy of the tibia and fibula at its middle third to correct excessive lateral tibiofibular torsion by internal fixation with plate and screws.

E. The crural fascia is divided longitudinally immediately lateral to the tibial crest. Anterior tibial muscles, the extensor digitorum longus, and the extensor hallucis longus are identified. The anterior tibial vessels and deep peroneal nerve lie in the interval between the anterior tibial muscle and extensor hallucis longus. Keep away from the neurovascular structures. Expose the periosteum of the tibia immediately lateral to the tibial crest, incise the periosteum longitudinally, and subperiosteally expose the medial and anterolateral surfaces of the tibia.

F. Determine the level of planned transverse osteotomy of the tibia. Place a six-hole AO compression plate in the wound, double-check the level of osteotomy, and mark it with an osteotome. Subperiosteally insert two large Chandler retractors on the posterior surface of the tibia.

An external fixator may be used for temporary fixation of the osteotomy and accurate determination of the degree of medial derotation. I often use the Wagner fixator because of its simplicity. First, one Schanz screw is inserted proximally at the upper diaphysis of the tibia, away from the upper end of the AO plate. Then a second Schanz screw is inserted distally at the desired degree. When the osteotomy is completed and the distal tibial fragment is rotated medially, the two Schanz screws will be parallel to each other.

A transverse osteotomy of the tibia is performed with an oscillating saw. Some surgeons may prefer drilling the cortices by multiple holes and performing a compatectomy without disturbing the intraosseous blood supply.

G. The distal tibial-fibular segments are rotated medially to the desired degree, the proximal and distal Schanz screws are aligned, and the Wagner external fixator is connected. The proximal and distal osteotomy fragments are compressed.

H. The six-hole AO plate is contoured to the lateral surface of the tibia by a plate bender. The curved AO compression plate is fixed to the tibia by screws.

I prefer an alternate method (not illustrated). First, perform an incomplete osteotomy (four fifths) of the tibial diaphysis on its anterolateral aspect. Next, the six-hole plate is fixed to the lateral surface of the upper tibial segment by three screws following routine AO technique. Then the osteotomy is completed with an osteotome, and the distal segment of the tibia is rotated medially to the desired degree and fixed to the plate with three screws. This technique makes the whole procedure very simple.

Radiograms in the anteroposterior and lateral projections of the tibia to include the knee and ankle joint are made. The tourniquet is released, and complete hemostasis is achieved. A prophylactic fasciotomy is performed, and a medium-sized Hemovac suction tube is inserted. The wound is closed in the usual fashion. An above-knee cast is applied with the knee in 45 degrees of flexion.

Postoperative Care. The cast and sutures are removed in three or four weeks. Radiograms are made, and if there is adequate healing, a below-knee cast is applied and the patient is allowed full weight-bearing. Complete consolidation of the osteotomy usually takes place in six to eight weeks.

Note: Preoperatively, it should be explained to the parents and patient that the plate will have to be removed in six to nine months. Following this, the patient will have to be in a below-knee cast until the screw holes are filled in to prevent refracture.

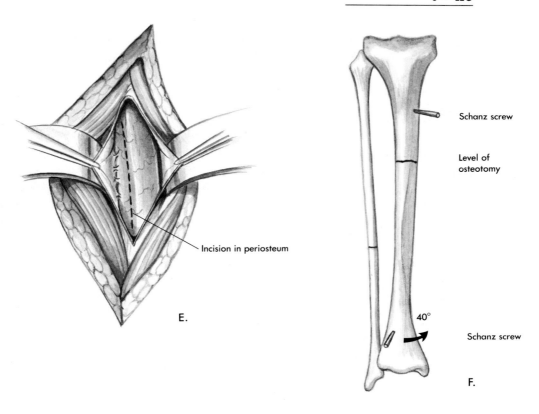

Incision in periosteum

E.

Schanz screw

Level of
osteotomy

40°

Schanz screw

F.

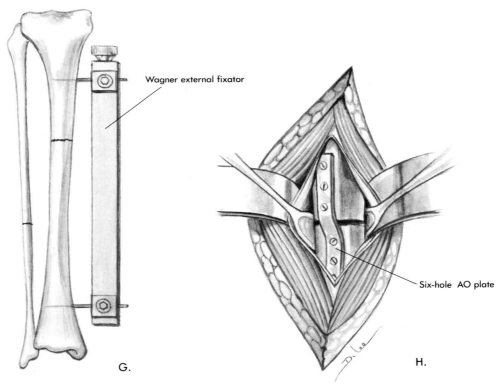

Wagner external fixator

G.

Six-hole AO plate

H.

Plate 166. (Continued)

PLATE 167 **Supramalleolar Rotation Osteotomy of the Distal Tibia and Fibula to Correct Excessive Lateral or Medial Tibial Torsion**

Indications. Severe rotational deformity of the tibia and fibula.

Radiographic Control. Image intensifier.

Patient Position. The patient is placed in supine position.

Operative Technique. First, an osteotomy of the distal fibular diaphysis is performed.

A. A longitudinal incision is made directly over the fibula beginning 2 cm. proximal to the tip of the lateral malleolus and extending proximally for a distance of 4 to 5 cm. The subcutaneous tissue is divided in line with the skin incision. The wound flaps are undermined and retracted, and the deep fascia is incised.

B. The peroneus longus and brevis tendons are retracted posteriorly and the peroneus tertius is retracted anteriorly, and a longitudinal "T" incision is made in the periosteum of the fibula.

C. The distal fibular shaft is exposed subperiosteally, and with the help of a power saw a transverse osteotomy is performed. Insert a straight osteotome into the osteotomy site to ensure that the cut is complete.

D. Next, make an oblique anterior incision in the distal one third of the leg. In a medial rotation osteotomy, the incision extends obliquely, and laterally. In a lateral rotation osteotomy, the incision extends obliquely and medially. Wound dehiscence is a problem, especially in the paralytic limbs of children with myelomeningocele. It is imperative that the incision be longitudinal and long enough. Avoid vigorous retraction of the wound flaps. For medial rotation osteotomy, begin the incision at the anterolateral part of the ankle joint immediately proximal to the ankle crease and extend it medially and proximally for a distance of 7 to 10 cm., ending at the crest of the tibia. Subcutaneous tissue is divided in line with the skin incision, and superficial and deep fasciae are incised.

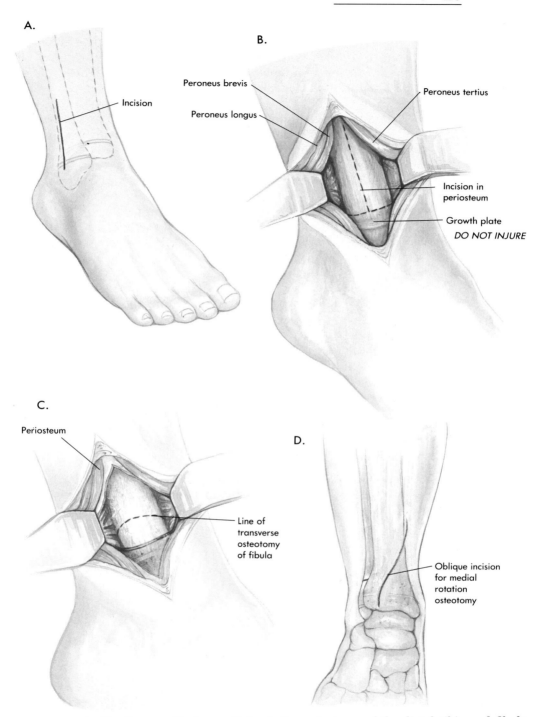

A.

Incision

B.

Peroneus brevis

Peroneus longus

Peroneus tertius

Incision in
periosteum

Growth plate
DO NOT INJURE

C.

Periosteum

Line of
transverse
osteotomy
of fibula

D.

Oblique incision
for medial
rotation
osteotomy

Plate 167. A.–D., Supramalleolar medial rotation osteotomy of the distal tibia and fibula
for correction of excessive lateral tibiofibular torsion. **E–I.,** Supramalleolar lateral rotation
osteotomy of the tibia-fibula to correct medial torsion.

E. The anterior tibial and extensor digitorum longus tendons with the intervening neurovascular bundle are retracted laterally, and the anterolateral surface of the tibia is exposed. With a Keith needle, the level of the distal tibial physis is determined with image-intensifier radiographic control. Then, make a T-incision in the periosteum with its transverse limb distal and 1 cm. proximal to the distal tibial physis.

F. With a power drill, holes are made in the medial and anterolateral cortices of the distal tibia at its mid-diaphyseal juncture. The drill tip should not penetrate the medullary cavity, thereby preventing damage to the marrow and intramedullary circulation.

The holes are connected with a sharp AO osteotome. The osteotome should not penetrate the marrow. With Chandler retractors protecting the soft tissues, the posterior surface of the tibia is osteotomized with a sharp AO osteotome.

G. Next, the tibia and fibula are rotated medially to the desired degree so that a plumb line from the proximal tibial tubercle will intersect the second ray of the foot with the foot and ankle in neutral position. Two criss-cross smooth Steinmann pins are inserted in a proximal to distal direction, stopping short of the growth plate for temporary fixation of the osteotomized fragments of the tibia. Radiograms are made to assess and determine the degree of correction of the deformity.

H. The osteotomy is fixed internally with a T-plate and screws. An alternate method of fixation is a staple or threaded Steinmann pins, especially in the skeletally immature child. The wound is closed in the usual fashion, and an above-knee cast is applied with the foot and ankle in neutral position.

I. For lateral derotation osteotomy, the incision begins immediately above the anteromedial corner of the ankle joint and extends proximally and laterally for a distance of 7 to 10 cm.

The other steps for surgery are similar to medial rotation osteotomy except that the ankle and foot are rotated laterally.

Postoperative Care. The cast is changed in three weeks, and a below-knee cast is applied if there is adequate healing and the patient has good knee control. The osteotomy usually heals in six to eight weeks.

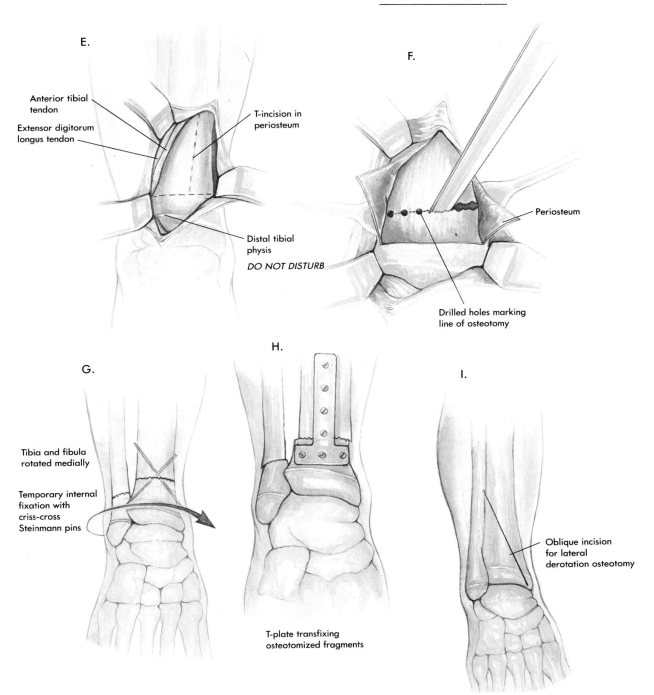

E.

Anterior tibial tendon

Extensor digitorum longus tendon

T-incision in periosteum

Distal tibial physis

DO NOT DISTURB

F.

Periosteum

Drilled holes marking line of osteotomy

G.

Tibia and fibula rotated medially

Temporary internal fixation with criss-cross Steinmann pins

H.

T-plate transfixing osteotomized fragments

I.

Oblique incision for lateral derotation osteotomy

Plate 167. (Continued)

PLATE 168 ### Osteotomy of the Distal Tibia and Fibula to Correct Ankle Valgus (Wiltse Technique)

Indications. Valgus tilt of the ankle of 20 degrees or more, such as in a paralytic limb, due to a high-riding fibula, congenital pseudarthrosis of the tibia or fibula, malunion of a fractured ankle, or multiple hereditary exostoses.

Principle. The technique designed by Wiltse is to resect a triangular segment of bone from the tibial diaphyseal-metaphyseal juncture with its apex pointing proximally and an oblique osteotomy of the fibula directed from distal-lateral to proximal-medial. The distal fragments of the tibia and fibula are rotated medially and shifted laterally, thereby producing normal alignment of the ankle without the unsightly prominence of the medial malleolus. The latter will result if a simple close-up wedge osteotomy of the distal tibia is performed.

Radiographic Control. Image intensifier.

Patient Position. The patient is placed in the supine position on a radiolucent operating table, and the surgery is performed with tourniquet ischemia.

Operative Technique

A. and **B.** In this simple closing wedge osteotomy for correction of ankle valgus, note the unsightly prominence of the medial malleolus with medial displacement of the ankle joint.

C. A longitudinal incision is made between the extensor digitorum longus laterally and the extensor hallucis longus medially; the incision begins immediately above the ankle joint and is extended proximally for a distance of 6 to 8 cm. Subcutaneous tissue is divided in line with the skin incision. The superficial fascia is incised, taking meticulous care not to injure the superficial peroneal nerve. The deep fascia and the transverse crural ligaments are incised vertically. The interval between the extensor digitorum longus laterally and the extensor hallucis longus medially is developed, and the anterior tibial vessels are exposed. The deep peroneal nerve lies lateral to the anterior tibial artery.

D. With a Keith needle, the distal tibial growth plate is identified under image-intensifier radiographic control.

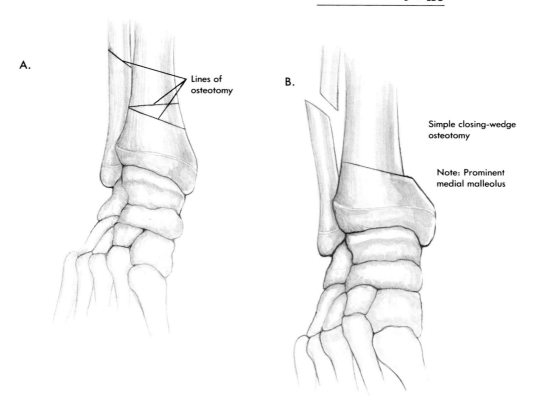

A.

Lines of osteotomy

B.

Simple closing-wedge osteotomy

Note: Prominent medial malleolus

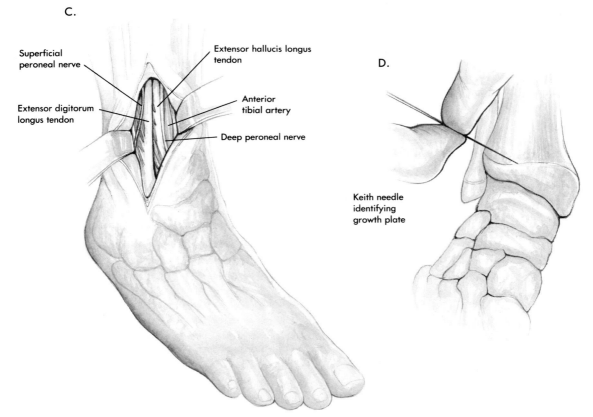

C.

Superficial peroneal nerve

Extensor digitorum longus tendon

Extensor hallucis longus tendon

Anterior tibial artery

Deep peroneal nerve

D.

Keith needle identifying growth plate

Plate 168. A.–H., Osteotomy of the distal tibia and fibula to correct ankle valgus (Wiltse technique).

E. and F. Next, the lower fibular shaft is exposed through a lateral incision beginning 3 cm. proximal to the tip of the lateral malleolus and extending cephalad for a distance of 5 cm. The subcutaneous tissue is divided in line with the skin incision. The wound flaps are developed and retracted. The superficial and deep fascia is incised and retracted with the skin. The peroneal tendons, which are posterior, are retracted out of harm's way, and the periosteum of the fibula is divided longitudinally and the fibular shaft is exposed.

With a power saw, an oblique osteotomy of the fibular shaft is made, extending distal-lateral to proximal-medial.

Through an H-shaped periosteal incision the distal tibial shaft and metaphysis are exposed subperiosteally. With the help of indelible ink the triangular segment of bone to be resected from the distal tibial diaphysis is outlined. The greater the degree of correction required, the more lateral the apex of the triangular bone.

Use image-intensifier control to ensure that the level of osteotomy is correct. Drill holes are made delineating the line of osteotomy.

With a power saw, the transverse line of osteotomy is made and then the triangular piece of bone is resected.

G. Apply traction to the ankle and foot, and medially rotate and laterally displace the distal tibial segment so that the medial surface of the distal segment is apposed against the lateral surface of the medial limb of the triangular cut.

H. Internal fixation is carried out either by criss-cross Steinmann pins, staples, or a plate and screws, depending on the preference of the surgeon. I recommend a compression plate and screw fixation in paralytic ankle valgus because the problem of delayed healing is higher than in normal bone in post-fracture ankle valgus. The wound is closed in the usual fashion. An above-knee cast is applied.

Postoperative Care. The cast is changed in three to four weeks, and if used, the Steinmann pins are removed. Another below-knee walking cast is applied for an additional three to four weeks. When a plate and screws are used for internal fixation, they are removed six to twelve months postoperatively.

REFERENCES

Wiltse, L. L.: Valgus deformity of the ankle as a sequel to acquired or congenital anomalies of the fibula. J. Bone Joint Surg., 54-A:595, 1972.

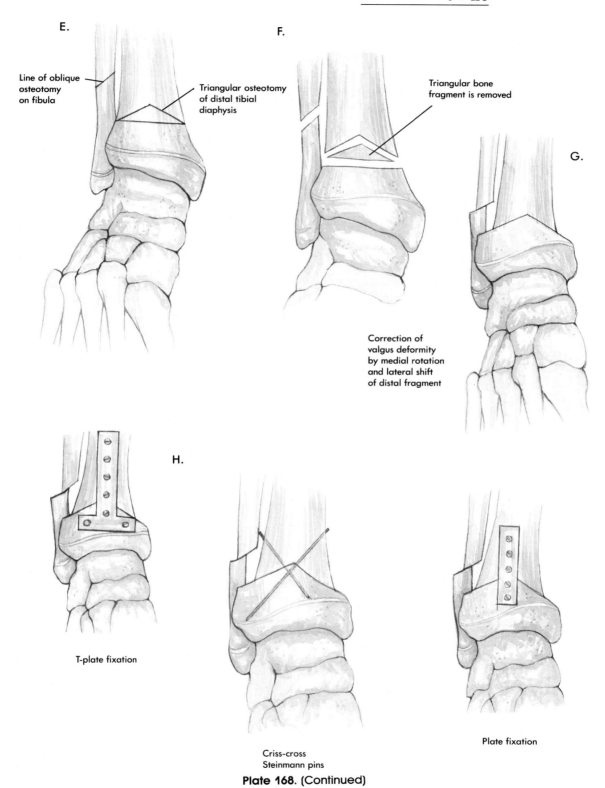

E.

Line of oblique osteotomy on fibula

Triangular osteotomy of distal tibial diaphysis

F.

Triangular bone fragment is removed

G.

Correction of valgus deformity by medial rotation and lateral shift of distal fragment

H.

T-plate fixation

Criss-cross Steinmann pins

Plate fixation

Plate 168. (Continued)

PLATE 169   ## Excision of the Physeal Bar of the Distal Tibial Growth Plate with Interposition of Fat (Langenskiöld-Peterson Technique)

Indications. Ankle varus due to premature closure of the growth plate with a bony bridge no greater than 50 per cent of the width of the physis.

Radiographic Control. Image intensifier.

Special Instrumentation. Dental burs and dental mirror.

Surgical Considerations. The surgical approach depends on the location and extent of the bar. Resection of the bony bar is indicated when the size of the bar is 50 per cent or less of the entire physis. Magnetic resonance imaging in the linear and transverse planes is the most accurate method to delineate the size, configuration, and anatomic location of the physeal bony bridge and the health of the noninvolved physis. Hypocycloidal tomograms can be used if magnetic resonance imaging is not available. The technique of Carlson and Wenger may be used to draw a schematic cross-sectional map on graph paper from the data obtained from biplane serial tomograms with cuts made 1 mm. thick. CT scanning does not determine the extent and site of the bony bridge because of the irregularity of the physis, but it is used to accurately determine the limb length. The skeletal age is determined by a radiogram of the left hand and wrist. It is important to know the remaining growth of the long bones and the potential for correction with longitudinal growth. There should be at least two years of further bone growth. When the angular deformity is greater than 20 degrees, osteotomy is ordinarily required to correct the deformity.

The type of surgical approach depends on the anatomic site of the physeal bony bridge. For centrally located bars, the transmetaphyseal approach is used. In this plate, the resection and fat interposition of a central bony bridge of the distal tibia is described and illustrated. The same principles and steps apply for excision of bars of other long bones, such as the femur, humerus, and radius.

Patient Position. Supine.

Operative Technique

A.–C. The elongated bars that extend from anterior to posterior surfaces depict a similar radiographic appearance in the anteroposterior projections; on the transverse sections, however, they have different contours.

D. The central physeal bony bridges with peripheral growth result in "tenting" or "cupping" of the physis.

E. When the bony bridge is asymmetrically located, varus or valgus deformity results. This diagram shows varus deformity of the ankle secondary to grade 2 supination-inversion fracture of the ankle. The medial part of the distal tibial physis is closed, and the lateral part of the distal tibial physis and the distal fibular physis continue to grow. First, insert one or two pins into the distal tibial physis at the bony bridge and determine the level of the physis by image-intensifier radiographic control.

The bony bar is exposed by removing a large window of cortical and cancellous bone through the distal tibial metaphysis. Avoid the pitfall of removing a small window and then enlarging the window piecemeal because of inadequate exposure. Next, with an electric oscillating saw, remove a window in the metaphysis of adequate size. Remove cancellous bone from the metaphysis to reach the level of the physis. Preserve the cortical wall of the metaphysis.

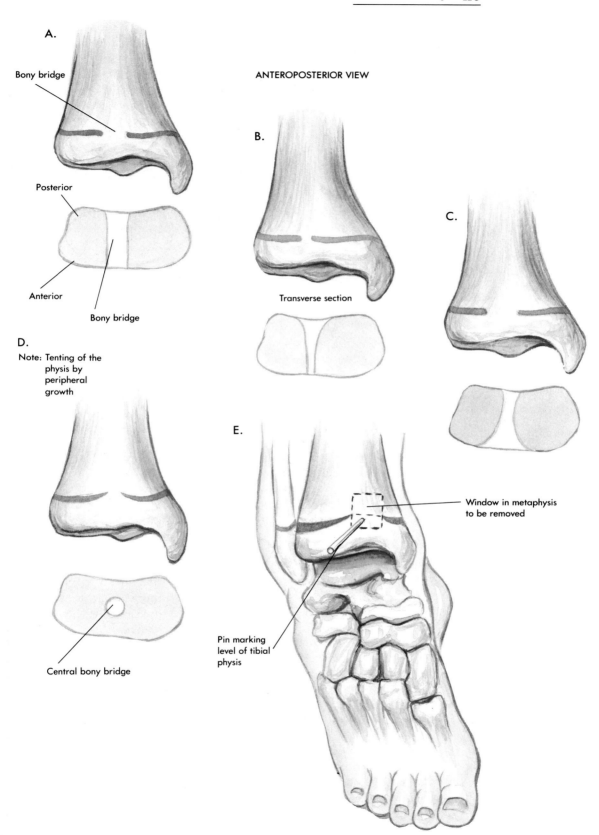

Plate 169. A.–J., Excision of the physeal bar of the distal tibial growth plate with interposition of fat (Langenskiöld-Peterson technique).

F. and G. With an electric bur, completely remove the bony bar from inside out until the normal cartilaginous growth plate is clearly visualized on all sides of the cavity. Use image-intensifier radiographic control in the anteroposterior, lateral, and oblique projections for accurate delineation of the depth and extent of the cavity. Do not transgress the subchondral bony plate of the epiphysis and enter the joint. Irrigate the cavity with normal saline, removing all osseous debris.

H. With a small dental mirror, inspect the cartilaginous cavity for thoroughness of resection of the bony bar and exposure of the cartilaginous growth plate.

I. Next, interposition material is inserted into the cavity across the physis to inhibit bone formation and prevent recurrence of the bony bridge. At present three materials are available: (1) polymeric silicone (Silastic); (2) methyl methacrylate without barium (Cranioplast); and (3) autogenous fat. This author prefers fat because it is biologically physiologic, nontoxic, and grows with the patient. Peterson recommends the use of Cranioplast because of the following advantages:

1. It is sterile and readily available without control of the Food and Drug Administration (as is Silastic).

2. There is no need for an extra skin incision and scar (as in fat).

3. It is easy to handle and mold into the desired size and shape.

4. It will firmly fill the cavity and achieve a certain degree of hemostasis by compression.

5. It is strong, and postoperative immobilization is ordinarily not required.

6. It has no apparent toxic effects.

Obtain fat of appropriate size from the gluteal region or lower abdomen. Fat migration is a problem. The interposition material should remain at the original site of the physeal bar and adjacent metaphysis-epiphysis. When the epiphysis grows away from the interposition material or the fat migrates, the likelihood of bony bridge re-formation across the physis increases.

This author recommends suturing the fat graft through drill holes made in the epiphysis and metaphysis surrounding the cavity. This step will ensure that the fat graft remains in the physis and adjacent epiphysis.

J. It is desirable to objectively measure and record the subsequent growth of the affected operated physis. Therefore, metal markers such as radiopaque vascular clips are placed in the cancellous bone proximally in the metaphysis and distally in the epiphysis. The metal markers should be in the same longitudinal direction. The remaining cavity superior to the fat graft is packed with cancellous bone graft, and the cortical wall of the window is firmly positioned into its original site. Radiograms in the anteroposterior, lateral, and oblique projection are made for radiographic documentation of the complete removal of the bony bridge and accurate placement of the fat, which is relatively radiolucent.

An alternate method is the use of Cranioplast as interposition material. The metaphyseal walls of the cavity are curetted so that it is flat and smooth. Through the walls of the cavity, drill holes are made into the epiphysis, and the epiphyseal walls are undermined with a right-angled curet. These steps ensure that the plug of Cranioplast will stay in the epiphysis and adjacent physis and will not displace proximally. Aspirate the liquid Cranioplast in a syringe with a short polyethylene tube, and inject the liquid Cranioplast into the cavity in the epiphysis and physis. Once the Cranioplast is partially set, it is carefully molded into the defect. There should be a minimal amount of the Cranioplast in the metaphysis. After the complete setting of the Cranioplast, the remaining metaphyseal cavity is packed with cancellous bone.

The tourniquet is removed, and complete hemostasis is achieved. The periosteum and wound are closed in the usual fashion.

Postoperative Care. When fat graft is used, I prefer immobilization in a below-knee cast with the ankle-foot in neutral position for three or four weeks. When Cranioplast is used, cast immobilization is usually not necessary. Active and passive exercises are performed for joint motion and motor strength.

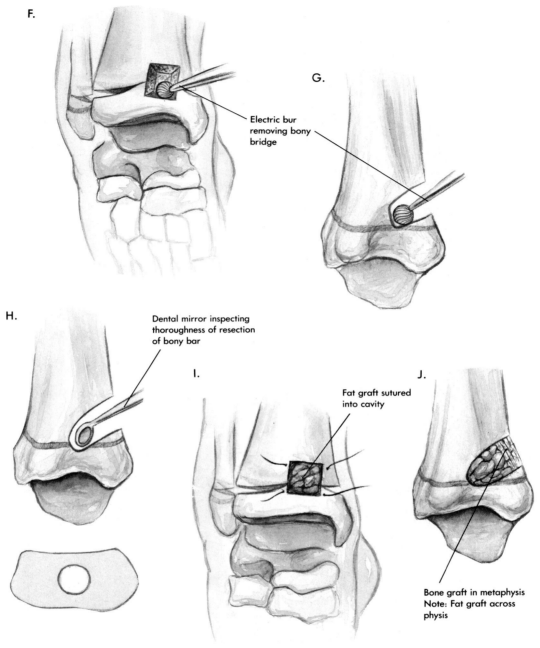

F.

G.

Electric bur
removing bony
bridge

H.

Dental mirror inspecting
thoroughness of resection
of bony bar

I.

Fat graft sutured
into cavity

J.

Bone graft in metaphysis
Note: Fat graft across
physis

Plate 169. (Continued)

REFERENCES

Bright, R. W.: Surgical correction of partial epiphyseal plate closure in dogs by bone bridge resection and use of silicone rubber implants. J. Bone Joint Surg., 54-A:1133, 1972.

Carlson, W. O., and Wenger, D. R.: A mapping method to prepare for surgical excision of a partial physeal arrest. J. Pediatr. Orthop., 4:232, 1984.

Langenskiöld, A.: An operation for partial closure of an epiphyseal plate in children and its experimental basis. J. Bone Joint Surg., 57-B:325, 1975.

Langenskiöld, A., Vidman, T., and Nevalainer, T.: The fate of fat transplants in operations for partial closure of the growth plate. Clinical examples and an experimental study. J. Bone Joint Surg., 68-B:234, 1986.

Peterson, H. A.: Review: Partial growth plate arrest and its treatment. J. Pediatr. Orthop., 4:246, 1984.

Peterson, H. A.: Partial growth plate arrest. *In*: Winter, R. B., and Lovell, W. W. (eds.): Pediatric Orthopaedics, 3rd ed. Philadelphia, J. B. Lippincott Co., 1990, pp. 1071–1089.

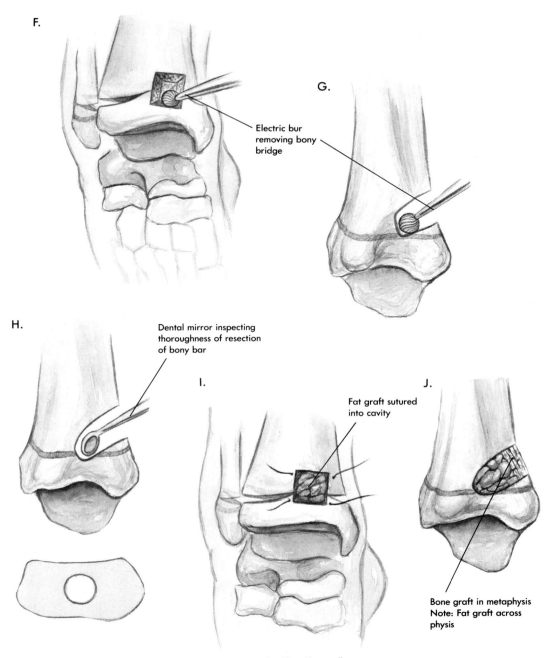

F.

G.

Electric bur
removing bony
bridge

H.

Dental mirror inspecting
thoroughness of resection
of bony bar

I.

Fat graft sutured
into cavity

J.

Bone graft in metaphysis
Note: Fat graft across
physis

Plate 169. (Continued)

PLATE 170   **Excision of Congenital Constriction Bands of the Leg**

Indications. Deep congenital constriction bands extending to the fascia and interfering with venous and lymphatic return, causing edema and enlargement of the distal part and neurovascular dysfunction.

Patient Position. Supine.

Operative Technique. The procedure is performed in two stages, including a Z-plasty each time. If the constricture is simply excised, it will recur. The following technique is adapted from Peet.

A. Two circumferential skin incisions are made ¼ inch proximal and distal to the constricting band. The distal incision is a serpentine line.

B. The incisions are carried through subcutaneous tissue down to deep fascia. The skin edges are undermined superiorly and inferiorly. The area to be excised is longitudinally divided.

C. The constriction band, the deep fascia, and the subcutaneous tissue and skin are excised by sharp dissection with a scalpel.

D. The wound edges are undermined and approximated with interrupted sutures except in one or two areas that are lengthened by Z-plasties.

E. The limbs of the Z-plasty are about ¾ inch long and at an angle of 45 to 60 degrees to the transverse incision line.

F. The triangular flaps are raised and transposed and sutured in position. The skin is closed with interrupted sutures. A compression dressing is applied, ensuring good circulation to the distal part.

Postoperative Care. Sutures are removed when the wound has healed—in about two or three weeks—and two or three months later the remaining area of constricture is excised and lengthened. If the constricture is very deep and circulation is precarious, the procedure is best performed in more than two stages.

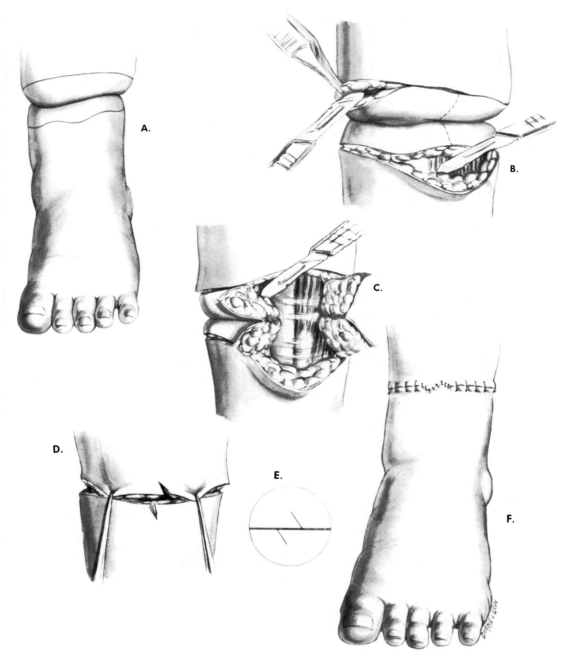

Plate 170. A.–F., Excision of congenital constriction bands of the leg.

PLATE 171   Syme's Amputation

Indications

1. Congenital deformity of the leg, such as complete congenital absence of the fibula, with poor function of the foot.
2. Malignant tumor of the foot.

Principle. The objective of Syme's amputation is to provide a good end-bearing stump. Correct placement of the skin incisions is vital. A single posterior heel flap is utilized. The heel pad resists pressure of the static force of body weight because of its specialized elastic adipose tissue consisting of dense septa of elastic fibrous tissue enclosing spaces filled with fat. Each loculus containing fat is separated and isolated from the adjacent loculi. This specialized subcutaneous tissue of the heel should be preserved when making incisions for Syme's amputation.

Patient Position. Supine.

Operative Technique

A. *Skin incisions:* A *dorsal incision* is made to open into the ankle joint; it extends from the inferior tip of the fibular malleolus, passes across the anterior aspect of the ankle joint at the level of the distal end of the tibia, and terminates 1.5 cm. distal to the tip of the medial malleolus. The *plantar incision* is carried vertically downward perpendicular to the sole of the foot and passes across the plantar aspect of the foot to join the medial and lateral dorsal starting points.

B. and **C.** The subcutaneous tissue on the front and sides of the ankle is divided in line with the skin incision. Subcutaneous veins are clamped and coagulated, and sensory nerves are divided with a sharp scalpel. The anterior tibial, long toe extensor, peroneal, and posterior tibial tendons are pulled down and sectioned to retract proximally. The anterior tibial vessels are isolated, ligated, and divided. The capsule of the ankle joint is divided anteriorly, medially, and laterally.

D. The foot is manipulated into marked plantar flexion, and the posterior part of the deltoid ligament is divided. A bone hook is placed on the posterior part of the dome of the talus, and the hindfoot is pulled into extreme equinus position. With a long knife the posterior capsule of the ankle joint is sectioned.

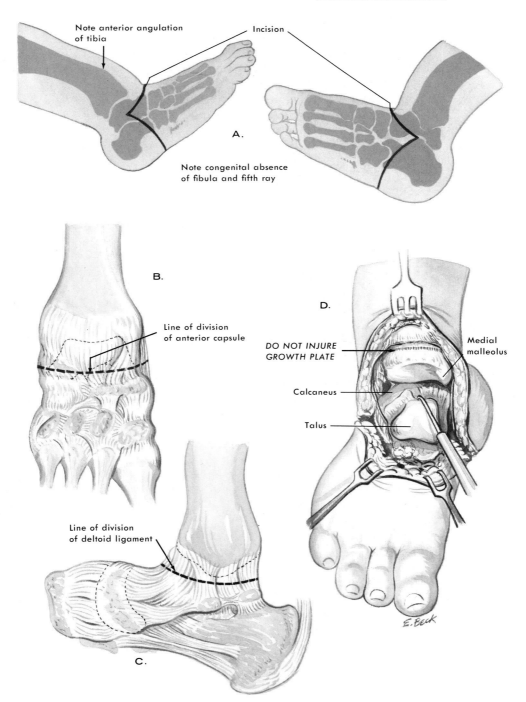

Note anterior angulation of tibia

Incision

A.

Note congenital absence of fibula and fifth ray

B.

Line of division of anterior capsule

D.

DO NOT INJURE GROWTH PLATE

Medial malleolus

Calcaneus

Talus

Line of division of deltoid ligament

C.

E. Beck

Plate 171. A.–H., Syme's amputation.

E. The Achilles tendon is identified and sectioned at its insertion in the posterior part of the calcaneus.

F. Next, a bone hook is placed on the back of the calcaneus, and the heel is pulled into plantar flexion. With a periosteal elevator, the calcaneus is dissected subperiosteally and the entire tarsus is removed, leaving the heel flap behind. Excision of the cartilaginous apophysis of the calcaneus should be complete. Do not leave behind any slivers of cartilage because as they ossify they will form painful ossicles that require excision.

G. The distal end of the tibia is exposed by retracting the heel flap posteriorly. The growth plate of the distal tibia is identified.

Caution! The growth plate should not be injured. Then, the articular end of the tibia is sectioned perpendicular to the weight-bearing line. The resected surface of the tibia should be parallel to the floor when the patient is standing. The medial and lateral plantar nerves are sharply divided. The posterior tibial vessels are isolated, ligated, and divided.

H. The heel flap is cleaned of all muscle. The tourniquet is released, and after complete hemostasis the wound is closed in the usual fashion over two catheters for Hemovac suction. A compression dressing is applied.

Postoperative Care. Complications in the immediate postoperative period are hematoma in the stump and ecchymosis in the skin flap. Hemostasis and closed suction should make it possible to avoid these problems. Slough may develop occasionally in the plantar flap, requiring skin grafting.

A definitive prosthesis is fitted within six to eight weeks. The prosthesis is end-bearing and has a flexible inner wall for suspension of a patellar tendon–bearing type of socket. A new prosthesis is usually required every one-and-one-half to two years by the growing child.

REFERENCES

Boyd, H. B.: Amputation of the foot with calcaneotibial arthrodesis. J. Bone Joint Surg., 21:997, 1939.

Eilert, R. E., and Jayakumar, S. S.: Boyd and Syme ankle amputations in children. J. Bone Joint Surg., 58-A:1138, 1976.

Harris, R. I.: Syme's amputation. The technical details essential for success. J. Bone Joint Surg., 38-B:614, 1956.

Harris, R, I.: The history and development of Syme's amputation. Artif. Limbs, 6:4, 1961.

Kruger, L. M., and Talbott, R. D.: Amputations and prosthesis as definitive treatment in congenital absence of the fibula. J. Bone Joint Surg., 43-A:625, 1961.

McCullough, N. C., Matthews, J. G., Traut, A., and Cowell, J.: Early opinions concerning the importance of bony fixation of the heel pad to the tibia in the juvenile amputee. N.Y.U. Inter-Clin. Inf. Bull., 3:1–16, August 1964.

Mazet, R., Jr.: Syme's amputation. A follow-up study of fifty-one adults and thirty-two children. J. Bone Joint Surg., 50-A:1549, 1968.

Syme, J.: Amputation at the ankle joint. London and Edinburgh, Month. J. Med. Sci., 3:93, 1843.

Westin, G. W., Sakai, D. N., and Wood, W. L.: Congenital longitudinal absence of the fibula: Treatment by Syme amputation. Indications and technique. J. Bone Joint Surg., 47-A:1159, 1963.

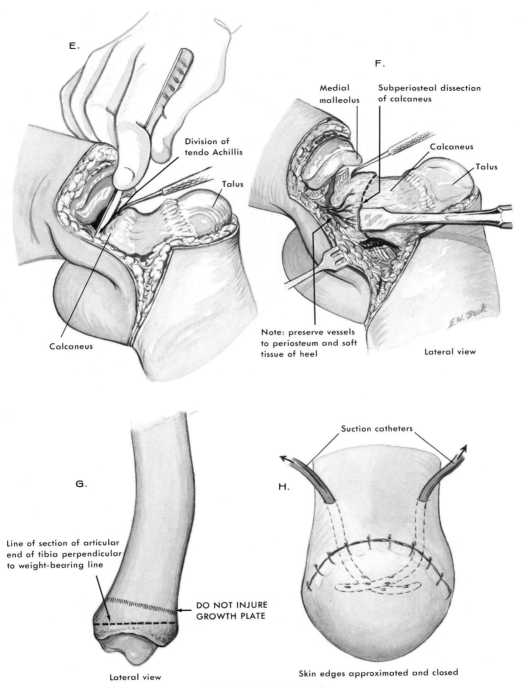

E.

Division of
tendo Achillis

Talus

Calcaneus

F.

Medial
malleolus

Subperiosteal dissection
of calcaneus

Calcaneus

Talus

Note: preserve vessels
to periosteum and soft
tissue of heel

Lateral view

E.W. Beck

G.

Line of section of articular
end of tibia perpendicular
to weight-bearing line

DO NOT INJURE
GROWTH PLATE

Lateral view

H.

Suction catheters

Skin edges approximated and closed

Plate 171. (Continued)

PLATE 172 **Exposure of the Angles of the Dome of the Talus for Excision of Osteochondritis Dissecans**

Indications. Osteochondritis dissecans that is detached.

Radiographic Control. Image intensifier.

Patient Position. Supine.

Operative Technique

Lateral Part of the Dome of the Talus

A. A curvilinear incision is made in front of the ankle, beginning at its medial margin and extending laterally; in front of the fibula it descends distally for a distance of 5 cm. The subcutaneous tissue and deep fascia are divided in line with the skin incision. The wound margins are elevated and retracted.

B. The long extensors are retracted medially and the peroneal tendons laterally. The capsule of the ankle joint is divided by a transverse incision.

C. Next, the talofibular ligament is identified and sectioned near its attachment to the talus. The ligament is tagged with a 00 Mersilene or Tycron whip suture for later attachment.

D. The hindfoot is inverted and plantar-flexed, exposing the lateral half of the dome of the talus. It is not necessary to osteotomize the distal fibula to expose the lateral compartment of the ankle joint. After excision of the osteochondritic fragment and drilling of its base, the talofibular ligament is repaired. The wound is closed, and a below-knee cast is applied for six weeks.

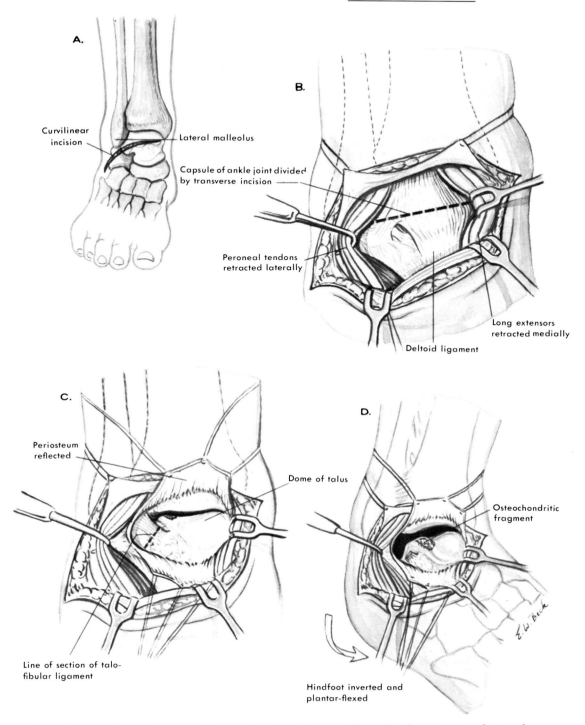

A. Curvilinear incision — Lateral malleolus — Capsule of ankle joint divided by transverse incision — Peroneal tendons retracted laterally — Long extensors retracted medially — Deltoid ligament

B.

C. Periosteum reflected — Dome of talus — Line of section of talofibular ligament

D. Osteochondritic fragment — Hindfoot inverted and plantar-flexed

E. W. Beck

Plate 172. A.–I., Exposure of the angles of the dome of the talus for excision of osteochondritis dissecans.

Medial Corner of the Dome of the Talus

To expose the medial corner of the dome of the talus, an osteotomy of the medial malleolus is required.

E. A medial incision about 7 to 9 cm. long is centered over the medial malleolus. The subcutaneous tissue and deep fascia are divided in line with the skin incision.

F. The level of the ankle joint and the tip of the medial malleolus are identified. If the *distal tibial physis* is still open, *it should not be injured*. The capsule of the ankle joint is opened by a transverse incision. The line of osteotomy of the medial malleolus is in line with the ankle joint.

G. The distal part of the medial malleolus is exposed subperiosteally. If the distal physis of the tibia is open, a transverse incision is made; if closed, a longitudinal incision is used.

H. Then a transverse osteotomy of the medial malleolus is performed at the level of the ankle joint. By rotating the medial malleolus downward 90 degrees and forcefully abducting the foot, the ankle joint and superior surface of the talus are visualized.

I. After excision of the osteochondritic fragment, the medial malleolus is anatomically reduced and internally fixed with two or three *smooth pins* when the distal tibial physis is open, or with a single metal screw in the skeletally mature ankle. The capsule of the ankle joint and the wound are closed. A below-knee cast is applied for six weeks. The healing of the osteotomized malleolus is not a problem.

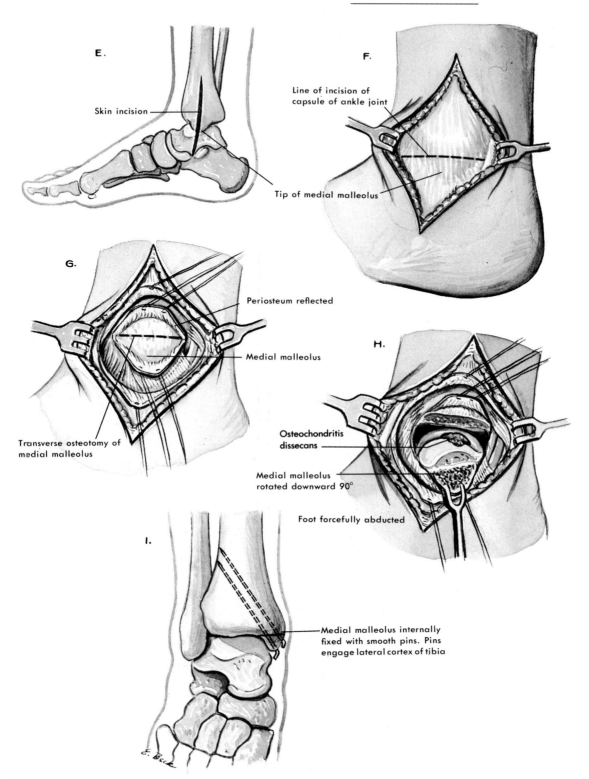

E.

Skin incision

F.

Line of incision of
capsule of ankle joint

Tip of medial malleolus

G.

Periosteum reflected

Medial malleolus

Transverse osteotomy of
medial malleolus

H.

Osteochondritis
dissecans

Medial malleolus
rotated downward 90°

Foot forcefully abducted

I.

Medial malleolus internally
fixed with smooth pins. Pins
engage lateral cortex of tibia

E. Beck

Plate 172. (Continued)

PLATE 173 ## Sliding Lengthening of the Heel Cord

Objectives

1. To correct a fixed myostatic contracture of the triceps surae, allowing a near-normal range of passive dorsiflexion of the ankle.

2. To establish a new tension-length relationship (Blix curve).

3. To alter the point at which the stretch reflex of the triceps surae is elicited.

4. To develop voluntary control and motor strength in the cerebral zero anterior tibial muscle.

5. To establish dynamic muscle balance between dorsiflexors and plantar flexors of the ankle.

Indications

1. Fixed equinus deformity of the foot-ankle with a toe-toe or toe-heel gait that is interfering with stability of stance and walking.

2. Failure to have an adequate period of nonsurgical management with excision, splinting, and stretching cast.

3. The development of fixed equinus or equinovalgus and rocker-bottom deformity.

4. Occasionally persisting functional equinus deformity of the foot-ankle in gait due to marked overactivity and stretch reflex of the gastrocnemius and soleus. This exists despite the fact that the foot can be passively dorsiflexed to neutral position.

Caution! In such an instance a prolonged period of conservative management should be attempted. The triceps surae should be good or better in motor strength. Do not overlengthen the heel cord!

The type of tendo Achillis lengthening does not make much difference—the results are similar. Equinus deformity may be caused by spasticity and contracture of both the soleus and gastrocnemius muscles or by contracture of gastrocnemius alone. Differentiate the two types of involvement by passive dorsiflexion of the ankle joint when the child is relaxed under general anesthesia, first with the knee flexed and then with it extended. The gastrocnemius is relaxed when the knee is flexed; therefore, when the equinus deformity is primarily due to contracture of the gastrocnemius, it disappears. In such an instance, Vulpius (see Plate 174) or Baker's tongue-in-groove lengthening of gastrocnemius aponeurosis (see Plate 175) is performed. When the position of the knee (flexed or extended) has no effect on the degree of equinus, both gastrocnemius and soleus are contracted; in such an instance, sliding lengthening of the heel cord is performed.

Requisites

1. Potential for independent or assisted gait is an absolute requisite. The child should be able to stand and walk, at least with the assistance of an orthosis.

2. Motor strength of triceps surae fair plus or better. When heel cord lengthening is performed on a weak triceps surae, the result will be calcaneus deformity, which is more disabling than equinus deformity. Perform multilevel simultaneous surgery with caution.

3. Absence of hip flexion deformity. Spasticity and contracture of hip flexors inhibit the action of the gluteus maximus, which is the most important antigravity muscle. The triceps surae can be hyperactive to compensate for hip extensor muscle weakness. Often equinus deformity is decreased following hip flexor release and acquisition of motor control over and strength of gluteus maximus. Correct hip flexion deformity prior to correction of equinus deformity. Perform multilevel simultaneous surgery with caution!

4. Feasibility of adequate postoperative care. Parents should understand that lengthening of triceps surae is the initial stage of treatment. Success of surgery depends on the adequacy of the postoperative care.

5. The patient should be at least three years of age. Do not perform tendo Achillis lengthening in a child with cerebral palsy younger than two years of age.

Patient Position. Supine or prone.

Operative Technique

A. With the patient preferably in prone position, a posteromedial incision about 5 to 7.5 cm. long is made 1 cm. medial to the tendo Achillis. The subcutaneous tissue and tendon sheath are divided in one plane so that the latter remains attached to subcutaneous tissue and can be reconstructed effectively later. It is not necessary to disturb the deep surface of the tendon or to dissect around the sheath.

B. The rotation of fibers of the tendo Achillis is studied next, as it varies greatly. The tendon usually rotates about 90 degrees on its longitudinal axis between its origin and insertion, so that the fibers that occupy a medial position proximally twist laterally as they approach their insertion on the calcaneus and are posterior to those fibers that proximally occupy a lateral position. Straight Keith needles may be used to mark rotation of fibers.

The Achilles tendon is then transversely sectioned at two levels. The site of division must be chosen according to the degree of rotation of fibers. Usually the anteromedial half to two thirds of the tendon is divided distally near its insertion and then the posteromedial half of its fibers is divided in the proximal end of the wound.

C. The foot is then passively dorsiflexed with the knee in extension. The medial portion of the tendon will slide on the lateral portion, lengthening the tendon in continuity. (A third incision, midway between the others, is indicated at times if stretching does not occur easily; its site can be readily determined by palpation.) There is no fraying of the tendon as in the Z-plasty type of tendon lengthening. The actual amount of lengthening depends on the degree of equinus deformity. At the end of the procedure the foot should rest comfortably in neutral position or 5 degrees of dorsiflexion. Correction beyond this point should be avoided, as it may cause calcaneus deformity. The pneumatic tourniquet is released, and all bleeding vessels are clamped and coagulated.

D. The sheath, including a small portion of the subcutaneous tissues, is meticulously closed over the lengthened Achilles tendon.

E. The lower limb is immobilized in a well-padded above-knee cast with the knee in full extension or 5 degrees of flexion (but no hyperextension) and the foot-ankle in neutral position or 5 to 10 degrees of dorsiflexion. It is essential to mold the plaster cast well, particularly at the ankle, heel, and knee.

Postoperative Care. The cast is removed three to four weeks following surgery, and a bivalved cast or splint is manufactured for night use. The foot should be in neutral position and the knee in 5 degrees of flexion. If there is any asymmetry or involvement of the trunk, it is best to manufacture a hip spica cast with the hips in 20 to 25 degrees of abduction and 5 degrees of lateral rotation and the knee-ankle-foot as above. Active and gentle passive exercises are performed to increase range of motion of the ankles, feet, and knees to develop motor strength of agonist and antagonist muscles, particularly the anterior tibial and triceps surae. When the joints have functional range of motion and the motor strength of the muscles is at least poor plus or, preferably, fair, the patient is allowed to ambulate, initially with support and then independently. It is vital that the knees not assume a flexion posture and that the hips be in extension and the trunk not carried forward. Calcaneus posture of the feet and ankles and crouch posture at the knees and hips should be avoided.

REFERENCES

Banks, H. H., and Green, W. T.: The correction of equinus deformity in cerebral palsy. J. Bone Joint Surg., 40-A:1359, 1958.

White, J. W.: Torsion of the Achilles tendon: Its surgical significance. Arch. Surg., 46:784, 1943.

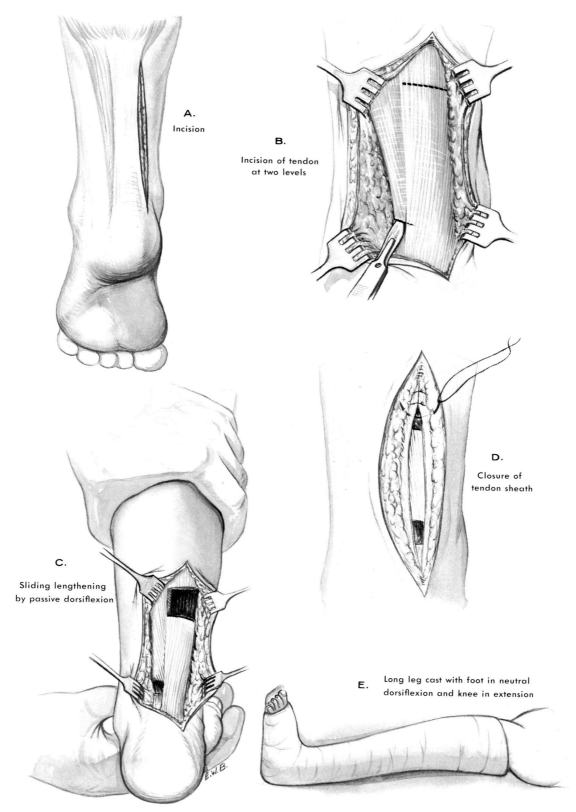

A.
Incision

B.
Incision of tendon
at two levels

C.
Sliding lengthening
by passive dorsiflexion

D.
Closure of
tendon sheath

E. Long leg cast with foot in neutral
dorsiflexion and knee in extension

Plate 173. A.–E., Sliding lengthening of the heel cord.

PLATE 174   Lengthening of the Gastrocnemius by the Vulpius Technique

Indications. Osteochondritis dissecans that is detached..

Patient Position. The patient is placed in the prone position.

Operative Technique

   A. A midline posterior, longitudinal incision is made, beginning at the juncture of the distal one fourth and proximal three fourths of the leg and extending proximally for a distance of 5 to 7 cm. The subcutaneous tissue and fascia are divided in line with the skin incision, and the wound flaps are retracted medially and laterally. Avoid injury to the sural nerve and saphenous veins.
   B. With a Freer elevator, the aponeurosis of gastrocnemius is separated from the underlying soleus muscle and one inverted-V or two inverted-V incisions are made 3 cm. apart.
   C. With the knee in extension, the foot is passively dorsiflexed, elongating the aponeurosis of gastrocnemius. Lengthen any taut aponeurotic fibers of the soleus deep in the wound.
   The tourniquet is released, and complete hemostasis is achieved. The wound is closed in the usual manner, and an above-knee cast is applied with the knee in neutral extension and the foot in 5 degrees of dorsiflexion.

Postoperative Care. The cast is removed three or four weeks following surgery, and a bivalved cast or splint is manufactured for night use. The foot should be in neutral position and the knee in 5 degrees of flexion. If there is any asymmetry or involvement of the trunk, it is best to manufacture a hip spica cast with the hips in 20 to 25 degrees of abduction and 5 degrees of lateral rotation and the knee-ankle-foot as described earlier. Active and gentle passive exercises are performed to increase the range of motion of the ankles, feet, and knees to develop motor strength of agonist and antagonist muscles, particularly the anterior tibial and triceps surae. When the joints have functional range of motion and the motor strength of the muscles is at least poor plus or, preferably, fair, the patient is allowed to ambulate, initially with support and then independently. It is vital that the knees do not assume a flexion posture and that the hips be in extension and the trunk not carried forward. Calcaneus posture of the feet and ankles and crouch posture at the knees and hips should be avoided.

REFERENCES

Vulpius, O., and Stoffel, A.: Orthopaedische Operationslehre, 2nd ed. Stuttgart, Ferdinand Enke, 1920.

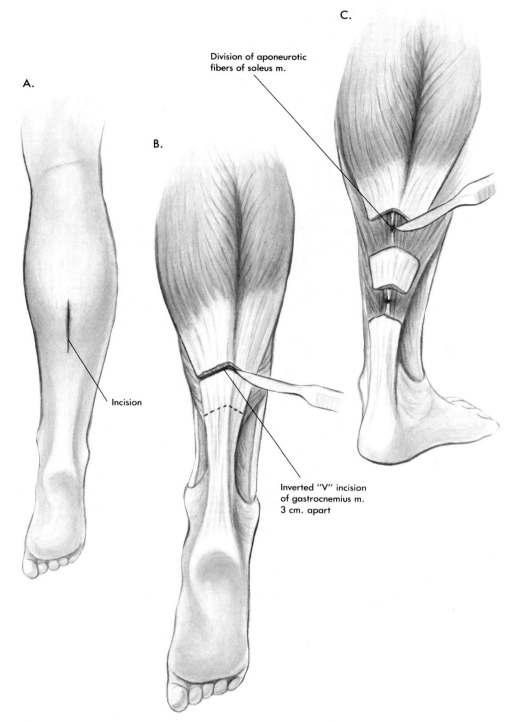

A.

Incision

B.

C.

Division of aponeurotic
fibers of soleus m.

Inverted "V" incision
of gastrocnemius m.
3 cm. apart

Plate 174. **A.–C.,** Lengthening of the triceps surae by the Vulpius technique.

<table>
<tr><td>PLATE 175</td><td></td></tr>
</table>

Baker's Technique of Tongue-in-Groove Lengthening of the Gastrocnemius Aponeurosis

Indications. Osteochondritis dissecans that is detached.

Patient Position. The procedure is performed with the patient in the prone position.

Operative Technique

A. A posterior longitudinal midline incision is made about 7.5 cm. long, extending from the lower border of the belly of the gastrocnemius muscle to the upper end of the Achilles tendon. The subcutaneous tissue is divided in line with the skin incision. Avoid injury to the sural nerve and the branches of the saphenous vein.

B. The deep fascia is divided in line with the skin incision, and the aponeurosis of the gastrocnemius muscle is exposed. An inverted-U incision (tongue-in-groove) is made in the central one half of the gastrocnemius aponeurosis, leaving the lateral and medial fourths of the gastrocnemius aponeurosis and the underlying soleus intact.

C. The middle portion, or tongue, of the gastrocnemius aponeurosis is dissected free from the soleus. Be sure there are no muscle fibers remaining attached to the tongue of the aponeurosis or the Achilles tendon. The distal attachments of the lateral and medial portions of the gastrocnemius aponeurosis are freed from the Achilles tendon. The dissection is carried out distally enough to permit full dorsiflexion of the ankle. Complete the dissection of the muscle fibers from the distal portion of the lengthened structures to avoid residual stretch reflex and clonus. The foot is dorsiflexed to 5 to 10 degrees beyond neutral. The central aponeurosis of the bipenniform soleus muscle is sectioned if necessary, if complete correction of equinus deformity cannot be obtained.

D. The four corners of the overlapping aponeurosis are sutured with 00 or 000 Tycron.

The tourniquet is released, complete hemostasis is achieved, and the wound is closed in the usual fashion. An above-knee cast is applied with the foot and ankle in 5 degrees of dorsiflexion and the knee in neutral extension.

Postoperative Care. (See Plate 173, p. 1002).

REFERENCES

Baker, L. D.: Triceps surae syndrome in cerebral palsy. Surgery, 68:216, 1954.
Baker, L. D.: Surgery in cerebral palsy. Arch. Phys. Med., 36:88, 1955.
Baker, L. D.: A rational approach to the surgical needs of the cerebral palsy patient. J. Bone Joint Surg., 38-A:313, 1956.
Baker, L. D., and Hill, L. M.: Foot alignment in the cerebral palsy patient. J. Bone Joint Surg., 46-A:1, 1964.

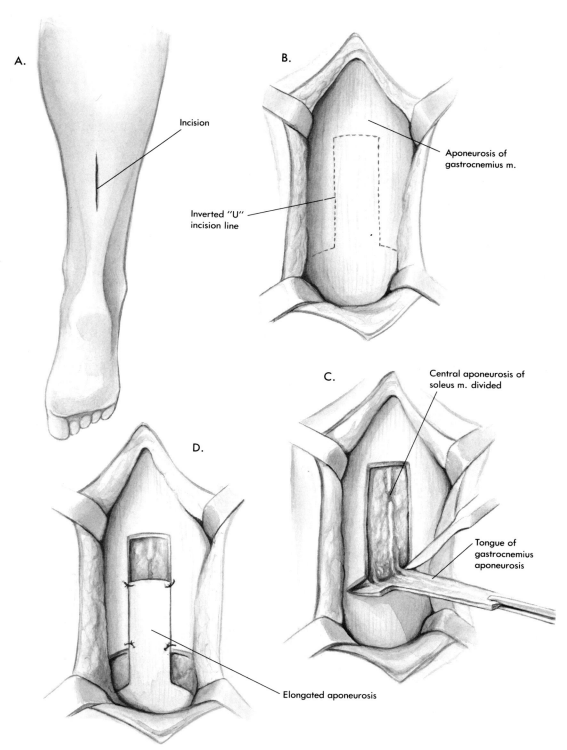

A.

Incision

B.

Aponeurosis of
gastrocnemius m.

Inverted "U"
incision line

C.

Central aponeurosis of
soleus m. divided

Tongue of
gastrocnemius
aponeurosis

D.

Elongated aponeurosis

Plate 175. A.–D., Baker's technique of tongue-in-groove lengthening of the gastrocnemius aponeurosis.

PLATE 176 **Z-Lengthening of the Tendo Achillis and Posterior Capsulotomy of the Ankle and Subtalar Joints**

Indications. Severe fixed equinus deformity of the ankle and subtalar joint, such as in arthrogryposis and other paralytic disorders.

Note: Sliding lengthening of the tendo Achillis should be performed whenever possible, as it preserves function of the triceps surae muscle; but if previous surgery has resulted in scarring of the Achilles tendon, a Z-plastic lengthening of the tendon is required.

Patient Position. Prone. The operation can be performed with the hip in flexion–abduction–lateral rotation.

Operative Technique

A. A longitudinal incision is made medial to the tendo calcaneus, beginning at the heel and extending proximally for a distance of 7 to 10 cm. The subcutaneous tissue and tendon sheath are divided in line with the skin incision, and the wound flaps are retracted, exposing the Achilles tendon.

B. Z-plastic lengthening is performed in the anteroposterior plane. With a knife the Achilles tendon is divided longitudinally into lateral and medial halves for a distance of 5 to 7 cm. The distal end of the medial half is detached from the calcaneus to prevent recurrence of varus deformity of the heel; the lateral half is divided proximally. Often posterior tibial tendon lengthening is required. Its technique is illustrated in Plate 180.

C. If the posterior capsules of the ankle and subtalar joints are contracted, a varying degree of equinus deformity will persist following sectioning of the tendo Achillis. Posterior capsulotomy of the ankle and subtalar joints is indicated if the foot cannot be dorsiflexed to 5 degrees beyond neutral. If in doubt, one should take radiograms to determine the exact degree of correction of the equinus deformity. The flexor hallucis longus tendon is retracted medially and the peroneal tendons are retracted laterally to expose the posterior part of the ankle and subtalar joints. Neurovascular structures behind the medial malleolus should be protected from injury.

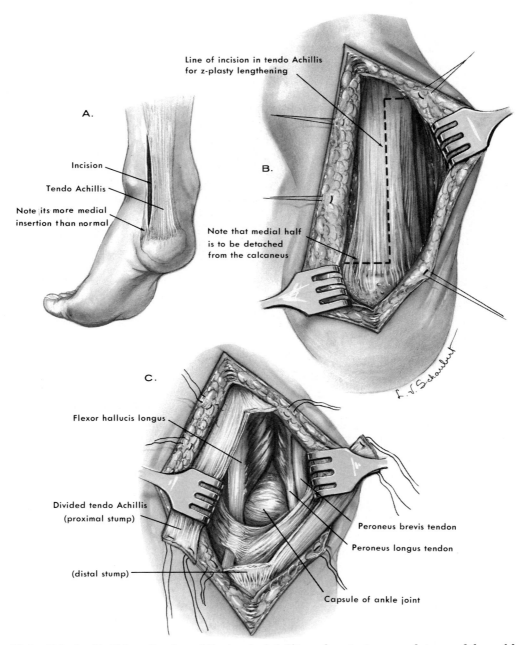

A.

Incision

Tendo Achillis

Note its more medial
insertion than normal

Line of incision in tendo Achillis
for z-plasty lengthening

B.

Note that medial half
is to be detached
from the calcaneus

C.

Flexor hallucis longus

Divided tendo Achillis
(proximal stump)

(distal stump)

Peroneus brevis tendon

Peroneus longus tendon

Capsule of ankle joint

Plate 176. A.–F., Z-lengthening of the tendo Achillis and posterior capsulotomy of the ankle
and subtalar joints.

D. Next, using Mayo or Metzenbaum scissors, completely divide the posterior capsules of the ankle and subtalar joints. A knife should not be used, as it may damage the articular cartilage.

Caution! The distal tibial epiphyseal plate must not be injured.

E. Laterally, section the calcaneofibular and talofibular ligaments, and take care not to injure the peroneal tendons. Medially, the posterior part of the deltoid ligament is divided immediately next to its attachment to the os calcis; in this way, the likelihood of injury to the posterior tibial vessels and tibial nerve is minimized. With a blunt periosteal elevator, free any remaining capsular fibers across the ankle and subtalar joints.

F. Next, lateral radiograms of the ankle and hindfoot are made with the foot held in maximal dorsiflexion to determine exactly the degree of correction achieved. Occasionally, fractional lengthening of the flexor hallucis longus and flexor digitorum longus may be required. The longitudinal halves of the tendo Achillis are sutured in the lengthened position. A Steinmann pin may be inserted transversely across the os calcis (I don't recommend its use). The tourniquet is released, and hemostasis is secured.

The edges of the skin are observed; if they are blanched and under tension when the foot is maximally dorsiflexed, initially the foot-ankle is immobilized in 15 to 20 degrees of plantarflexion. In 10 to 14 days, the cast is changed and the foot-ankle is manipulated into the desired degree of dorsiflexion.

An above-knee cast is applied in which the Steinmann pin (if used) is incorporated.

Postoperative Care. Change the cast 10 to 14 days postoperatively and manipulate the foot into further dorsiflexion. After four weeks, the Steinmann pin (if used) and sutures are removed, the foot is manipulated, and a new above-knee cast is applied for an additional two weeks. Prolonged immobilization in cast for three to four months is not recommended because of disuse atrophy and joint stiffness.

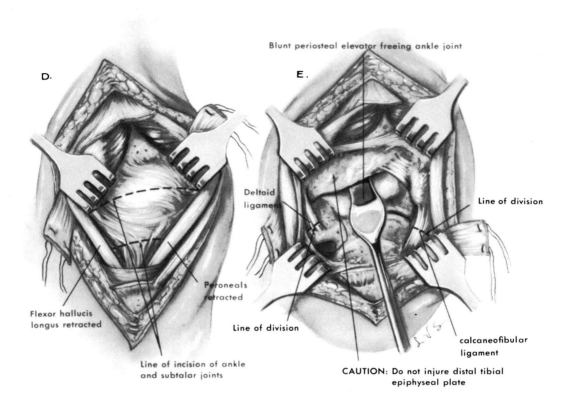

D.

E.

Blunt periosteal elevator freeing ankle joint

Deltoid ligament

Line of division

Peroneals retracted

Flexor hallucis longus retracted

Line of division

Line of incision of ankle and subtalar joints

calcaneofibular ligament

CAUTION: Do not injure distal tibial epiphyseal plate

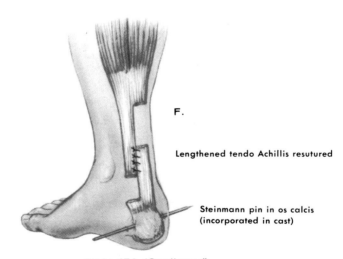

F.

Lengthened tendo Achillis resutured

Steinmann pin in os calcis (incorporated in cast)

Plate 176. (Continued)

PLATE 177 ### Correction of Severe Equinus with Flat-Top Talus and Ankle Joint Incongruity Using the Ilizarov Technique

Indications

In severe fixed equinus deformity of long-standing, untreated talipes equino-varus, the anterior one third of the articular surface of the dome of the talus is uncovered, and it is difficult or impossible to reposition the wider anterior part of the dome of the talus into the ankle mortise because there is insufficient space. A distinct ridge separates the anterior uncovered part from the posterior contained part. The dome of the talus that articulates with the tibia is flattened and incongruous. In such a severe deformity, it is best to perform an osteotomy through the body of the calcaneus and the neck of the talus and rotate the foot into dorsiflexion around the body of the talus with the Ilizarov external fixator. This bony procedure is combined with a posterior soft-tissue release in the form of tendo Achillis lengthening.

I prefer to treat moderate equinus deformities by extensive posterior soft-tissue release and tendo Achillis lengthening, posterior capsulotomy, and division of the posterior talofibular ligament, calcaneofibular ligament, and posterior one half of the deltoid ligament. Through a separate anterior surgical approach the anterior tibiofibular ligament and the lower end of the tibiofibular ligament are sectioned to widen the ankle mortise and make room for the talus.

Special Instrumentation. The following special instruments are used:

1. Ilizarov external fixator with complete set of all components.
2. Specially designed, mated, curved chisels with longitudinal grooves on the convex side of one chisel and on the concave side of the other and interlocking rims at their edges. Each chisel couples with its mate at the site of osteotomy.

Radiographic Control. Image intensifier.

Patient Position. Supine and tilted to the opposite side by a sandbag under the ipsilateral hip. The lower limb is prepped and draped sterile in the usual fashion, and the previously applied tourniquet is inflated.

Operative Technique. First, a Z-lengthening of the tendo Achillis is performed through a posteromedial incision.

A. and **B.** The frame is assembled (it is preferable to assemble it preoperatively). It consists of the following:

1. One or two ring fixators attached to the tibia with crossed wires.
2. A supporting foot frame with Ilizarov wires through the calcaneus and distal one third of the metatarsals. The foot frame is connected to the leg frame by hinged rods.

An Ilizarov wire will be inserted through the posterior part of the talus, which will be attached to the leg part of the apparatus by posts.

A lateral Ollier surgical approach is made, with the skin incision beginning 1 cm. distal and anterior to the tip of the lateral malleolus and curving dorsally and distally to end on the lateral aspect of the talonavicular joint. The long toe extensors are retracted dorsally and the extensor digitorum brevis is detached from its origin, elevated in one piece, and reflected distally. The peroneal tendons are retracted plantarward and posteriorly. The calcaneus, cuboid, navicular, and head of the talus are identified. The capsules of the talonavicular and calcaneocuboid joints are identified but not divided.

C. Next, under image-intensifier radiographic control, delineate the line of curved osteotomy through the neck of the talus and adjacent upper calcaneus.

D. An alternate method is a V osteotomy.

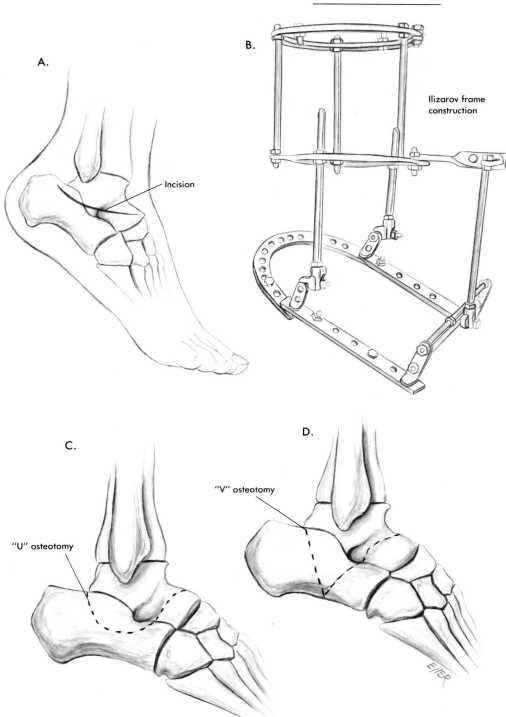

A.

Incision

B.

Ilizarov frame
construction

C.

"U" osteotomy

D.

"V" osteotomy

EIFER

Plate 177. A.–M., Correction of severe equinus with flat-top talus and ankle joint incongruity using the Ilizarov technique.

E. With a hammer, drive the first chisel with the grooves on the convex side and with its concavity plantarward across the proposed osteotomy site. The talar body and a small segment of the subjacent calcaneus with its articular surface are engaged by the first chisel. Verify the site and depth of the first chisel under image-intensifier radiogram.

F. The second chisel is driven in with a hammer directly beneath the first chisel.

G. and **H.** With the plantar surface of the forefoot pushed dorsally by an assistant, the second chisel is rotated in relation to the first chisel through the curved osteotomy site. The articular surface of talocalcaneal articulation with a small segment of the calcaneus is removed. The completeness of the osteotomy is checked with image-intensifier radiograms.

The pneumatic tourniquet is released, and complete hemostasis is achieved. The wound is drained with a medium-sized Hemovac drain, and closed in the usual fashion.

E.

First chisel is
hammered across
osteotomy site

F.

Second chisel with
grooves on convex side
is hammered in below
first chisel

Second chisel is
rotated upward

G.

Plantar surface of
foot pushed dorsally

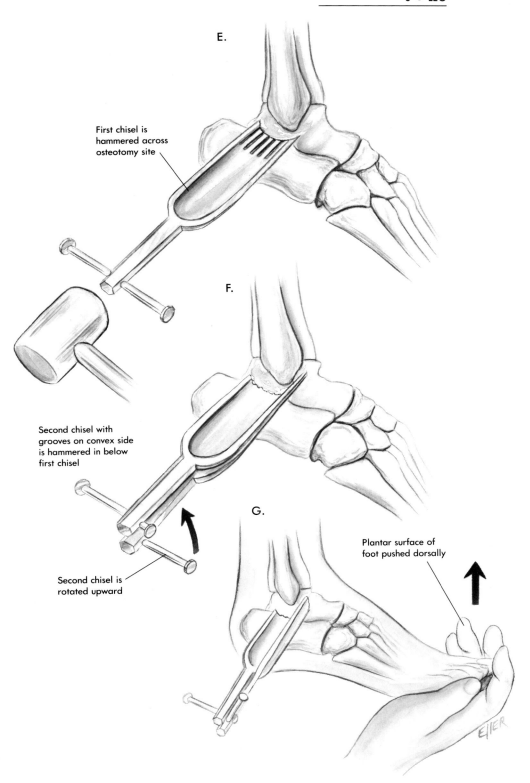

Plate 177. (Continued)

G. and H. With the plantar surface of the forefoot pushed dorsally by an assistant, the second chisel is rotated in relation to the first chisel through the curved osteotomy site. The articular surface of talocalcaneal articulation with a small segment of the calcaneus is removed. The completeness of the osteotomy is checked with image-intensifier radiograms.

The pneumatic tourniquet is released, and complete hemostasis is achieved. The wound is drained with a medium-sized Hemovac drain, and closed in the usual fashion.

I. and J. The Ilizarov wires are inserted and connected to the preassembled frame. Appropriate adjustments are made as required. The hinges should be at the correct level for rotation of the calcaneus, posterior talus, and midfoot and forefoot into dorsiflexion.

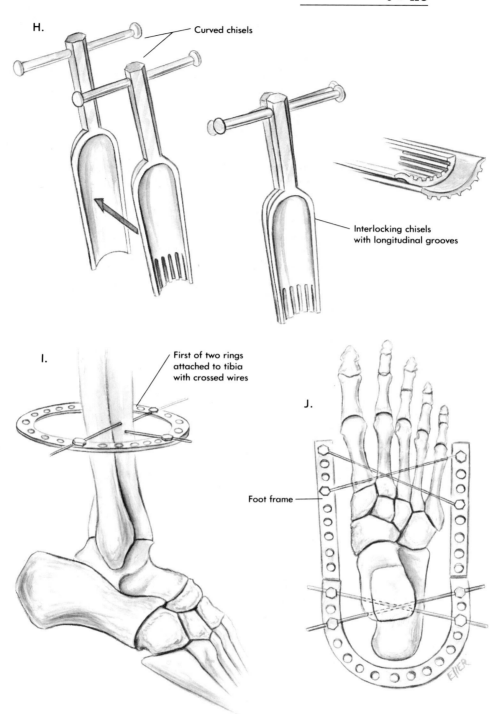

H. Curved chisels

Interlocking chisels with longitudinal grooves

I. First of two rings attached to tibia with crossed wires

J. Foot frame

Plate 177. (Continued)

K. Distraction posteriorly and compression anteriorly is commenced several days after operation, as soon as the patient is comfortable.

L. When equinus deformity of the ankle is combined with a supination-pronation deformity of the forefoot, midfoot hinges are incorporated into the anterior and posterior rods connecting the tibial frame to the foot assembly. Two-plane hinges provide rotational correction in both the sagittal and coronal planes.

In the illustrations J (preoperative) and K (postoperative) following correction, the assembly is illustrated after Ilizarov.

M. When ankle hindfoot equinus is combined with forefoot equinus (anterior cavus), anterior and posterior half rings are connected by a pair of threaded rods. This will distract and stretch the plantar soft tissues connecting the cavus deformity with the ankle equinus.

Postoperative Care. Ordinarily within four weeks the foot can be dorsiflexed to neutral position. The pins are removed and a below-knee walking cast is applied for an additional two or three weeks. The cast is then removed, and active and passive exercises are performed to restore motor strength of muscles controlling the foot and ankle and rays of the ankle and foot.

REFERENCES

Ilizarov, G. A.: Transosseous Osteosynthesis. Berlin, Springer-Verlag, 1992, pp. 583–585.

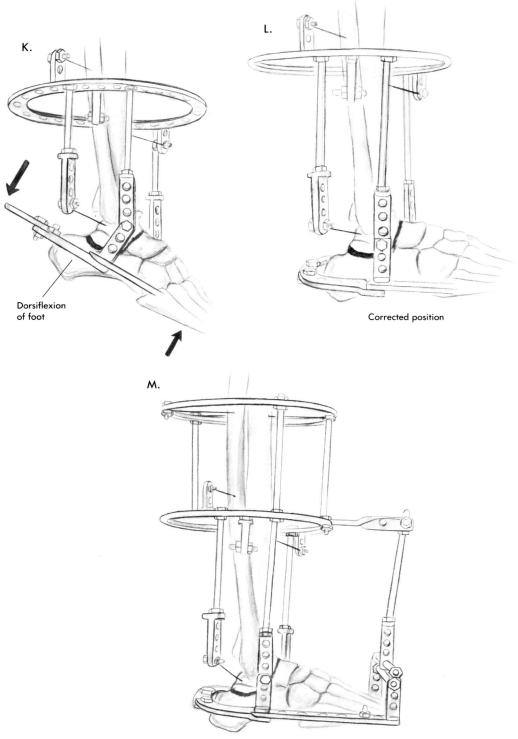

K.

Dorsiflexion
of foot

L.

Corrected position

M.

Plate 177. (Continued)

PLATE 178

Neurectomy of Motor Branches of the Tibial Nerve to the Gastrocnemius

Indications. Severe clonus on weight-bearing that interferes with walking.

Precautions

1. Neurectomy of motor branches of the tibial nerve produces fibrosis of the triceps surae muscle with consequent myostatic contracture and recurrence of fixed equinus deformity. After sectioning, reimplant the nerve into the muscle—this measure may prevent development of muscle fibrosis.

2. Do not lengthen the tendo Achillis simultaneously, because marked weakness of the triceps surae and calcaneus deformity may develop.

3. Distinguish the clonus caused by the gastrocnemius from that caused by the soleus. When it diminishes or disappears on flexion of the knee, the clonus is primarily caused by the gastrocnemius; when the clonus is unaltered by changes in the position of the knee, the soleus is the chief cause. Section the motor branches to the muscle that is causing the clonus.

Special Instrumentation. Nerve stimulator. Ask the anesthesiologist not to paralyze the patient.

Patient Position. The patient is placed in prone position with a pneumatic tourniquet on the proximal thigh.

Operative Technique

A. A transverse incision 5 to 7 cm. long is made immediately proximal to the popliteal crease in line with the flexion creases of the skin.

B. The deep fascia is divided and the tibial nerve, lying superficial to the vessels, is exposed. The first branch is cutaneous; it is not disturbed. The next two branches are the motor nerves to the gastrocnemius. One branch emerges from the medial side and enters the medial head close to its origin; just prior to disappearing into the muscle, it divides into three branches. The other branch emerges from the lateral side and similarly enters the lateral head close to its origin, but it divides into only two branches. The motor branch to the soleus muscle emerges distal to that of the gastrocnemius. It is best to stimulate each branch to determine which is the principal cause of clonus.

C. The appropriate motor branches are resected by dividing them proximally at their origin and distally at their entrance into the muscle. The wound is closed in layers in the usual manner. The limb is immobilized in an above-knee cast with the foot at 5 to 10 degrees of dorsiflexion at the ankle and with the knee in full extension.

Postoperative Care. The cast is removed in three weeks; the postoperative care is similar to that after heel cord lengthening. (Some surgeons apply only a pressure dressing and allow the patient to walk when he or she is comfortable and when the wound is healed.)

REFERENCES

Stoffel, A.: The treatment of spastic contractures. Am. J. Orthop. Surg., 10:611, 1913.

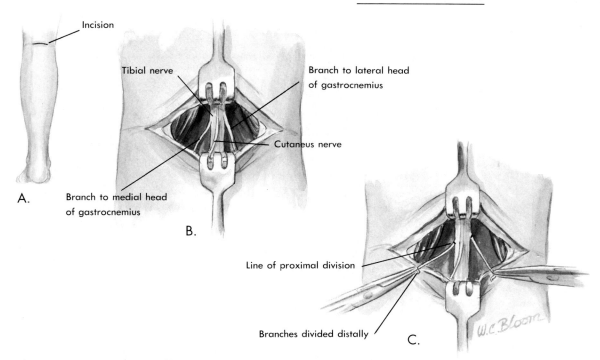

Plate 178. A.–C., Neurectomy of motor branches of the tibial nerve to the gastrocnemius.

PLATE   179   **Anterior Advancement of the Tendo Achillis for Correction of Spastic Equinus Deformity (Murphy's Technique)**

Indications. Equinus deformity in spastic paralysis when the triceps surae is fair minus or poor plus in motor strength.

A. and **B.** In this operation the tendo Achillis is detached from its insertion to the posterior tuberosity of the calcaneus and transferred to the dorsum of the calcaneus immediately posterior to the subtalar joint. It shortens the lever arm and weakens the triceps surae without changing its resting length.

The axis of ankle motion is the midportion of the body of the talus. The triceps surae muscle acts on the ankle joint and foot through a lever system, the fulcrum of which is located at point B in the midportion of the body of the talus. On anterior advancement of the heel cord from point C (the posterior tuberosity of the calcaneus) to point D (the upper surface of the calcaneus immediately behind the subtalar joint), the power of the triceps surae is diminished by 48 per cent according to the calculations of Pierrot and Murphy. On push-off the fulcrum in the foot moves distally to the first metatarsal head (point A), weakening the push-off power by the ratio of

$$\frac{CD}{AC} = 0.15 \pm 0.02$$

Therefore, the advantage of anterior advancement of the heel cord is that it decreases resistance to ankle dorsiflexion by 48 per cent.

Patient Position. The patient is placed in the prone position for this procedure.

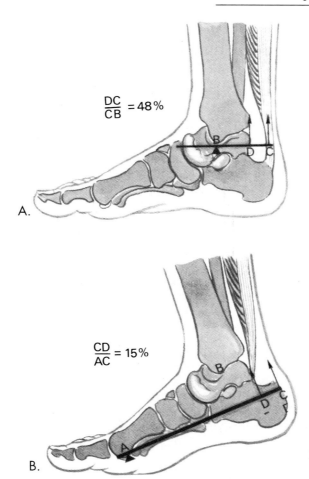

Plate 179. A.–F., Anterior advancement of the tendo Achillis for correction of spastic equinus deformity (Murphy's technique). (Redrawn from Pierrot, A. H., and Murphy, O. B.: Heel cord advancement—a new approach to the spastic equinus deformity. Orthop. Clin. North Am., 5:118, 1974.)

Operative Technique

C. A posteromedial incision is made about 1 cm. medial to the tendo Achillis; it begins at the os calcis and extends proximally for 7.5 to 10 cm. The subcutaneous tissue and tendon sheath are divided in one plane in line with the skin incision.

D. The Achilles tendon is identified and isolated by sharp and blunt dissection to its insertion. It is detached from the calcaneal tuberosity as far distally as possible to preserve length. Caution is exercised to avoid injury to the calcaneal apophysis.

E. Next, a Bunnell pull-out wire suture is placed on the distal end of the tendo Achillis. The flexor hallucis longus tendon is identified, mobilized, and retracted medially. The upper surface of the calcaneus is exposed. A 0.6-cm. drill hole is made from the superior part of the calcaneus immediately posterior to the subtalar joint to exit on the plantar aspect of the non–weight-bearing area of the calcaneus. With a curet the drill hole is enlarged, if necessary.

F. The pull-out wire and Achilles tendon are passed through the drill hole and are tied over a sterile, thick-felt pad and a button on the plantar aspect of the foot with the ankle in 15 degrees of plantar flexion. It is vital that the heel cord be routed anterior to the flexor hallucis longus. If attention is not paid to this important detail, the Achilles tendon will reattach itself to its original insertion. The tourniquet is released, and after complete hemostasis the wound is closed. An above-knee cast is applied with the ankle joint in 15 degrees of plantar flexion and the knee in 10 degrees of flexion.

Postoperative Care. The cast and pull-out wire are removed in four to six weeks. Physical therapy is begun to restore ankle motion and develop strength of the anterior tibial and triceps surae muscles. Other details of postoperative care follow the same principles outlined for tendo Achillis lengthening.

REFERENCES

Esteve, R.: Un procede d'equilibration des pieds spastique. Vie Med., 1:51, 1970.
Pierrot, A. H., and Murphy, O. B.: Heel cord advancement. Orthop. Clin. North Am., 5:117, 1975.

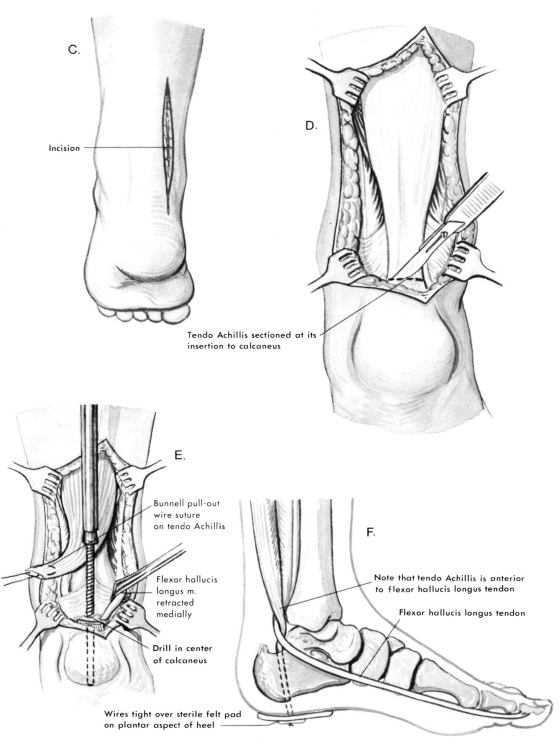

C.

Incision

Tendo Achillis sectioned at its insertion to calcaneus

D.

E.

Bunnell pull-out wire suture on tendo Achillis

Flexor hallucis longus m. retracted medially

Drill in center of calcaneus

F.

Note that tendo Achillis is anterior to flexor hallucis longus tendon

Flexor hallucis longus tendon

Wires tight over sterile felt pad on plantar aspect of heel

Plate 179. (Continued)

PLATE 180　　Musculotendinous Fractional Sliding Lengthening of the Posterior Tibial Tendon

Indications. Varus deformity of the hindfoot and midfoot caused by spasticity and contracture of posterior tibial tendon that has continuous abnormal activity in both stance and swing phases of walking as shown by dynamic electromyographic and gait analysis.

Precautions

1. Do not section and totally release the posterior tibial tendon because it may result in valgus deformity of the foot.

2. To prevent recurrence of deformity, it is crucial to splint at night for a prolonged period in the growing foot.

Patient Position. The patient is placed in the supine position with the hip laterally rotated and the knee flexed to 90 degrees.

Operative Technique

A. The posterior tibial tendon is exposed through a longitudinal incision immediately posterior to the medial border of the tibia. It begins 1 cm. proximal to the medial malleolus and extends superiorly for a distance of 5 to 6 cm. Subcutaneous tissue is divided in line with the skin incision, and the superficial fascia is incised.

B. The most superficial tendon immediately posterior to the medial border of the tibia is the flexor digitorum longus. It is identified by flexing and extending the lesser toes and then is retracted out of harm's way. Immediately deep to flexor digitorum longus is the posterior tibial tendon. With the help of Freer elevators, the tendon and posterior tibial muscle are retracted, and two incisions are made 5 cm. apart, well above the site where muscle fibers terminate on the tendon. The tendinous portion of the posterior tibial muscle is divided, but not the muscle fibers themselves. The proximal incision is transverse and the distal incision is oblique.

C. The sliding lengthening of the tendon is obtained by forcing the foot into valgus position and by gentle stretching of the muscle between two moist sponges.

The wound is closed in the usual fashion. An above- or below-knee cast is applied with the midfoot and hindfoot in valgus position and the ankle in slight dorsiflexion.

Postoperative Care. The cast is removed in three weeks, and active and passive exercises are performed to strengthen peroneal muscles and restore strength in the lengthened posterior tibial muscle.

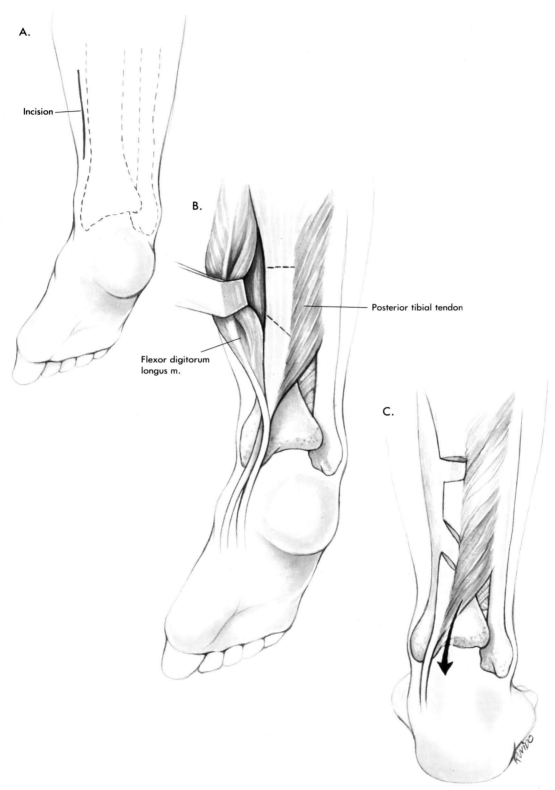

A.

Incision

B.

Posterior tibial tendon

Flexor digitorum
longus m.

C.

Plate 180. A.–C., Musculotendinous fractional sliding lengthening of the posterior tibial
tendon.

PLATE 181 **Extensor Hallucis Longus Rerouting Through the Anterior Tibial Tendon and Shortening of the Anterior Tibial Muscle**

Indications. Inability to develop voluntary control over a cerebral zero anterior tibial muscle one or two years following heel cord lengthening. The objective of surgery is reflex stimulation of the cerebral zero anterior tibial muscle by the contraction of a normal extensor hallucis longus.

An important part of the procedure is shortening of the stretched out and elongated anterior tibial muscle to establish normal tension-length (Blix) curve.

Requisites

1. The extensor hallucis longus must be normal or good in motor strength and neurophysiologically normal. The extensor hallucis brevis is of normal motor strength.

2. Absence of fixed equinus deformity. The ankle should passively dorsiflex 20 degrees beyond neutral with the knee in extension. If any equinus deformity is present, correct by below-knee, stretching, walking cast.

Disadvantages. Weakness of dorsiflexion of big toe. Patient may stub the big toe when walking. Interphalangeal joint fusion of the hallux may be required

Patient Position. Supine.

Operative Technique

A. A longitudinal incision about 7 cm. long is made over the dorsum of the foot. It starts at the base of the proximal phalanx of the big toe and extends proximally to the first cuneiform bone. Subcutaneous tissue is divided in line with the skin incision; wound margins are undermined and gently retracted. Injury to the superficial vessels and sensory nerves is avoided.

B. The extensor hallucis longus tendon is identified and detached from its insertion as far distally as possible. The stump is sutured to the tendon of the extensor hallucis brevis with the big toe held in marked dorsiflexion to prevent plantar drop of the hallux with the big toe held in marked dorsiflexion to prevent plantar drop of the hallux postoperatively. (It is described in Plate 218.) The tendon of the extensor hallucis longus is dissected free of its sheath as high as possible. Then a second incision is made over the course of the anterior tibial tendon in the distal third of the leg. The tendons of the extensor hallucis longus and the anterior tibial are identified. The extensor hallucis longus is pulled into the proximal wound by gentle traction.

C. With a scalpel, three slits of appropriate size are made in the anterior tibial tendon. The extensor hallucis longus tendon is rewound by passing it through these slits and is then delivered into the distal wound with an Ober tendon passer.

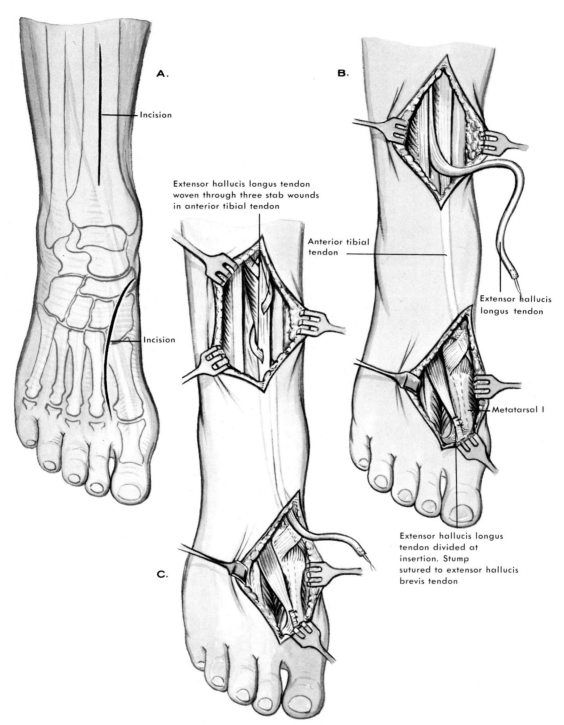

A.

Incision

B.

C.

Extensor hallucis longus tendon woven through three stab wounds in anterior tibial tendon

Anterior tibial tendon

Extensor hallucis longus tendon

Incision

Metatarsal I

Extensor hallucis longus tendon divided at insertion. Stump sutured to extensor hallucis brevis tendon

Plate 181. A.–E., Extensor hallucis longus rerouting through the anterior tibial tendon and shortening of the anterior tibial muscle.

D. The extensor hallucis longus tendon is sutured to the insertion of the anterior tibial muscle with the ankle in neutral position or 10 degrees of dorsiflexion. Any excess of the extensor hallucis longus tendon is either excised (as illustrated) or, if it is long enough, reattached to its insertion. Next, the lax anterior tibial tendon is shortened by plication and suturing to the capsule of the first metatarsal-cuneiform joint.

E. Another way of shortening the anterior tibial tendon is by excising an appropriate segment distally and suturing the cut ends together. The tourniquet is released, and after complete hemostasis the wound is closed in layers in the usual fashion. The foot and ankle are immobilized in a below-knee walking cast.

Postoperative Care. Three weeks after surgery the cast is removed and an above-knee splint is made that maintains the ankle at 5 to 10 degrees of dorsiflexion and the knee in neutral extension; the splint is worn at night. During the day a dorsiflexion-assist below-knee orthosis is used. Active assisted exercises are performed to develop function in and cerebral control over the cerebral zero anterior tibial muscle. Gentle passive exercises are carried out to maintain range of ankle motion. During the day periods of gait training without orthosis are carried out to activate the anterior tibial muscle function. The dorsiflexion-assist orthosis is gradually discontinued over a period of three to six months. Persistent and meticulous physical therapy and night splinting are vital.

REFERENCES

Tohen, A. Z., Carmona, J. P., and Barrera, J. R.: The utilization of abnormal reflexes in the treatment of spastic foot deformities. Clin. Orthop., 47:77, 1966.

D.

Anterior tibial tendon
plicated and sutured to
capsule with extensor hallucis
longus tendon

Tendon sutured with foot
in 10° dorsiflexion

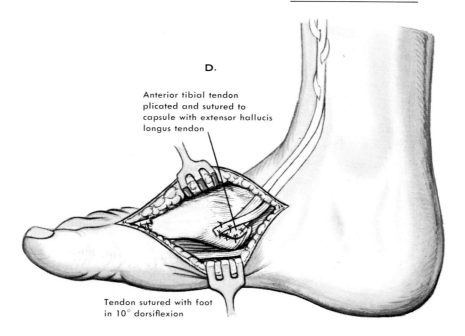

E.

If anterior tibial tendon
is lax, segment is removed
and cut ends are reunited

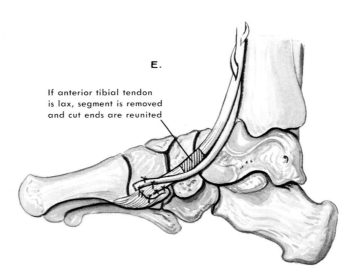

Plate 181. (Continued)

PLATE   182   ## Split Posterior Tibial Tendon Transfer

Indications. Varus deformity of the hindfoot and midfoot caused by spasticity and contracture of the posterior tibial muscle, which is diphasic as shown by dynamic electromyographic and gait analysis. The varus deformity is present during stance, and the posterior tibial is active during stance; the posterior tibial is also active during the swing phase of gait. If the posterior tibial is active throughout the gait cycle, it is lengthened and not transferred. The peroneal muscles are weak.

Requisites

1. Absence of fixed deformity. The varus should be dynamic and correctable by manipulation and soft-tissue procedures. When the deformity is fixed, some bony procedures are required for correction, such as closing lateral wedge Dwyer osteotomy and lateral displacement osteotomy of the calcaneus.

2. Absence of fixed equinus deformity—the ankle joint should passively dorsiflex 15 degrees beyond neutral. If fixed equinus deformity is present, correct it by heel cord lengthening. The procedure can be performed simultaneously.

3. Good or normal motor strength of posterior tibial muscle.

4. Anterior tibial muscle fair or less in motor strength and not a deforming varus force during swing phase of gait.

Patient Position. The patient is placed supine with the hip of the operated limb flexed, abducted, and laterally rotated.

Operative Technique

A. A posteromedial incision is made for exposure of the posterior tibial tendon. The incision begins 5 to 7 cm. proximal to the tip of the medial malleolus and 1 cm. behind the medial margin of the tibia. It extends distally to a point 1.5 cm. distal to the tip of the medial malleolus where it curves and extends distally and anteriorly to terminate 1 cm. distal to the tuberosity of the navicular.

An alternative method (not illustrated) is to make two incisions. One posterior incision begins 5 to 7 cm. proximal to the tip of the medial malleolus and 1 cm. posterior to the posteromedial border of the tibia and extending proximally. The second incision is made on the medial aspect of the foot beginning 1 cm. distal to the tuberosity of the navicular and extending posteriorly to a point 1 cm. anterior and 1 cm. distal to the tip of the medial malleolus. If necessary, these two incisions can be connected if difficulty is encountered in delivering the operated posterior tibial tendon from the distal to the proximal wound. Subcutaneous tissue and superficial and deep fascia are divided in line with the skin incision.

B. The posterior tibial tendon is identified behind the posteromedial margin of the tibia. The posterior tibial tendon lies deep to the flexor digitorum longus tendon. Double-check that the tendon is that of the posterior tibial by pulling on it. It will invert the midfoot, whereas the flexor digitorum longus tendon will flex the lesser toes. The sheath of the posterior tibial tendon is divided, and the plantar half of the posterior tibial tendon is sectioned at its insertion to the navicular and split longitudinally into two halves.

C. The posterior segment of the split tendon is pulled into the proximal wound. Do not injure the neurovascular bundle.

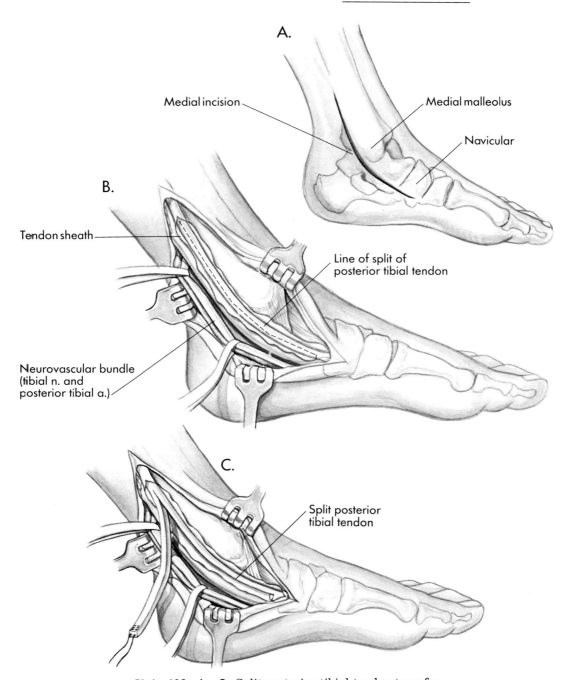

A.

Medial incision

Medial malleolus

Navicular

B.

Tendon sheath

Line of split of
posterior tibial tendon

Neurovascular bundle
(tibial n. and
posterior tibial a.)

C.

Split posterior
tibial tendon

Plate 182. **A.–J.,** Split posterior tibial tendon transfer.

D. Next, extend the hip and rotate it medially. Make an incision on the lateral aspect of the ankle extending from a point 3 cm. proximal to the tip of the lateral malleolus and 1.5 cm. posterior to the fibula and terminating at the base of the fifth metatarsal.

An alternative method (not illustrated, but preferred by this author) is to make two incisions. One is made behind the lateral malleolus and distal fibula, and the other extends from the base of the fifth metatarsal to a point 1 cm. distal and 1.5 cm. anterior to the tip of the lateral malleolus.

E. Subcutaneous tissue is divided in line with the skin incision, and the superficial and deep fascia are incised and the peroneal tendons are exposed.

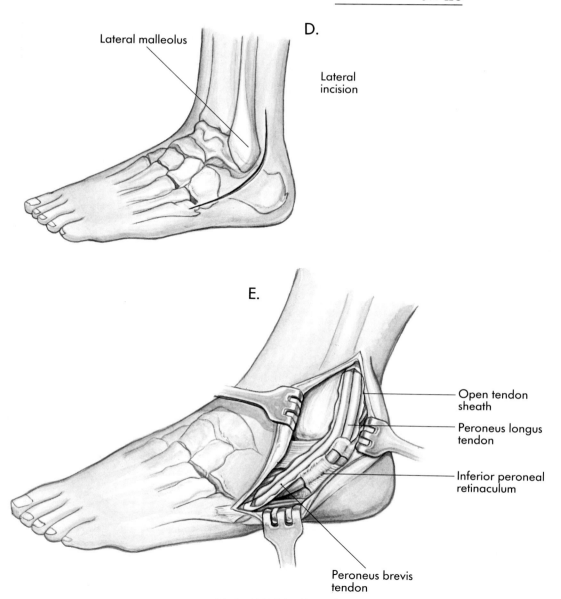

D.

Lateral malleolus

Lateral incision

E.

Open tendon sheath

Peroneus longus tendon

Inferior peroneal retinaculum

Peroneus brevis tendon

Plate 182. (Continued)

F. and **G.** With an Ober tendon passer, the split segment of the posterior tibial tendon is passed anterior to the neurovascular bundle and flexors of the toes behind the tibia from the medial to the lateral part of the wound.

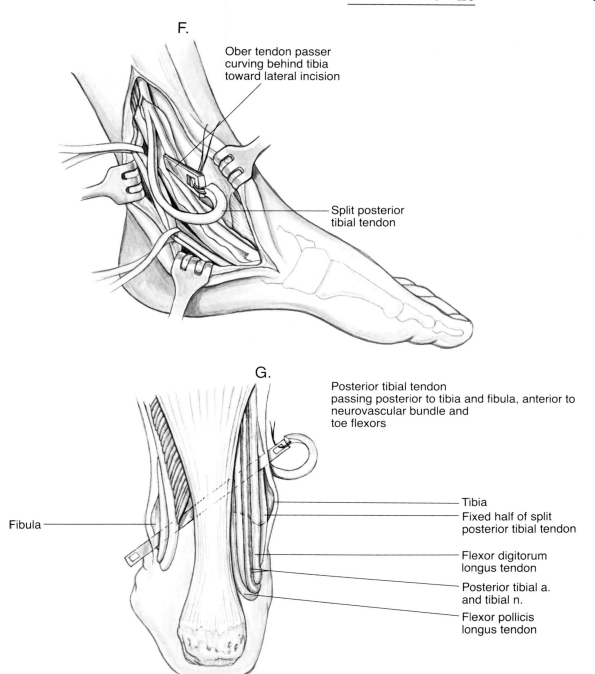

F.

Ober tendon passer
curving behind tibia
toward lateral incision

Split posterior
tibial tendon

G.

Posterior tibial tendon
passing posterior to tibia and fibula, anterior to
neurovascular bundle and
toe flexors

Fibula

Tibia

Fixed half of split
posterior tibial tendon

Flexor digitorum
longus tendon

Posterior tibial a.
and tibial n.

Flexor pollicis
longus tendon

Plate 182. (Continued)

H. Again, with an Ober tendon passer, the posterior tibial tendon is delivered from the leg wound to the distal wound on the lateral aspect of the foot.

I. Divide the sheath of the peroneus brevis. The split posterior tibial tendon is sutured with 00 Tycron to the peroneus brevis tendon under tension.

J. Posterior view of the ankle and hindfoot, showing the direction of the tendon transfer. It is oblique from its musculotendinous junction superiorly toward the tip of the lateral malleolus distally and laterally. The continuous contraction of the spastic posterior tibial tendon provides mechanical stability and control of the hindfoot in neutral position or 5 degrees of valgus inclination.

The tourniquet is released, and complete hemostasis is achieved. The wound is closed in the usual fashion. A below-knee cast is applied with the ankle in neutral position and the heel in about 5 degrees of eversion.

Postoperative Care. The cast is removed three or four weeks after operation, and active and passive range of motion exercises are performed.

REFERENCES

Green, N. E., Griffin, P. P., and Shiair, R.: Split posterior tibial transfer in cerebral palsy. J. Bone Joint Surg., 55-A:748, 1983.

Kling, T. F., Kaufer, H., and Hensinger, R. N.: Split posterior tibial-tendon transfers in children with cerebral spastic paralysis and equinovarus deformity. J. Bone Joint Surg., 67-A:186, 1985.

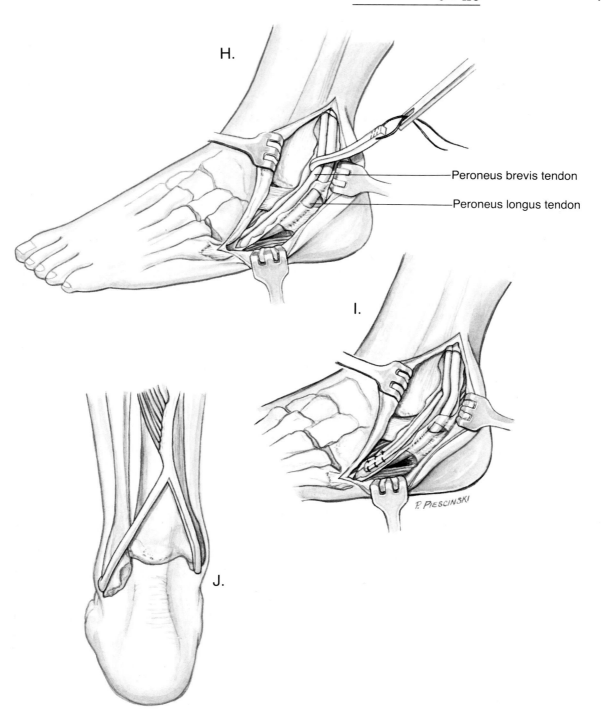

H.

Peroneus brevis tendon

Peroneus longus tendon

I.

P. PIESCINSKI

J.

Plate 182. (Continued)

PLATE 183 **Fractional Lengthening of the Peroneal Muscles at Their Musculotendinous Junction**

Indications. Mild or moderate valgus deformity of the hindfoot and midfoot in stance due to spasticity and contracture of peroneus brevis or longus, or both. The peroneal muscles should be active continuously through both the stance and the swing phases of the gait cycle as shown by dynamic electromyographic and gait analysis.

Requisites

1. A flexible hindfoot and midfoot with relative stability of the talocalcaneonavicular and calcaneocuboid joints. Unstable talocalcaneonavicular and calcaneocuboid joints with vertical or oblique talus require stabilization. Simple lengthenings of peroneal muscles will not correct the deformity.

2. Absence of equinus deformity with normal range of dorsiflexion of the ankle. If there is fixed equinus deformity, the peroneal lengthening is combined with sliding lengthening of the heel cord. Distally section the lateral half of tendo Achillis.

3. Failure to respond to an adequate period of trial of corrective therapy support of the foot with University of California Biomechanics Lab (UCBL) or supramalleolar ankle-foot orthosis (AFO). When the peroneus brevis is active only during the stance phase of gait (as shown by dynamic electromyographic and gait analysis), transfer of the peroneus brevis through the sheath of the posterior tibial to the navicular bone has been recommended by Perry and Hoffer. In my experience, results have been unsatisfactory; this procedure is not recommended and not illustrated.

Patient Position. Supine with a sandbag under the ipsilateral hip.

Operative Technique

A. Make a longitudinal incision 4 to 5 cm. long on the posterior one third of the lower leg at the juncture of the distal one fourth and proximal three fourths. Subcutaneous tissue is divided in line with the skin incision. Superficial and deep fasciae are incised.

B. The peroneus longus and brevis tendons are identified, and one or two transverse cuts are made on their tendons, leaving the overlying muscle intact.

C. The foot is inverted and tension is applied on the peroneals, and the divided tendinous segments are separated, thereby lengthening them at their musculotendinous juncture. The tourniquet is released, and complete hemostasis is achieved. The wound is closed in the usual fashion. A below- or above-knee cast is applied, depending on whether other surgical procedures have been performed simultaneously.

Postoperative Care. The cast is removed three weeks after surgery, and active and passive range of motion exercises are performed.

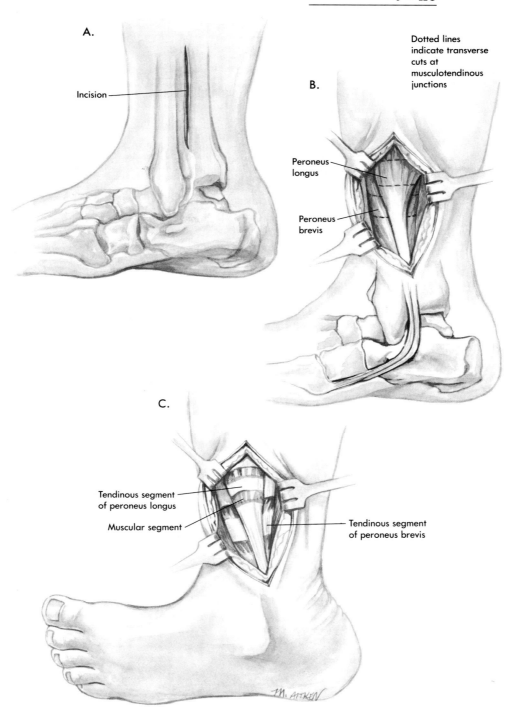

A.

Incision

Dotted lines
indicate transverse
cuts at
musculotendinous
junctions

B.

Peroneus
longus

Peroneus
brevis

C.

Tendinous segment
of peroneus longus

Muscular segment

Tendinous segment
of peroneus brevis

Plate 183. **A.–C.,** Fractional lengthening of the peroneal muscles at their musculotendinous junction.

PLATE 184   Arthrodesis of the Ankle Joint (Chuinard Technique)

Objective. To diminish the need for orthotic support.

Indications. Flail ankle with a foot that has normal alignment and adequate bony and ligamentous stability.

Requisites

1. The patient should be ten years of age or older. The physis of the distal tibia and fibula should not be disturbed.
2. Stability and adequate motor control of knee; the patient should be able to flex and extend the knee against gravity.
3. Gluteus maximus of four or better in motor strength.
4. Normal sensation of the foot and ankle, particularly on plantar surface.
5. Normal weight-bearing surface of the plantar surface of the foot—no varus or valgus deformity.

Precautions

1. Position of ankle fusion should not be more than 5 to 10 degrees of equinus. Make a lateral radiogram of the foot and ankle at the time of surgery. Excessive equinus results in increased pressure on the metatarsal heads with callosities and eventual ulceration of the skin.
2. Heel height should be adequate and even.

Radiographic Control. Image intensifier.

Patient Position. Supine.

Operative Technique

A. and **B.** A longitudinal skin incision is made, beginning 7 cm. proximal to the ankle joint between the extensor digitorum longus and extensor hallucis longus tendons; it extends distally across the ankle joint in line with the third metatarsal and ends 4 cm. distal to the ankle joint.

The subcutaneous tissue is divided, and the skin flaps are mobilized and retracted to their respective sides. The veins crossing the field are clamped, divided, and coagulated. The intermediate and medial dorsal cutaneous branches of the superficial peroneal nerve are identified and protected by retraction to one side of the wound.

C. The deep fascia and transverse crural and cruciate crural ligaments are divided in line with the skin incision. The ligaments are marked with 00 Tycron sutures for accurate closure later.

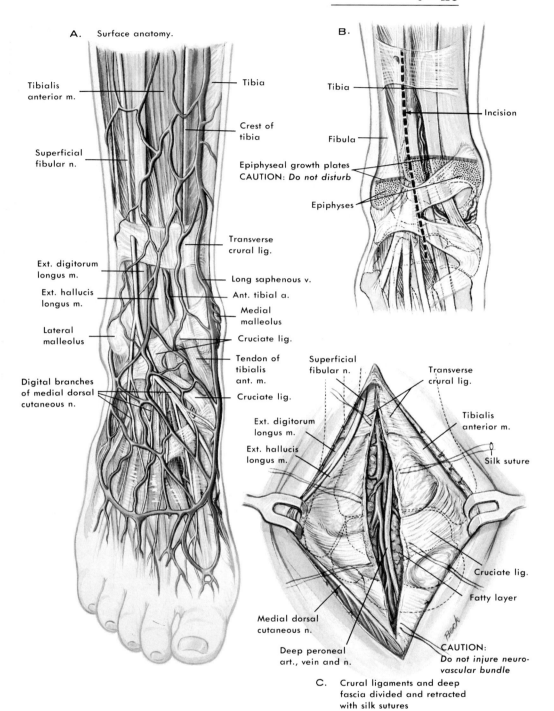

A. Surface anatomy.

Tibialis anterior m.

Tibia

Crest of tibia

Superficial fibular n.

Ext. digitorum longus m.

Ext. hallucis longus m.

Lateral malleolus

Digital branches of medial dorsal cutaneous n.

Transverse crural lig.

Long saphenous v.

Ant. tibial a.

Medial malleolus

Cruciate lig.

Tendon of tibialis ant. m.

Cruciate lig.

B.

Tibia

Incision

Fibula

Epiphyseal growth plates
CAUTION: *Do not disturb*

Epiphyses

Superficial fibular n.

Transverse crural lig.

Tibialis anterior m.

Silk suture

Ext. digitorum longus m.

Ext. hallucis longus m.

Cruciate lig.

Fatty layer

Medial dorsal cutaneous n.

Deep peroneal art., vein and n.

CAUTION:
Do not injure neuro-vascular bundle

C. Crural ligaments and deep fascia divided and retracted with silk sutures

Plate 184. A.–I ., Arthrodesis of the ankle joint (Chuinard technique).

D. The neurovascular bundle (deep peroneal nerve, anterior tibial—dorsalis pedis vessels) is identified, isolated, and retracted laterally with the extensor hallucis longus, extensor digitorum longus, and peroneus tertius tendons. The anterolateral malleolar and lateral tarsal arteries are isolated, clamped, divided, and ligated. The distal tibia, ankle joint, and talus are identified. A transverse incision is made in the capsule of the talotibial joint from the posterior tip of the medial malleolus to the lateral malleolus. The edges of the capsule are marked with 00 silk suture for meticulous closure later.

E.–G. The capsule is reflected and retracted distally on the talus and proximally on the tibia. The periosteum of the tibia should not be divided. The distal tibial and fibular epiphyseal plates should not be disturbed in growing children. With thin curved and straight osteotomes, the cartilage and subchondral bone are removed from the opposing articular surfaces of the distal tibia and proximal talus down to raw bleeding cancellous bone. Cartilage chips should not be left posteriorly.

H. Next, a large piece of bone for grafting is taken from the ilium and fashioned to fit snugly in the ankle joint. The graft should have both cortices intact and should be thicker at one end and wedge-shaped. The cortices of the graft are perforated with multiple tiny drill holes. The ankle joint is held in the desired position, and the bone graft is firmly fitted into the joint with an impacter. If any space is left on each side of the graft, it is packed with cancellous bone from the ilium. The graft in the ankle joint gives compressional force to the arthrodesis and adds to the height of the foot and ankle. The capsule of the ankle joint and the transverse crural and cruciate crural ligaments are closed carefully in layers. The deep fascia and the wound are closed in the usual manner. Radiograms are obtained in anteroposterior and lateral views to ensure that the ankle joint is in the desired position.

I. An above-knee cast is applied with the ankle joint in the desired position of plantar flexion (boys, 10 degrees; girls, 15 to 20 degrees) and the knee in 45 degrees of flexion.

Postoperative Care. Periodic radiograms are obtained to determine the position of the graft and the extent of healing. Eight to ten weeks after surgery, the solid cast is removed and radiograms are obtained with the cast off. Ordinarily, by this time, the fusion is solid and the patient is gradually allowed to be ambulatory. Full weight-bearing is begun two or three weeks later.

REFERENCES

Chuinard, E. G., and Peterson, R. E.: Distraction-compression bone-graft arthrodesis of the ankle. A method especially applicable for children. J. Bone Joint Surg., 45-A:481, 1963.

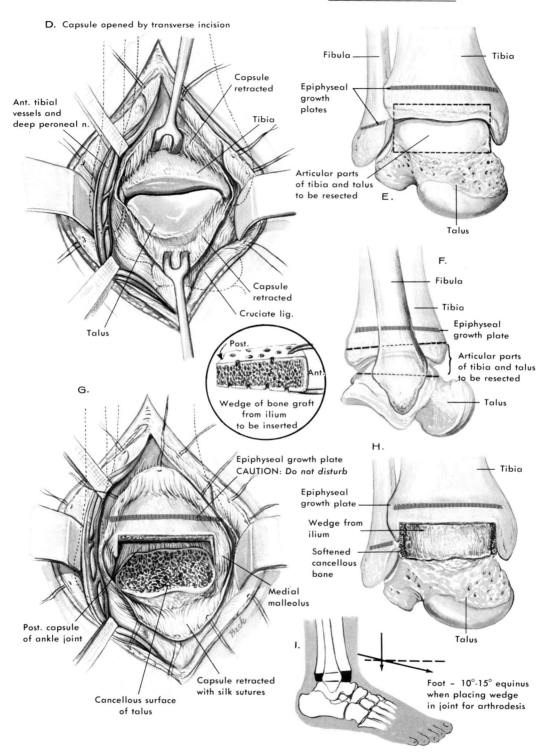

D. Capsule opened by transverse incision

Capsule retracted

Ant. tibial vessels and deep peroneal n.

Tibia

Capsule retracted

Cruciate lig.

Talus

Fibula

Tibia

Epiphyseal growth plates

Articular parts of tibia and talus to be resected

E.

Talus

Post.

Ant.

Wedge of bone graft from ilium to be inserted

F.

Fibula

Tibia

Epiphyseal growth plate

Articular parts of tibia and talus to be resected

Talus

G.

Epiphyseal growth plate CAUTION: Do not disturb

H.

Tibia

Epiphyseal growth plate

Wedge from ilium

Softened cancellous bone

Talus

Medial malleolus

Post. capsule of ankle joint

Cancellous surface of talus

Capsule retracted with silk sutures

I.

Foot – 10°-15° equinus when placing wedge in joint for arthrodesis

Plate 184. (Continued)

PLATE   185   ## Calcaneofibular Tenodesis

Indications. Relative shortening of the fibula with elevation of the lateral malleolus and valgus ankle with instability in a young child (between four and six years of age) with paralysis, such as that caused by poliomyelitis and myelomeningocele. Triceps surae is zero or trace in motor strength.

Radiographic Control. Image intensifier.

Patient Position. The patient is placed in the lateral position to facilitate the surgical exposure of the heel and lateral aspect of the ankle.

Operative Technique

A. A longitudinal incision is made immediately posterior to the fibula; it begins at the tip of the lateral malleolus and extends proximally for a distance of 7 to 10 cm.

B. The subcutaneous tissue is divided, and the wound flaps are undercut and reflected, exposing the tendo calcaneus and the lateral surface of the fibula. The Achilles tendon is sectioned transversely at its musculotendinous junction, as proximally as possible. Obtain adequate length of the tendon.

C. Next, the distal physis of the fibula is identified and marked with a Keith needle. Radiograms are made with the Keith needle in place to verify the site of the growth plate, which should not be disturbed. With a dental drill, a longitudinal slot about 3 cm. long and 0.5 to 0.75 cm. wide is made in the metaphyseal-diaphyseal area of the fibula. Its lower end should be 1 to 1.5 cm. proximal to the growth plate. The slot should be directed anteroposteriorly; do not break the lateral or medial cortex of the fibula.

D. The Achilles tendon is passed through the slot posteroanteriorly and sutured to itself under enough tension to hold the foot at an equinus angle of 15 to 20 degrees. The tendon is anchored to the periosteum of the fibula with additional sutures. Sometimes in the ankle of the child with myelomeningocele the fibula is so small and atrophied that it is safer to make a smaller slot, section the heel cord into halves, and pass only one half of the tendon through the slot and suture the other half to the fibular shaft through holes made with an electric drill. A calcaneofibular tenodesis may be combined with posterior transfer of the anterior tibial tendon to the os calcis through the interosseous route.

In calcaneus deformity secondary to overlengthening of the triceps surae in cerebral palsy, only the lateral half of the tendo calcaneus is attached to the fibula; its medial half is left continuous with the gastrocnemius-soleus muscle.

The tourniquet is released, and after complete hemostasis the wound is closed in the usual manner. An above-knee cast is applied with the ankle in 20 degrees of plantar flexion, but with the forefoot in neutral position. Avoid cavus deformity of the forefoot.

Postoperative Care. Four weeks following surgery the solid cast is removed and a new above-knee plastic splint is made to protect the limb, preventing forced dorsiflexion of the ankle and stretching of the tenodesis.

As soon as possible the child is fitted with an ankle-foot orthosis, in which a plantar flexion assist and stop at the ankle prevent dorsiflexion beyond −10 to −15 degrees. He or she is allowed to ambulate and bear weight with the support of crutches. The above-knee splint is worn at night. With the pull of the Achilles tendon the distal fibular epiphysis will grow, and gradually the lateral tilting of the ankle mortise will be corrected.

REFERENCES

Westin, G. W., and DiFore, R. J.: Tenodesis of the tendo Achillis to the fibula for paralytic calcaneus deformity. J. Bone Joint Surg., 56-A:1541, 1974.

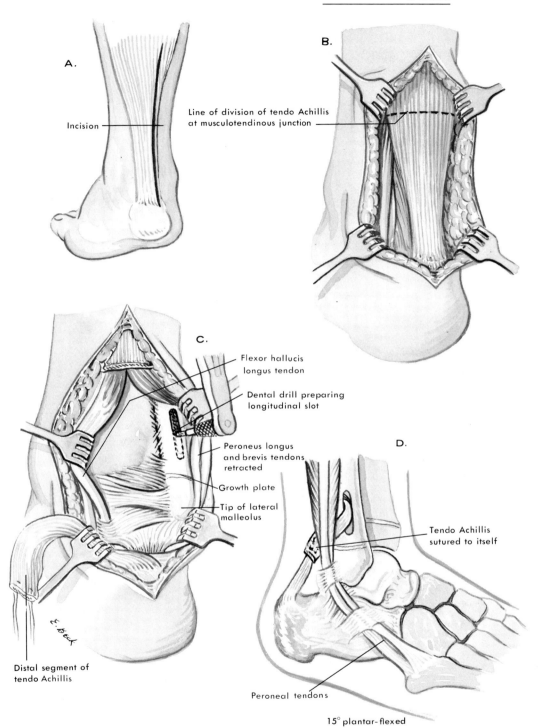

A.

Incision

B.

Line of division of tendo Achillis
at musculotendinous junction

C.

Flexor hallucis
longus tendon

Dental drill preparing
longitudinal slot

Peroneus longus
and brevis tendons
retracted

Growth plate

Tip of lateral
malleolus

Distal segment of
tendo Achillis

D.

Tendo Achillis
sutured to itself

Peroneal tendons

15° plantar-flexed

Plate 185. A.–D., Calcaneofibular tenodesis.

PLATE 186

Anterior Transfer of the Peroneus Longus Tendon to the Base of the Second Metatarsal

Indications. Paralysis of dorsiflexors of the ankle with drop foot gait and normal or good motor strength of the peroneus longus and brevis muscles.

Patient Position. The patient is placed in a semilateral position with a sandbag under the hip on the affected side.

Operative Technique

A. A 3- to 4-cm. incision is made over the lateral aspect of the foot, extending from the base of the fifth metatarsal to a point 1 cm. distal to the tip of the lateral malleolus. Subcutaneous tissue is divided, and the tendons of the peroneus longus and brevis are exposed. Then a second incision is made over the fibular aspect of the leg; it begins 3 cm. above the lateral malleolus and extends proximally for a distance of 7 cm. Subcutaneous tissue and deep fascia are incised, and the peroneal tendons are exposed by dividing their sheath. The peroneus longus tendon lies superficial to that of the peroneus brevis. The muscle is inspected to ensure that it is of normal gross appearance.

B. Next, the peroneus brevis muscle is detached from the base of the fifth metatarsal, and a whip suture is inserted into its distal end.

C. and D. The peroneus longus tendon is divided as far distally as possible. The peroneus brevis is sutured to the distal stump of the peroneus longus to preserve the longitudinal arch and depression of the first metatarsal.

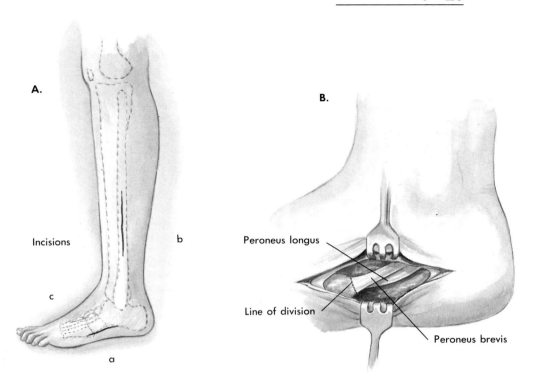

A.

Incisions

b

c

a

B.

Peroneus longus

Line of division

Peroneus brevis

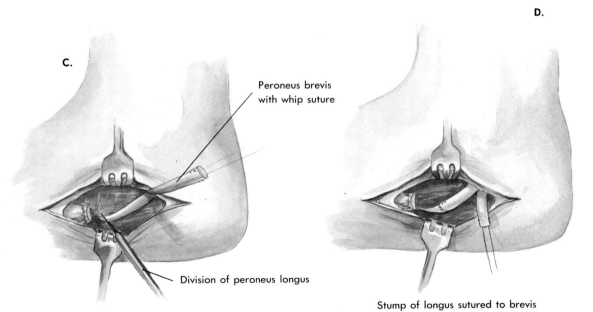

C.

Peroneus brevis
with whip suture

Division of peroneus longus

D.

Stump of longus sutured to brevis

Plate 186. **A.–J.,** Anterior transfer of the peroneus longus tendon to the base of the second metatarsal.

E. and **F.** The peroneus longus tendon is mobilized, and with the two-hand technique, it is gently pulled into the proximal wound in the leg. The origin of the peroneus brevis from the fibula should not be disrupted. An adequate opening is made in the intermuscular septum, taking care not to injure neurovascular structures.

G. and **H.** A 2- to 3-cm. longitudinal incision is made over the dorsum of the foot, centering over the base of the second metatarsal bone. The deep fascia is divided, and the extensor tendons are retracted to expose the proximal one fourth of the second metatarsal bone. The periosteum is divided longitudinally and the cortex of the recipient bone is exposed.

With an Ober tendon passer, the peroneus longus tendon along with its sheath is passed into the anterior tibial compartment, deep to the cruciate (crural) and tarsal ligaments, and delivered into the incision on the dorsum of the foot. The author does not recommend a subcutaneous route. A direct line of pull of the peroneus longus tendon from its origin to its insertion should be ensured.

I. and **J.** A drill hole is made in the base of the second metatarsal. A star-head hand drill is used to enlarge the hole to receive the tendon adequately. The peroneus longus tendon is passed through the recipient hole and sutured on itself under correct tension. If the peroneus longus tendon is not of adequate length, two small holes are made 1.5 cm. distal to the large hole at each side of the metatarsal shaft. The Tycron sutures at the end of the tendon are passed from the large central hole to the lateral distal small holes, and the tendon is securely sutured to the bone. The ankle joint should be in neutral position or 5 degrees of dorsiflexion. The pneumatic tourniquet is released and hemostasis is obtained. The wounds are closed in routine manner. A long leg cast is applied with the ankle in 5 degrees of dorsiflexion and the knee in 45 degrees of flexion.

Postoperative Care. Postoperative care follows the guidelines outlined in the section on principles of tendon transfer. The cast is removed four weeks following surgery. A night splint in the form of an AFO is manufactured to hold the foot-ankle in neutral position. Also, a day articulating AFO is made, allowing free dorsiflexion and limiting plantarflexion to neutral position. Active assisted exercises are performed several times a day to develop function of the transferred peroneals. Also, passive stretching exercises are performed to maintain range of dorsiflexion of the ankle.

Caution! Do not force the foot-ankle into marked plantarflexion. Gait training is crucial for developing a normal heel-toe gait pattern.

REFERENCES

Green, W. T.: Tendon transplantation in rehabilitation. J.A.M.A., 163:1235, 1957.
Green, W. T., and Grice, D. S.: The surgical correction of the paralytic foot. A.A.O.S. Instructional Course Lectures, 10:343, 1953.

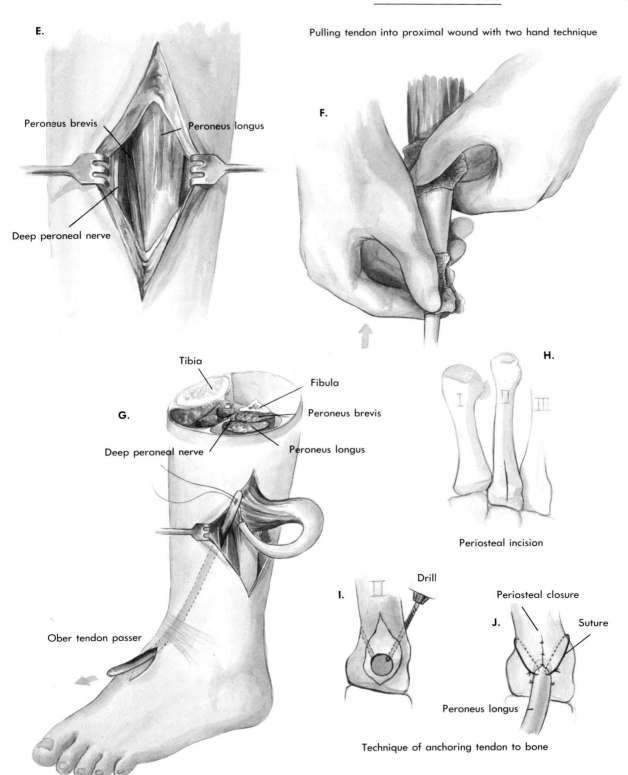

E.

Peroneus brevis

Peroneus longus

Deep peroneal nerve

Pulling tendon into proximal wound with two hand technique

F.

G.

Tibia

Fibula

Peroneus brevis

Deep peroneal nerve

Peroneus longus

Ober tendon passer

H.

Periosteal incision

I.

Drill

J.

Periosteal closure

Suture

Peroneus longus

Technique of anchoring tendon to bone

Plate 186. (Continued)

PLATE 187   ## Anterior Transfer of the Posterior Tibial Tendon Through the Interosseous Membrane

Indications. Poor or no motor strength of the ankle dorsiflexors with drop foot gait and a strong posterior tibial muscle.

Requisites

1. Normal or good motor strength of posterior tibial tendon.
2. Triceps surae of fair or better motor strength.
3. Normal range of dorsiflexion of ankle.
4. Stable ankle and subtalar joints.
5. A plantigrade foot with absence of fixed deformity.

Patient Position. Supine.

Operative Technique

A. A 4-cm. incision is made over the medial aspect of the foot, beginning posterior and immediately distal to the tip of the medial malleolus and extending to the base of the first cuneiform bone. A second longitudinal incision is made 1.5 cm. posterior to the subcutaneous medial border of the tibia, beginning at the center of the middle third of the leg and ending 3 cm. from the tip of the medial malleolus.

B. The posterior tibial tendon is identified at its insertion and its sheath is divided. The tendon is freed and sectioned at its attachment to the bone, preserving maximal length. The paratenon of the distal 3 cm. of the tendon is excised, and a Tycron 00 or 0 whip suture is inserted in its distal end.

C. The posterior tibial muscle is identified in the leg incision, and its sheath is opened and freed. Traction on the stump in the foot incision will aid in its identification. Moist sponges and the two-hand technique are used to deliver the posterior tibial tendon into the proximal wound. The muscle belly is freed well up the tibia. Be careful to preserve the nerve and blood supply to the posterior tibial muscle.

D. Next, a longitudinal skin incision is made anteriorly, one fingerbreadth lateral to the crest of the tibia, starting at the proximal margin of the cruciate ligament of the ankle and extending 7 cm. proximally. Then a 4-cm. longitudinal incision is made over the dorsum of the foot, centering over the base of the second metatarsal.

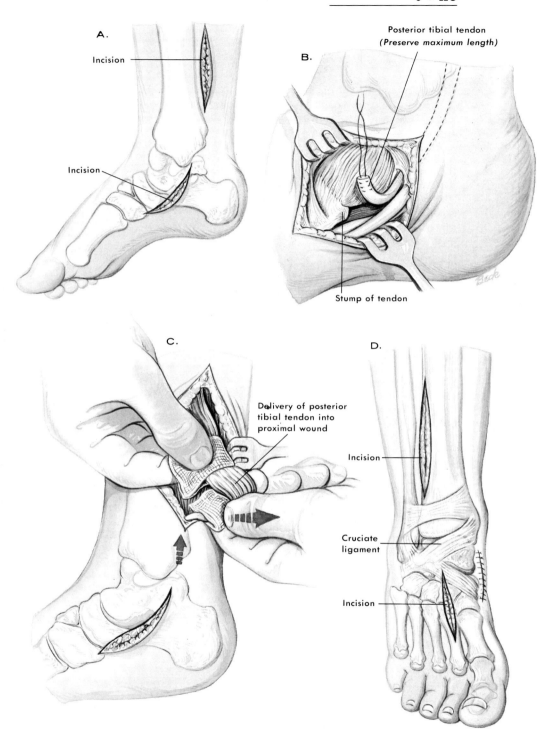

Plate 187. A.–G., Anterior transfer of the posterior tibial tendon through the interosseous membrane.

E. The anterior tibial muscle is exposed and elevated from the anterolateral surface of the tibia together with the anterior tibial artery and extensor hallucis longus muscle. It is retracted laterally, exposing the interosseous membrane. Next, a large rectangular window is cut in the interosseous membrane. Avoid stripping the periosteum from the tibia or fibula.

F. and **G.** Then, with an Ober tendon passer, the posterior tibial tendon is passed through the window in the interosseous membrane from the posterior into the anterior tibial compartment. Be careful not to twist the tendon or to damage its nerve or blood supply. Next, with the aid of an Ober tendon passer, the posterior tibial tendon is passed beneath the cruciate ligament and the extensors and delivered into the wound on the dorsum of the foot. It is anchored to the base of the second metatarsal bone according to the method described in anterior transfer of peroneal tendons (see Plate 186). The wounds are closed in layers in the usual manner. An above-knee cast is applied, holding the foot in neutral position at the ankle joint and the knee in 45 degrees of flexion.

Postoperative Care. The principles of postoperative care are the same as for any tendon transfer. The cast is removed four weeks following surgery. A night splint in the form of an AFO is manufactured to hold the foot-ankle in neutral position. Also, a day articulating AFO is made, allowing free dorsiflexion and limiting plantarflexion to neutral position. Active assisted exercises are performed several times a day to develop function of the transferred peroneals. Also, passive stretching exercises are performed to maintain range of dorsiflexion of the ankle.

Caution! Do not force the foot-ankle into marked plantarflexion. Gait training is crucial for developing a normal heel-toe gait pattern.

REFERENCES

Green, W. T.: Tendon transplantation in rehabilitation. J.A.M.A., 163:1235, 1957.
Green, W. T., and Grice, D. S.: The surgical correction of the paralytic foot. A.A.O.S. Instructional Course Lectures, 10:343, 1953.

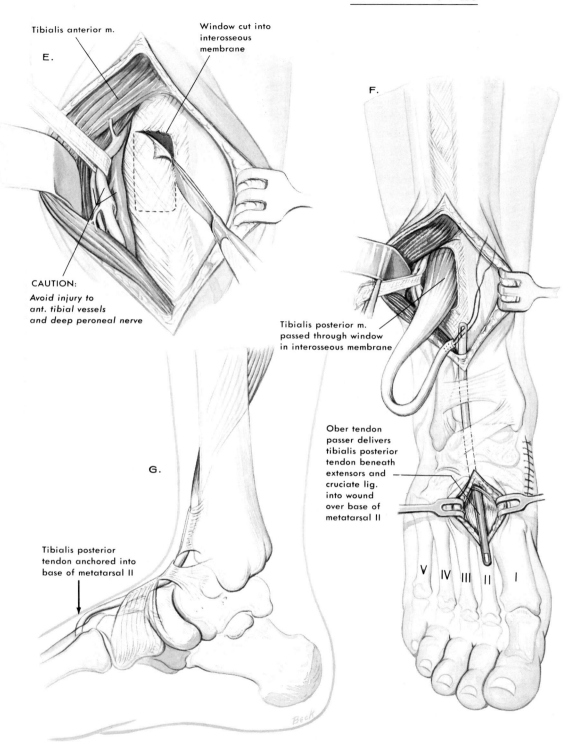

E.

Tibialis anterior m.

Window cut into interosseous membrane

CAUTION:

Avoid injury to ant. tibial vessels and deep peroneal nerve

F.

Tibialis posterior m. passed through window in interosseous membrane

Ober tendon passer delivers tibialis posterior tendon beneath extensors and cruciate lig. into wound over base of metatarsal II

V   IV   III   II   I

G.

Tibialis posterior tendon anchored into base of metatarsal II

Plate 187. (Continued)

PLATE 188

Open Reduction and Internal Fixation of a Triplane Fracture of the Ankle

Indications. Displaced triplane fracture of more than 2 mm.

Radiographic Control. Image intensifier.

Patient Position. Supine.

Operative Technique

A.–E. In this injury, the fracture occurs in three planes—sagittal, transverse, and coronal. It involves the articular surfaces of the epiphysis, physis, and metaphysis of the lower end of the tibia.

In the lateral projection, the radiographic appearance is that of a Salter-Harris II fracture, whereas in the anteroposterior projection it depicts as a Salter-Harris type III physeal injury. The triplane fracture results in a three-fragment fracture when the medial part of the distal tibial physis is open or in a two-fragment fracture when the medial part of the distal tibial physis is closed. If on the routine anteroposterior and lateral radiograms the fracture is displaced more than 2 mm. and the fibula is intact, closed reduction under general anesthesia is ordinarily required. Medial rotation of the heel on the leg usually is successful in reducing the fracture. Tomograms are made, if necessary, to delineate the accuracy of anatomic reduction. An associated greenstick or displaced fracture of the fibula may prevent reduction of the triplane fracture of the distal end of the tibia; the strong ligamentous attachments to the fibula and the lateral part of the tibia will maintain its angular deformity and the resultant shortening of the attached tibial fragment. Reduction of the triplane fracture cannot be accomplished until the fibular fracture is reduced.

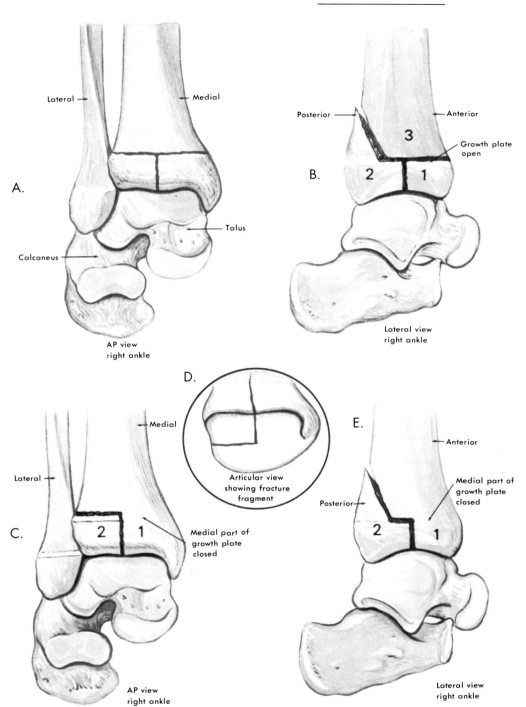

Plate 188. A.–H., Open reduction and internal fixation of a triplane fracture of the ankle.

F. First, the posterior fragment is reduced through a posteromedial approach. Make a longitudinal incision 1 to 2 cm. posterior to the medial border of the distal tibia, beginning at the tip of the medial malleolus and extending proximally for a distance of 5 cm. The subcutaneous tissue is divided in line with the skin incision. The wound flaps are elevated and retracted.

G. The flexor digitorum longus and posterior tibial tendon are identified; the sheaths are incised longitudinally, and the tendons with the neurovascular bundle are retracted posteriorly. With the heel rotated medially on the leg, the foot is dorsiflexed at the ankle and the posterior fragment of the fracture is reduced anatomically under image-intensifier radiographic control. The posterior fragment is fixed internally with two AO cannulated cancellous screws.

H. Anteroposterior and oblique radiograms of the ankle are made. If the vertical fracture line through the sagittal plane is 2 mm. or more in width, the fracture is exposed through an anterior approach to the ankle. The fracture fragments are exposed, anatomically reduced, and internally fixed with one transverse cannulated AO screw inserted transversely anterolaterally above the medial malleolus.

Avoid injury to the growth plate and penetration of the articular surface by the screw. Insert it under image-intensifier radiographic control.

The wounds are closed in the routine fashion. An above-knee cast is applied with the ankle-foot in neutral dorsiflexion and neutral rotation and the knee flexed 30 to 40 degrees.

Postoperative Care. The cast is removed in six weeks, and exercises are performed to restore range of ankle motion and motor strength of muscles controlling the foot and ankle.

REFERENCES

Clement, D. A., and Worlock, P. H.: Triplane fracture of the distal tibia. A variant in cases with an open growth plate. J. Bone Joint Surg., 69-B:412, 1987.

Cooperman, D. R., Spiegel, P. G., and Laros, G. S.: Tibial fractures involving the ankle in children. The so-called triplane epiphyseal fracture. J. Bone Joint Surg., 60-A:1040, 1978.

Dias, L. S., and Giegerich, C. R.: Fractures of the distal tibial epiphysis in adolescence. J. Bone Joint Surg., 65-A:438, 1983.

Karrholm, J., Hansson, L. I., and Laurin, S.: Computed tomography of intraarticular supination-eversion fractures of the ankle in adolescents. J. Pediatr. Orthop., 1:181, 1981.

Marmor, L.: An unusual fracture of the tibial epiphysis. Clin. Orthop., 73:132, 1970.

Von Laer, L.: Classification, diagnosis and treatment of transitional fractures of the distal part of the tibia. J. Bone Joint Surg., 67-A:687, 1985.

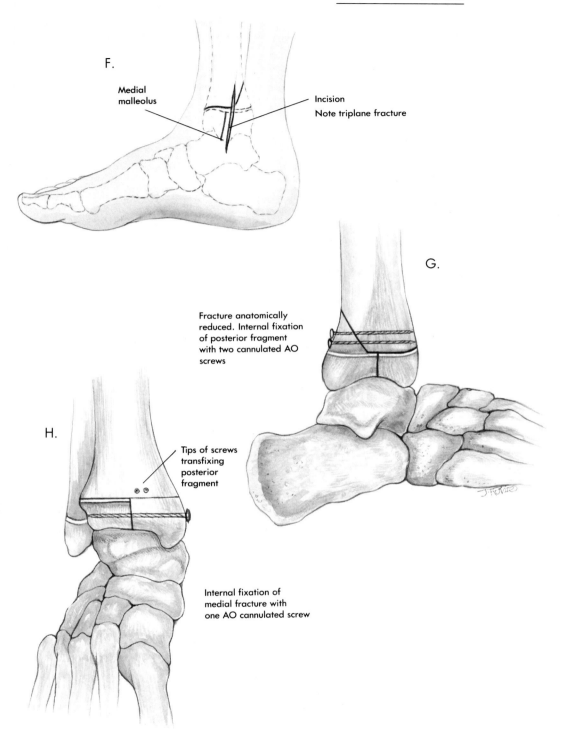

F.

Medial malleolus

Incision
Note triplane fracture

G.

Fracture anatomically
reduced. Internal fixation
of posterior fragment
with two cannulated AO
screws

H.

Tips of screws
transfixing
posterior
fragment

Internal fixation of
medial fracture with
one AO cannulated screw

Plate 188. (Continued)

PLATE 189 **Open Reduction and Internal Fixation of a Tillaux Fracture**

Indications. When the fracture is displaced more than 2 mm.

Radiographic Control. Image intensifier.

Patient Position. Supine.

Operative Technique

A. and **B.** This is a Salter-Harris type III physeal injury of the lateral part of the distal tibial epiphysis in the adolescent. The medial part of the distal tibial physis is closed, and the lateral part is open. The fracture is sustained by a lateral rotatory force, which exerts stress on the anterior talofibular ligament. The anterolateral fracture fragment is avulsed and displaced anterolaterally. The displacement of the fragment varies from minimal to marked. When the displacement is more than 1 to 2 mm., accurate anatomic open reduction and internal fixation with one cannulated screw or two smooth Kirschner wires are required.

C. An anterolateral incision is made beginning 4 to 5 cm. proximal to the ankle joint at the lateral border of the tibia and extending distally to terminate 1 to 2 cm. anterior to the lateral malleolus.

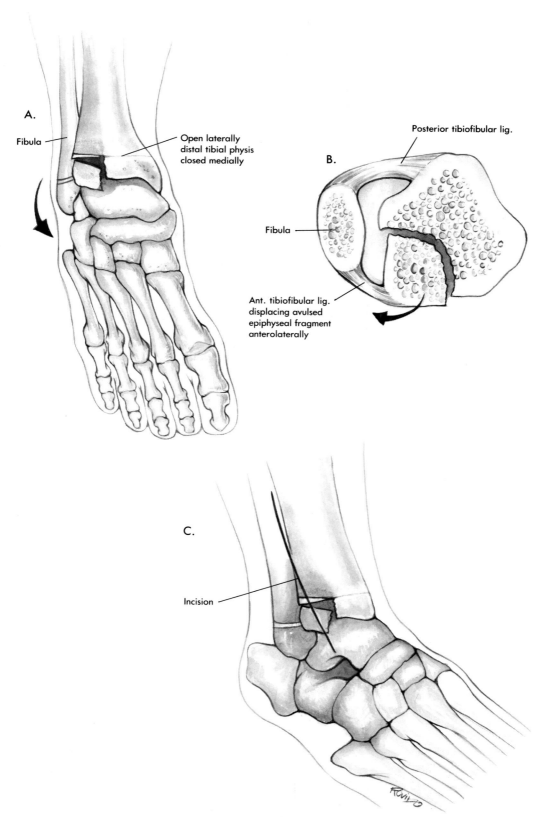

A.

Fibula

Open laterally
distal tibial physis
closed medially

Posterior tibiofibular lig.

B.

Fibula

Ant. tibiofibular lig.
displacing avulsed
epiphyseal fragment
anterolaterally

C.

Incision

Plate 189. A.–F., Open reduction and internal fixation of a Tillaux fracture.

D. Expose the fracture site by retracting the peroneal tendons posterolaterally and the extensor tendons and neurovascular bundle medially. Divide the ankle joint capsule transversely, and open the ankle joint.

E. and F. Reduce the fracture by applying longitudinal axial traction and, while maintaining the traction medially, rotate the hindfoot on the leg. With a Lewin bone clamp or similar bone holder, reduce the fracture anatomically and maintain the reduction. Do not strip and disrupt the periosteum.

Inspect the articular surface of the ankle joint. Be sure it is anatomically congruous. Internal fixation can be carried out by two pins; in the younger patient smooth pins are used: one pin perpendicular to the fracture and parallel to the ankle joint, and the other pin at a 45-degree angle to the first pin. The tips of the pins should penetrate the medial cortex of the tibia; the lateral ends are cut subcutaneously, bent, and buried into soft tissues.

An alternative method of internal fixation is by one small cannulated cancellous screw inserted transversely across the fracture line into the epiphysis; the screw should not penetrate the ankle joint or the open lateral growth plate.

First, insert the smooth pin and make radiograms of the ankle in the anteroposterior, oblique, and lateral projections to double-check the accuracy of anatomic reduction and position and length of the pin or pins. Then, insert the cannulated screw and take the pin out.

The tourniquet is released, and the wound is irrigated. After complete hemostasis, the torn periosteum is closed, if possible, by interrupted sutures. A medium Hemovac suction tube is inserted, and the wound is closed in the ordinary fashion. An above-knee cast is applied with the ankle-foot in neutral position and the knee flexed 40 degrees. In the cooperative, dependable patient, a below-knee cast can be applied.

Postoperative Care. Weight-bearing is not allowed for four to six weeks. Radiograms of the ankle out of cast are made at three and six months. When there is radiographic evidence of healing of the fracture, the smooth pins are removed and weight-bearing is permitted. When a cancellous screw is used for internal fixation, the screw is removed four to six months after surgery. The total period of cast immobilization is six to eight weeks, depending on the age of the child.

REFERENCES

Kleiger, B., and Mankin, H. J.: Fracture of the lateral portion of the distal tibial epiphysis. J. Bone Joint Surg., 46-A:25, 1964.

Kling, T. F., Jr., Bright, R. W., and Hensinger, R. N.: Distal tibial physeal fractures in children that may require open reduction. J. Bone Joint Surg., 66-A:647, 1984.

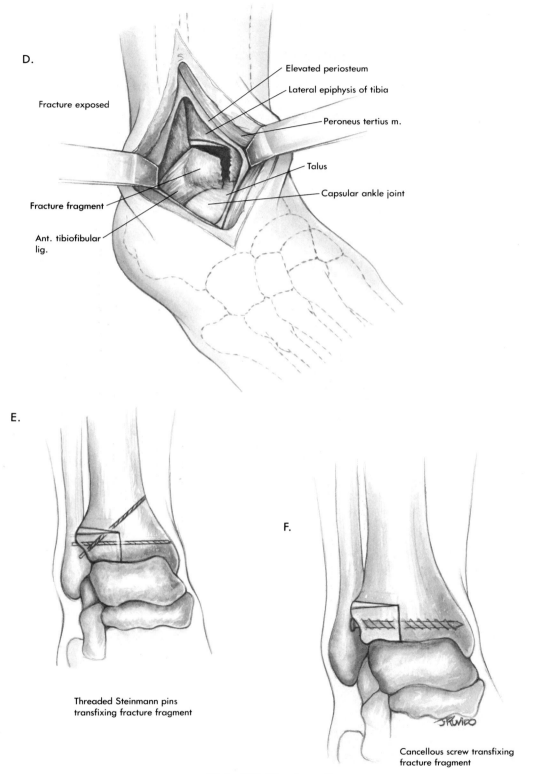

D.

Fracture exposed

Elevated periosteum

Lateral epiphysis of tibia

Peroneus tertius m.

Talus

Capsular ankle joint

Fracture fragment

Ant. tibiofibular
lig.

E.

Threaded Steinmann pins
transfixing fracture fragment

F.

Cancellous screw transfixing
fracture fragment

Plate 189. (Continued)

PLATE 190 **Anterior Release of Contracture of the Capsule of the Ankle Joint and Fractional Musculotendinous Lengthening of the Anterior Tibial and Long Toe Extensors**

Indications. Moderate to severe calcaneal deformity of the ankle and foot due to fibrosis and contracture of denervated anterior crural muscles or due to spasticity of the ankle dorsiflexors in myelomeningocele.

When the deformity is severe, anterior capsulotomy of the ankle may be required to correct the calcaneus deformity. An anterior approach is used to expose the lower leg and ankle.

Patient Position. Supine.

Operative Technique

A. A 6- to 7-cm. longitudinal incision is made in the anterolateral aspect of the ankle and lower leg; beginning at the ankle joint, it extends proximally for a distance of 4 to 5 cm. At the ankle joint it curves medially across the dorsum of the ankle and then extends distally for 2 cm. The subcutaneous tissue is divided in line with the skin incision. The wound flaps are undermined and elevated. Veins crossing the field are coagulated and divided. Sensory nerves are protected by retracting them out of harm's way.

B. When the calcaneovalgus defect is moderate and anterior capsulotomy of the ankle is not required to correct the contralateral deformity, one may make a 3- to 4-cm. transverse incision 2 to 3 cm. superior to the ankle joint for surgical exposure. This author prefers a longitudinal incision.

C. The superficial fascia and upper extensor retinaculum are divided. With sharp and dull dissection, the tendons of the anterior tibial, extensor hallucis longus, extensor digitorum longus, and peroneus tertius are identified from the medial to the lateral side.

Caution! Do not injure the deep peroneal (anterior tibial) nerve or the anterior tibial vessels; they lie between tibialis anterior and extensor hallucis longus tendons in the lower third of the leg; the nerve is situated on the lateral side of the vessels. Two cm. of each tendon is resected.

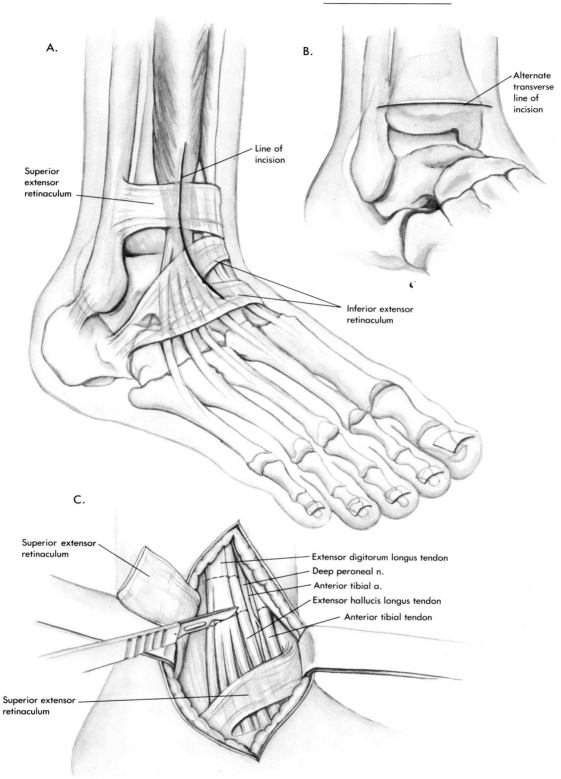

A.

Superior extensor retinaculum

Line of incision

Inferior extensor retinaculum

B.

Alternate transverse line of incision

C.

Superior extensor retinaculum

Extensor digitorum longus tendon
Deep peroneal n.
Anterior tibial a.
Extensor hallucis longus tendon
Anterior tibial tendon

Superior extensor retinaculum

Plate 190. A.–F., Anterior release of contracture of the capsule of the ankle joint and fractional musculotendinous lengthening of the anterior tibial and long toe extensors.

D. A longitudinal incision is made immediately posterior to the fibula; it begins 1 cm. above the tip of the lateral malleolus and extends proximally 4 to 5 cm. The subcutaneous tissue and deep fascia are divided in line with the skin incision. The peroneus longus and brevis tendons are identified; their sheath is opened and a 2 cm. segment of the tendons is resected.

E. Next, the ankle and foot are plantar-flexed and inverted. If the calcaneovalgus deformity is still present, an anterior capsulotomy of the ankle joint is performed. Retract the extensor digitorum longus with its neurovascular bundle medially and the peroneus tertius laterally.

F. Make a longitudinal incision in the capsule and open the ankle joint. Then make a transverse incision at the joint level.

The wound is closed, and a below-knee cast is applied with the foot-ankle in 15 to 20 degrees of plantar flexion and inversion.

Postoperative Care. The cast is removed in 10 to 14 days. Passive range of motion exercises are performed several times a day to maintain the degree of correction. An ankle-foot orthosis with the foot and ankle in neutral position is worn at night and during the day.

REFERENCES

Schafer, M. F., and Dias, L. S.: Myelomeningocele. Orthopaedic Treatment. Baltimore, Williams & Wilkins, 1983, pp. 197–202.

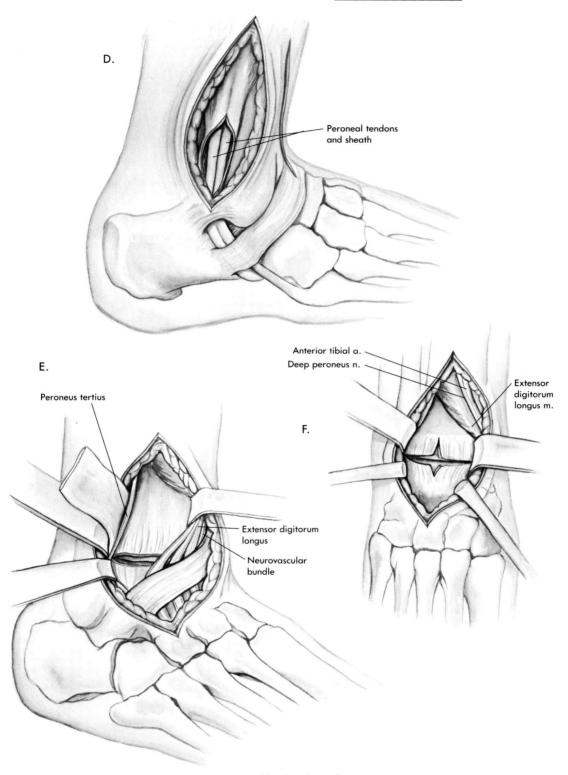

D.

Peroneal tendons
and sheath

E.

Peroneus tertius

Extensor digitorum
longus

Neurovascular
bundle

F.

Anterior tibial a.
Deep peroneus n.

Extensor
digitorum
longus m.

Plate 190. (Continued)

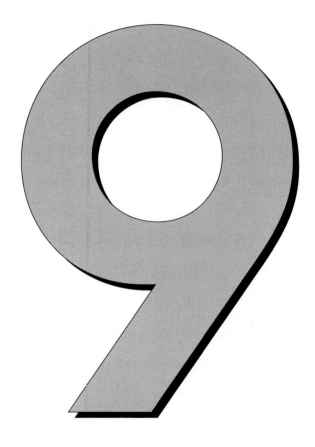

Foot

PLATE 191 ## Extra-articular Arthrodesis of the Subtalar Joint (Grice Procedure)

Indications. Severe valgus deformity of the hindfoot with oblique or vertical talus that interferes with shoe wear, balance, and locomotion.

Objective. To correct valgus deformity of the hindfoot and restore the height of the longitudinal arch.

Caution! The procedure does not (1) correct fixed valgus or varus deformity of the mid or forepart of the foot or (2) improve pes valgus due to ligamentous relaxation and sagging of the talonavicular and naviculocuneiform joints.

Advantage. Interferes minimally with growth of the foot because the graft is extra-articular.

Disadvantages

1. Causes loss of mediolateral mobility of the hindfoot and may cause difficulty in walking on rough terrain.

2. With fusion of the subtalar joint, excessive ligamentous stress is exerted on the ankle joint.

Requisites

1. Ability to restore the calcaneus to its normal position beneath the talus, as demonstrated on lateral radiograms of the foot–ankle made with the ankle in maximal plantar flexion and the foot in inversion.

2. Absence of equinus deformity. There should be normal range of ankle dorsiflexion. If fixed equinus deformity is present, correct it first by heel cord lengthening or stretching cast.

3. A stable ankle joint, as shown by anteroposterior weight-bearing stress radiograms of the ankle.

4. Absence of valgus deviation of the ankle joint. Normal anatomic level of fibular malleolus, with its physis level with the ankle joint. When there is marked valgus deformity of the ankle, it is corrected by supramalleolar osteotomy of the tibia.

5. Absence of invertor-evertor muscle imbalance of the foot and contractural deformity. If these are present, restore dynamic muscle balance by tendon transfers and correct contractural deformity by appropriate musculotendinous lengthenings.

Pitfalls to Avoid

1. Overcorrection. *Never fuse the hindfoot in varus!* Make intraoperative radiograms of the foot–ankle.

2. Shifting or malposition of the graft. When the graft is unstable, transfix the subtalar joint with a threaded Steinmann pin or AO cannulated screw.

Patient Position. Supine with a sandbag under the ipsilateral hip.

Operative Technique

A. A 5- to 6-cm.-long and slightly curved incision is made over the subtalar joint, centering over the sinus tarsi.

B. The incision is carried down to the sinus tarsi. The capsules of the posterior and anterior subtalar articulations are identified and left intact. The operation is extra-articular. If the capsule is opened inadvertently, it should be closed by interrupted sutures.

The periosteum on the talus corresponding to the lateral margin of the roof of the sinus tarsi is divided and reflected proximally. The fibrofatty tissue in the sinus tarsi with the periosteum of the calcaneus corresponding to the floor of the sinus tarsi and the tendinous origin of the short toe extensors from the calcaneus is elevated and reflected distally in one mass.

C. The remaining fatty and ligamentous tissue from the sinus tarsi is thoroughly removed with a sharp scalpel and a curet.

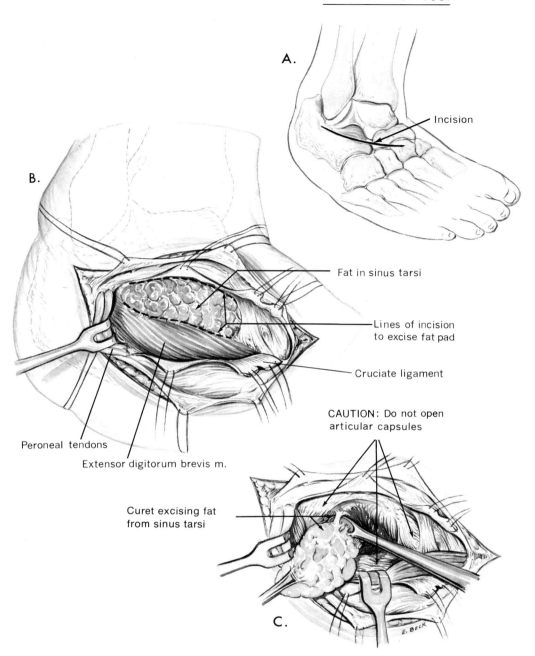

A.

Incision

B.

Fat in sinus tarsi

Lines of incision
to excise fat pad

Cruciate ligament

CAUTION: Do not open
articular capsules

Peroneal tendons

Extensor digitorum brevis m.

Curet excising fat
from sinus tarsi

C.

E. BECK

Plate 191. A.–F., Extra-articular arthrodesis of the subtalar joint (Grice procedure).

D. Next, the foot is manipulated into equinus position and inversion, rotating the calcaneus into its normal position beneath the talus and correcting the valgus deformity. Broad, straight osteotomes of various sizes (¾ to 1¼ inches or more) are inserted into the sinus tarsi, blocking the subtalar joint and determining the length and optimum position of the bone graft and the stability that it will provide. The long axis of the graft should be parallel with that of the leg when the ankle is dorsiflexed into neutral position, and the hindfoot should be in 5 degrees of valgus or neutral, but never of varus. Even a slight degree of varus deformity of the heel seems to increase with growth.

E. The optimum site of the bone graft bed is marked with the broad osteotome. A thin layer of cortical bone (⅛ to ³⁄₁₆ inch) is removed with a dental osteotome from the inferior surface of the talus (the roof of the sinus tarsi) and the superior surface of the calcaneus (the floor of the sinus tarsi) at the marked site for the bone graft. It is best to preserve the most lateral cortical margin of the graft bed to support the bone block and to prevent it from sinking into soft cancellous bone.

F. A bone graft of appropriate size can be taken from the anteromedial surface of the proximal tibial metaphysis as a single cortical graft, which is then cut into two trapezoidal bone grafts with their cancellous surfaces facing each other. The fibular shaft with the cortices intact is another source of bone graft; however, ankle valgus is a potential problem. I recommend the use of bicortical bone graft harvested from the iliac crest. The corners of the base of the graft are removed with a rongeur so that it is trapezoidal in shape and can be countersunk into cancellous bone, preventing lateral displacement after operation.

The bone graft is placed in the prepared graft bed in the sinus tarsi by holding the foot in varus position. An impactor may be used to fix the cortices of the graft in place. The longitudinal axis of the graft should be parallel with the shaft of the tibia with the ankle in neutral position.

With the foot held in the desired position, the distal soft-tissue pedicle of fibrofatty tissue of the sinus tarsi, the calcaneal periosteum, and the tendinous origin of the short toe extensors are sutured to the reflected periosteum from the talus. The subcutaneous tissue and skin are closed with interrupted sutures, and an above-knee cast is applied.

Postoperative Care. The cast is changed as necessary and it is removed eight to ten weeks after operation. Radiograms are taken; if there is solid healing of the graft, gradual weight-bearing is allowed with the protection of crutches. Active and passive exercises are performed to strengthen the muscles and to increase the range of motion of the ankle and knee.

REFERENCES

Chigot, P. L., and Sananes, P.: Arthrodèse de Grice. Rev. Chir. Orthop., 51:53, 1965.
Gresham, J. L.: Correction of flat feet in children. Grice-Green subastragalar arthrodesis. South. Med. J., 61:177, 1968.
Grice, D. S.: An extra-articular arthrodesis of the subastragalar joint for correction of paralytic flatfeet in children. J. Bone Joint Surg., 34-A:929, 1952.
Grice, D. S.: Further experience with extra-articular arthrodesis of the subtalar joint. J. Bone Joint Surg., 37-A:246, 1955.
Grice, D. S.: The role of subtalar fusion in the treatment of valgus deformities of the foot. A.A.O.S. Instructional Course Lectures, 16:127, 1959.
Romanini, L., Carfagni, A., and Amorese, V.: Grice's operation for spastic flat foot. Ital. J. Orthop. Traumatol., 9:439, 1983.
Vigliani, F., Maranzano, G., and Novati, G.: Grice-Green extra-articular subtalar arthrodesis in the treatment of infantile valgus pronated flat foot. Ital. J. Orthop. Traumatol., 9:411, 1983.
Weissman, S. L., Torok, G., and Kharmosh, O.: L'arthrodèse extraarticulaire avec transplantation tendineuse concommittante dans le traitement du pied plat valgus paralytique de jeune enfant. Rev. Chir. Orthop., 43:79, 1957.
Westin, G. W., and Hall, C. B.: Subtalar extra-articular arthrodesis. J. Bone Joint Surg., 39-A:501, 1957.

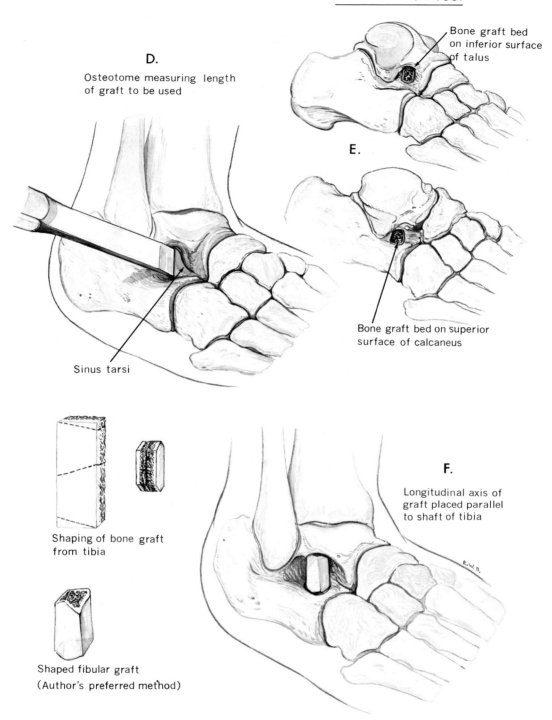

D.

Osteotome measuring length
of graft to be used

Sinus tarsi

Shaping of bone graft
from tibia

Shaped fibular graft
(Author's preferred method)

Bone graft bed
on inferior surface
of talus

E.

Bone graft bed on superior
surface of calcaneus

F.

Longitudinal axis of
graft placed parallel
to shaft of tibia

E.W.B.

Plate 191. (Continued)

PLATE 192 **Staple Arthroereisis Stabilization of the Subtalar Joint (Crawford Procedure)**

Indications. Flexible vertical talus in the child with cerebral palsy between the ages of three and eight years.

Requisites. Normal range of dorsiflexion of the ankle with dynamic balance between evertors and invertors of the foot. Postoperative support of the foot and ankle in an orthosis is mandatory.

Radiographic Control. Image intensifier.

Patient Position. The patient is supine with a sandbag under the ipsilateral hip so that the lower limb, foot, and ankle can be rotated medially.

Operative Technique

A. The subtalar joint is exposed through the lateral arm of a Cincinnati incision (Plate 203) or through a 5-cm.-long and slightly curved incision centered over the sinus tarsi, as described in the Grice procedure (see Plate 191).

B. The incision is carried down to the sinus tarsi. The periosteum on the talus corresponding to the lateral margin of the roof of the sinus tarsi is divided and reflected proximally. Excise the fibrofatty tissue in the sinus tarsi. Incise the periosteum of the calcaneus corresponding to the floor of the sinus tarsi. Elevate the tendinous origin of the extensor digitorum brevis from the calcaneus and reflect distally in one mass.

C. and D. Correct the dorsolateral subluxation of the talocalcaneal navicular joint by manipulation of the foot into equinus position and inversion, rotating the calcaneus into its normal position beneath the talus and correcting the valgus deformity. Insert a broad, straight osteotome of the appropriate size into the sinus tarsi, blocking the subtalar joint. Make radiograms to determine adequacy of reduction. If a normal anatomic relationship of the talocalcaneal navicular joint is achieved, I recommend transfixing the talus to the calcaneus with a threaded Steinmann pin drilled through a stab wound on the dorsum of the foot.

Anteroposterior and lateral radiograms are made again to assess adequacy of correction.

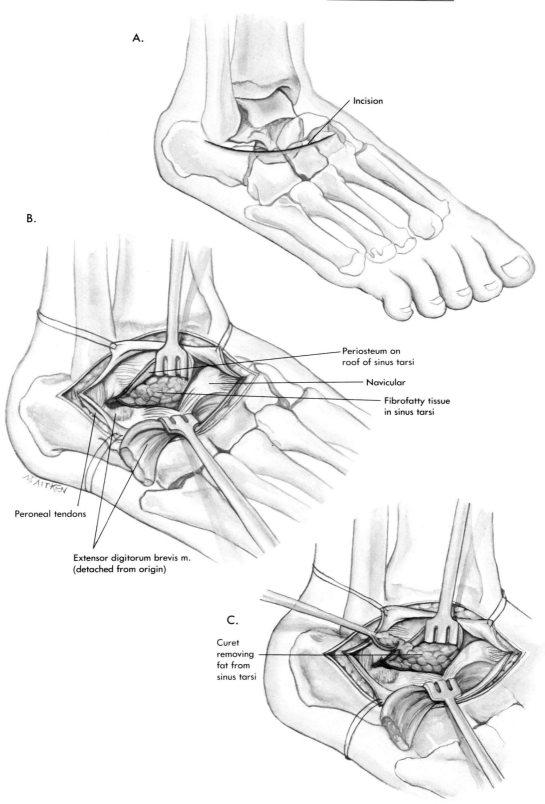

A.

Incision

B.

Periosteum on
roof of sinus tarsi

Navicular

Fibrofatty tissue
in sinus tarsi

Peroneal tendons

Extensor digitorum brevis m.
(detached from origin)

C.

Curet
removing
fat from
sinus tarsi

Plate 192. A.–F., Subtalar stabilization of the planovalgus foot by staple arthroereisis (Crawford procedure).

C. and **D.** Correct the dorsolateral subluxation of the talocalcaneal navicular joint by manipulation of the foot into equinus position and inversion, rotating the calcaneus into its normal position beneath the talus and correcting the valgus deformity. Insert a broad, straight osteotome of the appropriate size into the sinus tarsi, blocking the subtalar joint. Make radiograms to determine adequacy of reduction. If a normal anatomic relationship of the talocalcaneal navicular joint is achieved, I recommend transfixing the talus to the calcaneus with a threaded Steinmann pin drilled through a stab wound on the dorsum of the foot.

Anteroposterior and lateral radiograms are made again to assess adequacy of correction.

E. and **F.** A Vitallium staple is used for internal fixation. The staple should be aligned parallel to the tibia with the foot in 15 degrees of plantar flexion. It may be necessary to cut a small notch into the calcaneus because of the offset of the lateral margin of the calcaneus relative to the talus. This author finds simple drilling of the cortex of the lateral surface to be adequate. Next, the staple is driven into the calcaneus and the talus. Radiograms are made. Be sure that the staple is not in the ankle joint and that it is parallel to the longitudinal axis of the tibia. If, after correction of the talocalcaneal subluxation, the ankle joint is still in equinus, perform a tendo Achillis lengthening.

The wound is closed in the usual fashion, and an above-knee cast is applied with the foot and ankle in neutral position and the knee in 5 degrees of flexion.

Postoperative Care. Four weeks after surgery, the cast is removed and a polypropylene ankle-foot orthosis is used for support.

REFERENCES

Crawford, A. H., Kucharzyk, D., Roy, D. R., and Bilbo, J.: Subtalar stabilization of the planovalgus foot by staple arthroereisis in young children who have neuromuscular problems. J. Bone Joint Surg., 72-A:840, 1990.

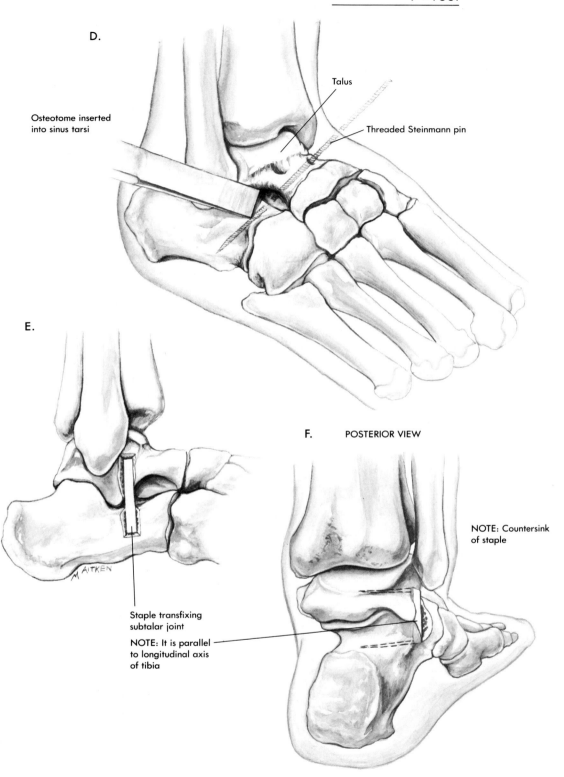

D.

Talus

Osteotome inserted
into sinus tarsi

Threaded Steinmann pin

E.

F.   POSTERIOR VIEW

M AITKEN

NOTE: Countersink
of staple

Staple transfixing
subtalar joint

NOTE: It is parallel
to longitudinal axis
of tibia

Plate 192. (Continued)

PLATE 193 ## Triple Arthrodesis

Objective. Fusion of the subtalar, calcaneocuboid, and talonavicular joints is designed to provide lateral stability to the hindfoot and to correct deformity by resection of the articular surfaces by pattern. The procedure was first described by Ryerson in 1923.

Indications

1. Instability of the foot as a result of paralysis of the muscles controlling the hindfoot and midfoot.
2. Pain due to arthritis—traumatic, infectious, or inflammatory.
3. Rigid deformity—varus, valgus, or calcaneal—in the skeletally mature foot.

Note: It is preferable to correct the deformity by osteotomy of the os calcis, cuboid, or navicular in order to preserve mobility of the subtalar and talonavicular or calcaneocuboid joints.

Requisites

1. Skeletally mature foot; growth of the foot should not be disturbed. Minimum age should be ten to 12 years in girls and 12 to 14 years in boys.
2. Stable ankle joint; test it clinically and by stress, anteroposterior, weight-bearing radiograms of the ankle; first with the hindfoot in forced, maximal eversion and abduction and then in forced inversion and adduction with the ankle in neutral dorsiflexion. There should be no lateral motion of the body of the talus in the ankle mortise. Triple arthrodesis is contraindicated in the presence of marked instability of the ankle.
3. Absence of fixed equinus deformity. The foot should be dorsiflexed at least to neutral position. If the fixed equinus deformity cannot be corrected by stretching cast, heel cord lengthening and posterior capsulotomy of the ankle and subtalar joints may be required. Prevent rocker-bottom deformity. Maintain function of the triceps surae as much as possible.
4. Absence of significant torsional or angular deformity of the tibia–fibula. If present, it should be corrected prior to surgery or subsequently. Align the foot with the ankle mortise and not with the knee.

Radiographic Control. Image intensifier.

Special Instrumentation. Staples when internal fixation is indicated.

Patient Position. A pneumatic tourniquet is placed on the proximal thigh, and the patient is positioned semilaterally with a large sandbag under the hip on the affected side.

Operative Technique

A. A curvilinear incision is made, centering over the sinus tarsi. It starts one fingerbreadth distal and posterior to the tip of the lateral malleolus and extends anteriorly and distally to the base of the second metatarsal bone.

B. Skin flaps should not be developed. The incision is carried to the floor of the sinus tarsi. By sharp dissection, with scalpel and periosteal elevator, the periosteum of the calcaneus, the adipose tissue contents of the sinus tarsi, and the tendinous origin of the exterior digitorum brevis are elevated in one mass from the calcaneus and lateral aspect of the neck of the talus and retracted distally. It is essential to provide a viable soft-tissue pedicle to obliterate the dead space remaining at the end of the operation.

An incision is made superiorly over the periosteum of the talus, and the head and neck of the talus are carefully exposed. The upper flap of the skin, subcutaneous tissue, and periosteum should be kept as thick as possible to avoid necrosis. Traction sutures are placed on the periosteum. At no time are the skin edges to

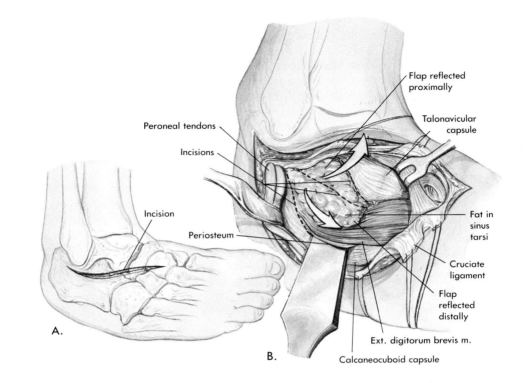

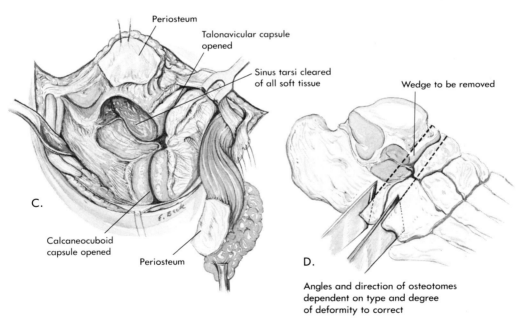

Plate 193. A.–T., Triple arthrodesis. I.–N., Correction of pes varus. O.–T., Correction of calcaneocavus deformity.

be retracted. It is not necessary to divide the peroneal tendons or their sheaths. By subperiosteal dissection, the peroneal tendons are retracted posteriorly for exposure of the subtalar joint.

C. and **D.** The capsules of the calcaneocuboid, talonavicular, and subtalar joints are incised. These joints are opened and their cartilaginous surfaces clearly visualized by turning the foot into varus position. A laminar spreader placed in the sinus tarsi aids in exposure of the posterior subtalar joint. Before excision of articular cartilaginous surfaces, review the deformity of the foot and decide on the wedges of bone to be removed to correct the deformity. Circulation of the talus and the complications of avascular necrosis of the talus and arthritis of the ankle following triple arthrodesis should always be kept in mind. The height of the foot is another consideration. A low lateral malleolus will cause difficulty with wearing shoes. At times, it is best to add a bone graft rather than resect wedges of bone.

Next, the articular cartilage surface of the talonavicular joint is exposed, the plane of osteotomy being perpendicular to the long axis of the neck of the talus and parallel to the calcaneocuboid joint. When the beak of the navicular is unduly prominent medially, or when, in a varus foot, one cannot obtain adequate exposure of the talonavicular joint without excessive retraction, I strongly recommend that a second dorsomedial incision be used to expose the talonavicular joint.

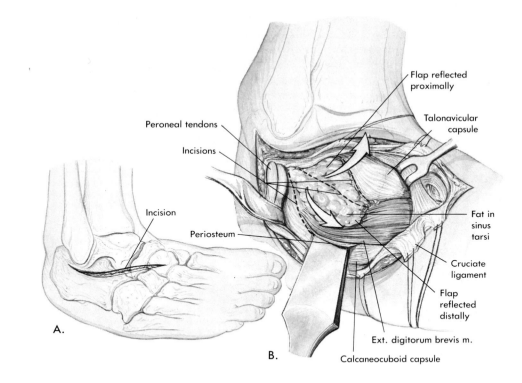

Flap reflected proximally

Talonavicular capsule

Peroneal tendons

Incisions

Incision

Periosteum

Fat in sinus tarsi

Cruciate ligament

Flap reflected distally

Ext. digitorum brevis m.

Calcaneocuboid capsule

A.

B.

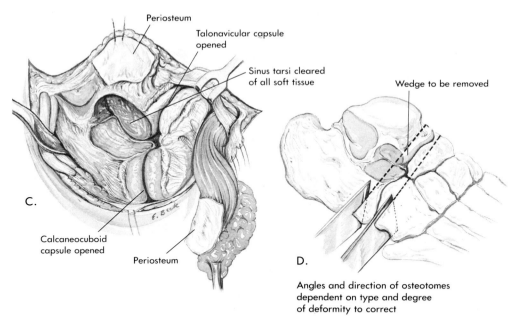

Periosteum

Talonavicular capsule opened

Sinus tarsi cleared of all soft tissue

Wedge to be removed

C.

Calcaneocuboid capsule opened

Periosteum

D.

Angles and direction of osteotomes dependent on type and degree of deformity to correct

Plate 193. (Continued)

E.–H. With a laminar spreader in the sinus tarsi, the subtalar joint is widely exposed and the cartilage of the anterior and posterior joints is excised.

Caution! Do not injure the neurovascular structures behind the medial malleolus. The wedges of bone that must be removed to correct the deformity are excised in one mass with the articular cartilage. It is of great help to leave the osteotome used on the opposing articular surface in place and held steady by the assistant as a second osteotome or gouge is used to take contiguous cartilage and bone. The divided articular surfaces of the joints to be arthrodesed are "fish-scaled" for maximum raw cancellous bony contact.

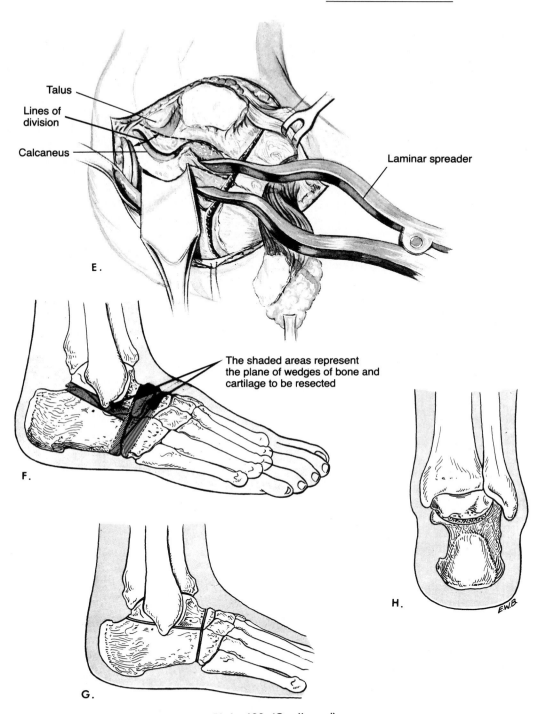

Talus

Lines of
division

Calcaneus

Laminar spreader

E.

The shaded areas represent
the plane of wedges of bone and
cartilage to be resected

F.

G.

H.

E.W.B.

Plate 193. (Continued)

Pes Varus

I.–K. The wedge of bone to be resected from the talonavicular and calcaneocuboid joints is based laterally. Lateral displacement of the forefoot is often prevented by the beak of the navicular, which projects posteriorly along the medial side of the head of the talus. Excise this beak flush with the main body of the navicular through the medial incision. The planes of the osteotomies of the talonavicular and calcaneocuboid joints should be parallel to each other in the vertical axis in order to have close apposition of bones. To correct varus deformity of the heel, resect a laterally based wedge from the subtalar joint. Remove most of the bone from the superior surface of the calcaneus. Only a minimal amount of bone should be excised from the talus. The hindfoot should be in 5 to 10 degrees of eversion. Such a slight degree of valgus position of the heel provides stability to the hindfoot. Do not accept a varus position of the heel.

L.–N. The tarsal bones are manipulated and apposed. At present, this author recommends staple fixation of the talonavicular joint medially and laterally and of the calcaneocuboid and subtalar joints laterally. Do not use staples with large-diameter limbs—they may split the navicular or cuboid. Pre-drill when the bones are hard.

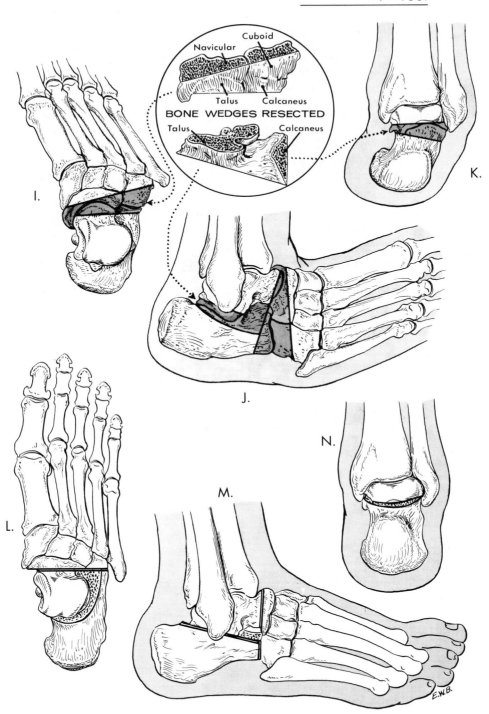

Navicular
Cuboid
Talus
Calcaneus
BONE WEDGES RESECTED
Talus
Calcaneus

I.

J.

K.

L.

M.

N.

E.W.B.

Plate 193. (Continued)

Calcaneocavus Deformity

O.–T. A wedge of bone based posteriorly is resected from the subtalar joint. Often, calcaneus deformity is associated with cavus deformity of the midfoot and forefoot. This is corrected by excising a wedge based dorsally from the talonavicular and calcaneocuboid joints. In correction of calcaneus deformity, it is important to displace the os calcis posteriorly to provide a longer lever arm. Sometimes the anterior capsule of the ankle joint is very contracted, and an anterior soft-tissue release of the ankle joint may be indicated.

The tarsal bones are manipulated and apposed. At present, this author recommends staple fixation of the talonavicular joint medially and laterally and of the calcaneocuboid and subtalar joints laterally.

Postoperative Care. The skin is closed with interrupted sutures. A well-molded above-knee cast is applied, holding the foot in the desired position. Weight-bearing is not allowed. The cast is changed in three to four weeks after surgery. If there is adequate healing, a below-knee cast is applied and partial weight-bearing with crutch support is permitted. The cast is removed when fusion has taken place, usually six to eight weeks postoperatively.

REFERENCES

Hallgrimsson, S.: Studies on reconstructive and stabilizing operations on the skeleton of the foot, with special reference to subastragalar arthrodesis in treatment of foot deformities following infantile paralysis. Acta Chir. Scand. (Suppl. 78), 88:1, 1943.

Hart, V. L.: Arthrodesis of the foot in infantile paralysis. Surg. Gynecol. Obstet., 64:794, 1937.

Ryerson, E. W.: Arthrodesing operations on the feet. J. Bone Joint Surg., 5:453, 1923.

Schwartz, R. P.: Arthrodesis of subtalus and midtarsal joint of the foot: Historical review, preoperative determinations, and operative procedures. Surgery, 20:619, 1946.

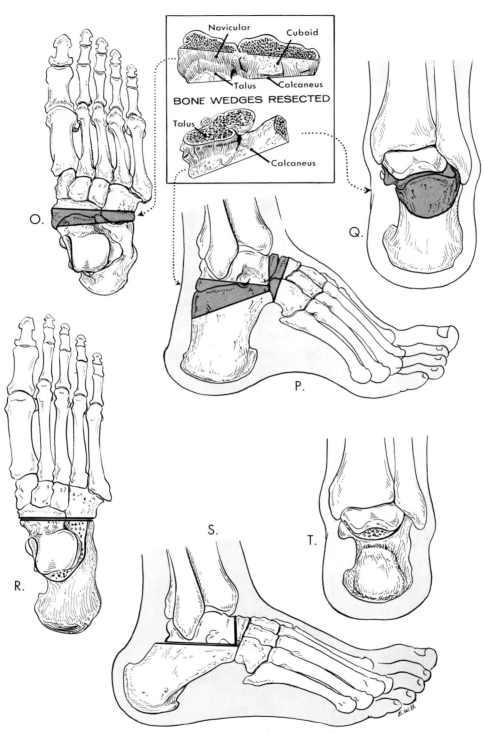

Navicular   Cuboid
Talus   Calcaneus

BONE WEDGES RESECTED

Talus

Calcaneus

O.

P.

Q.

R.

S.

T.

E.W.B.

Plate 193. (Continued)

PLATE 194 ### Triple Arthrodesis by Inlay Grafting (Williams and Menelaus Technique)

Indications. Severe, flexible valgus deformity of the foot seen in generalized ligamentous hyperlaxity in syndromes such as Marfan's and Down's. In these cases, resection of bone wedges with cartilage causes the foot to become floppy and shorter than its mate. In the Williams and Menelaus technique, the joints are undisturbed and the lateral inlay graft is inserted to achieve stabilization of the hindfoot and midfoot.

Requisites. No fixed deformity.

Radiographic Control. Image intensifier.

Patient Position. Supine with a sandbag under the ipsilateral hip.

Operative Technique

A. A curved longitudinal incision is made on the anterolateral aspect of the dorsum of the foot. It extends from immediately distal to the tip of the lateral malleolus to the second cuneiform. The subcutaneous tissue and deep fascia are divided in line with the skin incision.

B. The extensor digitorum brevis is elevated from its origin and reflected distally. The extensor digitorum longus tendons are retracted medially. The contents of the sinus tarsi and the capsules of the talonavicular, calcaneocuboid, and subtalar joints are excised.

C. Next, the foot is manipulated and securely held in the desired plantigrade position, with the valgus deviation corrected and a normal longitudinal arch. In the very flaccid foot, it is best to stabilize the tarsus by drilling two stout Kirschner wires longitudinally, one across the talonavicular and the other across the calcaneocuboid joint. A square or oblong trough is cut across the midfoot, extending across the talonavicular, anterior subtalar, calcaneocuboid, and naviculocuboid joints.

D. and **E.** A bone graft, slightly larger than the resected block, is taken from the upper third of the same tibia or the ilium and then hammered snugly into the trough in the tarsus.

With a gouge, the articular cartilage from the adjacent subtalar joint is removed and the defect is filled with the bone previously removed from the trough. The tourniquet is released, and after complete hemostasis the leg and foot wounds are closed in the usual fashion. The Kirschner wires are removed and an above-knee cast is applied with the foot–ankle in neutral position and the knee flexed 45 degrees.

Postoperative Care. The foot and leg are immobilized in a cast for a total period of three months. Bone healing is assessed clinically and radiologically. The cortical bone graft may appear dense initially, but in time it will become revascularized.

REFERENCES

Williams, P. F., and Menelaus, M. B.: Triple arthrodesis by inlay grafting—a method suitable for the undeformed or valgus foot. J. Bone Joint Surg., 59-B:333, 1977.

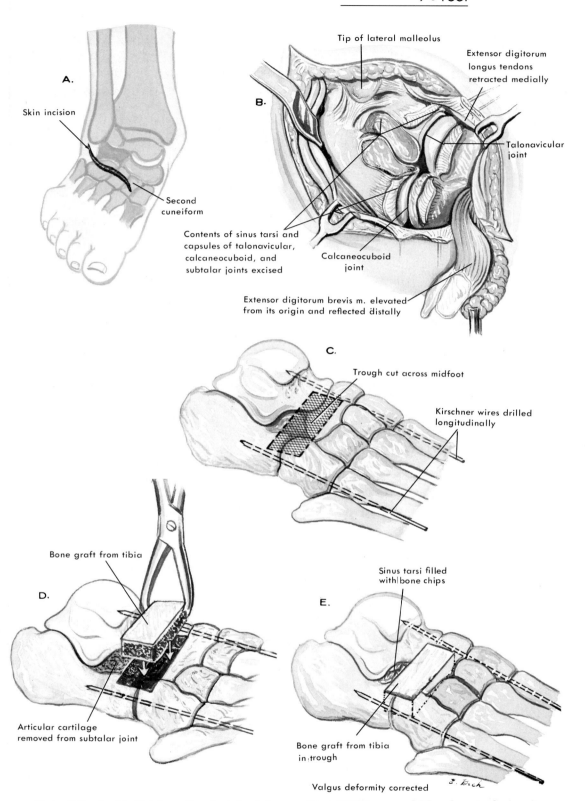

A.

Skin incision

Second cuneiform

B.

Tip of lateral malleolus

Extensor digitorum longus tendons retracted medially

Talonavicular joint

Contents of sinus tarsi and capsules of talonavicular, calcaneocuboid, and subtalar joints excised

Calcaneocuboid joint

Extensor digitorum brevis m. elevated from its origin and reflected distally

C.

Trough cut across midfoot

Kirschner wires drilled longitudinally

D.

Bone graft from tibia

Articular cartilage removed from subtalar joint

E.

Sinus tarsi filled with bone chips

Bone graft from tibia in trough

Valgus deformity corrected

Plate 194. A.–E., Triple arthrodesis by inlay grafting (Williams and Menelaus technique).

PLATE 195 **Correction of Pes Calcaneus and Ankle Valgus by Resection of Dorsal Wedge from the Calcaneus and Posterosuperior Displacement Osteotomy of the Calcaneus: Achilles Tendon Shortening and Tenodesis of Lateral Half of Achilles Tendon to Distal Fibular Metaphysis**

Indications. Severe, fixed calcaneus deformity of the hindfoot with a trace or zero triceps surae motor strength. An ankle valgus deformity of more than 20 degrees.

Radiographic Control. Image intensifier.

Patient Position. Prone.

Operative Technique

A. and **B.** The superolateral surface of the calcaneus is exposed as follows: A 5- to 7-cm.-long oblique incision is made on the lateral aspect of the heel parallel to and 1 cm. posterior and inferior to the peroneus longus tendon (see Plate 198). The subcutaneous tissue is divided in line with the skin incision. With skin hooks, the wound flaps are retracted. The saphenous nerve is identified and kept out of harm's way. The peroneal tendons are retracted dorsally, the calcaneofibular ligament is sectioned, and the periosteum is incised on the lateral surface of the calcaneus in line with the skin incision. The lateral surface of the calcaneus is subperiosteally exposed, and Chandler retractors are introduced on the plantar and superior aspects of the calcaneus. Be sure that the Achilles tendon is protected by the elevator.

With sharp osteotomes, mark the line of the wedge osteotomy based superiorly and medially (the base of the medial wedge depends on the degree of heel valgus to be corrected). With an oscillating power saw, the wedge of bone is resected. If there is varus deformity, the base of the wedge is wider laterally.

C. and **D.** The heel is manipulated, and the calcaneal bone fragments are approximated, correcting the calcaneus and valgus or varus deformity of the heel. One or two threaded Steinmann pins are used for transfixing the osteotomized fragments.

E. and **F.** Next, correct the associated valgus of the ankle. A tenodesis of the Achilles tendon to the distal fibular metaphysis is performed when the triceps surae is zero in motor strength (see Plate 185).

The tourniquet is released, and complete hemostasis is achieved. A medium-sized Hemovac suction tube is placed.

The wound is closed in the usual fashion, and an above-knee cast is applied, pushing the heel up into dorsiflexion and the forefoot into maximal dorsiflexion. Be sure the forefoot is not in equinus.

Postoperative Care. The cast is removed in four weeks, and the threaded Steinmann pins are removed. Another below-knee cast is applied, and the patient is allowed weight-bearing. The cast is removed in two to three weeks, and passive and active exercises are performed to restore range of motion of the ankle, subtalar, and midfoot. Orthotic support is provided, the type and extent depending on the severity and pattern of motor paralysis.

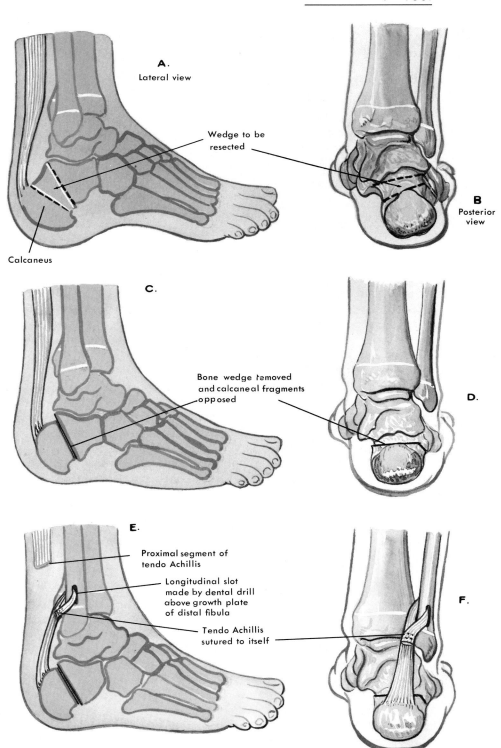

A. Lateral view

Wedge to be resected

Calcaneus

B Posterior view

C.

Bone wedge removed and calcaneal fragments opposed

D.

E.

Proximal segment of tendo Achillis

Longitudinal slot made by dental drill above growth plate of distal fibula

Tendo Achillis sutured to itself

F.

Plate 195. A.–F., Correction of pes calcaneus and ankle valgus by resection of dorsal wedge from the calcaneus and posterosuperior displacement osteotomy of the calcaneus; Achilles tendon shortening and tenodesis of the lateral half of the Achilles tendon to the distal fibular metaphysis.

PLATE 196 **Dwyer's Open-Up Medial Osteotomy of the Calcaneus with Bone Graft Wedge for Correction of Hindfoot Varus**

Indications. Hindfoot varus in a child eight years of age or older in whom the heel is small and short in height.

Disadvantages. Delayed wound healing, dehiscence, sloughing, and vascular compromise are serious problems of medial open-up osteotomy of the calcaneus. This author does not recommend this procedure for these reasons, but it is described in this atlas for the sake of completeness.

Radiographic Control. Image intensifier.

Patient Position. Supine with a sandbag under the ipsilateral hip.

Operative Technique

A. The skin incision begins at a point in the midline in the posterior prominence of the heel, along the skin creases, and extends distally to the anterior border of the insertion of the tendo Achillis; then it swings obliquely, dorsally, and distally to a point 2 cm. distal to the lower tip of the medial malleolus. This incision differs from that described by Dwyer; as the varus heel is corrected, the skin margins are pulled together rather than apart, thus preventing delayed wound healing and slough. The subcutaneous tissue is divided in line with the skin incision. The elevated wound flaps are retracted, and the plexus of veins is coagulated and divided to prevent bleeding later.

B. Next, the medial one third to one half of the insertion of the Achilles tendon to the calcaneus is sectioned. The laciniate ligament is divided near its insertion to the os calcis, at least 2.5 cm. inferior to the flexor hallucis longus tendon and neurovascular bundle. The medial surface of the calcaneus is subperiosteally exposed. The line of incision in the periosteum is 1.5 cm. inferior and in line with the flexor hallucis longus tendon. Avoid injury to the neurovascular structures. Chandler elevator retractors are used to partially expose the superior and inferior aspects of the calcaneus.

C.–E. With a wide osteotome, the calcaneus is sectioned just inferior to the flexor hallucis longus tendon. The lateral cortex of the calcaneus is left intact; however, its medial, inferior, and superior aspects should be completely divided.

With periosteal elevators and a laminectomy spreader, the site of the osteotomy is opened. The width of the bone graft wedge is determined by inserting osteotomes of various sizes between the fragments. An appropriate bone graft wedge is taken from the ilium and, with its base medially, is placed in the gap in the calcaneus. The author finds that bone grafts from the upper end of the tibia are usually inadequate and not sturdy enough. The tension of the tissues firmly holds the bone graft in position; ordinarily, internal fixation is not required. Radiograms are made in the operating room to ensure that the varus deformity of the hindfoot is corrected. The tourniquet is released and complete hemostasis is achieved. A small Hemovac suction tube is inserted for drainage. The wound is closed in the usual fashion. The skin is closed with interrupted sutures, and an above-knee cast is applied, holding the foot–ankle in neutral position and the knee in 30 to 45 degrees of flexion.

Postoperative Care. The cast and sutures are removed in two to three weeks, and a new above-knee cast is applied. Approximately ten weeks is required for the bone graft to consolidate. Early weight-bearing will result in collapse of the graft and loss of correction. The importance of protecting the foot until the bone graft is fully incorporated cannot be overemphasized.

REFERENCES

Dwyer, F. C.: The treatment of relapsed clubfoot by the insertion of a wedge into the calcaneum. J. Bone Joint Surg., 45-B:67, 1963.

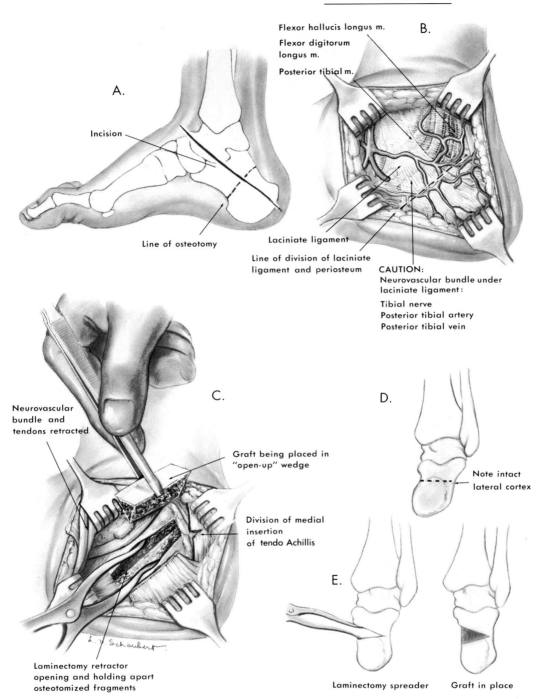

A.

Incision

Line of osteotomy

B.

Flexor hallucis longus m.

Flexor digitorum longus m.

Posterior tibial m.

Laciniate ligament

Line of division of laciniate ligament and periosteum

CAUTION:
Neurovascular bundle under laciniate ligament:

Tibial nerve
Posterior tibial artery
Posterior tibial vein

C.

Neurovascular bundle and tendons retracted

Graft being placed in "open-up" wedge

Division of medial insertion of tendo Achillis

Laminectomy retractor opening and holding apart osteotomized fragments

D.

Note intact lateral cortex

E.

Laminectomy spreader   Graft in place

Plate 196. A.–E., Dwyer's open-up medial osteotomy of the calcaneus with bone graft wedge for correction of hindfoot varus.

PLATE 197 **Dwyer's Lateral Wedge Resection of the Calcaneus for Correction of Hindfoot Varus**

Indications. Fixed varus deformity of the heel in the skeletally mature foot.

Close-up lateral wedge resection of the os calcis is designed to correct fixed varus deformity of the hindfoot in which the heel is of adequate height and size and the foot is skeletally mature.

Operative Technique

A. A 5-cm.-long oblique incision is made on the lateral aspect of the calcaneus parallel to, but 1.5 cm. posterior and inferior to, the peroneus longus tendon. The subcutaneous tissue is divided, and the wound flaps are retracted.

B. and **C.** The peroneal tendons are identified and retracted dorsally and distally. The periosteum is incised. The lateral surface of the calcaneus is subperiosteally exposed. Chandler elevator retractors are inserted subperiosteally on the posterosuperior aspect of the calcaneus and another Chandler retractor is inserted on its plantar aspect to protect the soft tissues. With a pair of sharp osteotomes of adequate width and an oscillating saw, a wedge of the os calcis with its base directed laterally is excised. The site of osteotomy is immediately inferior and posterior to the peroneus longus tendon. The medial cortex should be left intact. The width of the base of the wedge depends on the severity of the varus deformity of the heel.

D. Next, a Steinmann pin is inserted transversely across the posterior segment of the calcaneus. The forefoot is dorsiflexed, putting tension on the Achilles tendon, and, with the Steinmann pin serving as a lever, the bone gap is closed. The heel should be in 5 degrees of valgus. A large threaded Steinmann pin is inserted obliquely from the posteroplantar aspect of the os calcis across the calcaneal fragments and exits through the skin over the intermediate cuneiform bone. Radiograms are made, the transverse pin is removed, and the Steinmann pin transfixing the calcaneal fragments is cut subcutaneously at the calcaneus posteriorly and left protruding 1 cm. through the skin on the dorsum of the midfoot. The wound is closed, and an above-knee cast is applied. The knee is in 45 degrees of flexion.

Postoperative Care. The cast, pin, and sutures are removed in three to four weeks. A below-knee walking cast is applied for an additional two weeks, by which time the osteotomy should be healed.

REFERENCES

Dwyer, F. C.: Osteotomy of the calcaneum for pes cavus. J. Bone Joint Surg., 41-B:80, 1959.

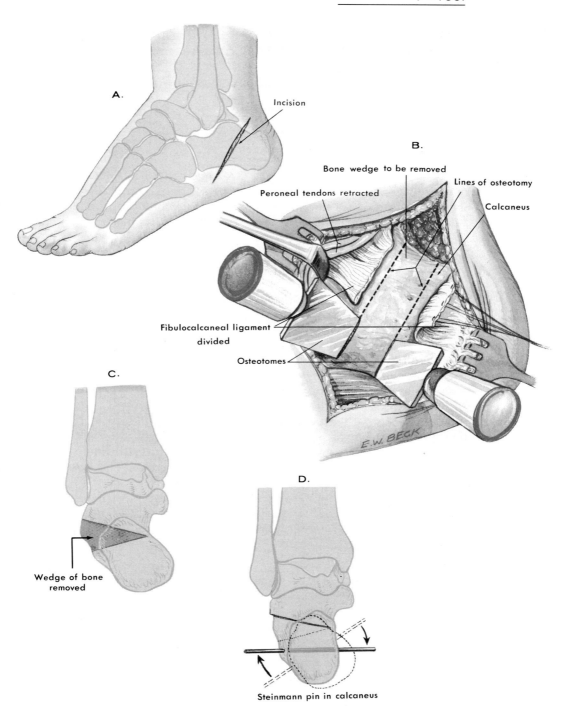

A.

Incision

B.

Bone wedge to be removed

Peroneal tendons retracted

Lines of osteotomy

Calcaneus

Fibulocalcaneal ligament
divided

Osteotomes

E.W. BECK

C.

Wedge of bone
removed

D.

Steinmann pin in calcaneus

Plate 197. **A.–D.,** Dwyer's lateral wedge resection of the calcaneus for correction of hindfoot varus.

PLATE 198 **Posterior and Superior Displacement Osteotomy of the Os Calcis for Correction of Pes Calcaneocavus**

Indications. Fixed calcaneus deformity of the hindfoot.

Radiographic Control. Image intensifier.

Patient Position. Prone. It can be performed in supine position.

Operative Technique

A. The entire lower limb is prepared and draped in the usual manner, and the operation is performed using tourniquet ischemia. An oblique lateral incision is made over the body of the calcaneus immediately plantar or inferior to the peroneal tendons and the subtalar joint. The upper end of the incision is 3 cm. posterior to its plantar end.

B. The subcutaneous tissue is divided in line with the skin incision. First, an extensive plantar release is performed. This is vital; otherwise, an adequate backward and upward displacement of the posterior segment of the calcaneus is not feasible. Mitchell uses a medial horizontal incision. This author carries out the plantar release as follows: the plantar fascia, abductor digiti quinti, and lateral part of the short plantar muscles are divided with scissors through the lateral incision. If one stays close to bone, this maneuver is relatively safe and neurovascular injury is avoided.

C. An alternative approach for plantar release is through a midline longitudinal plantar incision, 5 cm. long, made on the plantar aspect of the foot, in line with the second ray.

D. and E. With a periosteal elevator, the plantar fascia and short plantar muscles are stripped from the tuberosity of the calcaneus and elevated forward.

The short and long plantar ligaments, the plantar calcaneonavicular ligament, and the capsule of the calcaneocuboid joint are divided. The foot is manipulated to correct the cavus deformity as much as possible.

At this time, the lateral and plantar wounds are packed with hot, moist sponges and the tourniquet is released. In a few minutes, the packing is removed and the wounds are thoroughly inspected for bleeding. After complete hemostasis, the tourniquet is reinflated.

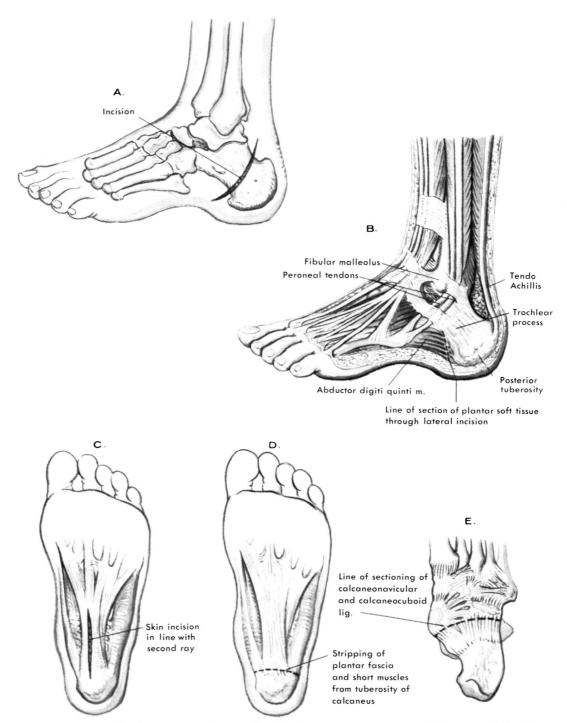

A.

Incision

B.

Fibular malleolus

Peroneal tendons

Tendo Achillis

Trochlear process

Abductor digiti quinti m.

Posterior tuberosity

Line of section of plantar soft tissue through lateral incision

C.

Skin incision in line with second ray

D.

Stripping of plantar fascia and short muscles from tuberosity of calcaneus

E.

Line of sectioning of calcaneonavicular and calcaneocuboid lig.

Plate 198. A.–N., Posterior and superior displacement osteotomy of the os calcis for correction of pes calcaneocavus.

F.–J. The lateral surface of the body of the calcaneus is exposed. The calcaneofibular ligament is sectioned and retracted. The peroneal tendons are pulled forward as far as possible, but there is no need to elevate them from their groove. Chandler elevators are placed on the superior and plantar surfaces of the calcaneus. The line of osteotomy is marked with multiple drill holes. Samilson makes a crescentic osteotomy (see **I.**, **J.**, and **K.**), whereas Mitchell's osteotomy is oblique transverse, inclining forward and plantarward (see **L.** and **M.**).

With an electric bone saw or a large, curved, sharp osteotome, the osteotomy is made.

K. A threaded Steinmann pin is inserted through the skin into the center of the apophysis of the calcaneus and the posterior bone segment. By manipulation and by using the Steinmann pin as a lever, the posterior fragment is displaced backward and upward, reducing the calcaneocavus deformity. The degree of correction obtained is checked on stress-lateral radiograms of the foot. The calcaneal pitch should be 10 to 20 degrees. (The calcaneal pitch is the angle formed between the sole line—joining the plantar aspects of the metatarsal heads and the calcaneal tuberosity—and the plantar calcaneal line—drawn between the posterior and anterior calcaneal tuberosities.) If correction is satisfactory, the Steinmann pin is drilled into the anterior part of the os calcis, transfixing the osteotomized bones securely. This author prefers that the threaded Steinmann pin exit through the skin over the dorsolateral aspect of the midfoot and remain subcutaneous or flush with the calcaneus posteriorly.

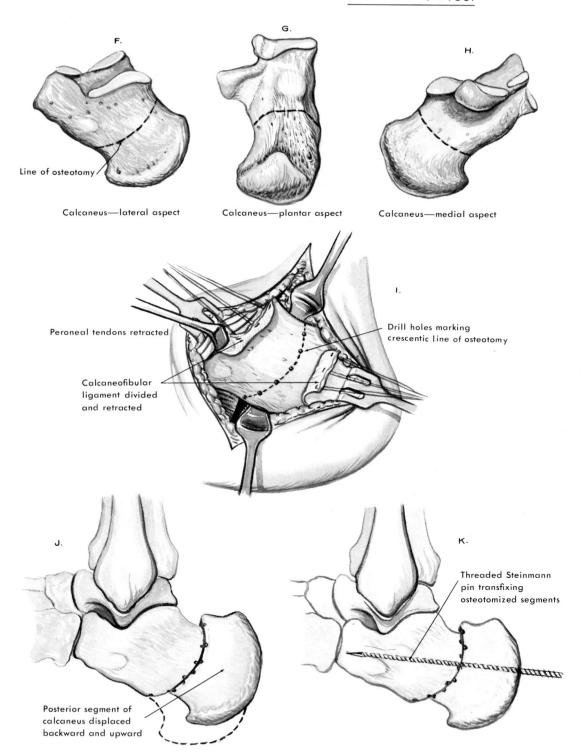

F.

G.

H.

Line of osteotomy

Calcaneus—lateral aspect

Calcaneus—plantar aspect

Calcaneus—medial aspect

I.

Peroneal tendons retracted

Drill holes marking
crescentic line of osteotomy

Calcaneofibular
ligament divided
and retracted

J.

K.

Threaded Steinmann
pin transfixing
osteotomized segments

Posterior segment of
calcaneus displaced
backward and upward

Plate 198. (Continued)

Oblique Transverse Osteotomy According to the Technique of Mitchell

L.–N. The line of osteotomy from the superior part inclines downward and forward. Drill holes are not made in the soft cancellous bone. The osteotomy is performed with a wide, straight osteotome. The foot is manipulated; with the leverage of the Steinmann pin, the posterior fragment is displaced backward and upward. This is easily done if all plantar soft tissues attached to the posterior tuberosity of the calcaneus are divided.

The wound is closed in the usual manner. A below-knee cast is applied, incorporating the pin in the cast. I prefer an above-knee cast with the knee flexed 45 degrees and do not recommend incorporation of the pin in the cast.

Postoperative Care. Weight-bearing is not allowed for three to four weeks, at which time the first cast and pin are removed. A new below-knee walking cast is applied for another two to three weeks. Weight-bearing is then permitted.

REFERENCES

Mitchell, G. P.: Posterior displacement osteotomy of the calcaneus. J. Bone Joint Surg., 59-B:233, 1977.
Samilson, R. L.: Crescentic osteotomy of the os calcis for calcaneocavus feet. In: Bateman, J. E. (ed.): Foot Science. Philadelphia, W. B. Saunders Co., 1976, pp. 18–25.

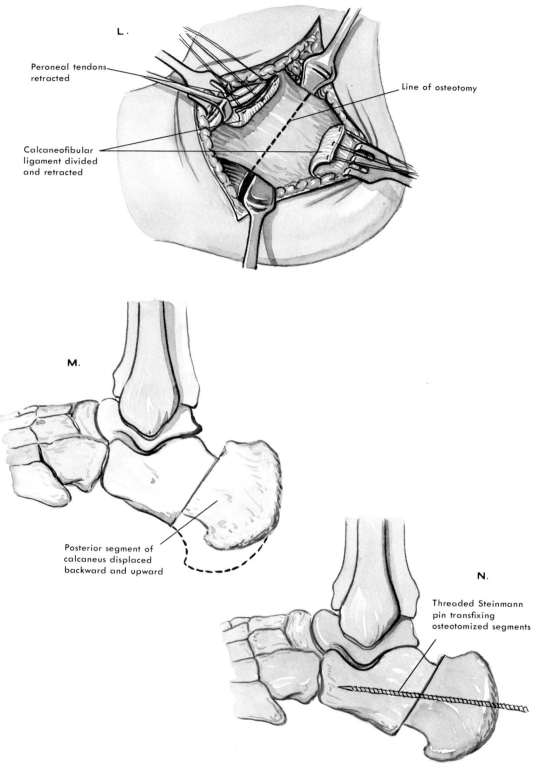

L.

Peroneal tendons retracted

Line of osteotomy

Calcaneofibular ligament divided and retracted

M.

Posterior segment of calcaneus displaced backward and upward

N.

Threaded Steinmann pin transfixing osteotomized segments

Plate 198. (Continued)

PLATE 199 **Fasciotomy of the Foot for Decompression in Compartment Syndrome**

Indications. Acute compartment syndrome with increased tissue pressure and compromise of circulation and viability of the contents in the compartments of the foot. Causes are crush injury of the foot, fractures and fracture dislocation of the forefoot or midfoot, and following routine surgery of the foot, such as osteotomy of the metatarsals and tarsal bones for correction of deformities with or without the use of internal fixators.

Patient Position. Supine.

Operative Treatment. Prior to treatment of compartment syndrome of the foot, it is essential to have a detailed knowledge of the anatomy of the foot, particularly its plantar aspect from skin to bone. According to Henry, the muscles in the plantar aspect of the foot can be grouped in four layers.

A. and B. *Layer I* consists of a triad of muscles: (1) abductor hallucis, (2) flexor digitorum brevis, and (3) abductor digiti quinti.

A.

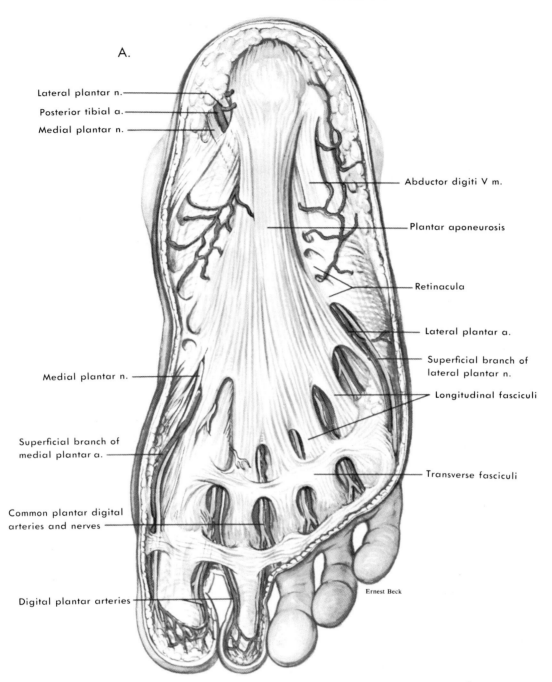

Lateral plantar n.

Posterior tibial a.

Medial plantar n.

Abductor digiti V m.

Plantar aponeurosis

Retinacula

Lateral plantar a.

Superficial branch of
lateral plantar n.

Medial plantar n.

Longitudinal fasciculi

Superficial branch of
medial plantar a.

Transverse fasciculi

Common plantar digital
arteries and nerves

Digital plantar arteries

Ernest Beck

Plate 199. A.–Q., Fasciotomy of the foot for decompression in compartment syndrome.
    A. and **B.,** Layer I.
    C., Dissection of plantar aspect of right foot.
    D., Second layer of plantar muscles of right foot.
    E., Third layer of plantar muscles.
    F., Deep dissection of the plantar aspect of the right foot.
    G., Ligaments on the plantar aspect of the right foot.
    H., Cross section of the right foot.

A. and **B.** *Layer I* consists of a triad of muscles: (1) abductor hallucis, (2) flexor digitorum brevis, and (3) abductor digiti quinti.

B.

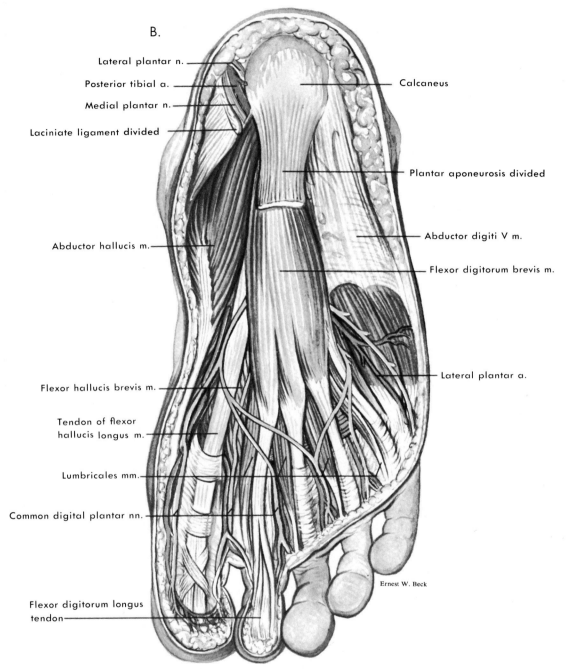

Lateral plantar n.

Posterior tibial a.

Medial plantar n.

Laciniate ligament divided

Calcaneus

Plantar aponeurosis divided

Abductor hallucis m.

Abductor digiti V m.

Flexor digitorum brevis m.

Flexor hallucis brevis m.

Tendon of flexor hallucis longus m.

Lumbricales mm.

Lateral plantar a.

Common digital plantar nn.

Flexor digitorum longus tendon

Ernest W. Beck

Plate 199. (Continued)

C. and **D.** *Layer II* (a tetrad) is composed of two long tendons—(1) flexor hallucis longus and (2) flexor digitorum longus—and two short muscles—(3) quadratus plantae and (4) lumbricals.

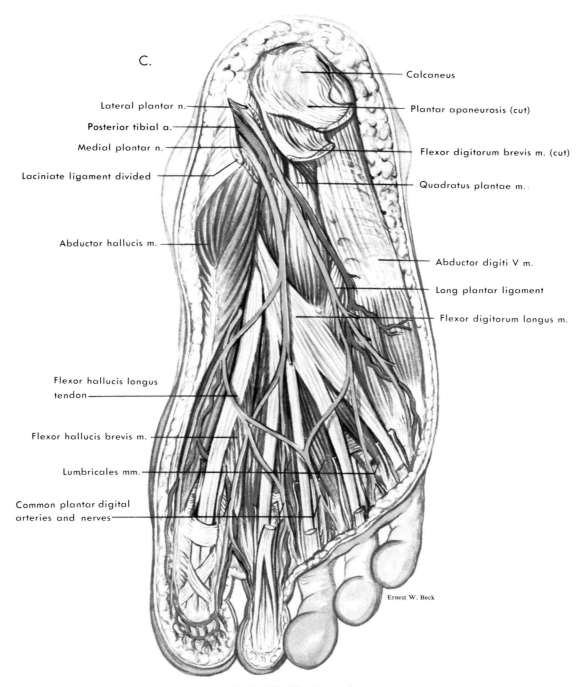

C.

Lateral plantar n.

Posterior tibial a.

Medial plantar n.

Laciniate ligament divided

Abductor hallucis m.

Flexor hallucis longus tendon

Flexor hallucis brevis m.

Lumbricales mm.

Common plantar digital arteries and nerves

Calcaneus

Plantar aponeurosis (cut)

Flexor digitorum brevis m. (cut)

Quadratus plantae m.

Abductor digiti V m.

Long plantar ligament

Flexor digitorum longus m.

Ernest W. Beck

Plate 199. (Continued)

C. and **D.** *Layer II* (a tetrad) is composed of two long tendons—(1) flexor hallucis longus and (2) flexor digitorum longus—and two short muscles—(3) quadratus plantae and (4) lumbricals.

D.

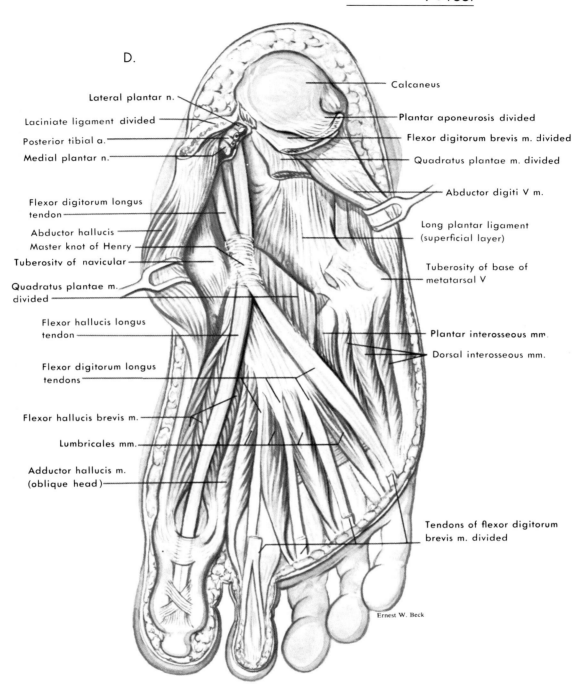

Lateral plantar n.

Laciniate ligament divided

Posterior tibial a.

Medial plantar n.

Flexor digitorum longus tendon

Abductor hallucis

Master knot of Henry

Tuberosity of navicular

Quadratus plantae m. divided

Flexor hallucis longus tendon

Flexor digitorum longus tendons

Flexor hallucis brevis m.

Lumbricales mm.

Adductor hallucis m. (oblique head)

Calcaneus

Plantar aponeurosis divided

Flexor digitorum brevis m. divided

Quadratus plantae m. divided

Abductor digiti V m.

Long plantar ligament (superficial layer)

Tuberosity of base of metatarsal V

Plantar interosseous mm.

Dorsal interosseous mm.

Tendons of flexor digitorum brevis m. divided

Ernest W. Beck

Plate 199. (Continued)

E. *Layer III* consists of a triad of muscles: (1) flexor hallucis brevis, (2) adductor hallucis, and (3) flexor digiti minimus.

E.

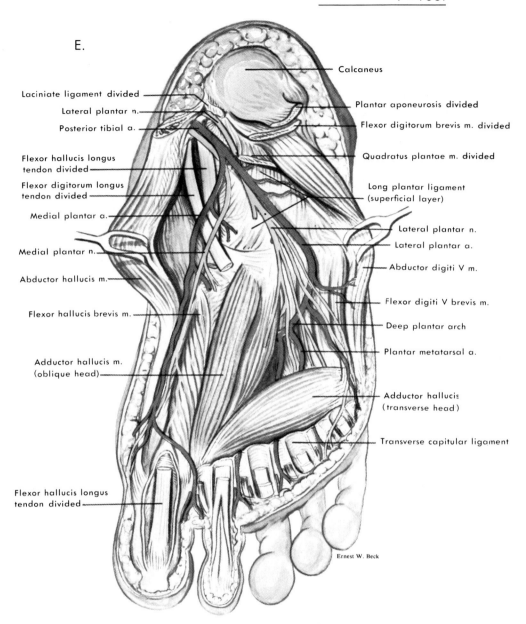

Calcaneus

Laciniate ligament divided

Lateral plantar n.

Posterior tibial a.

Plantar aponeurosis divided

Flexor digitorum brevis m. divided

Flexor hallucis longus
tendon divided

Flexor digitorum longus
tendon divided

Quadratus plantae m. divided

Long plantar ligament
(superficial layer)

Medial plantar a.

Lateral plantar n.

Medial plantar n.

Lateral plantar a.

Abductor hallucis m.

Abductor digiti V m.

Flexor hallucis brevis m.

Flexor digiti V brevis m.

Deep plantar arch

Adductor hallucis m.
(oblique head)

Plantar metatarsal a.

Adductor hallucis
(transverse head)

Transverse capitular ligament

Flexor hallucis longus
tendon divided

Ernest W. Beck

Plate 199. (Continued)

F. and **G.** *Layer IV* is composed of the long tendons of the peroneus longus and tibialis posterior and the interossei.

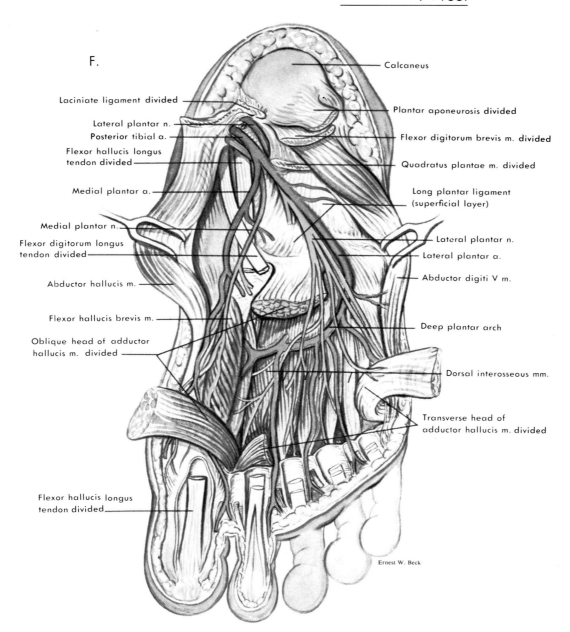

F.

Laciniate ligament divided

Lateral plantar n.

Posterior tibial a.

Flexor hallucis longus tendon divided

Medial plantar a.

Medial plantar n.

Flexor digitorum longus tendon divided

Abductor hallucis m.

Flexor hallucis brevis m.

Oblique head of adductor hallucis m. divided

Flexor hallucis longus tendon divided

Calcaneus

Plantar aponeurosis divided

Flexor digitorum brevis m. divided

Quadratus plantae m. divided

Long plantar ligament (superficial layer)

Lateral plantar n.

Lateral plantar a.

Abductor digiti V m.

Deep plantar arch

Dorsal interosseous mm.

Transverse head of adductor hallucis m. divided

Ernest W. Beck

Plate 199. (Continued)

F. and **G.** *Layer IV* is composed of the long tendons of the peroneus longus and tibialis posterior and the interossei.

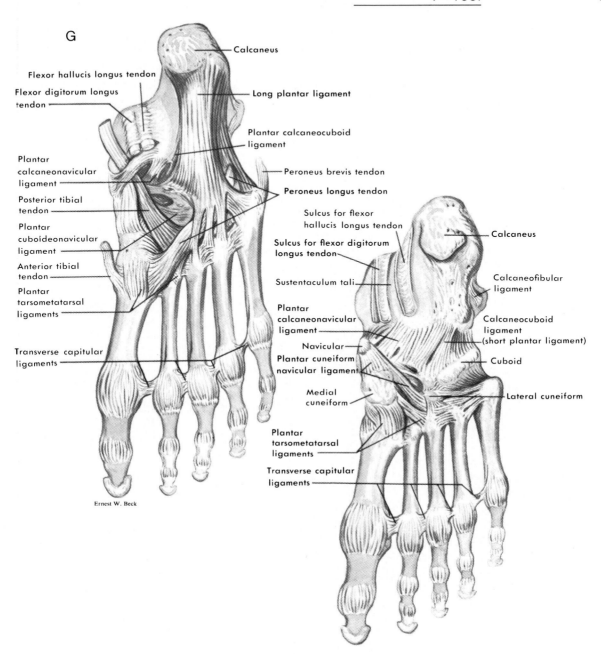

G

Flexor hallucis longus tendon
Flexor digitorum longus tendon
Calcaneus
Long plantar ligament
Plantar calcaneocuboid ligament
Plantar calcaneonavicular ligament
Posterior tibial tendon
Plantar cuboideonavicular ligament
Anterior tibial tendon
Plantar tarsometatarsal ligaments
Transverse capitular ligaments
Peroneus brevis tendon
Peroneus longus tendon
Sulcus for flexor hallucis longus tendon
Sulcus for flexor digitorum longus tendon
Sustentaculum tali
Plantar calcaneonavicular ligament
Navicular
Plantar cuneiform navicular ligament
Medial cuneiform
Plantar tarsometatarsal ligaments
Transverse capitular ligaments
Calcaneus
Calcaneofibular ligament
Calcaneocuboid ligament (short plantar ligament)
Cuboid
Lateral cuneiform

Ernest W. Beck

Plate 199. (Continued)

H. A cross section of the right foot at various levels: at Chopart's joint, at Lisfranc's joint, at the midtarsal joint, and at the metatarsophalangeal joints.

H.

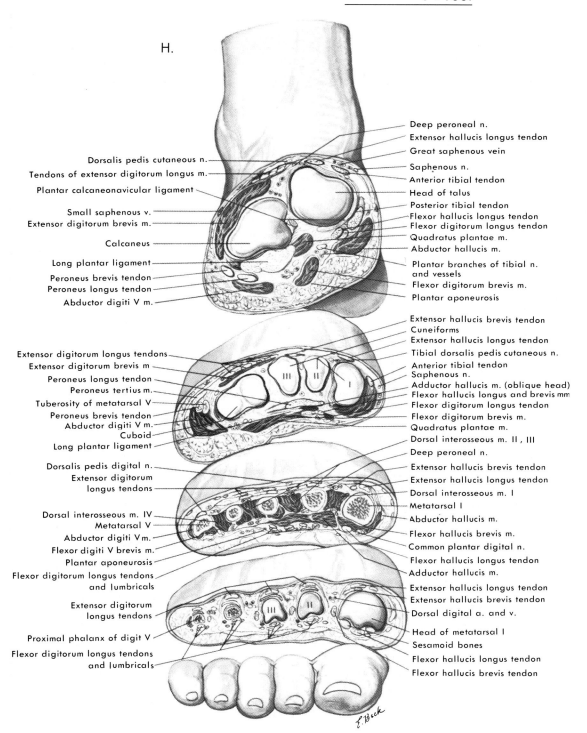

Dorsalis pedis cutaneous n.
Tendons of extensor digitorum longus m.
Plantar calcaneonavicular ligament
Small saphenous v.
Extensor digitorum brevis m.
Calcaneus
Long plantar ligament
Peroneus brevis tendon
Peroneus longus tendon
Abductor digiti V m.

Deep peroneal n.
Extensor hallucis longus tendon
Great saphenous vein
Saphenous n.
Anterior tibial tendon
Head of talus
Posterior tibial tendon
Flexor hallucis longus tendon
Flexor digitorum longus tendon
Quadratus plantae m.
Abductor hallucis m.
Plantar branches of tibial n. and vessels
Flexor digitorum brevis m.
Plantar aponeurosis

Extensor digitorum longus tendons
Extensor digitorum brevis m
Peroneus longus tendon
Peroneus tertius m.
Tuberosity of metatarsal V
Peroneus brevis tendon
Abductor digiti V m.
Cuboid
Long plantar ligament

Extensor hallucis brevis tendon
Cuneiforms
Extensor hallucis longus tendon
Tibial dorsalis pedis cutaneous n.
Anterior tibial tendon
Saphenous n.
Adductor hallucis m. (oblique head)
Flexor hallucis longus and brevis mm
Flexor digitorum longus tendon
Flexor digitorum brevis m.
Quadratus plantae m.
Dorsal interosseous m. II, III
Deep peroneal n.

Dorsalis pedis digital n.
Extensor digitorum longus tendons

Dorsal interosseous m. IV
Metatarsal V
Abductor digiti V m.
Flexor digiti V brevis m.
Plantar aponeurosis
Flexor digitorum longus tendons and lumbricals

Extensor digitorum longus tendons

Proximal phalanx of digit V

Flexor digitorum longus tendons and lumbricals

Extensor hallucis brevis tendon
Extensor hallucis longus tendon
Dorsal interosseous m. I
Metatarsal I
Abductor hallucis m.
Flexor hallucis brevis m.
Common plantar digital n.
Flexor hallucis longus tendon
Adductor hallucis m.

Extensor hallucis longus tendon
Extensor hallucis brevis tendon
Dorsal digital a. and v.

Head of metatarsal I
Sesamoid bones
Flexor hallucis longus tendon
Flexor hallucis brevis tendon

E. Beck

Plate 199. (Continued)

I. The foot can be divided into four separate compartments, according to Mubarak, Hargens, and Shereff:

1. The *medial compartment* is bounded dorsally by the inferior surface of the first metatarsal, medially and inferiorly by the plantar aponeurosis, and laterally by the medial intermuscular septum. It contains the (a) abductor hallucis muscle, (b) flexor hallucis muscle, and (c) flexor hallucis longus tendon. The medial compartment also contains the insertion of the tendons of peroneus longus and posterior tibial.

2. The *central compartment* is bounded dorsally by the interosseous fascia, inferiorly by the plantar aponeurosis, and medially and laterally by distinct intermuscular septa. The contents of the central compartment from plantar to dorsal are (a) flexor digitorum brevis, (b) flexor digitorum longus tendon, (c) lumbrical muscles, and (d) adductor hallucis. The tendon of peroneus longus and posterior tibial traverse this compartment.

3. The *lateral compartment* is bounded by the fifth metatarsal shaft dorsally, the lateral intermuscular septum medially, and the plantar aponeurosis and its dorsolateral extension inferiorly and laterally. It contains the abductor digiti quinti, the flexor digitorum brevis muscle to the fifth toe, and the opponens digiti quinti.

4. The *interosseous compartment* is bounded dorsally by the metatarsals and dorsal interosseous fascia, medially by the lateral aspect of the first metatarsal shaft, laterally by the medial aspect of the fifth metatarsal shaft and intermuscular septum, and inferiorly by the plantar interosseous fascia. The interosseous compartment contains the dorsal and plantar interossei and the plantar arterial arches and digital nerves.

The compartments of the foot can be decompressed either by Henry's medial approach to the foot, which utilizes a single incision to decompress all four compartments and is indicated when compartment syndrome of the foot is not associated with fractures; or through a double dorsal incision, recommended when compartment syndrome of the foot is associated with fractures of the metatarsals and tarsal bones and when internal fixation of the fracture or fracture-dislocation is indicated. The dorsal approach is technically simpler than the medial approach.

Decompression Through Henry's Plantar Medial Approach

J. The foot is positioned on its lateral border with the knee flexed 45 to 60 degrees. A curvilinear incision is made beginning at the medial aspect of the first metatarsal head and extending proximally and posteriorly toward the tuberosity of the navicular and the calcaneus 2 cm. distal to the tip of the medial malleolus. The subcutaneous tissue is divided along the skin incision.

K. The medial extension of the plantar aponeurosis and fascia over the abductor hallucis and flexor digitorum brevis is divided longitudinally throughout its extent, thereby decompressing the medial compartment.

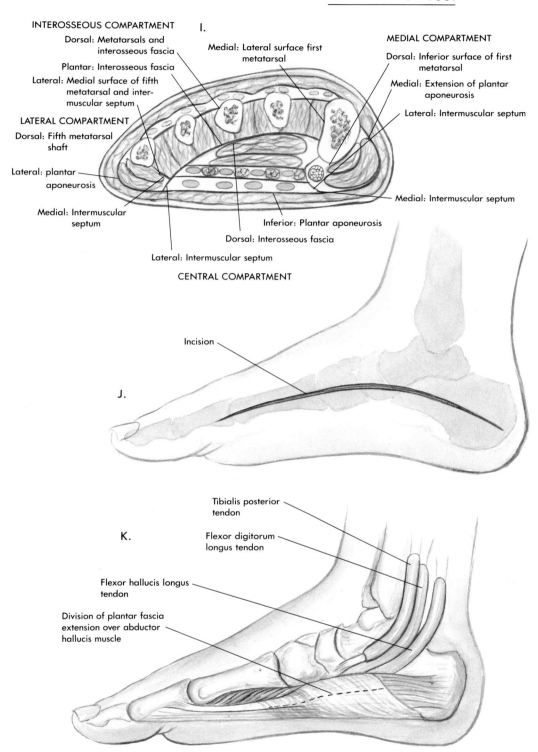

INTEROSSEOUS COMPARTMENT
Dorsal: Metatarsals and interosseous fascia
Plantar: Interosseous fascia
Lateral: Medial surface of fifth metatarsal and intermuscular septum

I.

Medial: Lateral surface first metatarsal

MEDIAL COMPARTMENT
Dorsal: Inferior surface of first metatarsal
Medial: Extension of plantar aponeurosis
Lateral: Intermuscular septum

LATERAL COMPARTMENT
Dorsal: Fifth metatarsal shaft
Lateral: plantar aponeurosis
Medial: Intermuscular septum

Medial: Intermuscular septum

Lateral: Intermuscular septum

Inferior: Plantar aponeurosis

Dorsal: Interosseous fascia

CENTRAL COMPARTMENT

J.

Incision

K.

Tibialis posterior tendon

Flexor digitorum longus tendon

Flexor hallucis longus tendon

Division of plantar fascia extension over abductor hallucis muscle

Plate 199. (Continued)

L. and **M.** Decompress the central compartment by dividing the intermuscular septa medially and laterally and the interosseous fascia dorsally.

Detach the abductor hallucis from its origin, and elevate and reflect it with the flexor digitorum brevis muscle plantarward. Incise the plantar interosseous fascia dorsal to the quadratus plantae muscle to decompress the interosseous compartment. Deepen the interval between the quadratus plantae muscle and lumbricals and make a second incision in the interosseus fascia.

N. By blunt dissection, develop the plane between the lumbrical muscles and the flexor digitorum brevis and incise the lateral intermuscular septum, thereby decompressing the lateral compartment.

The wound is thoroughly irrigated with normal saline and left open with Xeroform dressings.

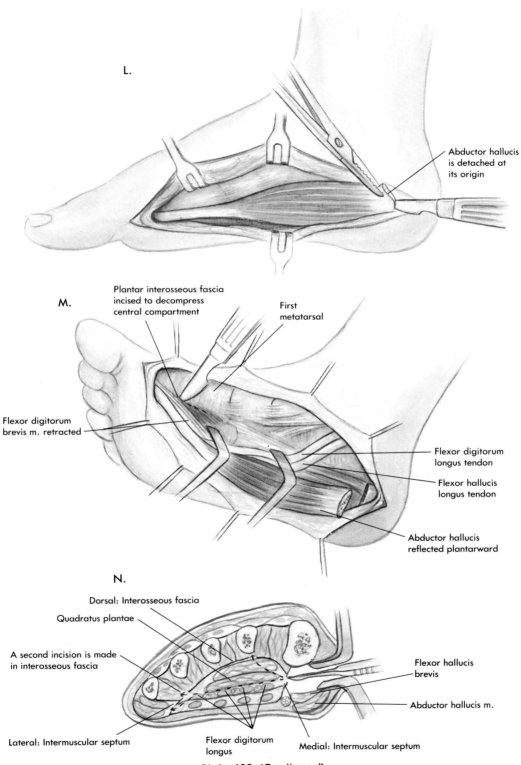

L.

Abductor hallucis is detached at its origin

M.

Plantar interosseous fascia incised to decompress central compartment

First metatarsal

Flexor digitorum brevis m. retracted

Flexor digitorum longus tendon

Flexor hallucis longus tendon

Abductor hallucis reflected plantarward

N.

Dorsal: Interosseous fascia

Quadratus plantae

A second incision is made in interosseous fascia

Flexor hallucis brevis

Abductor hallucis m.

Lateral: Intermuscular septum

Flexor digitorum longus

Medial: Intermuscular septum

Plate 199. (Continued)

Decompression Through Two Longitudinal Dorsal Incisions

O. Make two longitudinal incisions over the dorsum of the foot, one centered between the first and second metatarsals and the other over the lateral border of the fourth metatarsal. The incisions begin distally at the head of the metatarsals and terminate proximally at the metatarsocuneiform joint. The subcutaneous tissue is divided in line with the skin incision.

P. The wound flaps are retracted on either side with the extensor longus and brevis tendons and the digital vessels and nerves. The dorsal interosseous fascia is incised between the first and second metatarsals and also between the third and fourth metatarsals.

Q. By blunt dissection, the plantar interosseous fascia is exposed on either side of the metatarsals. Begin the dissection distally near the web between the base of the digits and then proceed proximally. Divide the interosseous fascia in the first web space, continue the dissection medially, and incise the intermuscular septum to decompress the *medial compartment*.

The *central compartment* is decompressed by incising the plantar interosseous fascia and intermuscular septum between the second and third metatarsals.

The *lateral compartment* is decompressed by dividing the intermuscular septum plantar to the fifth metatarsal.

The wounds are left open, and a sterile dressing is applied.

Postoperative Care. Following decompression, there should be dramatic relief of pain. Passive dorsiflexion and plantar flexion of the toes will become painless. The degree of return of motor and sensory function depends on the extent of damage to muscles and nerves.

The dressings are changed daily for five to seven days. Antibiotics are given to prevent infection. A split-thickness graft is applied whenever the tissues appear healthy.

Physical therapy in the form of gentle passive and active exercises is performed several times a day. The foot and leg are elevated. Ambulation is allowed when local swelling and wound conditions permit, initially non–weight-bearing and then gradually progressing to partial weight-bearing with three-point crutch gait and to full weight-bearing.

REFERENCES

Bonutti, P. M., and Bell, G. R.: Compartment syndrome of the foot. A case report. J. Bone Joint Surg., 68-A:1449, 1986.

Grodinsky, M.: A study of the fascial spaces of the foot and their bearing on infections. Surg. Gynecol. Obstet., 49:737, 1929.

Henry, A. K.: Extensile Exposures, 2nd ed. Baltimore, Williams & Wilkins, 1957, p. 300.

Mubarak, S. J., and Hargens, A. R.: Compartment Syndromes and Volkmann's Contracture. Philadelphia, W. B. Saunders Co., 1981, pp. 147–165.

Myerson, M.: Acute compartment syndromes of the foot. Bull. Hosp. Joint Dis. Orthop. Inst., 47:251, 1987.

Myerson, M. S.: Experimental decompression of the fascial compartments of the foot: The basis for fasciotomy in acute compartment syndrome. Foot Ankle, 8:308, 1988.

Sarrafian, S. K.: Anatomy of the Foot and Ankle. Philadelphia, J. B. Lippincott, 1983.

Shereff, M.: Compartment syndromes of the foot. A.A.O.S. Instructional Course Lectures, 39:127, 1990.

O.

DORSAL APPROACH

P.

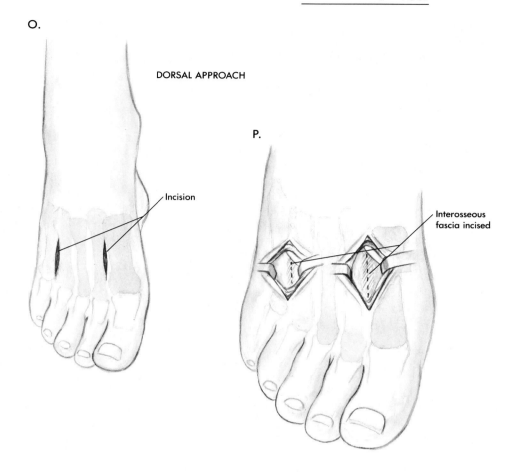

Incision

Interosseous
fascia incised

CROSS SECTION

Q.

Blunt dissection of
interosseous fascia

Interosseus m.

Dorsal interosseous fascia

Plantar interosseous fascia

Adductor hallucis m.

Flexor hallucis brevis m.

Abductor hallucis m.

Medial
intermuscular
septum

Intermuscular septum

Quadratus plantae m.

Abductor digiti
minimi m.

Flexor digiti
minimi brevis m.

Flexor digitorum
brevis m.

Flexor digitorum longus m.

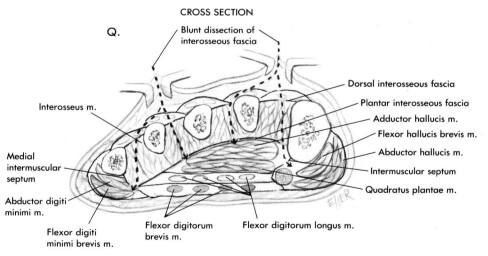

Plate 199. (Continued)

PLATE 200   ## Medial Displacement Osteotomy of the Calcaneus for Severe, Flexible Pes Planovalgus

Indications. Severe hindfoot valgus causing pain and difficulty with walking and shoe wear.

Radiographic Control. Image intensifier.

Patient Position. Preferably prone; it can be performed supine.

Operative Technique

A. In the normal foot, the biomechanical axis of weight-bearing forces of the body is transmitted through the talus into the center of the calcaneus.

B. In flexible pes planovalgus, the line along which body weight is transmitted through the talus passes medial to the calcaneus.

C. The objective of the operation is to displace the posterior part of the calcaneus medially, thereby restoring the normal weight-bearing mechanical line.

Medial Displacement Osteotomy of the Calcaneus for Treatment of Hindfoot Valgus in Severe Pes Planovalgus

D. The patient is placed in prone position with the knee flexed 30 to 45 degrees by a sterile sandbag under the lower leg. An oblique incision is made on the lateral aspect of the body of the calcaneus, parallel and immediately posterior to the peroneal tendons. It extends proximally from the lateral margin of the tendo Achillis to the plantar aspect of the heel, terminating at the calcaneocuboid joint. The subcutaneous tissue is divided in line with the skin incision.

E. The wound margins are undermined, elevated, and held apart by self-retaining retractors. Avoid damage to the sural nerve. The peroneal tendons are identified, and the deep fascia is incised immediately posterior to the peroneal tendons. Ordinarily, it is not necessary to divide the sheath of the peroneal tendons. The superior and inferior peroneal retinaculi are sectioned near their attachment to the os calcis. Two Chandler elevator retractors are inserted, one on the superior and the other on the inferior surface of the os calcis, exposing its dorsal and lateral surfaces.

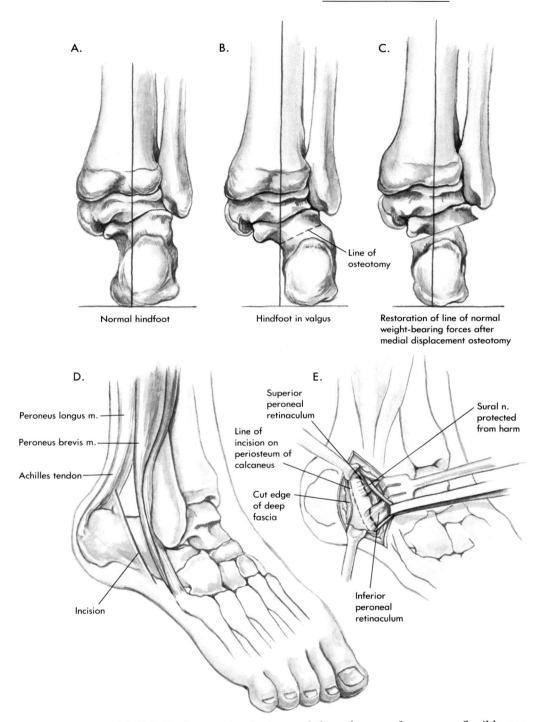

A. Normal hindfoot

B. Hindfoot in valgus — Line of osteotomy

C. Restoration of line of normal weight-bearing forces after medial displacement osteotomy

D.
Peroneus longus m.
Peroneus brevis m.
Achilles tendon
Incision

E.
Superior peroneal retinaculum
Line of incision on periosteum of calcaneus
Cut edge of deep fascia
Sural n. protected from harm
Inferior peroneal retinaculum

Plate 200. A.–I., Medial displacement osteotomy of the calcaneus for severe, flexible pes planovalgus.

F. The peroneal tendons are retracted anteriorly, and the periosteum is incised in line with the skin incision immediately posterior to the peroneal tendons. The incised periosteum on the lateral surface of the calcaneus is elevated anteriorly and posteriorly.

Do not violate the subtalar joint! The two Chandler elevator retractors are removed and replaced subperiosteally on the posterosuperior and inferolateral corners of the os calcis. Be sure to be anterior and deep to the Achilles tendon.

G. With a wide osteotome, mark the line of osteotomy. With an electric oscillating saw, the calcaneus is sectioned. Saw in and out and not sideways in order to prevent damage to neurovascular structures on the medial aspect of the calcaneus. The calcaneal segments are spread open, first with a wide osteotome and then with a large periosteal Cobb elevator. A laminectomy spreader may be used for adequate exposure if it is necessary to strip the periosteum on the medial aspect of the calcaneus. Sometimes the taut plantar soft tissues are sectioned to achieve sufficient medial displacement.

H. Next, the posterior fragment of the calcaneus is displaced medially until its medial margin is in line with the sustentaculum tali. It is usually necessary to displace one third to one half of the width of the calcaneus.

I. The calcaneal fragments are transfixed by one large threaded Steinmann pin, inserted obliquely from the posteroplantar aspect of the os calcis. The pin exits through the skin over the intermediate cuneiform and should be subcutaneous or flush with the calcaneus posteriorly. Avoid injury to the dorsalis pedis artery anteriorly.

Anteroposterior, lateral, and tangential views of the foot and os calcis are made to determine the degree of correction and position of the pins. The tourniquet is released, and complete hemostasis is achieved. A Hemovac suction tube is placed, the wound is closed in the usual fashion, and a well-padded above-knee cast is applied with the ankle in neutral position and the knee in 35 degrees of flexion.

Postoperative Care. Three to four weeks after the operation, the cast is changed. The threaded Steinmann pin and the sutures are removed. By then, bony union has usually taken place. A below-knee walking cast is applied for an additional two weeks. Following removal of the cast, a UCBL (University of California Biomechanics Laboratory) foot orthosis is worn for six to 12 months to maintain the hindfoot in neutral position and to support the medial longitudinal arch. Tiptoe exercises are performed several times a day to strengthen the triceps surae.

REFERENCES

Koutsogiannis, E.: Treatment of mobile flat foot by displacement osteotomy of a calcaneus. J. Bone Joint Surg., 53-B:96, 1971.

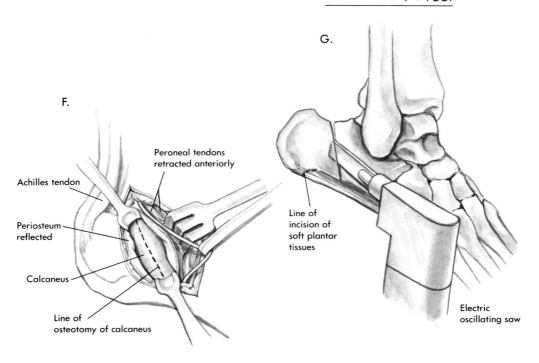

G.

Line of
incision of
soft plantar
tissues

Electric
oscillating saw

F.

Achilles tendon

Peroneal tendons
retracted anteriorly

Periosteum
reflected

Calcaneus

Line of
osteotomy of calcaneus

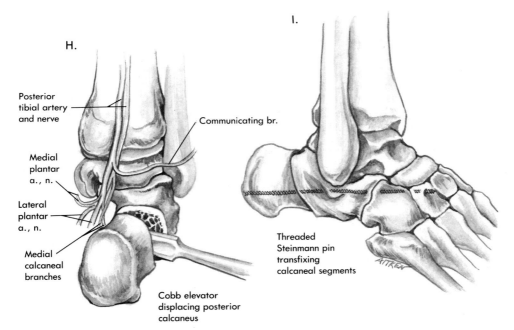

H.

Posterior
tibial artery
and nerve

Communicating br.

Medial
plantar
a., n.

Lateral
plantar
a., n.

Medial
calcaneal
branches

Cobb elevator
displacing posterior
calcaneus

I.

Threaded
Steinmann pin
transfixing
calcaneal segments

Plate 200. (Continued)

PLATE 201 ## Posterior Tendon Transfer to the Os Calcis for Correction of Calcaneal Deformity (Green-Grice Procedure)

Indications. Progressive calcaneus deformity of the hindfoot due to muscle imbalance with zero or poor strength of the triceps surae and normal or good motor strength of the anterior tibial, toe extensors, and peroneals.

Requisites

1. Adequate motor strength of the long toe extensors to be able to dorsiflex the foot against gravity.
2. Age of patient between three and six years at time of surgery.
3. Adequate range of plantar flexion of the ankle (at least 15 to 20 degrees).

Patient Position. It is best to place the patient in the prone position to facilitate the surgical exposure of the heel. The posterior tibial and peroneus longus and brevis tendons are divided distally at their insertion and delivered into the proximal wound following the technique and steps described in Plate 186. When the flexor hallucis longus tendon is to be transferred, its distal portion is sutured to the flexor hallucis brevis muscle. The anterior tibial tendon is delivered into the calf and heel through the interosseous route.

Operative Technique

A. A 5-cm.-long posterior transverse incision is made around the heel along one of the skin creases in the part that neither presses the shoe nor touches the ground.

B. The skin and subcutaneous flaps are undercut and reflected, exposing the os calcis and the insertion of the tendo calcaneus. An L-shaped cut is made in the lateral two thirds of the insertion of the tendo calcaneus. The divided portion is reflected proximally, exposing the apophysis of the os calcis.

C. Next, with a ⁹⁄₆₄-inch drill, a hole is made through the calcaneus, beginning in the center of the apophysis and extruding laterally at its plantar aspect. With a diamond-head hand drill and curet, the hole is enlarged to receive all the transferred tendons.

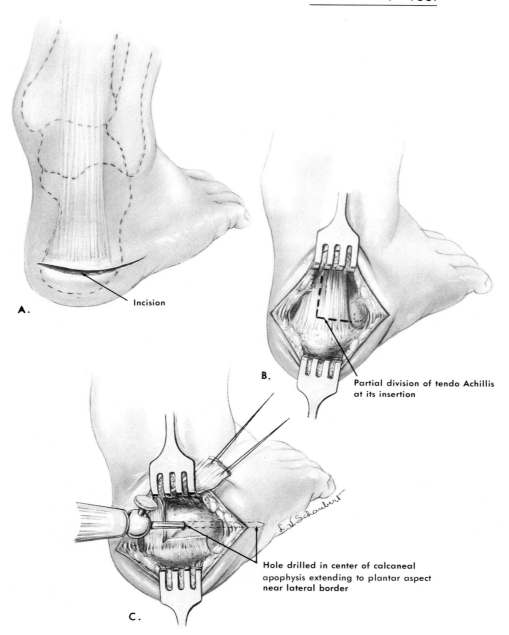

Plate 201. A.–G., Posterior tendon transfer to the os calcis for correction of calcaneal deformity (Green-Grice procedure).

D. Through a lateral incision, the intermuscular septum is widely divided between the lateral and posterior compartments. An Ober tendon passer is inserted through the wound and directed anterior to the tendo calcaneus into the transverse incision over the os calcis. The threads of the whip sutures at the ends of the peroneal tendons are passed through the hole in the tendon passer, and the tendons are delivered at the heel. The posterior tibial tendon is delivered at the heel by a similar route, through an incision in the intermuscular septum between the medial and posterior compartments and anterior to the tendo calcaneus. Next, with a twisted wire probe, the tendons are inserted in the hole and pulled through the tunnel in the calcaneus.

E. At their point of exit on the lateral aspect of the calcaneus, the tendons are sutured to the periosteum and ligamentous tissues. The tendons are sutured under enough tension to hold the foot in 15 degrees of equinus when the remaining ankle dorsiflexors are fair in motor strength, and in 30 degrees of equinus if they are good or normal. The tendons are sutured to each other and to the periosteum of the apophysis of the calcaneus at the posterior end of the tunnel.

F. and G. The divided portion of the tendo calcaneus is resutured in its original position posterior to the transferred tendons.

The wounds are closed and a long leg cast is applied, the knee in 45 to 60 degrees of flexion, the hindfoot in 15 to 30 degrees of equinus, but the forefoot in neutral position. Cavus deformity of the forefoot should be avoided.

Postoperative Care. Three to four weeks following surgery, the solid cast is removed and a new above-knee bivalved cast is made to protect the limb at all times when exercises are not being performed. It is imperative to prevent forced dorsiflexion of the ankle and stretching of the transferred tendons.

Exercises are first performed with the patient side-lying and with gravity eliminated and then in prone position against gravity. To teach the patient the new action of the transferred muscle, he or she is asked to move the foot in the direction of a component of the original action of the muscle and then to plantarflex the foot. For example, when the peroneals are transferred, the patient is asked to evert and plantarflex the foot; or when the anterior tibial is transferred, to invert and plantarflex the foot. Soon, under supervision, guided dorsiflexion of the foot is performed along with plantar flexion. It is important to develop reciprocal motion and motor strength of agonists and antagonist muscles. Weight-bearing is not allowed. Ambulation is permitted in the above-knee bivalved cast with crutches.

In about four to six weeks, when the transferred tendons are fair in motor strength, the patient is allowed to stand on both feet. The heel of the foot that was operated on rests on a 3-cm.-thick block to prevent stretching of the transferred tendons. Bearing partial weight on the foot, the patient should rise up on the tiptoes while holding on to a table with the hands or using two crutches.

When the transplant functions effectively on tiptoe standing, walking with crutches is begun with three-point gait and partial weight-bearing on the affected limb. The heel of the shoe is elevated with a 1- to 1.5-cm. lift that tapers in front (toward the toes). Walking periods are gradually increased. When the transplant works effectively in gait and take-off has been developed in walking, standing tiptoe-rising exercises are started without the support of crutches. The knee should not be flexed, and the patient should not lean forward while rising up on the toes at least three times. This may take a long time (as much as a year or more), but it is a very important phase of postoperative management.

A plantarflexion spring orthosis or an orthosis with a posterior elastic is worn when the patient is uncooperative in the use of crutches or when muscular control of the knee and hip is poor because of extensive paralysis. A stop at the ankle prevents dorsiflexion of the ankle beyond neutral position.

REFERENCES

Green, W. T., and Grice, D. S.: The management of calcaneus deformity. A.A.O.S. Instructional Course Lectures, 13:135, 1959.

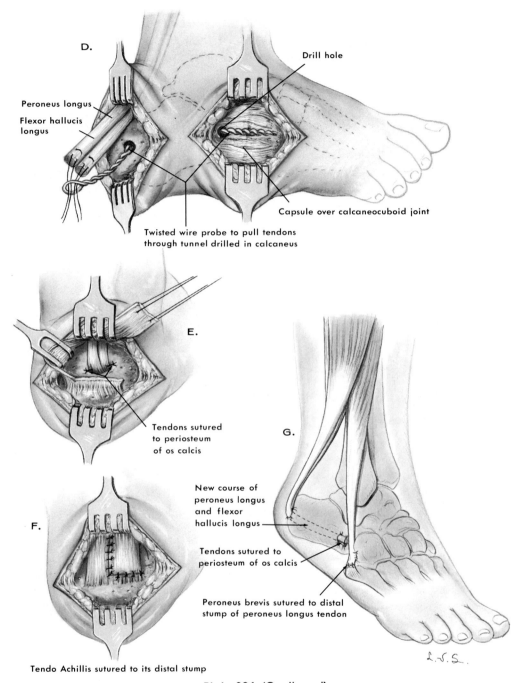

D.

Drill hole

Peroneus longus

Flexor hallucis longus

Capsule over calcaneocuboid joint

Twisted wire probe to pull tendons through tunnel drilled in calcaneus

E.

Tendons sutured to periosteum of os calcis

G.

New course of peroneus longus and flexor hallucis longus

Tendons sutured to periosteum of os calcis

Peroneus brevis sutured to distal stump of peroneus longus tendon

F.

Tendo Achillis sutured to its distal stump

L.S.S.

Plate 201. (Continued)

PLATE 202 ### Open Reduction of the Talocalcaneonavicular and Calcaneocuboid Joints by Complete Subtalar Release in Talipes Equinovarus by Posteromedial and Lateral Surgical Approach

Objectives

1. To achieve concentric reduction of the displacement or subluxation of the talocalcaneonavicular and calcaneocuboid joints.
2. To maintain the reduction.
3. To restore normal articular alignment of the tarsus and the ankle.
4. To establish muscle balance between the evertors and invertors and the dorsiflexors and plantar flexors.
5. To provide a mobile foot with normal function and weight-bearing.

Indications. Failure to achieve reduction of the displaced talocalcaneonavicular and calcaneocuboid joints by manipulation and casts.

The probability of successful closed manipulative reduction is minimal, probably 5 to 10 per cent, and this is in mild cases. Closed methods of treatment are primarily performed to elongate the contracted soft tissues and skin as a preliminary step to open surgical reduction. Persistent forceful manipulation and prolonged cast immobilization do more harm than good. Because the articular cartilage, physis, and bones are "soft," they will be damaged before the ligaments and capsule will yield to stretching. Rigidity of joints, fibrosis of soft tissues, and disuse atrophy of muscles will develop. Conservative treatment of the rigid intrinsic talipes equinovarus is by open surgery.

Requisites

1. Age of patient: minimum of eight to 12 weeks.
2. Adequate size of the foot (at least 10 cm.). The smaller the foot, the greater the risk of iatrogenic trauma.
3. Experienced pediatric orthopedic surgeon. The novice should beware!

The surgery should be systematic and performed in sequential steps. Employ a progressive approach. In order to achieve corrective reduction, all obstacles to reduction should be corrected. The structures to be sectioned or lengthened are listed in Table 9–1.

The order of specific surgical steps to obtain correction varies, depending on the surgical approach and the surgeon's concept of the pathoanatomy of talipes equinovarus. In this atlas, three surgical approaches are described and illustrated: (1) posteromedial and lateral, (2) Cincinnati, and (3) Carroll. The technique utilized depends on the surgeon's training and experience.

In the severely deformed foot with marked equinus, in which skin necrosis is likely to develop by the transverse Cincinnati incision, this author recommends two incisions: posteromedial and lateral that extends proximally behind the lateral malleolus.

Table 9–1. Structures Divided or Lengthened in the Treatment of Talipes Equinovarus

A. **Muscles–Tendons**
  1. *Achilles*
       Always; common technique is Z-lengthening with division of distal part medially; McKay
           lengthens in coronal plane
       Pitfall to avoid—do not overlengthen
  2. *Posterior tibial*
       Always lengthen; supramalleolar level; preserve tendon sheath and canal; maintain
           function; never section; do not transfer primarily, except in paralytic clubfoot
  3. *Abductor hallucis*
       Always; most surgeons recess at origin; this author recommends excision
  4. *Flexor hallucis longus and flexor digitorum longus*
       Lengthen when toes are flexed and cannot be straightened when the ankle is dorsiflexed to
           neutral position at the end of surgery
       Recommended musculotendinous recession at two or three sites to obtain desired amount of
           lengthening; when tendon lengthening, preserve sheath; prevent scarring, especially at
           Henry's knot
  5. *Flexor digitorum brevis, abductor digiti quinti,* and *quadratus plantae* with plantar aponeurosis
       and long plantar ligament—from calcaneal origin
B. **Capsule–Ligaments**
  1. *Talonavicular*
       Always: medial, dorsal, plantar, and lateral
  2. *Subtalar*
       Always: medial, anterior, lateral, and posterior
  3. *Calcaneocuboid joint*
       Medial, plantar, and dorsal—always
       Lateral—this author always sections
  4. *Ankle capsule*
       Posterior: always
       Medial: preserve integrity of deep part of deltoid ligament
       Lateral: divide if necessary, preferably partially
       Anterior: only if contracted, limiting plantar flexion; should be staged
  5. *Contracted ligaments on posterolateral aspect of ankle and subtalar joint*
       Always section:
       a. Calcaneofibular ligament
       b. Posterior talofibular ligament
       c. Superior peroneal retinaculum
  6. *Interosseous talocalcaneal ligament*
       Divide partially or completely when medial rotation of the calcaneus at the subtalar joint
           cannot be corrected

Radiographic Control. Yes.

Patient Position. The operation is performed in a bloodless field obtained by exsanguinating the limb with an Esmarch bandage and inflating the pneumatic tourniquet to 200 to 250 mm. Hg. The posture of the patient is supine. The lower limb is washed with povidone-iodine (Betadine) soap, painted with Betadine solution, and draped with the knee free. The patella and proximal tibial tubercle are marked with indelible ink to facilitate determination of appropriate realignment of the foot in relation to the knee.

Operative Technique

Surgical Approach: Skin Incisions

A. In the surgical approach described in this plate, two separate incisions are made—a posteromedial and a lateral. (The lateral incision is not illustrated.)

The *posteromedial incision* is curvilinear, beginning 7 to 10 cm. proximal to the medial malleolus, passing 1 cm. behind the posterior margin of the tibia, and extending inferiorly to a point 1.5 cm. distal to the tip of the medial malleolus, where it is gently curved distally and anteriorly along the sustentaculum tali to terminate at the base of the first metatarsal bone. It is important to keep one fingerbreadth of skin intact behind the medial malleolus and not to cross the posterior and plantar skin creases.

The *lateral skin incision* starts at the base of the fourth metatarsal, 1.5 to 2.0 cm. dorsal to the plantar border of the bone (not the sole, which is quite thick in the infant). Palpate the bone! The skin incision then extends posteriorly to a point 1 cm. distal to the tip of the lateral malleolus, and then it curves and extends proximally for a distance of 2 to 3 cm. This provides access to the calcaneofibular ligament and superior peroneal retinaculum. Posteriorly, there should be adequate width of intact skin between the two incisions.

The incised skin margins are elevated with skin hooks, and subcutaneous tissues are divided in line with the skin incision. Superficial blood vessels are clamped and coagulated; if possible, preserve the venous drainage of the foot and leg. Injury to the cutaneous nerves should be avoided. The sural nerve is identified, mobilized, and protected during surgery.

Dissection and Elongation of the Tendons–Muscles on the Posteromedial Aspect of the Ankle and Foot and Dissection and Mobilization of the Medial Neurovascular Bundle and Its Branches

B. and **C.** First, identify the Achilles tendon and dissect it free from the soft tissues on its posterior, medial, and lateral aspects. The paratenon of the triceps surae is divided longitudinally at the medial margin of the tendo Achillis. Inadvertent injury to the neurovascular bundle should be avoided. The tendon is freed of the fibrofatty tissue anterior to it. A tongue blade is passed deep to the Achilles tendon.

Lengthening of the tendo Achillis by Z-plasty is performed in the anteroposterior (sagittal) plane. With a knife, divide the Achilles tendon longitudinally into lateral and medial halves for a distance of 5 to 7 cm. The distal end of the medial half is detached from the calcaneus to prevent recurrence of varus deformity of the heel; the lateral half is divided proximally. The medial segment of the divided tendon is reflected proximally, and the lateral segment is reflected distally to its insertion at the calcaneal apophysis.

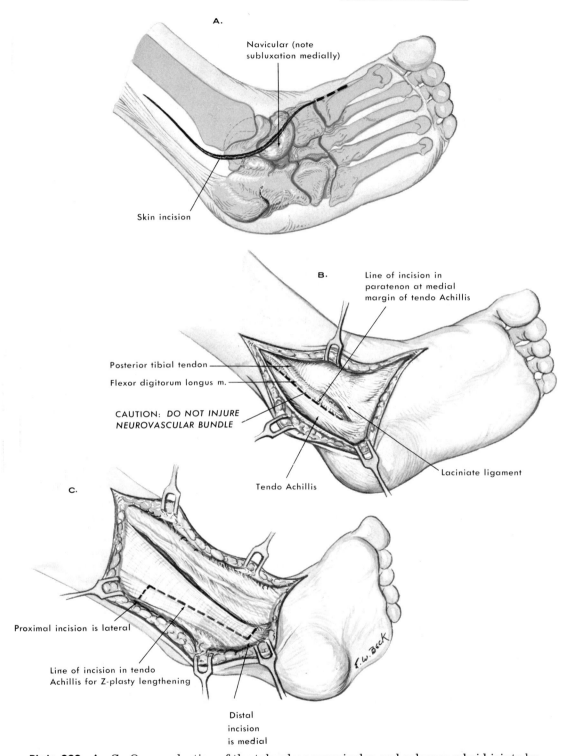

A.

Navicular (note subluxation medially)

Skin incision

B.

Line of incision in paratenon at medial margin of tendo Achillis

Posterior tibial tendon

Flexor digitorum longus m.

CAUTION: *DO NOT INJURE NEUROVASCULAR BUNDLE*

Tendo Achillis

Laciniate ligament

C.

Proximal incision is lateral

Line of incision in tendo Achillis for Z-plasty lengthening

Distal incision is medial

F. W. Beck

Plate 202. A.–S., Open reduction of the talocalcaneonavicular and calcaneocuboid joints by complete subtalar release in talipes equinovarus by posteromedial and lateral surgical approach.

D. and **E.** Next, identify and dissect free the *posterior tibial tendon*. In the distal part of the leg, it lies immediately posterior to the tibia; it is deep to the flexor digitorum longus tendon. Pulling on the posterior tibial tendon will invert the midfoot.

Identify and dissect free the *flexor digitorum longus* tendon. It is the most superficial tendon on the posteromedial border of the tibia. Pulling the flexor digitorum tendon will flex the toes. A length of white Silastic tubing is placed around the posterior tibial tendon and another around the flexor digitorum longus tendon for gentle traction.

The *medial neurovascular bundle* (posterior tibial vessels and tibial nerve) is identified above the medial malleolus; it lies between the flexor digitorum longus and flexor hallucis longus. With a nerve dissector, the neurovascular bundle is dissected free and mobilized with its sheath distally to the canal beneath the laciniate ligament (flexor retinaculum). A piece of yellow silicone (Silastic) tubing is passed around the neurovascular bundle for protection.

With a curved hemostat, locate and identify the *flexor hallucis longus tendon.* It is lateral and deep to the medial neurovascular bundle. Dissect the tendon free from the level of the ankle joint to its canal beneath the talus and pass white Silastic tubing around the tendon.

The *laciniate ligament* is a strong, fibrous band extending from the medial malleolus above to the calcaneus below. It is the "door" to the plantar aspect of the foot, converting a series of bony grooves into four canals for the passage of tendons and the neurovascular bundle. Enumerated anteroposteriorly, these canals transmit (1) the tendon of the tibialis posterior; (2) the tendon of the flexor digitorum longus; (3) the posterior tibial vessels and tibial nerve (neurovascular bundle); and (4) the tendon of the flexor hallucis longus (the last-named canal is partly formed by the talus).

The *abductor hallucis longus* muscle fibers take origin from the lower border of the laciniate ligament. With sharp and dull dissection, the abductor hallucis muscle is freed from its extensive origin—the navicular bone, sustentaculum tali, medial process of the calcaneal tuberosity, first metatarsal, and other structures on the medial aspect of the foot. The abductor hallucis is then elevated and reflected distally and plantarward. The nerve supply to the abductor hallucis muscle (medial plantar nerve) should be preserved.

In the moderately to severely deformed paralytic or arthrogrypotic type of clubfoot, this author excises the abductor hallucis from its tendinous, distal one fourth to its origin. Excision of abductor hallucis facilitates exposure of the medial and plantar aspects of the foot for deep dissection, makes skin closure easier with less tension, and diminishes the likelihood of metatarsus adductus as a postoperative problem. This author has not encountered hallux valgus as a sequela to excision of abductor hallucis.

A Freer elevator or a blunt probe is inserted beneath the superior edge of the laciniate ligament to protect the neurovascular bundle. The *laciniate ligament* is sectioned over the blunt probe near its attachment to the medial malleolus.

Caution! Do not injure the neurovascular bundle as it enters the plantar aspect of the foot!

The *medial neurovascular bundle* is traced to the plantar aspect of the foot; its branches (the medial and lateral plantar vessels and nerves and the calcaneal branches) are dissected free, and yellow Silastic tubing is passed around each branch. It is important to be meticulous in freeing and mobilizing the medial neurovascular bundle and all its branches.

D.

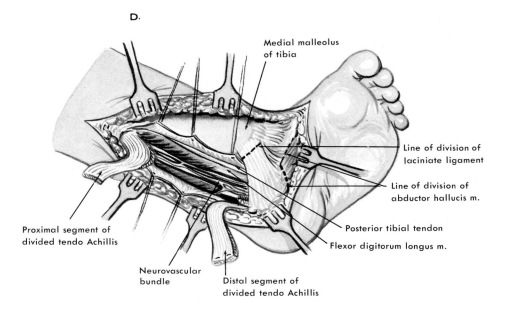

Medial malleolus
of tibia

Line of division of
laciniate ligament

Line of division of
abductor hallucis m.

Posterior tibial tendon

Flexor digitorum longus m.

Proximal segment of
divided tendo Achillis

Neurovascular
bundle

Distal segment of
divided tendo Achillis

E.

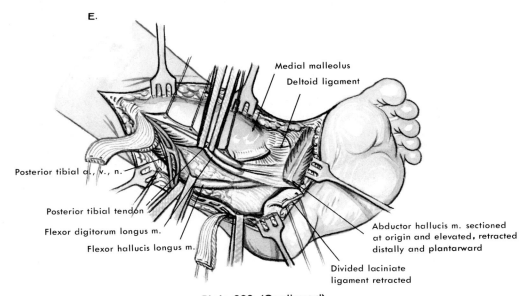

Medial malleolus

Deltoid ligament

Posterior tibial a., v., n.

Posterior tibial tendon

Flexor digitorum longus m.

Flexor hallucis longus m.

Abductor hallucis m. sectioned
at origin and elevated, retracted
distally and plantarward

Divided laciniate
ligament retracted

Plate 202. (Continued)

F. The posterior tibial tendon is lengthened by Z-plasty above the medial malleolus. The tendon sheath of the posterior tibial muscle behind the medial malleolus is left intact because the posterior tibial muscle is an important dynamic force in supporting the medial longitudinal arch of the foot, and its function should be preserved. This author does not section and discard the posterior tibial tendon because overcorrection and pes valgus are definite complications.

Release of Dorsal and Medial Aspects of the Talonavicular Joint and Dissection of Master Knot of Henry

G. and **H.** The proximal segment of the posterior tibial tendon is tagged with 000 or 00 Tycron or similar nonabsorbable suture. Insert a blunt probe of small diameter into the canal of the posterior tibial tendon from above the ankle. The tip of the probe is directed toward the navicular, which in severe talipes equinovarus abuts the medial malleolus. Make a small incision (1 to 2 cm.) on the tendon sheath, over the tip of the probe parallel to the course of the tendon and immediately proximal to the tendon's insertion at the navicular. The distal segment of the posterior tibial tendon is pulled out of its sheath distally into the medial part of the foot.

Note: At the end of the surgery, the distal segment of the posterior tibial tendon will be reinserted through its canal and sutured to the proximal segment in elongated position. This technique, in contrast to replacing the tendon in its open sheath, prevents formation of fibrous adhesions and allows gliding of the tendon through the pulley and maintains function of the posterior tibial muscle. The suture on the distal stump of the posterior tibial tendon may be left in the sheath of the tendon; this facilitates redirection and passage of the posterior tibial tendon through its sheath.

The distal segment of the tendon is pulled out of its sheath distally into the medial part of the foot. Traction on the distal posterior tibial stump serves as a guide in locating the navicular bone and talonavicular joint. The navicular is found distally medially and plantarward tethered to the medial malleolus and the sustentaculum tali by a dense mass of thick, fibrous tissue. The navicular bone lies almost parallel to the long axis of the foot. The joint lines are obscured, making it easy to damage articular cartilage and bone. In order to avoid injury, dissection should proceed distally, not laterally. Sectioning of the neck or head of the talus and the sustentaculum tali should be avoided.

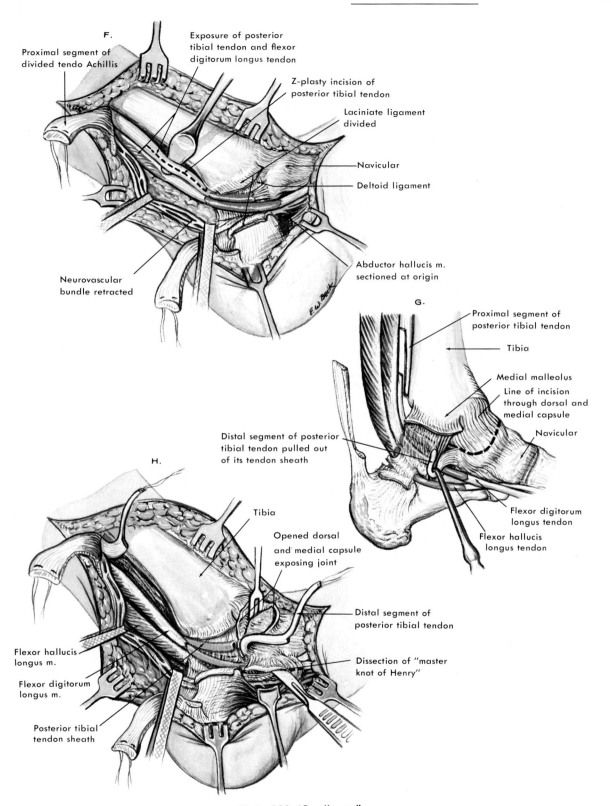

F.

Proximal segment of divided tendo Achillis

Exposure of posterior tibial tendon and flexor digitorum longus tendon

Z-plasty incision of posterior tibial tendon

Laciniate ligament divided

Navicular

Deltoid ligament

Abductor hallucis m. sectioned at origin

Neurovascular bundle retracted

F.W. Beck

G.

Proximal segment of posterior tibial tendon

Tibia

Medial malleolus

Line of incision through dorsal and medial capsule

Navicular

Distal segment of posterior tibial tendon pulled out of its tendon sheath

Flexor digitorum longus tendon

Flexor hallucis longus tendon

H.

Tibia

Opened dorsal and medial capsule exposing joint

Distal segment of posterior tibial tendon

Dissection of "master knot of Henry"

Flexor hallucis longus m.

Flexor digitorum longus m.

Posterior tibial tendon sheath

Plate 202. (Continued)

Insert a small Chandler retractor on the dorsum of the talus deep to the toe extensor tendons, the anterior tibial tendon, and the dorsalis pedis vessels. With a two-pronged sharp skin hook, pull the navicular distally and section the thick tibionavicular ligament (anterior tibionavicular ligament or anterior part of the deltoid) immediate to the navicular. This is a thickened band that extends from the medial malleolus to the tuberosity of the navicular. By gentle traction on the posterior tibial tendon, the talonavicular joint is identified. With a double skin hook, pull the navicular distally and medially and section the dorsal-medial parts of the talonavicular capsule. It is important to perform an adequate dorsal release in order to get the navicular down from its tethered position. Compromise of dorsal blood supply to the talus (i.e., the leash of vessels that pass from the dorsalis pedis to the talar neck) is avoided by staying distal; section tissues near the navicular. Keep as far distally on the talar head as possible. The capsule of the naviculocuneiform is left intact.

The flexor digitorum and flexor hallucis longus tendons are traced and mobilized from above the ankle to the medial-plantar aspect of the foot.

Distal to the anterior end of the sustentaculum tali, the flexor digitorum longus tendon crosses the flexor hallucis longus tendon from the lateral to the medial side in an oblique course dorsal (i.e., deep) to it. At the crossing point, the flexor hallucis longus and the flexor digitorum longus tendons are bound together by a strong, fibrous band—the master knot of Henry—which is attached to the plantar surface of the navicular. With sharp scissors, the master knot of Henry is divided and the long flexor tendons are dissected free, mobilized, and retracted plantarward with the neurovascular bundle. Ordinarily, the long flexor tendons and flexor hallucis longus muscles have a fair amount of excursion and are not markedly contracted; therefore, routine lengthening of the flexor tendons is not indicated. However, when the foot is dorsiflexed to neutral position at the ankle and the toes are still flexed and cannot be passively straightened into full extension, the flexor digitorum longus and flexor hallucis longus are fractionally lengthened at their musculotendinous junction behind the ankle and lower leg. It is best to perform flexor tendon lengthening at the end of the procedure, as traction on the lengthened tendons may cause their discontinuity. It is important not to open the sheaths of the flexor tendons and not to perform Z-lengthening on the medial aspect of the foot, as it may result in adherence of the lengthened tendons to scar tissue. Attention to these details prevents development of hammertoe and dorsal bunion.

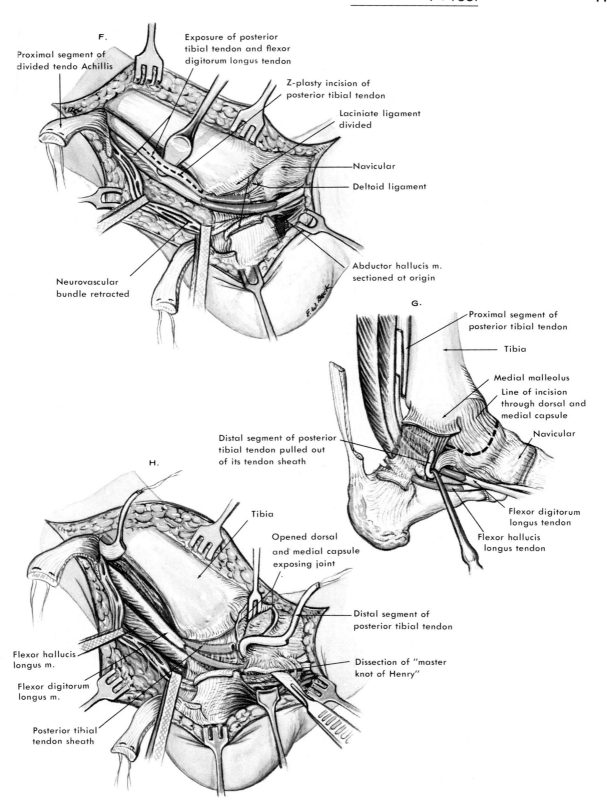

F.

Proximal segment of divided tendo Achillis

Exposure of posterior tibial tendon and flexor digitorum longus tendon

Z-plasty incision of posterior tibial tendon

Laciniate ligament divided

Navicular

Deltoid ligament

Abductor hallucis m. sectioned at origin

Neurovascular bundle retracted

G.

Proximal segment of posterior tibial tendon

Tibia

Medial malleolus

Line of incision through dorsal and medial capsule

Navicular

Distal segment of posterior tibial tendon pulled out of its tendon sheath

Flexor digitorum longus tendon

Flexor hallucis longus tendon

H.

Tibia

Opened dorsal and medial capsule exposing joint

Distal segment of posterior tibial tendon

Dissection of "master knot of Henry"

Flexor hallucis longus m.

Flexor digitorum longus m.

Posterior tibial tendon sheath

Plate 202. (Continued)

Release of the Ligamentous and Capsular Tether on the Plantar and Lateral Sides of the Articulations Between the Talus, Navicular, Calcaneus, and Cuboid

I. This step entails division of (1) plantar and lateral parts of the talonavicular capsule; (2) plantar calcaneonavicular ligament; (3) calcaneonavicular limb of the bifurcate ligament; and (4) calcaneocuboid limb of the bifurcate ligament.

The goal of release of these structures is to enable lateral translation of the talonavicular and calcaneocuboid joints and also to correct posterior cavus (fixed equinus) at the talonavicular and calcaneocuboid joints.

The plantar aspect of the foot is visualized. The *plantar calcaneonavicular ligament* (spring ligament) is a thick band connecting the anterior margin of the sustentaculum tali of the calcaneus to the plantar surface of the navicular. It is shortened and is a fixed obstacle to reduction of the talocalcaneonavicular joint; it should be divided after adequate exposure. Normally, the plantar surface of the spring ligament is supported by the posterior tibial tendon medially and the flexor hallucis longus and flexor digitorum longus tendons laterally. (The posterior tibial tendon has already been divided and dissected free to its insertion.)

At this point, the neurovascular bundle and long toe flexors and flexor hallucis longus tendons are retracted inferiorly, and the *plantar calcaneonavicular ligament* and the *plantar and lateral parts of the capsule of the talonavicular joint* are sectioned. With medial displacement of the navicular, the lateral talonavicular ligament becomes adherent to the anterolateral part of the anterior end of the talus. It is important to release the lateral talonavicular joint capsule for lateral translation of the calcaneocuboid joint.

Next, the *calcaneonavicular limb of the bifurcate ligament* is sectioned; it attaches the calcaneus to the lateral side of the navicular and, if shortened, will check lateral mobility of the navicular. If on manipulation the cuboid does not translate horizontally, the calcaneocuboid limb of the bifurcate ligament and medial plantar capsule of the calcaneocuboid joint are also sectioned.

Inadvertent division of the peroneus longus tendon should be avoided. Identify the anterior tibial tendon insertion to the base of the first metatarsal; using it as a guide, locate the peroneus longus tendon, which is immediately plantar and lateral to the insertion of the anterior tibial tendon. Divide the sheath of the peroneus longus tendon, and retract it out of the way with a long, narrow, right-angle retractor (an instrument referred to by pediatric surgeons as an infantile rectal retractor).

This author finds it much simpler to release the calcaneocuboid joint through the lateral incision. Should the lateral-dorsal capsule of the calcaneocuboid joint be opened? Yes! It is true that the lateral column of the foot is longer than the medial column of the foot in talipes equinovarus and the lateral capsule of the calcaneocuboid joint is overlengthened; however, it is not loose, and the lateral and dorsal parts of the calcaneocuboid joint become adherent to the anterolateral part of the anterior part of the talus, similar to the lateral talonavicular ligament.

Through the lateral incision, the inferior extensor retinaculum is divided. With scalpel and periosteal elevator, the tendinous origin of the extensor digitorum brevis is elevated from the anterolateral part of the calcaneus. The calcaneocuboid joint is exposed. By subperiosteal dissection, the peroneus longus tendon is retracted plantarward. The dorsal, lateral, and plantar parts of the capsule of the calcaneocuboid joint are divided. Next, a Freer elevator is inserted into the calcaneocuboid joint lateral to the medial aspect, and all ligamentous tissue on the medial aspect of the calcaneocuboid joint is sectioned. On manipulation, the cuboid should translate laterally on the anterior end of the calcaneus.

J. Use the flexor hallucis longus tendon as the guide to the sustentaculum tali. Identify the tibiocalcaneal, or middle, fibers of the superficial deltoid ligament and section them near the calcaneus; they descend almost perpendicularly to the

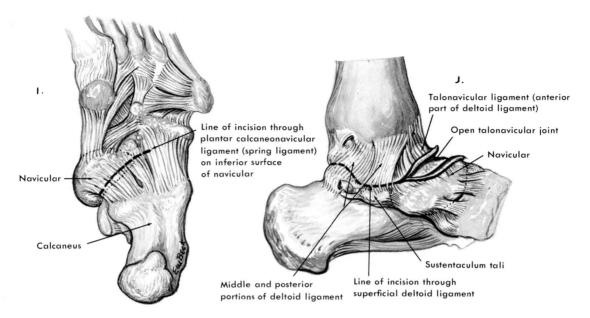

I.

Navicular

Line of incision through plantar calcaneonavicular ligament (spring ligament) on inferior surface of navicular

Calcaneus

Middle and posterior portions of deltoid ligament

Plantar aspect of foot

J.

Talonavicular ligament (anterior part of deltoid ligament)

Open talonavicular joint

Navicular

Sustentaculum tali

Line of incision through superficial deltoid ligament

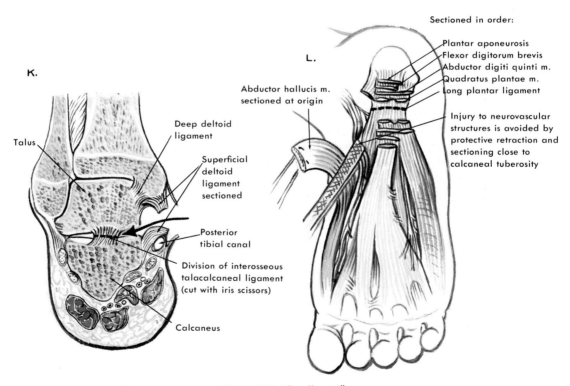

K.

Talus

Deep deltoid ligament

Superficial deltoid ligament sectioned

Posterior tibial canal

Division of interosseous talacalcaneal ligament (cut with iris scissors)

Calcaneus

L.

Abductor hallucis m. sectioned at origin

Sectioned in order:

Plantar aponeurosis
Flexor digitorum brevis
Abductor digiti quinti m.
Quadratus plantae m.
Long plantar ligament

Injury to neurovascular structures is avoided by protective retraction and sectioning close to calcaneal tuberosity

Plate 202. (Continued)

whole length of the sustentaculum tali of the calcaneus. Medially, the subtalar joint runs a sinusoidal course; take care not to damage articular cartilage. The posterior fibers of the superficial deltoid ligament (posterior tibiotalar), which passes backward and laterally to the medial side of the talus and its medial tubercle, are divided.

K. The deep portion of the deltoid that inserts to the nonarticular portion of the body of the talus must be left intact, because if it is divided, the body of the talus will tilt laterally and cause valgus deviation of the ankle. If necessary, in the older child or in the infant with very severe rigid deformity, the hindfoot is everted and the interosseous talocalcaneal ligament (located above the sustentaculum tali) is sectioned under direct vision. Release of the talocalcaneal interosseous ligament is a controversial issue. Its indication is failure of correction of subtalar calcaneal rotation. Therefore, it should *not* be performed at this phase of surgery. It should be left to be done toward the end of surgery. If, after complete subtalar release, full correction can be achieved, as documented by intraoperative radiography, the interosseous ligament is retained.

When the interosseous ligament is sectioned, the problem is overcorrection and valgus deformity of the talonavicular and subtalar joints. Therefore, it is important to position the tarsal bones in concentric reduction and internally fix the talocalcaneal joint with one, or preferably two, threaded Kirschner wires.

Plantar Release

L. By blunt dissection, develop the space around the medial calcaneal nerve and the lateral plantar vessels and nerve. Insert a blunt instrument or Freer nerve dissector in the axilla and enlarge the aperture. Next, insert a long, narrow, right-angle retractor (infantile rectal retractor) in the aperture and dorsally retract the neurovascular bundle with the tendons of the flexor digitorum longus and flexor hallucis longus; place the blades of a Metzenbaum or Mayo scissors next to the os calcis as follows: The plantar blade of the scissors is superficial to the plantar fasciae and the dorsal blade next to bone, with the retractor separating it from the neurovascular bundle. Double check the position of the blades and feel the opposite side on the lateral side of the heel with your fingers. Section from their origin at the tuberosity of the calcaneus: (1) plantar fascia, (2) flexor digitorum brevis, (3) quadratus plantae, (4) long plantar ligament, (5) abductor digiti quinti, and (6) remnants of the deep head of the abductor hallucis. By staying close to bone, one can avoid injury to the neurovascular structures.

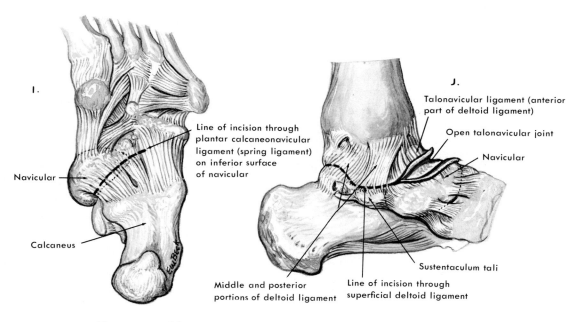

I.

Navicular

Calcaneus

Line of incision through plantar calcaneonavicular ligament (spring ligament) on inferior surface of navicular

Plantar aspect of foot

J.

Talonavicular ligament (anterior part of deltoid ligament)

Open talonavicular joint

Navicular

Sustentaculum tali

Middle and posterior portions of deltoid ligament

Line of incision through superficial deltoid ligament

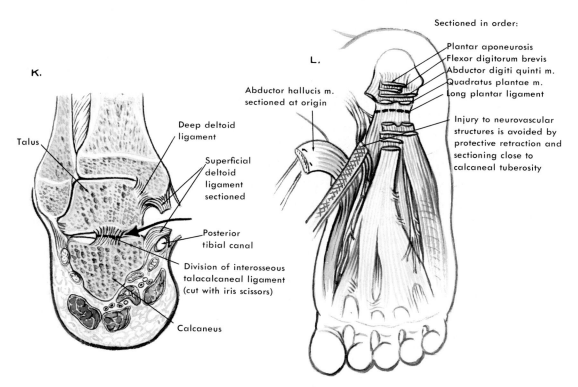

K.

Talus

Deep deltoid ligament

Superficial deltoid ligament sectioned

Posterior tibial canal

Division of interosseous talacalcaneal ligament (cut with iris scissors)

Calcaneus

L.

Abductor hallucis m. sectioned at origin

Sectioned in order:

Plantar aponeurosis
Flexor digitorum brevis
Abductor digiti quinti m.
Quadratus plantae m.
Long plantar ligament

Injury to neurovascular structures is avoided by protective retraction and sectioning close to calcaneal tuberosity

Plate 202. (Continued)

Posterior Capsulotomy of the Subtalar and Ankle Joints

M. First, incise the superior peroneal retinaculum—this is a ligamentous tissue that runs in the same direction as the calcaneofibular ligament. Identify but do not open the peroneal sheaths at this level. This detail of technique prevents anterior displacement of the peroneal tendons over the lateral malleolus. Locate the flexor hallucis longus tendon; it lies on the medial side of the subtalar joint and serves as a guide to locating the subtalar joint.

The posterior part of the capsule of the tibiotalar and talocalcaneal joints is exposed by retracting the flexor hallucis longus tendon medially and the peroneal tendons laterally. A Chandler elevator or Davis retractor is used to retract the peroneal tendons and protect them from inadvertent injury. The neurovascular structures behind the medial malleolus are retracted forward. Next, with sharp tenotomy or Metzenbaum scissors, completely divide the posterior capsule of the ankle joint by a horizontal incision, and the subtalar joint capsule by a sinusoidal cut. Do not use a knife, as it may damage the articular cartilage. Caution must be exercised so as not to injure the distal tibial physis. If in doubt, use radiographic control. Posterior capsulotomy of the ankle joint is carried out; it starts laterally at the peroneal tendon sheath and extends medially to the edge of the posterior tibial tendon sheath.

I strongly recommend that the deep deltoid (tibiotalar) ligament not be divided, as the ankle joint will become unstable and valgus ankle deformity may develop. The tibiotalar ligament divided inadvertently or by plan (as in the Goldner technique) should be repaired.

Posterolateral Release

N. Dissection of the posterolateral aspect of the foot is carried out, and the following contracted soft-tissue structures between the fibula, os calcis, and talus are released: (1) calcaneofibular ligament, (2) posterolateral talocalcaneal ligament, (3) posterior talofibular ligament, and (4) thickened superior peroneal retinaculum and thick peroneal sheath. These tethers hold the calcaneus close to the lateral malleolus and checkrein rotation of the calcaneus, and they also prevent rotation and posterior movement of the talus in the ankle mortise. The fibula should be free to rotate for the talus to move.

1. Divide the sheath of the peroneus longus and brevis tendons laterally at the level of the lateral subtalar joint. (As stated, if the peroneal tendon sheaths are divided proximally at the level of the ankle joint, the peroneal tendon may subluxate anteriorly.) Meticulous care is exercised not to section the peroneal tendon inadvertently. Next, the peroneal tendons are mobilized and retracted posteriorly and anteriorly, and the *peroneal tendon sheaths* are completely excised circumferentially.

2. The peroneal tendons and sural nerve are retracted anteriorly, and the thickened short calcaneofibular ligament is exposed. Insert a Freer elevator or a hemostat beneath the calcaneofibular ligament in a posteroanterior direction and divide the ligament close to the calcaneus. McKay cuts the calcaneofibular ligament in an oblique fashion in order to provide a larger surface area and facilitate proper healing and reattachment of the ligament to the calcaneus.

3. Retract the peroneal tendon laterally and excise the previously incised thickened fibrous band of *superior peroneal retinaculum.*

4. Section the posterolateral part of the talocalcaneal capsule.

5. Identify and vertically section the posterior talofibular ligament, which holds the talus in plantar flexion. McKay prefers to preserve the posterior talofibular ligament; this author finds that in the rigid clubfoot, it is difficult to position the talus in the ankle mortise when the posterior talofibular ligament is intact.

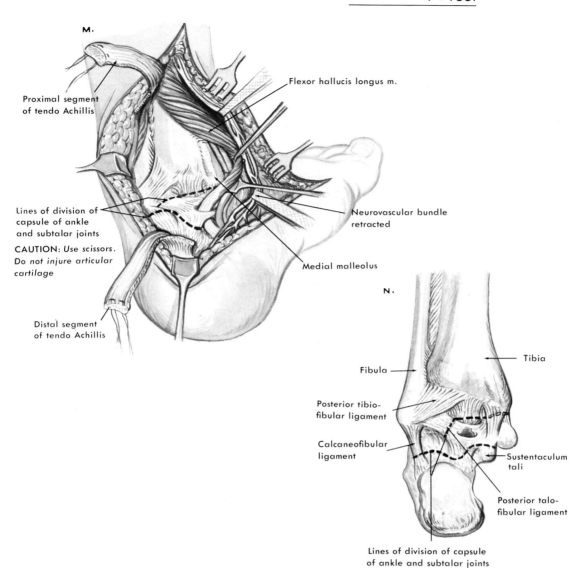

M.

Proximal segment
of tendo Achillis

Flexor hallucis longus m.

Lines of division of
capsule of ankle
and subtalar joints

CAUTION: *Use scissors.
Do not injure articular
cartilage*

Neurovascular bundle
retracted

Medial malleolus

Distal segment
of tendo Achillis

N.

Fibula

Tibia

Posterior tibio-
fibular ligament

Calcaneofibular
ligament

Sustentaculum
tali

Posterior talo-
fibular ligament

Lines of division of capsule
of ankle and subtalar joints

Plate 202. (Continued)

Lateral Release

O1.–O3. With the peroneal tendons retracted posteriorly, the lateral talocalcaneal ligament and joint capsule are completely sectioned.

By blunt dissection through the lateral part of the wound, the lateral part of the talonavicular joint is exposed and the capsule is divided from its inferior lateral aspect to the dorsum of the foot. Again, meticulous care is exercised in order not to injure blood vessels on the dorsum of the talus. The release of dorsal, medial, lateral, and plantar capsules of the calcaneocuboid joint has already been described in **N.** Next, determine whether the anterior portion of the calcaneus rotates laterally. If subtalar calcaneal rotation cannot be corrected, division of the interosseous ligament is performed.

O₁.

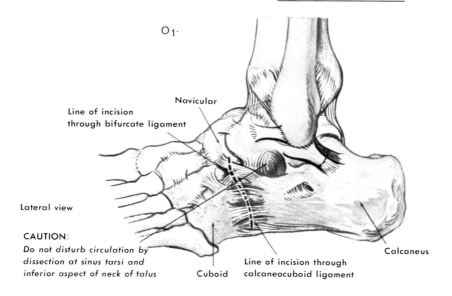

Line of incision
through bifurcate ligament

Navicular

Lateral view

CAUTION:
Do not disturb circulation by
dissection at sinus tarsi and
inferior aspect of neck of talus

Cuboid

Line of incision through
calcaneocuboid ligament

Calcaneus

O₂.

Freer elevator checking
thoroughness of release of
talonavicular and calcaneocuboid joints

O₃.

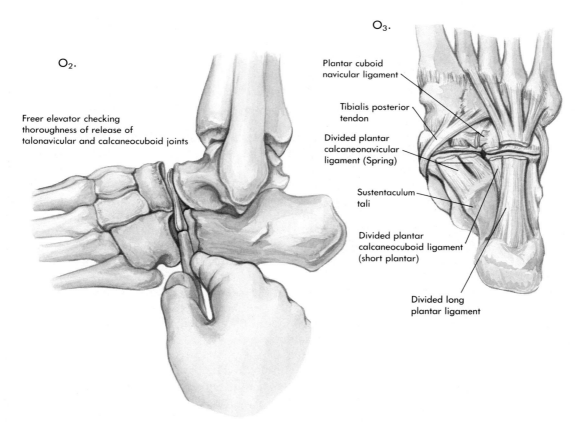

Plantar cuboid
navicular ligament

Tibialis posterior
tendon

Divided plantar
calcaneonavicular
ligament (Spring)

Sustentaculum
tali

Divided plantar
calcaneocuboid ligament
(short plantar)

Divided long
plantar ligament

Plate 202. (Continued)

Concentric Reduction of the Talocalcaneonavicular and Calcaneocuboid Joint by Repositioning of the Bones and Internal Fixation with Threaded Pins

P1.–P3. and Q. The foot and ankle are gently manipulated into increasing dorsiflexion. The dome of the talus should be repositioned in the ankle mortise, and, on dorsiflexion of the ankle, the posterior surface of the body of the talus should be visualized. In severe fixed equinus deformity, one may have to section the distal tibiofibular syndesmosis. Fractional lengthening of the flexor hallucis longus and flexor digitorum longus muscles at their musculotendinous junction may be required if the toes are acutely flexed upon neutral dorsiflexion of the ankle. In very severe flexion deformity of the hallux, Z-lengthening of the flexor hallucis longus is performed on the plantar aspect of the foot; the problem with Z-lengthening at the level of the master knot of Henry is scarring of the elongated tendon with resultant deformities of clawing of the great toe and dorsal bunion. Whenever possible, it is best to lengthen at the musculotendinous junction by recession; section at two or three sites to obtain the desired length.

Through the medial part of the wound, the navicular is displaced laterally; and, through the lateral part of the wound, the head of the talus is displaced medially.

Reduction is facilitated by insertion of a threaded Kirschner wire (0.062 or 0.045 cm. in diameter in infants) in the longitudinal axis of the talus from the posterior aspect of its body. The point of entry of the Kirschner wire is immediately lateral to the posterior ridge of the talus; the wire is directed to emerge at the center of the anterior end of the talus. It is vital to use a threaded wire. Smooth pins may migrate, causing loss of alignment and making pin removal very difficult.

The leverage of the pin is used to rotate the anterior end of the talus medially and that of the calcaneus laterally, obtaining normal talocalcaneal divergence in the anteroposterior plane. Then distal traction is applied on the forefoot, the navicular pushed laterally, and the anterior end of the calcaneus rotated laterally, achieving concentric reduction of the talocalcaneonavicular joint.

Prior to inserting the pin into the navicular, carefully inspect the relationship of the navicular to the anterior end, "the head" of the talus. The use of two small Chandler elevator retractors—one dorsal and the other plantar to the talonavicular articulation—will assist proper visualization and palpation of the repositioned bony structures. The medial side of the navicular normally protrudes slightly medially beyond the edge of the talar head and should not be plantar-flexed with respect to the navicular; nor should the navicular be displaced superiorly in relationship to the talar head. The lateral side of the talonavicular joint also should be palpated carefully to ensure that there is no lateral step-off at the level of the joint. The relationship of the repositioned bone is determined visually by manual palpation and with an instrument. Overcorrection, a common error after extensive soft-tissue release, should be avoided. The threaded pin is then drilled distally across the talonavicular joint.

Inspection of the position of the foot is necessary before the pin is drilled through the dorsum of the forefoot. The long axis of the foot should be in approximately 10 degrees of lateral rotation with respect to the previously marked tibial tubercle. The foot must not be supinated and must not be translated or tilted laterally into a valgus position. If the position is not satisfactory, the talonavicular pin is withdrawn from the navicular, the navicular is repositioned, and the talonavicular pin is reinserted. It is vital that the position of the talonavicular joint and the foot be correct and precise in relation to the leg–knee. The importance of concentric reduction and alignment cannot be overemphasized.

Avoid multiple drilling of the talus and navicular. Fracture of these bones will create a very difficult problem of fixation.

When the deformity is severe with marked medial subluxation of the calcaneocuboid joint following concentric reduction, the calcaneocuboid joint is also fixed internally with one threaded Steinmann pin.

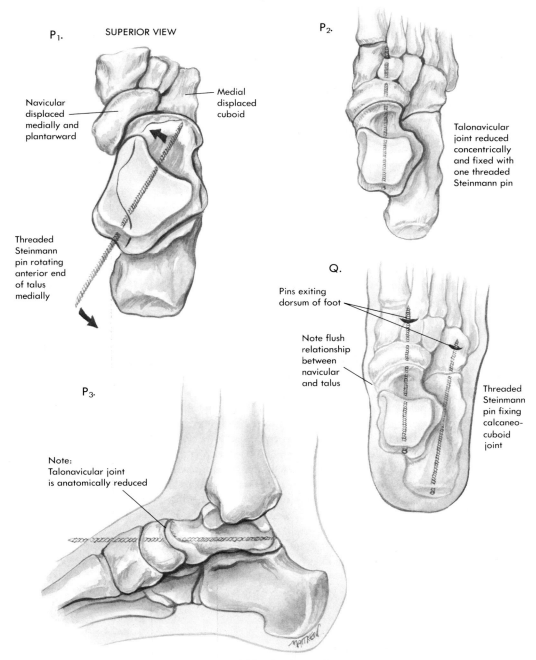

P₁.   SUPERIOR VIEW

Navicular displaced medially and plantarward

Medial displaced cuboid

Threaded Steinmann pin rotating anterior end of talus medially

P₂.

Talonavicular joint reduced concentrically and fixed with one threaded Steinmann pin

Q.

Pins exiting dorsum of foot

Note flush relationship between navicular and talus

Threaded Steinmann pin fixing calcaneo-cuboid joint

P₃.

Note: Talonavicular joint is anatomically reduced

Plate 202. (Continued)

Internal Fixation of Talocalcaneal Joint and Repair of Tendons

R. and **S.** If the interosseous ligament is sectioned, it is best to fix the calcaneus to the talus with one or two threaded Steinmann pins to maintain corrected subtalar rotation. The pins are inserted from the plantar surface of the calcaneus and up through the talus, but not protruding through the ankle joint. When the talocalcaneal pins are inserted, the subtalar joint should be closed. Anteroposterior and lateral radiograms of the foot and ankle are made in the corrected position to verify concentricity of reduction of the talocalcaneonavicular joint. The value of intraoperative radiograms cannot be overemphasized. If reduction is concentric, the talonavicular pin is drilled out through the dorsum of the forefoot. The drill is changed to the anterior end of the pin, and the pin is withdrawn so that its posterior end is flush with the back of the talus. The protruding anterior end of the pin is cut off subcutaneously or protruding through the skin 1 cm. The talocalcaneal pins are cut protruding 1 cm. out of the sole of the heel.

Anteroposterior and lateral radiograms of the foot are made to determine the position of the pins and concentricity of reduction.

In the severely deformed foot with fixed forefoot varus, capsulotomy of the first metatarsal cuneiform joint and osteotomy of the base of the second metatarsal may be indicated. The wounds are irrigated, a compression bandage is applied, and the tourniquet is released. After a few minutes, the compression bandage is removed and complete hemostasis is obtained.

The distal segment of the posterior tibial tendon is introduced through its canal behind the medial malleolus, delivered into the back of the ankle, and resutured to its proximal segment.

The tendo Achillis is resutured with proper tension with the ankle at only 5 degrees of dorsiflexion. Avoid overlengthening of the triceps surae muscle. The skin margins are observed for adequacy of circulation; they may be blanched from tension when the ankle is maximally dorsiflexed. The foot is plantar-flexed 10 degrees farther from the position of the foot at which capillary refill of the skin margin is complete. The subcutaneous tissue is closed with absorbable sutures, and the skin with subcuticular or 00 nylon sutures.

A bulky sterile dressing and sheet wadding are applied and reinforced with an above-knee, well-padded plaster of Paris cast. The ankle joint is immobilized in plantar flexion as described above to relax the tension of the skin edges; the knee is in 45 degrees of flexion. If there is any question about circulation to the skin, the cast is omitted and only a Jones compression dressing with a posterior splint is applied.

Postoperative Care. Ten to 14 days after surgery, the patient is taken back to the operating room on an outpatient basis, and under general anesthesia, the dressing is removed and wound healing is assessed. *The sutures and pins are not removed.* The foot is repeatedly manipulated into maximal plantar flexion and neutral dorsiflexion. This manipulation of the foot into plantar flexion is performed in order to prevent contracture of the anterior capsule of the ankle joint. Another above-knee cast is applied with the ankle in neutral or 5 degrees of dorsiflexion. The second cast is removed in two weeks, at which time the pins and sutures are also removed. Again, the ankle joint is manipulated into plantar flexion and dorsiflexion; and another above-knee cast (the third) is applied for an additional period of two weeks. The total period of cast immobilization is about six weeks.

After removal of the cast, the foot and ankle are held at night in a slightly overcorrected position in an above-knee posterior splint made of polypropylene or some other plastic. The purpose of this retentive apparatus is to maintain correction; it is worn only at night and at naptime. It is used for 6 to 12 months until skeletal growth remodels and straightens the medial and plantar tilting of the head and neck of the talus and normal articular relationships are restored. The decreased angle of declination of the talus may be compared with excessive femoral

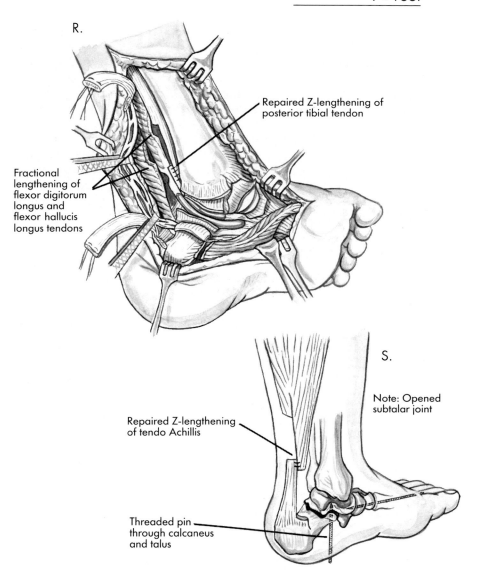

R.

Repaired Z-lengthening of
posterior tibial tendon

Fractional
lengthening of
flexor digitorum
longus and
flexor hallucis
longus tendons

S.

Note: Opened
subtalar joint

Repaired Z-lengthening
of tendo Achillis

Threaded pin
through calcaneus
and talus

Plate 202. (Continued)

antetorsion in developmental dislocation of the hip; the same principles should be applied.

The Denis Browne splint (with a 10- to 23-cm. everting crossbar between the feet) is not recommended, as it is ineffective in controlling the ankle and hindfoot and may cause genu valgum and exaggerated lateral tibiofibular torsion.

Passive stretching exercises are performed by the parents on the child's foot and leg two to three times a day, each session consisting of 25 to 40 manipulations of the ankle into dorsiflexion and plantar flexion, heel eversion, forefoot abduction, and stretching of plantar contracted soft tissues. Active exercises are performed by the older child to develop motor function in the triceps surae, posterior tibial, and peroneal muscles. In the infant and young child, muscle stimulation techniques are utilized to develop motor power. Children with clubfoot should be observed at periodic intervals until the foot is skeletally mature.

REFERENCES

Turco, V. J.: Surgical correction of the resistant club foot. One-stage posteromedial release with internal fixation: A preliminary report. J. Bone Joint Surg., 53-A:477, 1971.

Turco, V. J.: Surgical corrections of the resistant congenital club-foot—one-stage release with internal fixation. Chicago, A.A.O.S. Film Library, 1980.

Turco, V. J.: Resistant congenital club foot—one-stage posteromedial release with internal fixation. A follow-up report of a fifteen-year experience. J. Bone Joint Surg., 61-A:805, 1979.

Turco, V. J.: Clubfoot. In: Current Problems in Orthopaedics. New York, Churchill Livingstone, 1981.

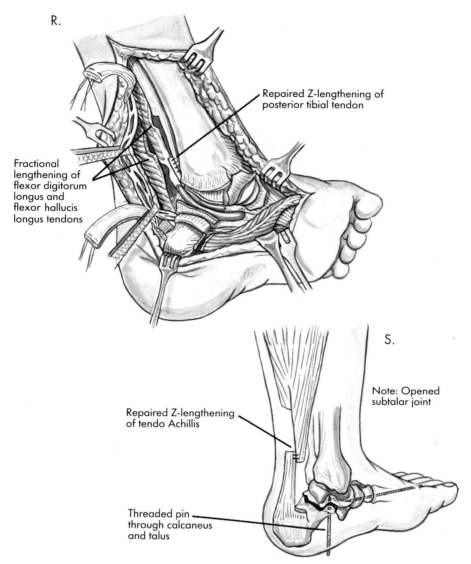

R.

Repaired Z-lengthening of posterior tibial tendon

Fractional lengthening of flexor digitorum longus and flexor hallucis longus tendons

S.

Repaired Z-lengthening of tendo Achillis

Note: Opened subtalar joint

Threaded pin through calcaneus and talus

Plate 202. (Continued)

PLATE 203

Open Reduction of the Talocalcaneonavicular Joint (Cincinnati Approach)

Indications. See Plate 202.

Patient Position. The patient is placed in prone position with a pneumatic tourniquet on the proximal thigh. After preparation and draping of the patient in routine fashion, the patella and proximal tibial tubercle are marked with an indelible pen for orientation of rotation of the foot after complete subtalar release.

Operative Technique

A.–D. The Cincinnati incision is used for surgical exposure. Make a transverse incision, beginning at the base of the first metatarsal and extending posteriorly 5 mm. superior to the heel crease under the medial malleolus and then posterolaterally to the tip of the lateral malleolus and distally and anteriorly to the cuboid fifth metatarsal joint. If necessary, the medial incision can extend more distally for adequate release of the abductor hallucis. Subcutaneous tissue is divided in line with the skin incision and spread apart by sharp, pointed tenotomy scissors inserted perpendicular to the wound.

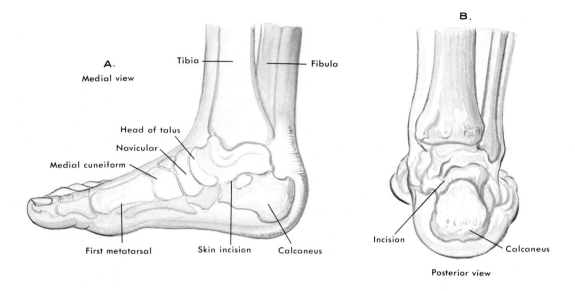

A.
Medial view

Tibia — Fibula

Head of talus
Navicular
Medial cuneiform

First metatarsal   Skin incision   Calcaneus

B.

Incision   Calcaneus

Posterior view

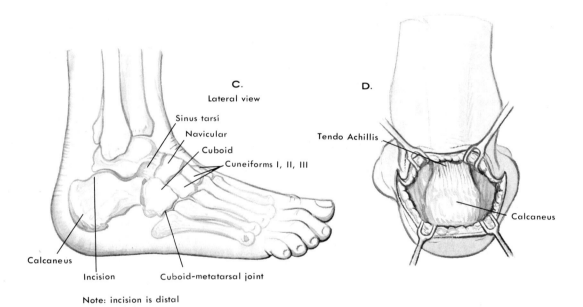

C.
Lateral view

Sinus tarsi
Navicular
Cuboid
Cuneiforms I, II, III

Calcaneus

Incision   Cuboid-metatarsal joint

Note: incision is distal
to sinus tarsi

D.

Tendo Achillis

Calcaneus

Plate 203. A.–U., Open reduction of the talocalcaneonavicular joint (Cincinnati approach).

E. The abductor hallucis is detached from its origin and reflected plantarward and distally. The dorsal and posterior wound flap is elevated and retracted proximally.

Next, identify the laciniate ligament (flexor retinaculum); it is the door to the plantar aspect of the foot. Deep to it passes the neurovascular bundle, which is located between the tendons of the flexor digitorum longus and flexor hallucis longus. Pass a Freer or a scored Frazier dural elevator deep to the flexor retinaculum over the neurovascular bundle, and incise the laciniate ligament. The neurovascular bundle is gently dissected, and Silastic tubing is passed around it. Distally, in the hindfoot, the neurovascular bundle overlies the flexor hallucis longus tendon, which, in turn, overlies the subtalar joint underneath the sustentaculum tali. Identify the calcaneal branch of the nerve and preserve it. In about 1 to 2 per cent of clubfoot cases, the blood supply of the foot is anomalous. If you have difficulty finding the vessels, it is best to deflate the tourniquet to bring the vascular bundle into view. In rare cases, the anomalous vessels originate from the deep peroneal vessel crossing obliquely over the lower end of the flexor hallucis longus tendon.

F. Identify the flexor digitorum longus tendon and incise its sheath longitudinally as far proximally as the skin incision will allow and as far distally as the master knot of Henry.

Caution! Do not injure the plantar nerve, which is in close proximity to the sheath of the flexor digitorum longus in its distal one third.

Pass Silastic tubing around the flexor digitorum longus tendon. Identify the posterior tibial tendon and open its sheath distally to the level of the ankle joint, but not distal to it. Then perform a Z-lengthening of the posterior tibial tendon at the supramalleolar level.

Next, identify and free the flexor hallucis longus tendon.

Caution! Do not injure the neurovascular bundle.

G. In the posterior dissection, first the Achilles tendon is lengthened. Divide the distal part medially and the proximal part laterally. Lengthen enough to allow adequate correction of equinus.

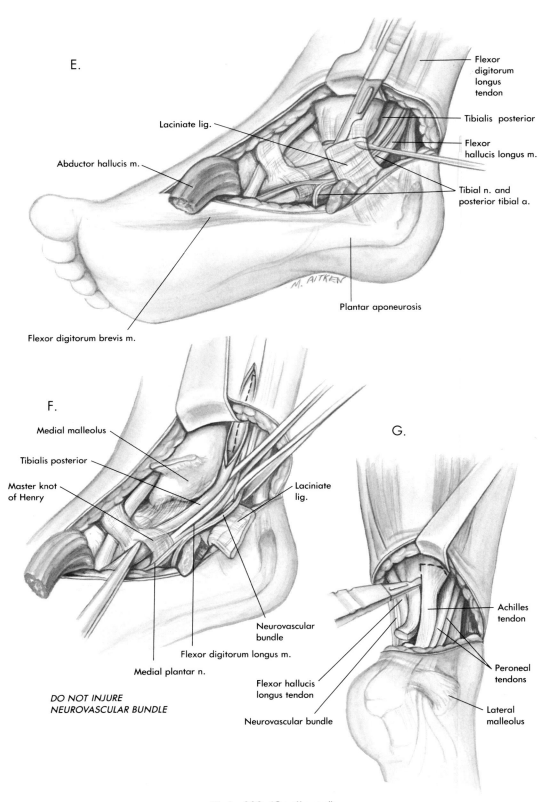

E.

Flexor digitorum longus tendon

Tibialis posterior

Flexor hallucis longus m.

Tibial n. and posterior tibial a.

Laciniate lig.

Abductor hallucis m.

Plantar aponeurosis

Flexor digitorum brevis m.

F.

Medial malleolus

Tibialis posterior

Master knot of Henry

Laciniate lig.

Neurovascular bundle

Flexor digitorum longus m.

Medial plantar n.

*DO NOT INJURE
NEUROVASCULAR BUNDLE*

G.

Achilles tendon

Peroneal tendons

Lateral malleolus

Flexor hallucis longus tendon

Neurovascular bundle

Plate 203. (Continued)

H. Expose the posterior part of the capsule of the tibiotalar and talocalcaneal joints by retracting the flexor hallucis longus tendon medially and the peroneal tendons laterally. Keep the neurovascular bundle out of harm's way by retracting it anteriorly.

Determine the level of the ankle joint by plantarflexion and dorsiflexion of the ankle. Make a small horizontal incision with a scalpel.

Caution! Do not injure the posterior part of the distal tibial growth plate.

With a tenotomy scissors, divide the capsule of the ankle joint, beginning laterally at the peroneal tendons and extending anteromedially to the posterior tibial sheath. The subtalar joint is also divided.

Caution! Do not injure the deep deltoid ligament.

Divide the posterior talofibular ligament vertically.

I. and J. The lateral side of the hindfoot is exposed by dissection of the wound flap dorsally and plantarward. Identify the sural nerve and retract it out of harm's way with Silastic tubing. Identify the peroneal tendons, incise the sheaths, and retract the tendons posteriorly. The subtalar joint is anterior to the peroneal tendons. With a pair of sharp dissecting scissors, incise the capsule of the talocalcaneal joint posteriorly and laterally. Identify the calcaneofibular ligament. Retract the peroneal tendons and sural nerve anteriorly, and divide the calcaneofibular ligament.

H.

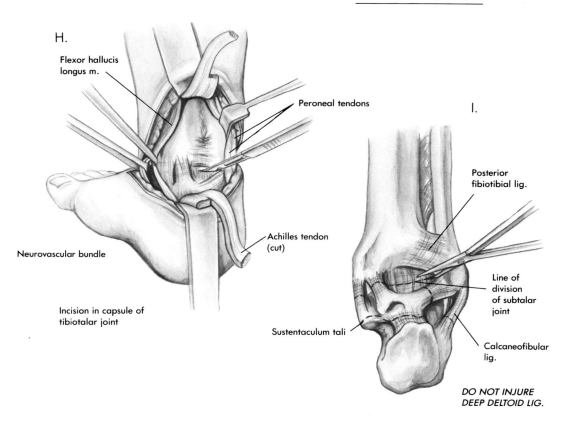

Flexor hallucis
longus m.

Peroneal tendons

Neurovascular bundle

Achilles tendon
(cut)

Incision in capsule of
tibiotalar joint

I.

Posterior
fibiotibial lig.

Line of
division
of subtalar
joint

Sustentaculum tali

Calcaneofibular
lig.

*DO NOT INJURE
DEEP DELTOID LIG.*

J.

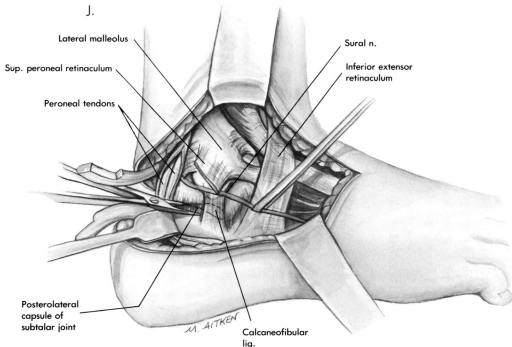

Lateral malleolus

Sup. peroneal retinaculum

Peroneal tendons

Sural n.

Inferior extensor
retinaculum

Posterolateral
capsule of
subtalar joint

Calcaneofibular
lig.

M. AITKEN

Plate 203. (Continued)

K. The calcaneocuboid joint is subluxated medially and plantarward, and the capsule is contracted on its medial and plantar aspect. The calcaneocuboid joint is circumferentially sectioned on its dorsal, lateral, medial, and plantar aspects.

L. Next, perform deep medial release. Insert a probe in the canal of the distal segment of the posterior tibial tendon sheath, and make a longitudinal incision over the tip of the probe. The distal segment of the posterior tibial tendon is delivered through the aperture of the sheath, preserving a part of the posterior tendon sheath to act as a pulley.

Apply gentle traction on the posterior tibial tendon, pulling it distally. Commonly, the navicular is displaced proximally and medially, abutting the medial malleolus and forming a tibionavicular pseudoarticulation. Make an incision in the contracted soft tissues medially and in the tibionavicular ligament dorsally. With the help of a double skin hook, pull the navicular distally, and with the help of a scalpel and sharp scissors inserted in a horizontal direction, perform a capsulotomy of the talonavicular joint medially, dorsally, and plantarward. At this point, a probe is inserted between the talonavicular and the calcaneocuboid joints to ensure complete release of these articulations. There should be no tethering structures, and the talonavicular and calcaneocuboid joints should be readily translated laterally.

M. Next, incise the medial capsule of the subtalar joint. The talocalcaneal articulation is easily located from its posterior aspect. With the help of sharp scissors, divide the capsule from inside out.

N. Insert a Freer elevator across the talonavicular and calcaneocuboid joints to double-check complete release.

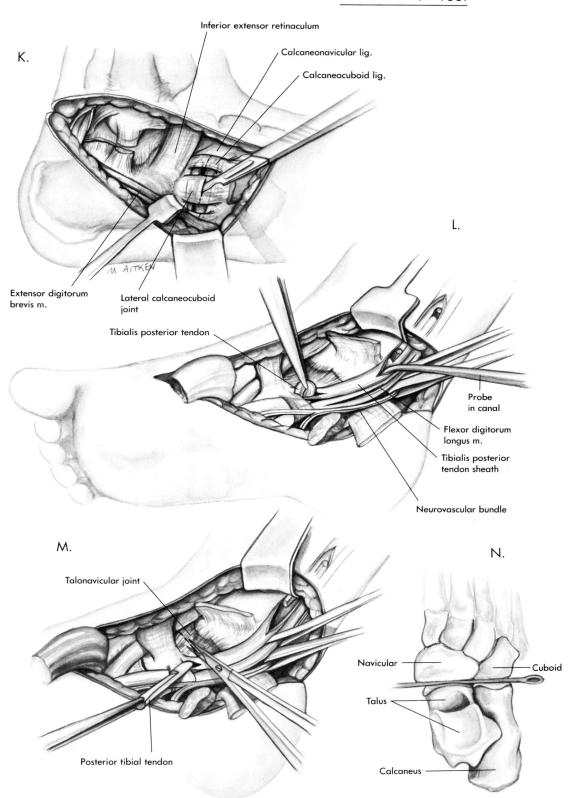

K.

Inferior extensor retinaculum

Calcaneonavicular lig.

Calcaneocuboid lig.

M AITKEN

Extensor digitorum brevis m.

Lateral calcaneocuboid joint

L.

Tibialis posterior tendon

Probe in canal

Flexor digitorum longus m.

Tibialis posterior tendon sheath

Neurovascular bundle

M.

Talonavicular joint

Posterior tibial tendon

N.

Navicular

Cuboid

Talus

Calcaneus

Plate 203. (Continued)

O. When the medial subtalar spin cannot be corrected the interosseous talocalcaneal ligament is sectioned.

P. and **Q.** Perform a plantar release through the posterior part of the medial wound. Make a small incision in the subcutaneous tissue deep to the skin, adjacent to the calcaneal nerve. Insert a pair of tenotomy scissors into the subcutaneous tissue superficial to the plantar fascia. Spread the points of the scissors and retract the neurovascular bundle anteriorly and distally and insert a Metzenbaum scissors. With one blade superficial to the plantar fascia and the other blade immediately next to the anterior part of the calcaneus, divide the plantar aponeurosis, flexor digitorum brevis, abductor digiti quinti, quadratus plantaris, and long plantar ligament.

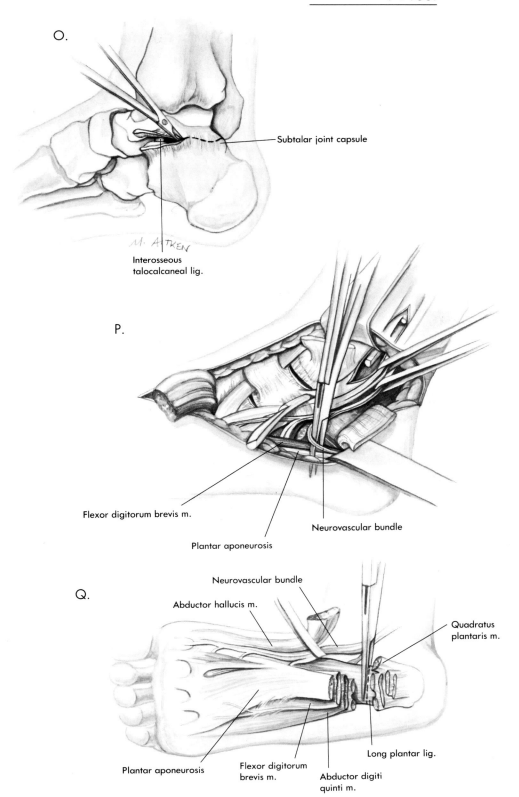

O.

Subtalar joint capsule

M. AITKEN

Interosseous
talocalcaneal lig.

P.

Flexor digitorum brevis m.

Neurovascular bundle

Plantar aponeurosis

Q.

Neurovascular bundle

Abductor hallucis m.

Quadratus
plantaris m.

Plantar aponeurosis

Flexor digitorum
brevis m.

Abductor digiti
quinti m.

Long plantar lig.

Plate 203. (Continued)

R.–U. Concentric reduction of the talonavicular, talocalcaneal, and calcaneocuboid joints is performed by repositioning of the foot and internal fixation with two or three threaded Steinmann pins. In the older age group, if the calcaneocuboid joint is released completely and the clubfoot deformity is severe, it is best to fix the calcaneocuboid joint first. Drill a pin from the posterior aspect of the calcaneus across the cuboid to exit on the dorsolateral aspect of the foot. Be sure that the calcaneocuboid joint is anatomically aligned and not displaced dorsally or plantarward. Double-check the position of the calcaneocuboid joint by radiograms.

Next, the talonavicular joint is transfixed with a threaded Steinmann pin. Simons prefers to put the pin into the center of the talar head and drill it to emerge posteriorly on the posterolateral ridge of the talus. At this point, the flexor tendons and neurovascular bundles are retracted toward the medial part of the foot. Then the pin is drilled farther until it protrudes several inches posteriorly. The drill bit is disengaged from the anterior end of the pin and attached to the posterior part of the pin, and the pin is then drilled posteriorly until the anterior tip is buried immediately beneath the head of the talus.

Next, the navicular bone is positioned on the head of the talus. The navicular should not be flush with the medial aspect of the talar head; it should protrude slightly medially. The dorsal surface of the navicular should be flush with the dorsal surface of the talar head. The longitudinal axis of the talus should be aligned with the navicular and the midfoot. The pin is then inserted across the talonavicular joint slowly to exit on the dorsum of the foot.

Check the position of the foot clinically. Flex the patient's knee 90 degrees, and hold the foot at right angles to the leg. The foot should not be supinated or pronated and should not be translated or tilted into valgus position; it should be perfectly plantigrade and in 5 to 10 degrees of lateral rotation in relation to the proximal tibial tubercle. Place a pin across the calcaneotalar joint by inserting it across the plantar surface of the calcaneus, across the subtalar joint and into the talus, but not into the ankle joint. Be sure that the calcaneus is not tilted into varus or valgus.

Final true anteroposterior and lateral radiograms are made to determine the accuracy of the placement of the pins.

The tourniquet is released, and complete hemostasis is achieved. If the flexor hallucis longus and flexor digitorum longus muscles are very taut and the toes are held rigidly in flexion, the toe flexors are lengthened either by Z-lengthening or by fractional lengthening at their musculotendinous juncture. The wound is closed in the usual fashion with a small Hemovac drain placed in the medial and lateral aspects of the wound. The pins are cut subcutaneously, and either a posterior mold or a very well-padded, loose cast is applied with the knee in 50 degrees of flexion and the ankle in 20 degrees of plantarflexion.

Postoperative Care. The postoperative care is the same as for open reduction of the talocalcaneonavicular-calcaneocuboid joint through the medial and lateral approach.

REFERENCES

Crawford, A. H., Marxsen, J. L., and Osterfeld, D. L.: The Cincinnati incision: A comprehensive approach for surgical procedures for the foot and ankle in childhood. J. Bone Joint Surg., 64-A:1355, 1982.

McKay, D. W.: New concept of and approach to clubfoot treatment: Section I—Principles and morbid anatomy. J. Pediatr. Orthop., 2:347, 1982.

McKay, D. W.: New concept of and approach to clubfoot treatment: Section II—Correction of the clubfoot. J. Pediatr. Orthop., 3:10, 1983.

McKay, D. W.: New concept of and approach to clubfoot treatment: Section III—Evaluation and results. J. Pediatr. Orthop., 3:141, 1983.

Simons, G. W.: Complete subtalar release in club feet: Part I. A preliminary report. J. Bone Joint Surg., 67-A:1044, 1985.

Simons, G. W.: Complete subtalar release in club feet: Part II. Comparison with less extensive procedures. J. Bone Joint Surg., 67-A:1056, 1985.

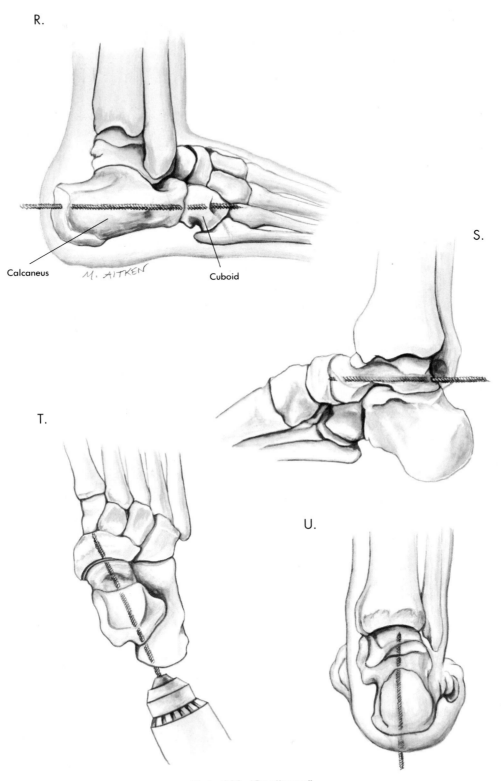

R.

Calcaneus
M. AITKEN
Cuboid

S.

T.

U.

Plate 203. (Continued)

PLATE 204   Carroll's Technique of Open Reduction of the Talocalcaneonavicular and Calcaneocuboid Joints for Correction of Talipes Equinovarus

Indications. See Plate 202.

Patient Position. The patient is in the prone position. First, apply a pneumatic tourniquet on the proximal thigh with the patient in supine position. To prevent distal slipping of the tourniquet on the conical-shaped proximal thigh, pull the soft tissues of the upper thigh distally and then wrap it with flannelette; this measure changes the shape of the upper thigh from conical to cylindrical. The tubes of the tourniquet should be posteriorly placed. Then the patient is turned over into prone position. After routine preparation and draping, the tourniquet is inflated to 100 mm. above the systolic pressure of the patient.

Operative Technique

   A. and **B.** In the Carroll technique, two incisions are made: (1) a curvilinear medial and (2) an oblique posterolateral. For the *medial incision* (see **A.**), the following anatomic structures are marked: (1) the anterior margin of the tip of the medial malleolus, (2) the center of the medial surface of the heel, and (3) the base of the first metatarsal. These three points form a triangle. The *midpart* of the incision parallels the sole of the foot; the *posterior limb* of the incision curves in a plantar direction toward the center of the heel; and the *anterior limb* extends distally around the dorsum of the foot.

   The vertical posterolateral incision runs longitudinally between the Achilles tendon and the lateral malleolus; it begins 2 cm. distal of the tip of the lateral malleolus and extends obliquely upward to the midline of the calf at the juncture of the lower one third and proximal two thirds of the calf.

   C. The posterior limb of the medial incision exposes the plantar structures, and the dorsoanterior part of the medial incision exposes the talonavicular joint. The subcutaneous tissue and superficial fasciae are divided in line with the skin incision. The abductor hallucis is exposed. Note that it takes its origin from the distal border of the laciniate ligament. The abductor hallucis is gently elevated and detached with sharp dissection from its extensive attachments: the navicular bone, sustentaculum tali, medial process of the calcaneal tuberosity, first metatarsal, and other structures on the medial aspect of the foot. Elevate the abductor hallucis muscle and reflect it distally and plantarward, taking care not to injure its nerve supply (medial plantar nerve).

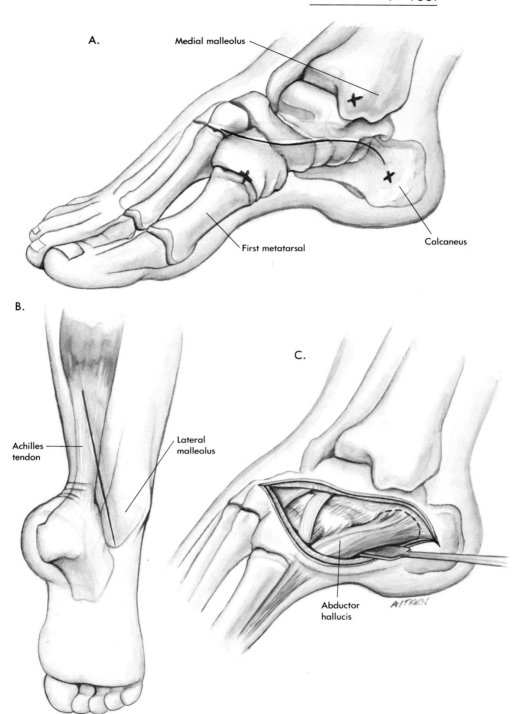

A.
Medial malleolus
First metatarsal
Calcaneus

B.
Achilles tendon
Lateral malleolus

C.
Abductor hallucis

AITKEN

Plate 204. A.–R., Open reduction of the talocalcaneonavicular and calcaneocuboid joints for correction of talipes equinovarus (Carroll technique).

D. The deep accessorius fasciae is incised and opened to expose the medial plantar vessels and nerve and the lateral plantar vessels and nerve.

E. Develop a plane between the plantar fascia and the fat beneath the sole of the foot; identify the tunnel through which the lateral plantar vessels and nerve pass toward the lateral side of the foot. Insert one blade of a Metzenbaum scissors in the tunnel for the lateral plantar vessels and nerve and the other blade superficial to the plantar fascia and section the following structures from their calcaneal origin: plantar fascia, flexor digitorum brevis, and abductor digiti minimi pedis. The quadratus plantae is in the second layer of muscles in the sole of the foot and deep to the lateral nerve and artery. The Metzenbaum scissors divides just the first layer plantar fascia, flexor digitorum brevis, and the abductor digiti quinti.

F. Identify the sheath of flexor digitorum longus below the medial malleolus. Open its sheath and follow its tendon distally to the master knot of Henry, where the flexor hallucis longus tendon is identified.

Section the thickened fibrous sheath of the master knot of Henry and pass a Silastic tube around the flexor hallucis longus and flexor digitorum longus tendons, protecting them from inadvertent injury.

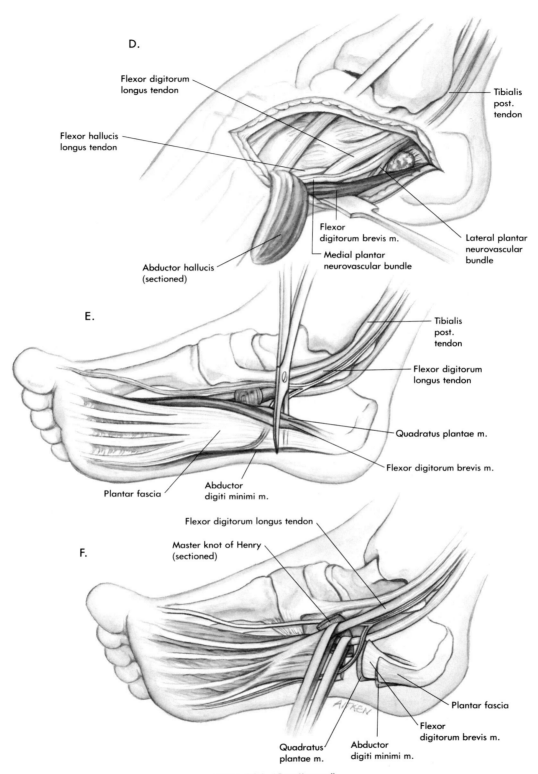

D.

Flexor digitorum longus tendon

Flexor hallucis longus tendon

Tibialis post. tendon

Flexor digitorum brevis m.

Medial plantar neurovascular bundle

Lateral plantar neurovascular bundle

Abductor hallucis (sectioned)

E.

Tibialis post. tendon

Flexor digitorum longus tendon

Quadratus plantae m.

Flexor digitorum brevis m.

Plantar fascia

Abductor digiti minimi m.

F.

Flexor digitorum longus tendon

Master knot of Henry (sectioned)

Plantar fascia

Flexor digitorum brevis m.

Quadratus plantae m.

Abductor digiti minimi m.

Plate 204. (Continued)

G. On the dorsum of the foot, identify the tibialis anterior tendon and trace it to the base of the first metatarsal.

H1. and **H2.** The neurovascular bundles and the flexor hallucis longus and flexor digitorum longus tendons are retracted plantarward, and under the proximal metatarsal, the peroneus longus tendon is exposed. The sheath of the peroneus longus tendon is incised and is traced proximally to the point at which it curves around the lateral border of the foot.

Protect the peroneus longus tendon with a slender, right-angle retractor, and section the long and short plantar ligaments.

I. Identify the calcaneocuboid joint, and divide its medial and plantar thickened capsule.

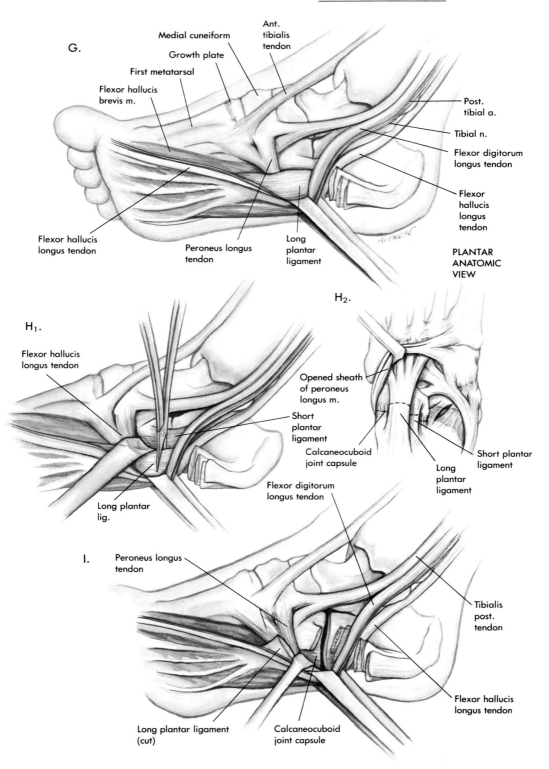

G.

Medial cuneiform

Ant. tibialis tendon

Growth plate

First metatarsal

Flexor hallucis brevis m.

Post. tibial a.

Tibial n.

Flexor digitorum longus tendon

Flexor hallucis longus tendon

Flexor hallucis longus tendon

Peroneus longus tendon

Long plantar ligament

PLANTAR ANATOMIC VIEW

H₁.

Flexor hallucis longus tendon

Short plantar ligament

Long plantar lig.

H₂.

Opened sheath of peroneus longus m.

Calcaneocuboid joint capsule

Flexor digitorum longus tendon

Short plantar ligament

Long plantar ligament

I.

Peroneus longus tendon

Tibialis post. tendon

Flexor hallucis longus tendon

Long plantar ligament (cut)

Calcaneocuboid joint capsule

Plate 204. (Continued)

J. Next, the subcutaneous tissue and superficial fascia are incised through the posterior skin incision. Identify the sural nerve and saphenous veins, and protect them by retracting them laterally.

Dissect the tendo Achillis free, and perform a Z-lengthening in the sagittal plane by sectioning its distal medial half from the os calcis and its proximal lateral part from the triceps surae.

K. In the lateral part of the posterior wound, identify the peroneal tendons and retract them laterally to expose the posterior calcaneofibular ligament. On the medial side of the posterior wound, the flexor digitorum longus and tibialis posterior tendons are identified and their fasciae are opened.

Divide the deep fascia overlying the flexor hallucis longus and neurovascular bundle. Dissect and free the neurovascular bundle and the flexor hallucis longus tendon to the level of the subtalar joint.

L. The posterior tibial tendon is lengthened by a long Z-plasty. Tag its distal stump with a suture.

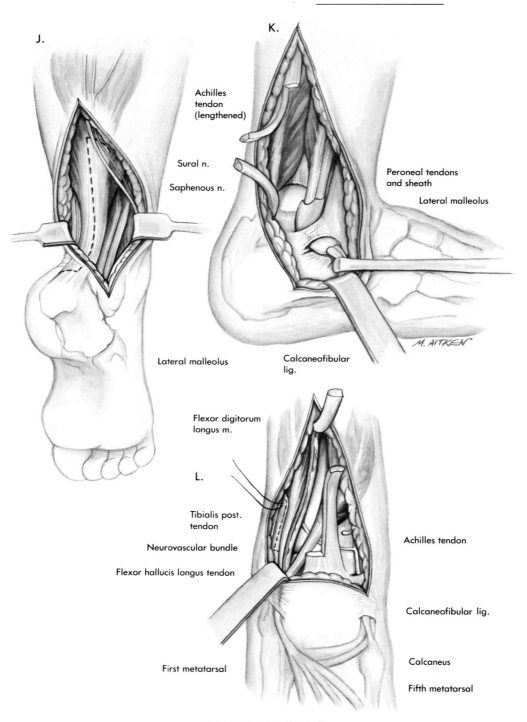

J.

Achilles
tendon
(lengthened)

Sural n.

Saphenous n.

Lateral malleolus

K.

Peroneal tendons
and sheath

Lateral malleolus

Calcaneofibular
lig.

M. AITKEN

Flexor digitorum
longus m.

L.

Tibialis post.
tendon

Neurovascular bundle

Flexor hallucis longus tendon

First metatarsal

Achilles tendon

Calcaneofibular lig.

Calcaneus

Fifth metatarsal

Plate 204. (Continued)

M. Insert a narrow, long retractor underneath the flexor hallucis longus, neurovascular bundle, and flexor digitorum longus, and its tip should protrude through the medial incision.

N. Divide the posterior capsules of the ankle and subtalar joints and the posterior talofibular and calcaneofibular ligaments. The posterior portion of the deltoid ligament posterior to the flexor digitorum longus is divided in order to reduce the body of the talus into the ankle mortise.

O. Through the medial incision, pull the distal segment of the posterior tibial tendon distally through its sheath. Identify the navicular, and dissect it free from the medial malleolus. Grasp the distal portion of the tibialis posterior, and pull the navicular distally and laterally. One can also use a second suture through the posterior tibial navicular junction. Section the anterior tibionavicular ligament and all thickened fibrous tissue between the medial malleolus and the navicular.

Completely divide the capsule of the talonavicular joint, the extensions of the posterior tibial tendon and the calcaneonavicular ligament (spring ligament). Insert a Freer elevator in both the talonavicular and the calcaneocuboid joints, and section any contracted soft tissues (bifurcated ligament) between the dorso-medial portion of the calcaneus and the navicular.

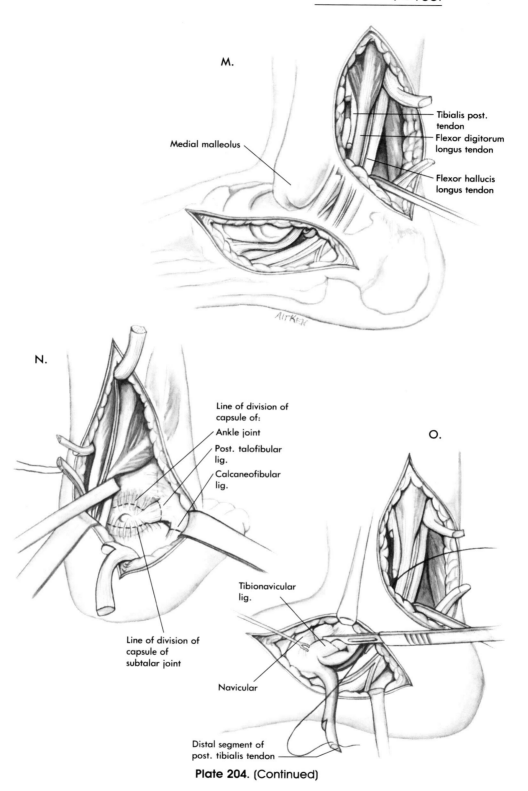

M.

Medial malleolus

Tibialis post. tendon

Flexor digitorum longus tendon

Flexor hallucis longus tendon

N.

Line of division of capsule of:

Ankle joint

Post. talofibular lig.

Calcaneofibular lig.

Line of division of capsule of subtalar joint

O.

Tibionavicular lig.

Navicular

Distal segment of post. tibialis tendon

Plate 204. (Continued)

P. and **Q.** Through the posterior incision, place a Kirschner wire in the laterally rotated body of the talus, rotating it medially in the ankle mortise as the calcaneus is rotated laterally. This maneuver restores the normal anatomic relationship between the calcaneus and the talus.

The navicular is reduced over the anterior end of the talus, and the Kirschner wire is advanced distally across the reduced talonavicular joint through the cuneiform to exit through the skin on the dorsum of the forefoot proximal to the metatarsophalangeal joints. In the severely deformed foot, especially in the older child, a second Kirschner wire is inserted across the calcaneocuboid joint. If it is difficult to restore the divergence between the talus and the os calcis, spread open the subtalar joint and divide the anterior ligament of the subtalar joint, but preserve the interosseous ligament.

At this point, assess the concentricity of reduction of the talocalcaneonavicular and calcaneocuboid joints. The heel must align with the longitudinal axis of the tibia, the lateral border of the foot must be straight, and the equinus of the forefoot and midfoot must be completely corrected. Be sure that the navicular is not riding up into dorsiflexion over the head of the talus and that the navicular is not laterally displaced on the head of the talus, as it will result in an overcorrected valgus foot.

R. Anteroposterior and lateral radiograms of the foot and ankle are made to assess the adequacy of reduction and the position of the pin or pins. If the correction is satisfactory, the pin is advanced so that its posterior part is flush with the cartilage on the back of the talus, and the distal end of the Kirschner wire is cut against the retracted skin on the dorsum of the foot.

If the flexor hallucis longus and flexor digitorum longus muscles are taut and the great toe and lesser toes are flexed, perform a lengthening of the tendons by making a two-level incision at their intermuscular portion. The tibialis posterior is pulled back through its sheath and sutured to its proximal segment under normal physiologic tension. The tendo Achillis is repaired with the foot in plantigrade neutral position. A small Hemovac drain is placed in the medial incision, and the wounds are closed in the usual fashion. The tourniquet is released, and pressure is held on the wounds for five minutes. A Jones-type compression dressing is applied, keeping the knee in extension in order to facilitate venous drainage.

Postoperative Care. The child is returned to the operating room in 7 to 10 days, and a below-knee cast is applied. Carroll recommends cast immobilization and internal fixation with pins for eight weeks, with a cast change at four weeks. The child is then fitted with an ankle-foot orthosis, which is worn 18 hours of the day. Passive stretching and active exercises are performed by the parents several times a day. The orthosis is worn until the child walks with a plantigrade or heel-toe gait.

REFERENCES

Carroll, N. C.: Pathoanatomy and surgical treatment of the resistant clubfoot. A.A.O.S Instructional Course Lectures, 37:93, 1988.

Carroll, N. C.: Pathoanatomy and treatment of talipes equinovarus. In: Symposium: Current Practices in the Treatment of Idiopathic Club Foot in the Child Between Birth and Five Years of Age. Parts I and II. Contemp. Orthop., 1 and 2, 1988.

Carroll, N. C.: Clubfoot. In: Morrissy, R. T. (ed.): Lovell and Winter's Pediatric Orthopaedics. Philadelphia, J. B. Lippincott Co., 1990, pp. 927–956.

Carroll, N. C., McMurtry, R., and Leete, S. F.: The pathoanatomy of congenital clubfoot. Orthop. Clin. North Am., 9:225, 1978.

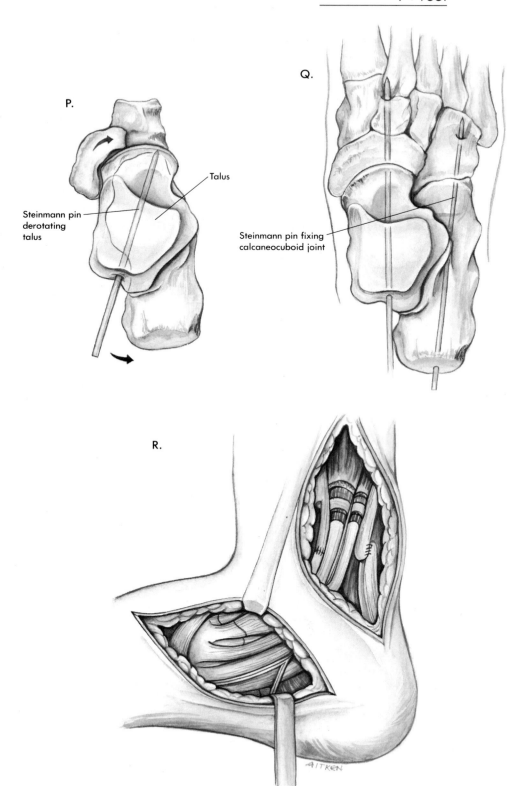

P.

Steinmann pin derotating talus

Talus

Q.

Steinmann pin fixing calcaneocuboid joint

R.

AITKEN

Plate 204. (Continued)

PLATE 205

Open Reduction of Dorsolateral Subluxation of the Talocalcaneonavicular and Calcaneocuboid Joints (Congenital Convex Pes Valgus)

Indications. Rigid congenital convex pes valgus deformity with dorsolateral displacement of the talocalcaneonavicular and calcaneocuboid joints.

Requisites. Adequate size of the foot and four to six months of age or older.

Patient Position. Supine. (Prone if the surgeon prefers.)

Operative Technique

A. A longitudinal incision is made lateral to the tendo calcaneus, beginning at the heel and extending proximally for a distance of 7 to 10 cm. The subcutaneous tissue and tendon sheath are divided in line with the skin incision, and the wound flaps are retracted, exposing the Achilles tendon.

B. Z-plastic lengthening is performed in the anteroposterior plane. With a knife, divide the Achilles tendon longitudinally into lateral and medial halves for a distance of 5 to 7 cm. The distal end of the lateral half is detached from the calcaneus to prevent recurrence of valgus deformity of the heel; the medial half is divided proximally. When the equinus deformity is not marked, sliding lengthening of the heel cord is performed.

C. and **D.** Perform a posterior capsulotomy of the ankle and subtalar joint if necessary. The calcaneofibular ligament is sectioned. The thickened capsule of the calcaneocuboid joint and the bifurcated ligament are divided through a separate lateral incision. The Cincinnati transverse incision, shown in Plate 203, is an alternative surgical approach; it is preferred by this author. When the Cincinnati approach is used, the posterior release is performed through the posterior limb of the incision.

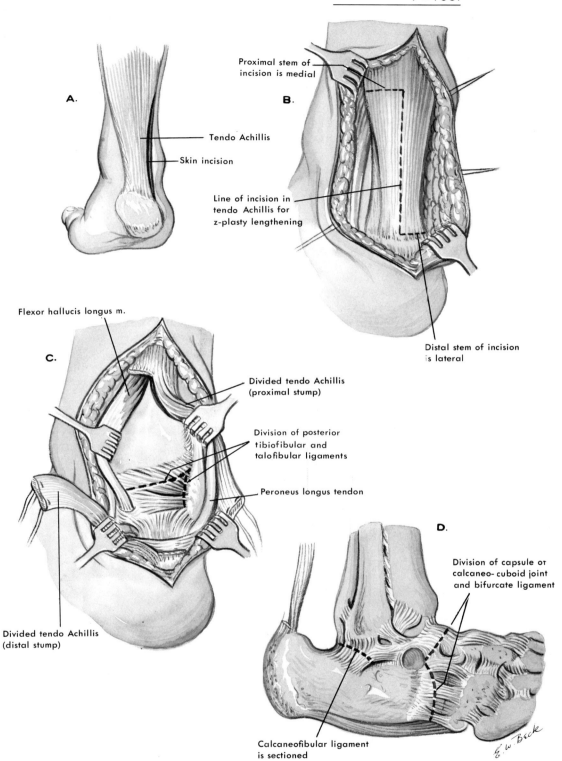

A.

Tendo Achillis

Skin incision

B.

Proximal stem of incision is medial

Line of incision in tendo Achillis for z-plasty lengthening

Distal stem of incision is lateral

C.

Flexor hallucis longus m.

Divided tendo Achillis (proximal stump)

Division of posterior tibiofibular and talofibular ligaments

Peroneus longus tendon

Divided tendo Achillis (distal stump)

D.

Division of capsule oτ calcaneo- cuboid joint and bifurcate ligament

Calcaneofibular ligament is sectioned

E.W.Beck

Plate 205. A.–K., Open reduction of dorsolateral subluxation of the talocalcaneonavicular and calcaneocuboid joints (congenital convex pes valgus).

E. The medial skin incision begins at a point 2 cm. posterior and 1 cm. distal to the tip of the medial malleolus and extends distally to the base of the first metatarsal. The subcutaneous tissue is divided. The skin margins are mobilized and retracted to expose the dorsal, medial, and plantar aspects of the tarsus.

F. and **G.** The posterior tibial tendon is identified, dissected, and divided at its insertion to the tuberosity of the navicular. The end of the tendon is marked with 0 or 00 Tycron suture for later reattachment. The articular surface of the head of the talus points steeply downward and medially to the sole of the foot and is covered by the capsule and ligament. The navicular is found against the dorsal aspect of the neck of the talus, locking it in vertical position. The pathologic anatomy of the ligaments and capsule is noted and the incisions planned so that a secure capsuloplasty can be performed and the talus maintained in its normal anatomic position. Circulation to the talus is another important consideration; it should be disturbed as little as possible by exercising great care and gentleness during dissection. Avascular necrosis of the talus is always a potential serious complication of open reduction. The plantar calcaneonavicular ligament is identified and divided distally from its attachment to the sustentaculum tali, and a 00 Tycron suture is inserted in its end for later reattachment. The talonavicular articulation is exposed by a T-incision. The transverse limb of the T is made distally over the tibionavicular ligament (the anterior portion of the deltoid ligament) and over the dorsal and medial portions of the talonavicular capsule. A cuff of capsule is left attached to the navicular for plication on completion of surgery. The longitudinal limb of the incision is made over the head and neck of the talus inferiorly.

The articular surface of the head of the talus is identified, and a large threaded Kirschner wire is inserted in its center. With a periosteal elevator and the leverage of the Kirschner wire, the head and neck of the talus are lifted dorsally and the forefoot is manipulated into plantar flexion and inversion, bringing the articular surfaces of the navicular and head of the talus into normal anatomic position.

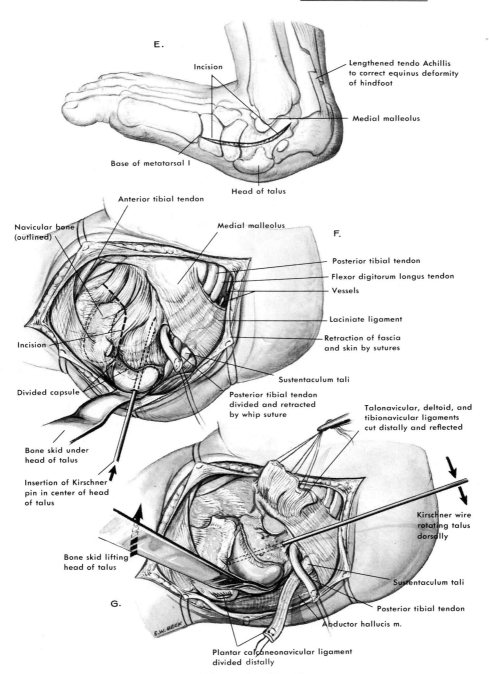

E.

Incision

Lengthened tendo Achillis
to correct equinus deformity
of hindfoot

Medial malleolus

Base of metatarsal I

Head of talus

Anterior tibial tendon

Navicular bone
(outlined)

Medial malleolus

F.

Posterior tibial tendon

Flexor digitorum longus tendon

Vessels

Laciniate ligament

Retraction of fascia
and skin by sutures

Incision

Sustentaculum tali

Divided capsule

Posterior tibial tendon
divided and retracted
by whip suture

Bone skid under
head of talus

Talonavicular, deltoid, and
tibionavicular ligaments
cut distally and reflected

Insertion of Kirschner
pin in center of head
of talus

Kirschner wire
rotating talus
dorsally

Bone skid lifting
head of talus

Sustentaculum tali

Posterior tibial tendon

G.

Abductor hallucis m.

E.W. BECK

Plantar calcaneonavicular ligament
divided distally

Plate 205. (Continued)

H. The Kirschner wire is drilled retrograde into the navicular, cuneiform, and first metatarsal bones, maintaining the reduction. Radiograms of the foot are taken at this time to verify the reduction.

In the older child, the calcaneocuboid and talocalcaneal interosseous ligaments may prevent reduction of the laterally subluxated Chopart's and subtalar joints. If necessary, they are divided through a separate anterolateral incision. The anterior tibial, extensor hallucis longus, extensor digitorum longus, and peroneal muscles may also be so shortened that they prevent reduction; if so, they are lengthened. I prefer fractional lengthening of these muscles through a separate longitudinal incision over the anterior tibial compartment. Others prefer to lengthen them by a Z-plasty over the dorsum of the foot.

I. and **J.** A careful capsuloplasty is very important for maintaining the reduction and the normal anatomic relationship of the talus and navicular. The redundant inferior part of the capsule should be tightened by plication and overlapping of its free edges. First, the plantar-proximal segment of the T of the capsule is pulled dorsally and distally and sutured to the dorsal corner of the inner surface of the distal capsule. Next, the dorsoproximal segment of the T is brought plantarward and distally over the plantar-proximal segment of the capsule and sutured to the plantar corner on the inner surface of the distal capsule. Interrupted sutures are then used to tighten the capsule on its plantar and medial aspects by bringing the distal segment over the proximal segments.

The plantar calcaneonavicular ligament is sutured under tension to the base of the first metatarsal. To tighten the posterior tibial tendon under the head of the talus, it is advanced distally and sutured to the inferior surface of the first cuneiform.

The anterior tibial may be transferred to provide additional dynamic force for maintaining the navicular in correct relationship to the talus. The tendon is detached from its insertion to the medial cuneiform and first metatarsal bone and is dissected free proximally and medially for a distance of 5 cm. Then it is redirected to pass along the medial aspect of the neck of the talus and beneath the head of the talus, where it is fixed to the inferior aspects of the talus and navicular with 00 Tycron sutures. Normally the lower end of the anterior tibial tendon may be split near its insertion. Often I leave intact the attachment to the first metatarsal, dividing only the insertion to the medial cuneiform. The tendon is split (if not normally bifurcated), and the portion to the medial cuneiform bone is transferred to the head of the talus and the navicular. Sometimes, following adequate capsuloplasty, the reduction of the talonavicular joint is so stable that anterior tibial transfer is not necessary to restore support to the head of the talus.

K. The wounds are then closed in routine fashion. The Kirschner wire across the talonavicular joint is cut subcutaneously. To maintain the normal anatomic relationship of the os calcis to the talus, a Kirschner wire is inserted transversely in the os calcis and incorporated into the cast. An alternate method is to pass the wire from the sole of the foot upward through the calcaneus into the talus. I prefer the former, as it controls the heel in the cast and prevents recurrence of both equinus deformity and eversion of the hindfoot. An above-knee cast is applied, with the knee in 45 degrees of flexion, the ankle in 10 to 15 degrees of dorsiflexion, the heel in 10 degrees of inversion, and the forefoot in plantar flexion and inversion. The longitudinal arch and the heel in the cast are well molded.

Postoperative Care. The Kirschner wires are removed in six weeks, but the foot and ankle are immobilized in a solid above-knee cast for an additional two to three weeks. After removal of the cast, an above-knee polypropylene splint is worn at night for one to two years. In the splint, the knee is held in 50 to 60 degrees of flexion, the ankle in neutral dorsiflexion, the heel inverted, and the forefoot plantarflexed and inverted. Passive exercises to develop and maintain range of joint motion and active exercises to develop muscle function are performed several times a day.

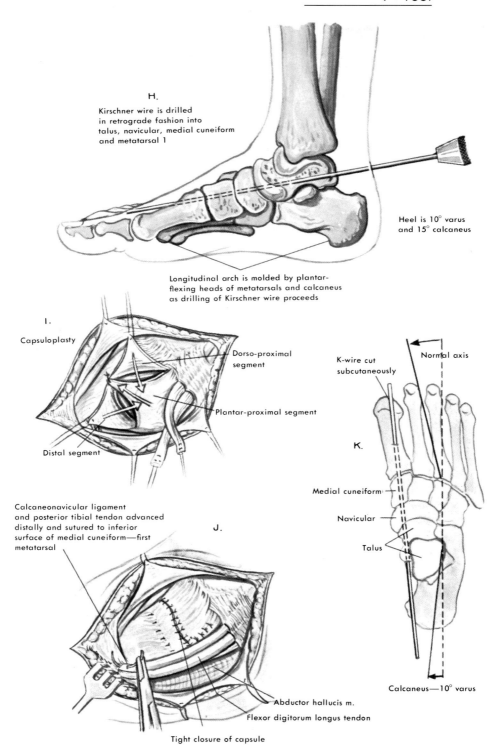

H.

Kirschner wire is drilled
in retrograde fashion into
talus, navicular, medial cuneiform
and metatarsal 1

Heel is 10° varus
and 15° calcaneus

Longitudinal arch is molded by plantar-
flexing heads of metatarsals and calcaneus
as drilling of Kirschner wire proceeds

I.

Capsuloplasty

Dorso-proximal
segment

Plantar-proximal segment

Distal segment

K.

K-wire cut
subcutaneously

Normal axis

Medial cuneiform

Navicular

Talus

Calcaneus—10° varus

Calcaneonavicular ligament
and posterior tibial tendon advanced
distally and sutured to inferior
surface of medial cuneiform—first
metatarsal

J.

Abductor hallucis m.

Flexor digitorum longus tendon

Tight closure of capsule

Plate 205. (Continued)

REFERENCES

Coleman, S. S., Martin, A. F., and Jarrett, J.: Congenital vertical talus: Pathogenesis and treatment. J. Bone Joint Surg., 48-A:1442, 1966.

Coleman, S., Stelling, F. H., and Jarrett, J.: Pathomechanics and treatment of congenital vertical talus. Clin. Orthop., 70:62, 1970.

Storen, H.: On the closed and open correction of congenital convex pes valgus with a vertical astragalus. Acta Orthop. Scand., 36:352, 1965.

Storen, H.: Congenital convex pes valgus with vertical talus. Acta Orthop. Scand., Suppl. 94:1, 1967.

Tachdjian, M. D.: Congenital convex pes valgus. Orthop. Clin. North Am., 3:131, 1972.

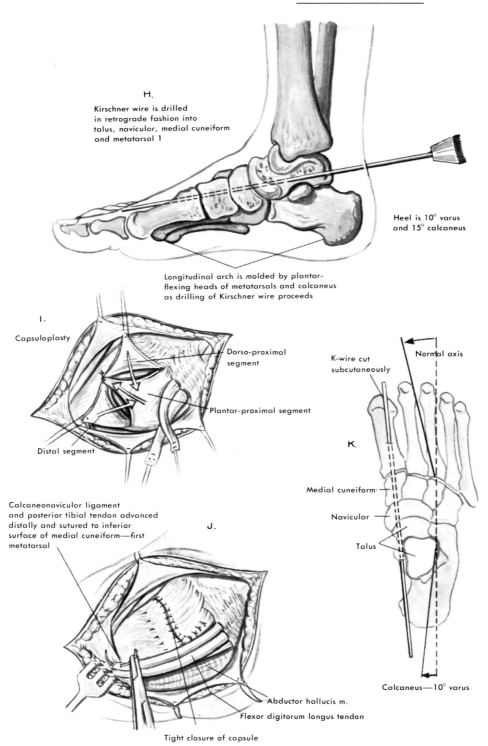

H.

Kirschner wire is drilled
in retrograde fashion into
talus, navicular, medial cuneiform
and metatarsal 1

Heel is 10° varus
and 15° calcaneus

Longitudinal arch is molded by plantar-
flexing heads of metatarsals and calcaneus
as drilling of Kirschner wire proceeds

I.

Capsuloplasty

Dorso-proximal
segment

Plantar-proximal segment

Distal segment

K.

K-wire cut
subcutaneously

Normal axis

Medial cuneiform

Navicular

Talus

Calcaneus—10° varus

Calcaneonavicular ligament
and posterior tibial tendon advanced
distally and sutured to inferior
surface of medial cuneiform—first
metatarsal

J.

Abductor hallucis m.

Flexor digitorum longus tendon

Tight closure of capsule

Plate 205. (Continued)

PLATE 206   ## Medial Plantar Release for Correction of Pes Cavus

Indications. Fixed cavovarus deformity caused by contracted, taut plantar fascia and short plantar muscles and plantar ligaments.

Patient Position. The patient is placed in supine position with the knee flexed and the hip rotated laterally.

Operative Technique

A. A curvilinear incision is made over the medial aspect of the foot; it begins over the posterior tuberosity of the calcaneus in line with skin creases, extends dorsally and anteriorly to a point 1 cm. inferior to the medial malleolus, and then extends distally to terminate at the middle one third of the first metatarsal. Subcutaneous tissues are divided in line with the skin incision. The wound edges are undermined, elevated, and retracted.

B. The abductor hallucis muscle is identified, separated from the flexor hallucis brevis muscle, and detached distally. It is elevated and dissected proximally. In severe cavovarus deformity, this author recommends excision of the abductor hallucis muscle; it facilitates surgical exposure and closure of the wound. An alternate method is to detach the abductor hallucis from its extensive origin and elevate and reflect it distally and plantarward.

C. The flexor digitorum longus and flexor hallucis longus tendons are identified distally, and the master knot of Henry is sectioned. The flexor tendons are mobilized and retracted dorsally.

D. Next, the laciniate ligament is identified and sectioned near its attachment to the calcaneus.

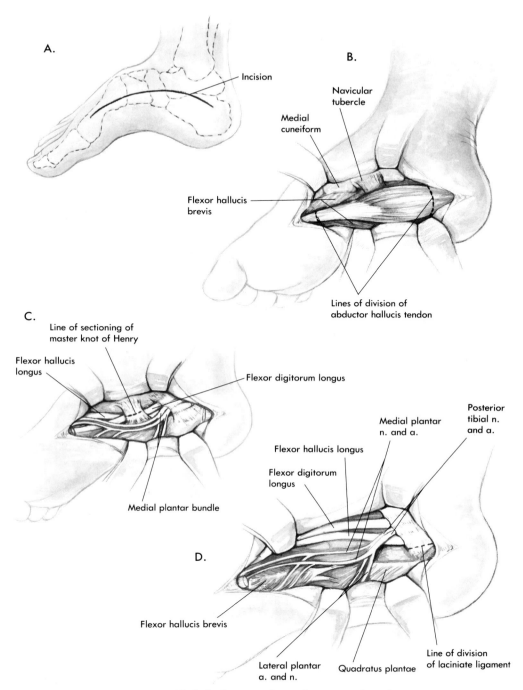

A.

Incision

B.

Navicular
tubercle

Medial
cuneiform

Flexor hallucis
brevis

Lines of division of
abductor hallucis tendon

C.

Line of sectioning of
master knot of Henry

Flexor hallucis
longus

Flexor digitorum longus

Medial plantar bundle

Medial plantar
n. and a.

Posterior
tibial n.
and a.

Flexor hallucis longus

Flexor digitorum
longus

D.

Flexor hallucis brevis

Lateral plantar
a. and n.

Quadratus plantae

Line of division
of laciniate ligament

Plate 206. A.–L., Medial plantar release for correction of pes cavus.

E. With a Freer elevator, the neurovascular bundle is identified, mobilized, and then retracted dorsally.

F. A 1-cm.-long incision is made in the subcutaneous tissue superficial to the plantar fascia near its origin from the tuberosity of the calcaneus.

G. and **H.** With dull, pointed Metzenbaum scissors, the aperture in the subcutaneous tissue is enlarged. A long, narrow retractor pulls the neurovascular bundle dorsally and distally; with a Freer elevator, make an aperture in the soft tissues immediately next to bone anterior to the tuberosity of the calcaneus. Stay close to bone to keep out of trouble. Insert one blade of a Metzenbaum or Mayo scissors in the aperture between the plantar fascia and the subcutaneous tissue, and insert the other blade into the hole made by the Freer elevator immediately next to the calcaneus.

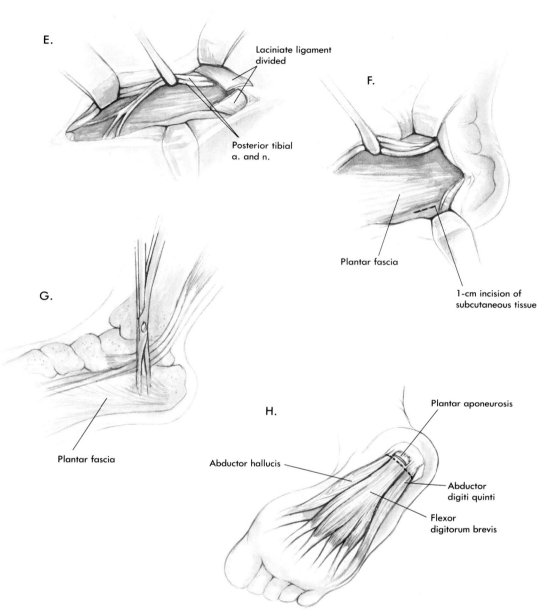

E.

Laciniate ligament divided

Posterior tibial a. and n.

F.

Plantar fascia

1-cm incision of subcutaneous tissue

G.

Plantar fascia

H.

Plantar aponeurosis

Abductor hallucis

Abductor digiti quinti

Flexor digitorum brevis

Plate 206. (Continued)

I.–K. Section the taut soft-tissue structures from their calcaneal origin: the plantar fascia, plantar aponeurosis, flexor digitorum brevis, quadratus plantae, abductor digiti quinti, and long plantar ligament. With a periosteal elevator, the sectioned plantar muscles and ligaments are extraperiosteally elevated from their calcaneal origin and reflected distally.

L. Elevate the forefoot. If the capsule of the first metatarsal cuneiform and naviculocuneiform joints are contracted, they are sectioned on their medial and plantar aspects. If necessary, the contracted tendinous expansions of the posterior tibial tendon are also divided at their metatarsal and cuneiform attachments because they fix the first metatarsal in equinus posture.

The wound is packed, and the tourniquet is released. After complete hemostasis, the wound is closed in the usual fashion and closed Hemovac suction tubes are placed. A below-knee cast is applied with the forefoot in maximal dorsiflexion. There should be adequate padding on the medial and plantar aspects of the foot. The patient is allowed partial to full weight-bearing as soon as he or she is comfortable.

Postoperative Care. The cast is changed at biweekly intervals. The total period of immobilization is about six weeks.

REFERENCES

Bost, F. C., Schottstaedt, E. R., and Larsen, L. J.: Plantar dissection. An operation to release the soft tissues in recurrent or recalcitrant talipes equinovarus. J. Bone Joint Surg., 42-A:151, 1960.
Sherman, F. C., and Westin, G. W.: Plantar release in the correction of deformities of the foot in childhood. J. Bone Joint Surg., 63-A:1382, 1981.
Steindler, A.: Operative treatment of pes cavus. Surg. Gynecol. Obstet., 24:612, 1917.
Steindler, A.: Stripping of the os calcis. J. Orthop. Surg., 2:8, 1920.
Steindler, A.: The treatment of pes cavus. Arch. Surg. (Chicago), 2:325, 1921.

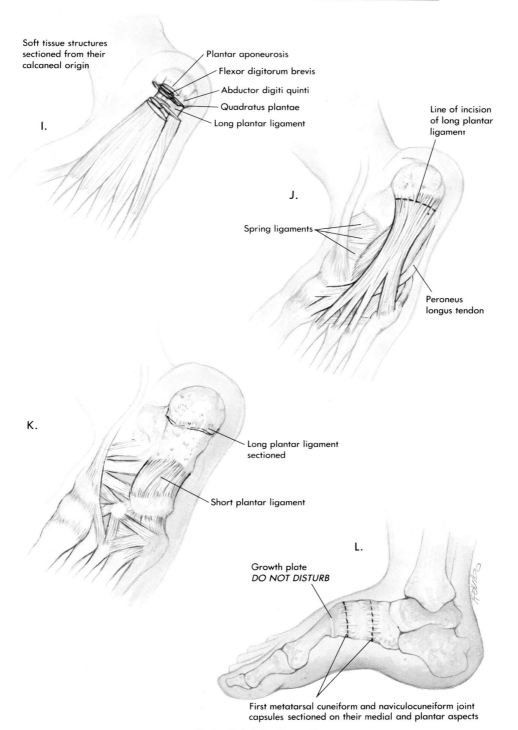

Soft tissue structures
sectioned from their
calcaneal origin

Plantar aponeurosis
Flexor digitorum brevis
Abductor digiti quinti
Quadratus plantae
Long plantar ligament

I.

Line of incision
of long plantar
ligament

J.

Spring ligaments

Peroneus
longus tendon

K.

Long plantar ligament
sectioned

Short plantar ligament

L.

Growth plate
DO NOT DISTURB

First metatarsal cuneiform and naviculocuneiform joint
capsules sectioned on their medial and plantar aspects

Plate 206. (Continued)

PLATE 207   **Dorsal Wedge Resection for Pes Cavus**

Indications. Cavus deformity with equinus taking place at the midfoot in the skeletally mature foot.

Radiographic Control. Image intensifier.

Patient Position. Supine.

Operative Technique. The dorsal aspect of the tarsal bones may be exposed by several means. Cole and Japas make a single dorsal longitudinal incision approximately 6 to 8 cm. long in the midline of the foot, centering over the midtarsal arch (naviculocuneiform junction). Subcutaneous tissue is divided, and the long toe extensors are identified and separated. The plane between the long extensor tendons of the second and third toes is developed, and the extensor digitorum brevis muscle is identified, elevated, and retracted laterally with the peroneus brevis tendon. The anterior tibial tendon and the long extensor tendons of the second and big toes are retracted medially. The periosteum is incised, longitudinally elevated, and retracted medially and laterally.

Méary makes two longitudinal incisions, each about 5 to 6 cm. in length, on the dorsum of the foot. The medial incision is parallel to the longitudinal axis of the second metatarsal and is centered over the intermediate cuneiform bone. The extensor hallucis longus tendon, dorsalis pedis vessels, and anterior tibial tendon are identified, dissected free, and retracted medially. The lateral incision is about 3 cm. long and is centered over the cuboid bone. The peroneus brevis is identified and retracted laterally.

This author uses two longitudinal incisions, one dorsolateral and the other medial.

A. and **B.** Two longitudinal skin incisions are made. The medial incision, about 5 cm. long, is over the medial aspect of the navicular and first cuneiform bones in the interval between the anterior tibial and the posterior tibial tendons. The subcutaneous tissue is divided. The anterior tibial tendon is retracted dorsally; the posterior tibial tendon is partially detached from the tuberosity of the navicular and is retracted plantarward to expose the medial and dorsal aspects of the navicular and first cuneiform bones. The dorsolateral incision, about 4 cm. long, is centered over the cuboid bone. The extensor brevis muscle is identified, elevated, and retracted distally and laterally with the peroneus brevis tendon. The long toe extensors are retracted medially.

C. Through the medial wound, the capsule and periosteum of the navicular and first cuneiform bones are incised and elevated. The soft tissues are retracted dorsally and plantarward with Chandler elevator retractors. The capsule of the talonavicular joint should not be disturbed. If in doubt, one should take radiograms to identify the tarsal bones with certainty.

D. and **E.** With osteotomes, a wedge of bone is excised, including the naviculocuneiform articulation. The base of the wedge is dorsal, its width depending on the severity of the forefoot equinus deformity to be corrected. Through the dorsolateral incision, the wedge osteotomy of the cuboid is completed.

F. The forefoot is then manipulated into dorsiflexion. If the plantar fascia is contracted, a plantar fasciotomy is performed. In severe cases, the short plantar muscles are also sectioned. The first cuneiform bone should be dorsally displaced over the navicular bone. Two Steinmann pins are inserted to transfix the tarsal osteotomy. The medial pin is inserted into the shaft of the first metatarsal, directed posteriorly through the first cuneiform, across the osteotomy site into the navicular and the head of the talus. The lateral pin is started posteriorly along the longitudinal axis of the calcaneus, across the calcaneocuboid joint, into the cuboid and the base of the fifth metatarsal. (Méary uses staples to maintain position of the osteotomy.) Radiograms are taken to verify the position of the pins and the

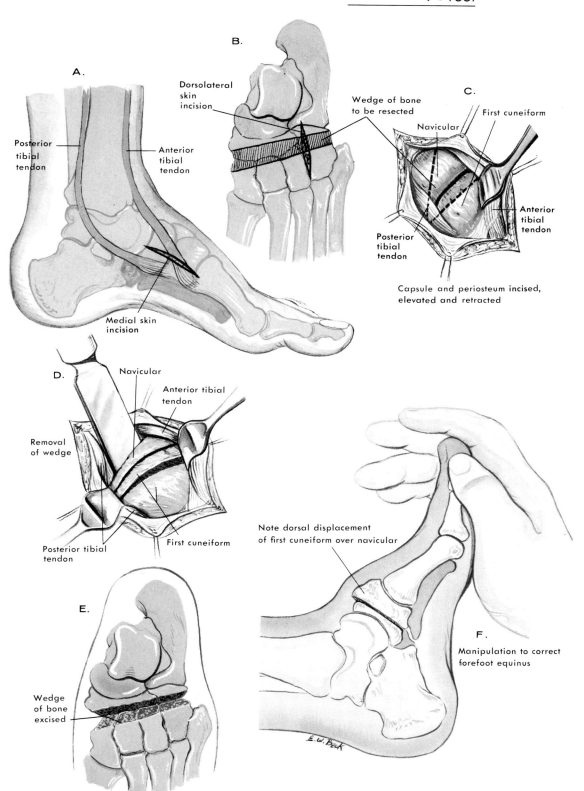

Plate 207. A.–F., Dorsal wedge resection for pes cavus.

maintenance of correction of forefoot equinus deformity. The tourniquet is released, and complete hemostasis is obtained. The incisions are closed. The pins are cut subcutaneously, and a below-knee cast is applied.

Postoperative Care. The foot and leg are immobilized for six weeks, at which time the cast, pins, and sutures are removed. A new below-knee walking cast is given—to be worn for another two to four weeks.

REFERENCES

Cole, W. H.: The treatment of claw-foot. J. Bone Joint Surg., 22:895, 1940.

Japas, L. M.: Surgical treatment of pes cavus by tarsal V-osteotomy. Preliminary report. J. Bone Joint Surg., 50-A:927, 1968.

Méary, R.: Le pied creux essentiel. Symposium. Rev. Chir. Orthop., 53:389, 1967.

Méary, R., Mattei, C. R., and Tomeno, B.: Tarsectomie antérieure pour pied creux. Indications et results lointains. Rev. Chir. Orthop., 62:231, 1976.

Saunders, J. T.: Etiology and treatment of clawfoot. Arch. Surg. (Chicago), 30:179, 1935.

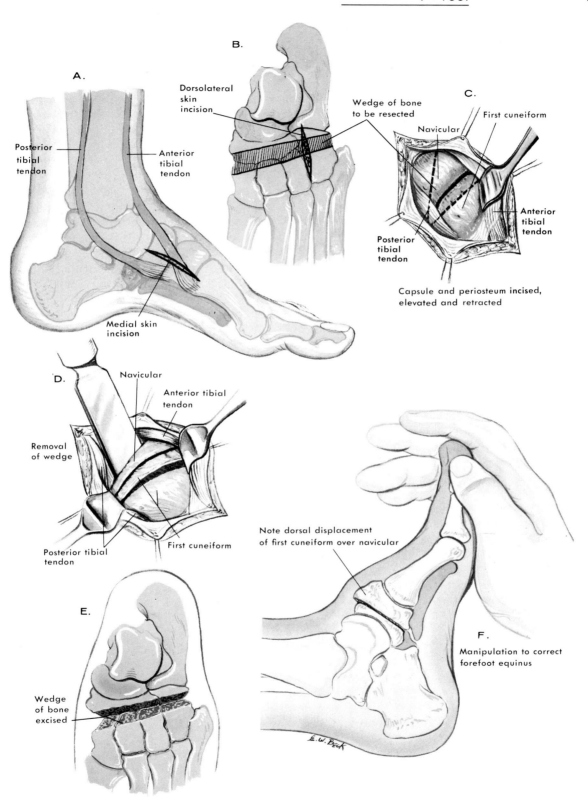

A.

Posterior tibial tendon

Anterior tibial tendon

Medial skin incision

B.

Dorsolateral skin incision

Wedge of bone to be resected

C.

Navicular

First cuneiform

Anterior tibial tendon

Posterior tibial tendon

Capsule and periosteum incised, elevated and retracted

D.

Navicular

Anterior tibial tendon

Removal of wedge

Posterior tibial tendon

First cuneiform

E.

Wedge of bone excised

F.

Note dorsal displacement of first cuneiform over navicular

Manipulation to correct forefoot equinus

E.W. Beck

Plate 207. (Continued)

PLATE 208   ## Japas V-Osteotomy of the Tarsus

Indications. Cavus deformity with equinus taking place at the midfoot in the skeletally mature foot.

This procedure does not shorten the foot. The forefoot is elevated by displacing the base of the distal segment plantarward.

Radiographic Control. Image intensifier.

Patient Position. Supine.

Operative Technique

A. The dorsal aspect of the tarsal bones is exposed by a longitudinal incision 6 to 8 cm. long in the midline of the foot, i.e., between the second and third rays; it is centered over the midtarsal area at the naviculocuneiform junction.

B. and **C.** The subcutaneous tissue is divided. The superficial nerves are isolated and protected. The long toe extensor tendons are identified and separated, and the plane between those of the second and third toes is developed. The extensor digitorum brevis muscle is identified, extraperiosteally elevated, and retracted laterally with the peroneal tendons. The extensor hallucis longus tendon, dorsalis pedis vessels, and anterior tibial tendon are identified, dissected free, and retracted medially. The osteotomy site is exposed extraperiosteally.

The talonavicular joint is identified next.

Caution! Do not injure the midtarsal joint and compromise its function.

If bony landmarks are distorted, radiograms are made for proper orientation. Inadvertent partial ostectomy of the head of the talus will result in aseptic necrosis and traumatic arthritis. The V line of the osteotomy is marked; its apex is located in the midline of the foot at the height of the arch of the cavus deformity; its medial limb extends to the middle of the medial cuneiform, exiting proximal to the cuneiform–first metatarsal joint, and its lateral limb extends to the middle of the cuboid, emerging proximal to the cuboid–fifth metatarsal joint. The V is often shallow, i.e., shaped more like a dome.

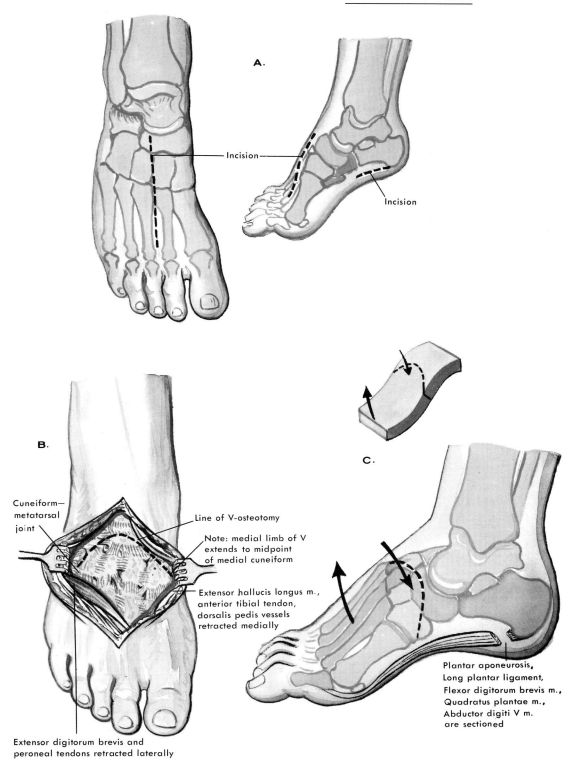

Incision
Incision

B.

Cuneiform— metatarsal joint

Line of V-osteotomy

Note: medial limb of V extends to midpoint of medial cuneiform

Extensor hallucis longus m., anterior tibial tendon, dorsalis pedis vessels retracted medially

Extensor digitorum brevis and peroneal tendons retracted laterally

C.

Plantar aponeurosis, Long plantar ligament, Flexor digitorum brevis m., Quadratus plantae m., Abductor digiti V m. are sectioned

Plate 208. A.–F., Japas V-osteotomy of the tarsus.

D. and **E.** The osteotomy is begun with an oscillating bone saw and is completed with an osteotome. Splintering of the ends of the medial and lateral limbs should be avoided. Next, a curved periosteal elevator is inserted into the osteotomy site, manual traction is applied on the forefoot, and, with the elevator used as a lever, the base of the distal fragment is depressed plantarward. This maneuver corrects the cavus deformity and lengthens the concave plantar surface of the foot. The foot is not shortened, as it would be by resection of a bone wedge, and any abduction or adduction deformity can be corrected if necessary.

F. Once desired alignment is achieved, a single Steinmann pin is inserted through the distal part of the first metatarsal and directed posteriorly and laterally to terminate in the lateral part of the calcaneus or the cuboid. Radiograms are made to verify the completeness of correction. Then the tourniquet is removed, hemostasis obtained, and the wound closed with interrupted sutures. The pin is cut subcutaneously, and a below-knee cast is applied.

Postoperative Care. Two weeks after surgery, a walking heel is placed posteriorly—under the long axis of the tibia—and gradual partial weight-bearing is permitted with crutches. Three to four weeks after surgery, the cast, sutures, and Steinmann pin are removed. Radiograms are made. Another below-knee cast is applied for an additional two to three weeks; full weight-bearing is allowed.

REFERENCES

Japas, L. M.: Surgical treatment of pes cavus by tarsal V-osteotomy. Preliminary report. J. Bone Joint Surg., 61-A:1096, 1979.

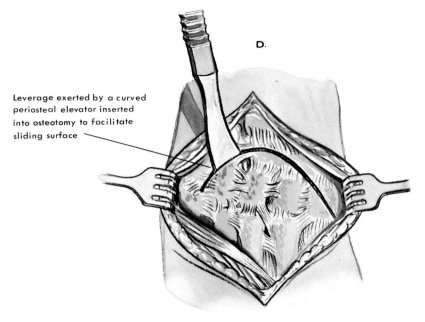

D.

Leverage exerted by a curved periosteal elevator inserted into osteotomy to facilitate sliding surface

E.

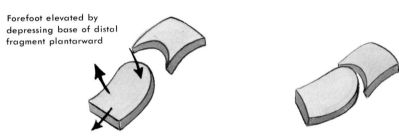

Forefoot elevated by depressing base of distal fragment plantarward

Distal traction applied on forefoot

F.

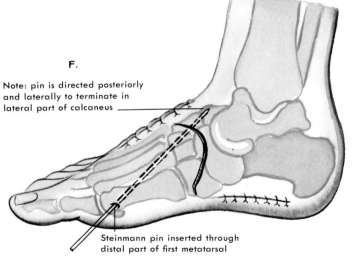

Note: pin is directed posteriorly and laterally to terminate in lateral part of calcaneus

Steinmann pin inserted through distal part of first metatarsal

Plate 208. (Continued)

PLATE 209   Lengthening of the Lateral Column of the Foot with Open-Up Osteotomy of the Cuboid with an Iliac Bone Graft

Indications. Valgus deformity of the midfoot and forefoot with lateral subluxation of the talonavicular joint without lateral tilting of the calcaneocuboid joint. When there is lateral tilting of the calcaneocuboid joint, a reverse Evans operation is performed (see Plate 214).

Patient Position. Supine.

Radiographic Control. Image intensifier.

Operative Technique

   A. The cuboid bone and calcaneocuboid joint are exposed through a 5-cm.-long dorsolateral incision centered over the cuboid. The calcaneocuboid joint is identified, and the cuboid bone is subperiosteally exposed, as described in the reverse Evans operation (see Plate 214). The cuboid bone is subperiosteally exposed. A Chandler elevator retractor is placed on the plantar aspect of the cuboid bone. The dorso-medial wound flap is retracted medially with a rake. With an electric oscillating saw, a vertical osteotomy is made in the middle of the cuboid.

   B. First, a broad osteotome and then a large Cobb periosteal elevator are inserted into the osteotomy site, and the osteotomized cuboid segments are pried apart. A laminectomy spreader may be used if necessary. The width of the bone graft is measured with an osteotome. An autogenous bone graft of appropriate size with a wedge based laterally is taken from the ilium; it is trimmed and inserted into the osteotomy site.

   C. Radiograms are made in anteroposterior, lateral, and oblique projections. If the correction is satisfactory, criss-cross threaded Steinmann pins are used for internal fixation.

   The tourniquet is released. The wound is irrigated, and after complete hemostasis the wound is closed in the usual fashion and a below-knee cast applied. Weight-bearing is not permitted.

Postoperative Care. The cast and pins are removed in three to four weeks postoperatively. Another below-knee walking cast is applied for three additional weeks. Full weight-bearing is allowed.

REFERENCE

Evans, D. C.: Calcaneovalgus deformity. J. Bone Joint Surg., 57-B:270, 1975.

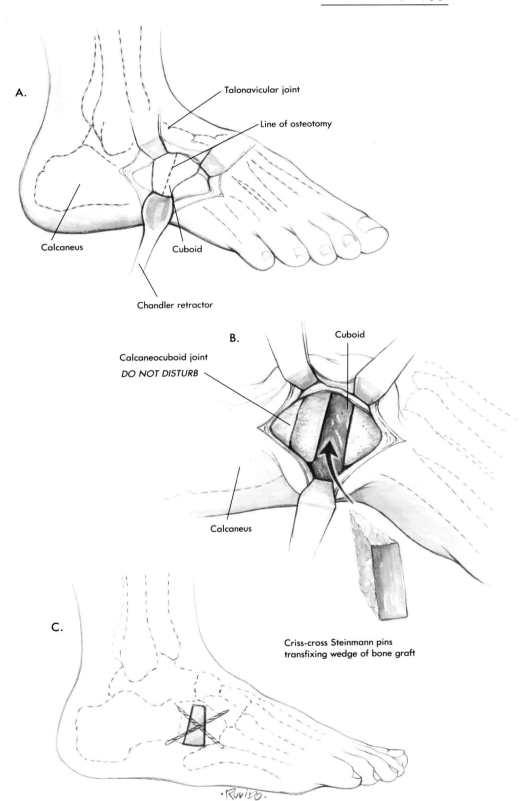

A.

Talonavicular joint

Line of osteotomy

Calcaneus

Cuboid

Chandler retractor

B.

Cuboid

Calcaneocuboid joint
DO NOT DISTURB

Calcaneus

Criss-cross Steinmann pins
transfixing wedge of bone graft

C.

·Ruvido·

Plate 209. A.–C., Lengthening of the lateral column of the foot with open-up osteotomy of the cuboid with an iliac bone graft.

PLATE 210   Shortening of the Lateral Column of the Foot

Indications. Fixed convexity of the lateral column of the foot with a short medial column of the foot in rigid intrinsic talipes equinovarus. Several procedures are described in the literature. Each has its indications (see **A.**).

Radiographic Control. Image intensifier.

Patient Position. Supine.

Operative Technique

A1. When the calcaneocuboid joint is tilted medially, a vertical osteotomy of the anterior part of the calcaneus is performed with a wedge of bone resected, based laterally. The calcaneocuboid joint is left intact.

A2. In the Lichtblau procedure, the anterior end of the calcaneus is resected, including its articular cartilage. This procedure is indicated when the lateral column of the foot is relatively long with no malalignment of the calcaneocuboid joint.

A3. In the Evans operation, the calcaneocuboid joint is resected with a wedge based laterally and fused. It is indicated in paralytic clubfoot in which stability of the lateral column of the foot is desired. It is contraindicated in a child younger than eight years of age because of potential complications of overcorrection and valgus deformity.

A4. A wedge resection and partial decancellation of the cuboid bone (Ogston procedure) is performed when there is fixed varus inclination of the midfoot only.

B. A longitudinal incision about 4 cm. long is made, centering over the dorsolateral aspect of the cuboid bone. Subcutaneous tissue and deep fascia are divided in line with the skin incision. The peroneus brevis tendon is identified and retracted plantarward. The extensor digitorum brevis muscle is elevated off the cuboid bone and retracted dorsally and medially. Be careful not to injure the sural nerve.

C. *Simons procedure.* When the level of the osteotomy is at the anterior part of the calcaneus, identify the calcaneocuboid joint by inspection and palpation and verify its location with the help of image intensifier or routine radiograms. Do not disturb the capsule or the articular cartilage of the calcaneocuboid joint. With a Chandler retractor on the plantar aspect of the foot protecting the peroneal tendons and with retractors on the dorsum of the foot pulling the extensor digitorum brevis dorsally, using a power saw and sharp osteotomes, resect a wedge ⅜ inch wide based laterally. Be sure that the center of the wedge is even on its dorsal and plantar surfaces. The foot is manipulated, and two staples or threaded Kirschner wires are used for internal fixation. If a staple is used, the limbs of the staple should be in the cuboid and calcaneus.

D. *Lichtblau procedure.* Identify the calcaneocuboid joint, and with the help of sharp osteotomes excise the anterior ¼ to ⅜ inch of the calcaneus, including its articular cartilage.

Caution! Do not damage the hyaline cartilage of the cuboid bone.

E. *Evans procedure.* The calcaneocuboid joint and cuboid bone and anterior one half of the calcaneus are subperiosteally exposed, and, with the help of a power saw and sharp osteotomes, a laterally based wedge of calcaneocuboid joint is excised. The foot is manipulated, and internal fixation is achieved with two threaded Steinmann pins or staples.

F. When there is varus inclination of the midfoot only, a cuboid decancellation is performed. With an osteotome, a wedge of bone based laterally is excised from the cuboid bone; with a sharp curet, most of the cancellous bone from the cuboid bone is removed. The foot is then manipulated, bringing the forepart into marked abduction. This author does not recommend the use of staples.

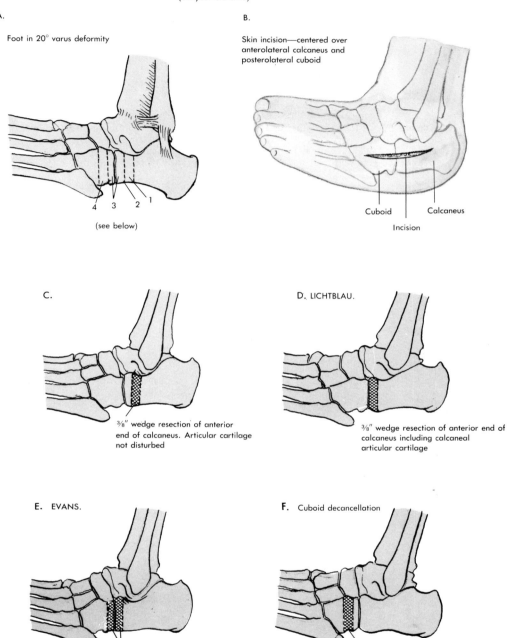

SHORTENING OF LATERAL COLUMN OF FOOT
(Six-year-old child)

A.

Foot in 20° varus deformity

4 3 2 1

(see below)

B.

Skin incision—centered over
anterolateral calcaneus and
posterolateral cuboid

Cuboid   Calcaneus

Incision

C.

3/8" wedge resection of anterior
end of calcaneus. Articular cartilage
not disturbed

D. LICHTBLAU.

3/8" wedge resection of anterior end of
calcaneus including calcaneal
articular cartilage

E. EVANS.

Resection and fusion of calcaneocuboid joint.

F. Cuboid decancellation

Wedge to be
resected

Plate 210. A.–F., Shortening of the lateral column of the foot.

The wound is closed, and a below-knee cast is applied, holding the forepart of the foot in marked abduction.

Postoperative Care. After three weeks, the cast and pins are removed, the foot is manipulated into corrected position, and a new cast is applied. The foot is immobilized for a total period of six weeks.

REFERENCES

Abrams, R. C.: Relapsed club foot. The early results of an evaluation of Dillwyn Evans' operation. J. Bone Joint Surg., 51-A:270, 1969.

Evans, D.: Relapsed club foot. J. Bone Joint Surg., 43-B:722, 1961.

Evans, D.: Treatment of unreduced or lapsed clubfoot in older children. Proc. R. Soc. Med., 61:782, 1968.

Lichtblau, S.: A medial and lateral release operation for clubfoot. A preliminary report. J. Bone Joint Surg., 55-A:1377, 1973.

Ogston, A.: A new principle of curing club-foot in severe cases in children a few years old. Br Med. J., 1:1524, 1902.

Simons, G. W.: Complete subtalar release in club feet: Part I. A preliminary report. J. Bone Joint Surg., 67-A:1044, 1985.

Simons, G. W.: Complete subtalar release in club feet: Part II. Comparison with less extensive procedures. J. Bone Joint Surg., 67-A:1056, 1985.

SHORTENING OF LATERAL COLUMN OF FOOT
(Six-year-old child)

A.

Foot in 20° varus deformity

(see below)

B.

Skin incision—centered over
anterolateral calcaneus and
posterolateral cuboid

Cuboid   Calcaneus

Incision

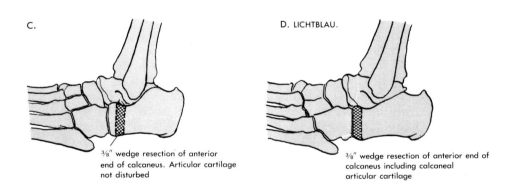

C.

⅜" wedge resection of anterior
end of calcaneus. Articular cartilage
not disturbed

D. LICHTBLAU.

⅜" wedge resection of anterior end of
calcaneus including calcaneal
articular cartilage

E. EVANS.

Resection and fusion of calcaneocuboid joint.

F. Cuboid decancellation

Wedge to be
resected

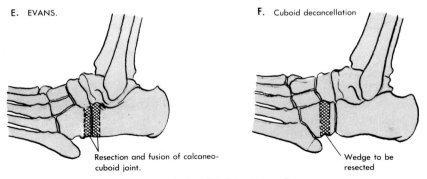

Plate 210. (Continued)

PLATE 211 ## Correction of Midfoot Varus by Open-Up Osteotomy of the Medial Cuneiform and Closing-Wedge Osteotomy of the Cuboid

Indications. Fixed midfoot varus deformity with relative overgrowth of the lateral column of the foot in talipes equinovarus.

Radiographic Control. Image intensifier.

Patient Position. Supine.

Operative Technique

A. A slight, dorsally curved incision is made on the medial aspect of the foot; it begins immediately posterior to the tuberosity of the navicular and extends distally to end at the proximal one fourth of the first metatarsal. The subcutaneous tissue is divided in line with the skin incision, and the wound margins are undermined, elevated, and gently retracted.

B. Identify the medial cuneiform, navicular, and base of the first metatarsal. The posterior tibial tendon inserts into the tuberosity of the navicular, and the anterior tibial tendon into the base of the first metatarsal. Detach abductor hallucis from its origin and elevate and reflect it plantarward. An alternate method is to divide the abductor hallucis muscle distally, reflect it proximally, and excise a segment, exposing the medial cuneiform, navicular, and base of the first metatarsal.

Caution! Do not inadvertently divide the flexor hallucis brevis muscle.

Use image intensifier radiographic control, if necessary, to identify the medial cuneiform. Do not disturb the capsules of the naviculocuneiform and cuneiform–first metatarsal joints. Insert a Homan or Chandler retractor dorsally, deep to the extensor hallucis longus and neurovascular bundle, and another Homan or Chandler retractor immediately posterior to the medial cuneiform bone to protect the flexor hallucis longus and neurovascular bundle. With a power saw, perform a vertical osteotomy of the medial cuneiform, leaving its lateral cortex intact.

C. A longitudinal lateral incision about 4 to 5 cm. long is made centered over the dorsolateral aspect of the cuboid bone. Subcutaneous tissue and deep fascia are divided in line with the skin incision.

Caution! Do not injure the sural nerve.

The peroneus longus and brevis tendons are identified and retracted plantarward, and a Chandler retractor is inserted on the plantar surface of the cuboid bone. Dorsally, the extensor digitorum brevis is elevated off the cuboid bone and retracted dorsally and medially.

D. Identify the cuboid bone; if in doubt, use radiographic control. With a sharp osteotome or power saw, a wedge of bone, based laterally, of the required width is excised from the cuboid bone.

E. The foot is manipulated by bringing the midfoot and forefoot into abduction, correcting the varus deformity. The osteotomy site of the medial cuneiform is opened up with an osteotome. The wedge of bone taken from the cuboid bone is inserted into the medial cuneiform and firmly impacted.

F. The osteotomized fragments of cuboid bone should be closely apposed, and this author recommends two staples or criss-cross pins for internal fixation. It is also best to fix the medial cuneiform osteotomy internally with criss-cross pins. Radiograms are made in the anteroposterior and lateral plane to determine the degree of correction.

The tourniquet is released, and complete hemostasis is achieved. The wound is closed in the usual fashion, and a below-knee cast is applied.

Postoperative Care. The cast is changed in three weeks. The sutures and pins are removed. If staples are used for internal fixation, they are left in place for three to six months. Another below-knee cast is applied for three weeks, upon which the patient is allowed to bear weight.

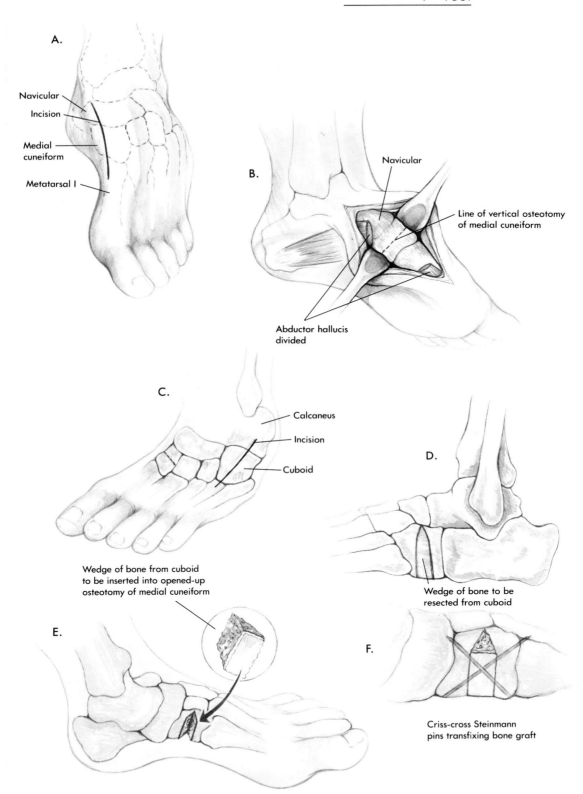

A.

Navicular

Incision

Medial
cuneiform

Metatarsal I

B.

Navicular

Line of vertical osteotomy
of medial cuneiform

Abductor hallucis
divided

C.

Calcaneus

Incision

Cuboid

Wedge of bone from cuboid
to be inserted into opened-up
osteotomy of medial cuneiform

D.

Wedge of bone to be
resected from cuboid

E.

F.

Criss-cross Steinmann
pins transfixing bone graft

Plate 211. A.–F., Correction of midfoot varus by open-up osteotomy of the medial cuneiform and closing-wedge osteotomy of the cuboid.

REFERENCES

Coleman, S. S.: Complex Foot Deformities in Children. Philadelphia: Lea & Febiger, 1983.

McHale, K. A., and Lenhart, M. K.: Treatment of residual clubfoot deformity—the "bean-shaped" foot—by opening wedge medial cuneiform osteotomy and closing wedge cuboid osteotomy. Clinical review and cadaver correlations. J. Pediatr. Orthop., 11:374, 1991.

Schoenecker, P. L., Anderson, D. J., Blair, V. P., and Capelli, A. M.: Combined lateral column shortening and medial column lengthening in the treatment of severe forefoot adductus. In Simons, G. W. (ed.): The Clubfoot: The Present and a View of the Future. New York: Springer-Verlag, 1993, pp. 412–416.

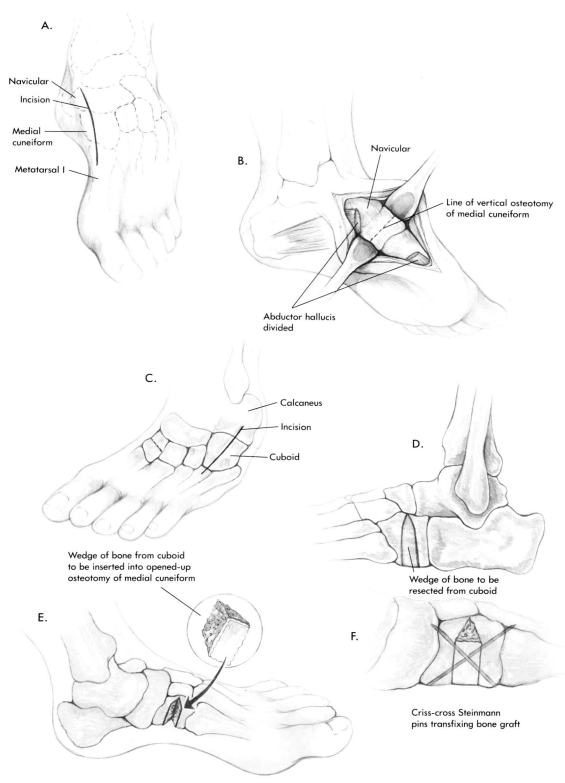

A.

Navicular

Incision

Medial
cuneiform

Metatarsal I

B.

Navicular

Line of vertical osteotomy
of medial cuneiform

Abductor hallucis
divided

C.

Calcaneus

Incision

Cuboid

Wedge of bone from cuboid
to be inserted into opened-up
osteotomy of medial cuneiform

D.

Wedge of bone to be
resected from cuboid

E.

F.

Criss-cross Steinmann
pins transfixing bone graft

Plate 211. (Continued)

PLATE 212 **Resection of the Calcaneonavicular Coalition with Interposition of the Extensor Digitorum Brevis Muscle or Adipose Tissue**

Indications. Calcaneonavicular coalition causing persisting pain, muscle spasm, and loss of subtalar motion.

Requisites

1. No degenerative changes in the talonavicular joint.
2. Younger than 14 years of age. An attempt may be made in the older age group, provided that there are no degenerative changes in the tarsal joints. If there is degenerative arthritis and severe pain, triple arthrodesis should be the primary procedure of choice.

Radiographic Control. Image intensifier.

Patient Position. Supine with sandbag under ipsilateral hip.

Operative Technique

A. A lateral Ollier approach is made. The incision starts immediately below the lateral malleolus and curves upward to end on the lateral aspect of the talonavicular joint.

B. The peroneal tendons are retracted posteriorly, and the long toe extensors are retracted dorsally. The origin of the extensor digitorum brevis muscle is detached and elevated in one piece and reflected distally.

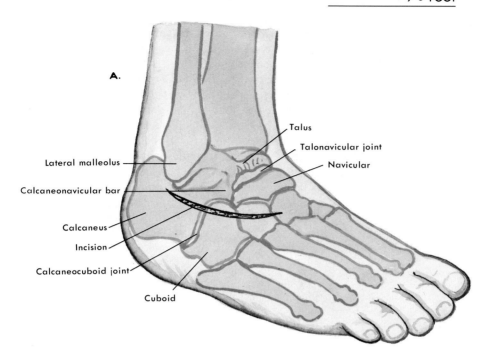

A.

Lateral malleolus

Calcaneonavicular bar

Calcaneus

Incision

Calcaneocuboid joint

Cuboid

Talus

Talonavicular joint

Navicular

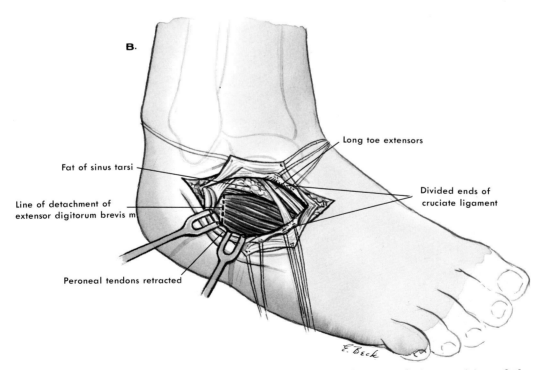

B.

Fat of sinus tarsi

Line of detachment of
extensor digitorum brevis m

Peroneal tendons retracted

Long toe extensors

Divided ends of
cruciate ligament

E. Beck

Plate 212. A.–F., Resection of the calcaneonavicular coalition with interposition of the extensor digitorum brevis muscle or adipose tissue.

C. The calcaneus, cuboid, and navicular bones are identified. The capsule of the calcaneocuboid joint is incised to facilitate exposure of the calcaneonavicular bar. Do not divide the talonavicular capsule, or dorsal subluxation of the navicular on the head of the talus may result. The boundaries of the bar are determined with two smooth Kirschner wires drilled under image intensifier radiographic control: One wire marks the calcaneal attachment of the bar and the other the navicular part. Next, the entire bar is resected as a rectangle, not a wedge, with two straight osteotomes. The osteotome for the calcaneal portion of the bar is directed almost horizontally, whereas the one for the navicular portion is angled plantarward. An oscillating electric saw may be used if preferred.

D. It is imperative to remove the bar adequately, with generous portions of the calcaneal and navicular components. The plantar aspects of the navicular and the talar head should be level. The raw cancellous bleeding bases of the excised bar are coagulated.

Caution! Do not disturb the circulation between the talus and the navicular.

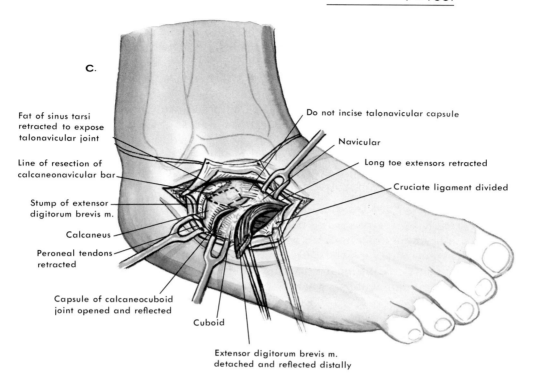

C.

Fat of sinus tarsi retracted to expose talonavicular joint

Line of resection of calcaneonavicular bar

Stump of extensor digitorum brevis m.

Calcaneus

Peroneal tendons retracted

Capsule of calcaneocuboid joint opened and reflected

Cuboid

Extensor digitorum brevis m. detached and reflected distally

Do not incise talonavicular capsule

Navicular

Long toe extensors retracted

Cruciate ligament divided

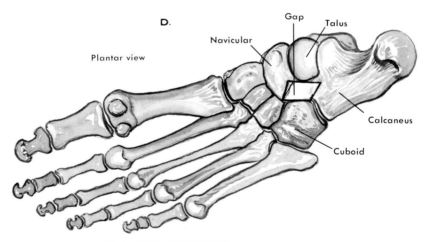

D.

Plantar view

Navicular

Gap

Talus

Calcaneus

Cuboid

Plate 212. (Continued)

E. In Cowell's technique, the entire origin of the extensor digitorum brevis muscle is placed in the defect and secured with a chromic suture. Two Keith needles are used, one on each end of the suture; they are pulled out on the medial side of the foot, where the suture is tied over a well-padded button or over a rectangular piece of sterile felt.

F. The author prefers to place adipose tissue from the gluteal area in the gap created by excision of the bar to obliterate dead space and prevent new bone formation. The fat spacer is sutured on the medial aspect of the foot with absorbable sutures such as 00 Vicryl. This measure will prevent migration of the fat. The extensor digitorum brevis is sutured back to its origin. The wound is closed, and the foot and ankle are immobilized in a below-knee cast.

Postoperative Care. In about ten days, the cast is bivalved and passive and active exercises are performed to develop inversion and eversion of the hindfoot. The foot and ankle are supported in neutral position in a posterior splint made of polypropylene or other plastic material. Full weight-bearing is not permitted; the splint support is continued until the patient obtains adequate active subtalar motion. Usually eight to ten weeks is required.

REFERENCES

Badgley, C. E.: Coalition of the calcaneus and the navicular. Arch. Surg., 15:75, 1927.

Bentzon, P. G. K.: Coalitio calcaneo-navicularis, mit besondere Bezugnahme auf die operative Behandlung des durch diese Anomalie bedingten Plattfusses. Verh. Dtsch. Orthop. Ges., 23:269, 1929.

Bentzon, P. G. K.: Bilateral congenital deformity of the astragalo-calcaneal joint—bony coalescence between os trigonum and the calcaneus? Acta Orthop. Scand., 1:359, 1930.

Cowell, H. R.: Extensor brevis arthroplasty. J. Bone Joint Surg., 52-A:820, 1970.

Cowell, H. R.: Talocalcaneal coalition and new causes of peroneal spastic flatfoot. Clin. Orthop., 85:16, 1972.

Cowell, H. R.: Diagnosis and management of peroneal spastic flatfoot. A.A.O.S. Instructional Course Lectures, 24:94, 1975.

Cowell, H. R., and Elener, V.: Rigid painful flatfoot secondary to tarsal coalition. Clin. Orthop., 177:54, 1983.

Mitchell, G. P., and Gibson, J. M. C.: Excision of calcaneonavicular bar for painful spasmodic flat foot. J. Bone Joint Surg., 49-B:281, 1967.

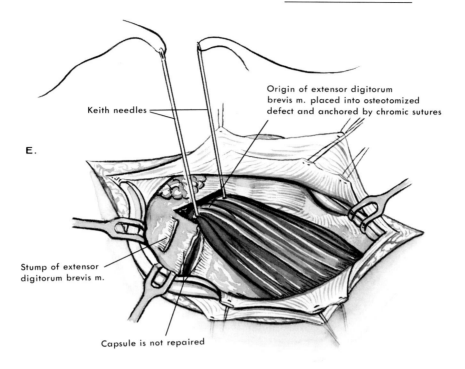

E.

Keith needles

Origin of extensor digitorum
brevis m. placed into osteotomized
defect and anchored by chromic sutures

Stump of extensor
digitorum brevis m.

Capsule is not repaired

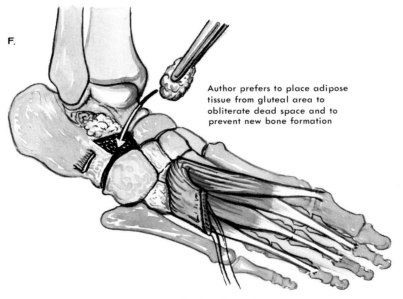

F.

Author prefers to place adipose
tissue from gluteal area to
obliterate dead space and to
prevent new bone formation

Plate 212. (Continued)

PLATE 213   ## Split Anterior Tibial Tendon Transfer

Indications. Supination deformity of the midfoot and forefoot caused by dynamic imbalance between the anterior tibial and the peroneus longus. The split lateral half of the anterior tibial is transferred to the base of the cuboid bone, leaving its medial half intact and attached to its insertion; thereby, some function of the anterior tibial tendon as a dorsiflexor of the first metatarsal is preserved, balancing its antagonist, the peroneus longus muscle, as a plantar flexor of the first metatarsal.

Requisites. Normal range of passive pronation of the forefoot. If there is fixed supination deformity of the forefoot and midfoot, a soft-tissue release in the form of capsulotomy of the first metatarsocuneiform joint and osteotomy of the bases of the second and third metatarsals is performed. For the split anterior tibial tendon transfer to function actively, the forepart of the foot should passively pronate 20 to 30 degrees.

Patient Position. Supine.

Operative Technique

A. A 5-cm.-long incision is made over the dorsomedial aspect of the foot centered over the medial cuneiform. The subcutaneous tissue is divided in line with the skin incision. The skin margins are retracted. A second longitudinal incision, 5 to 7 cm. long, is made over the anterior aspect of the distal one third of the leg lateral to the crest of the tibia. The subcutaneous tissue is divided, and the anterior tibial tendon is identified at the musculotendinous juncture.

B. The anterior tibial tendon is identified with its sheath and carefully dissected to its insertion into the medial plantar aspect of the base of the first metatarsal.

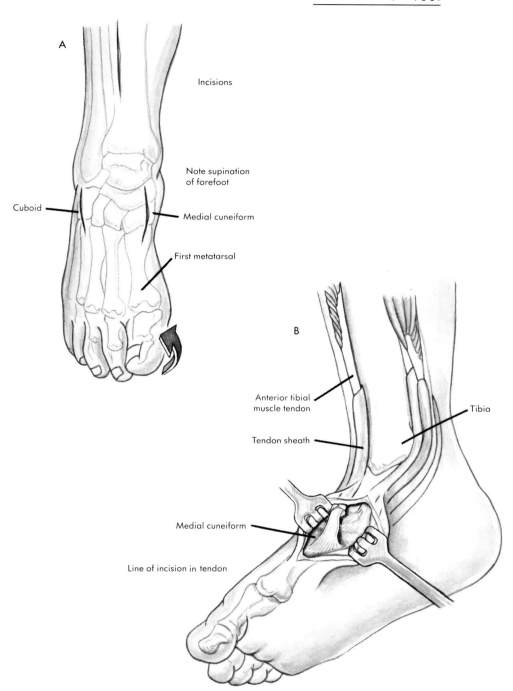

A

Incisions

Note supination
of forefoot

Cuboid

Medial cuneiform

First metatarsal

B

Anterior tibial
muscle tendon

Tibia

Tendon sheath

Medial cuneiform

Line of incision in tendon

Plate 213. A.–I., Split anterior tibial tendon transfer.

C. The anterior tibial tendon is split into two halves. The lateral half of the tendon is sectioned near its insertion to the base of the first metatarsal, with meticulous care taken not to injure the growth plate of the first metatarsal. The lateral half of the tendon is tagged with 00 Tycron suture.

D. and **E.** An Ober tendon passer is inserted into the tendon shaft of the anterior tibial tendon, and the split lateral half of the tendon is delivered into the proximal wound.

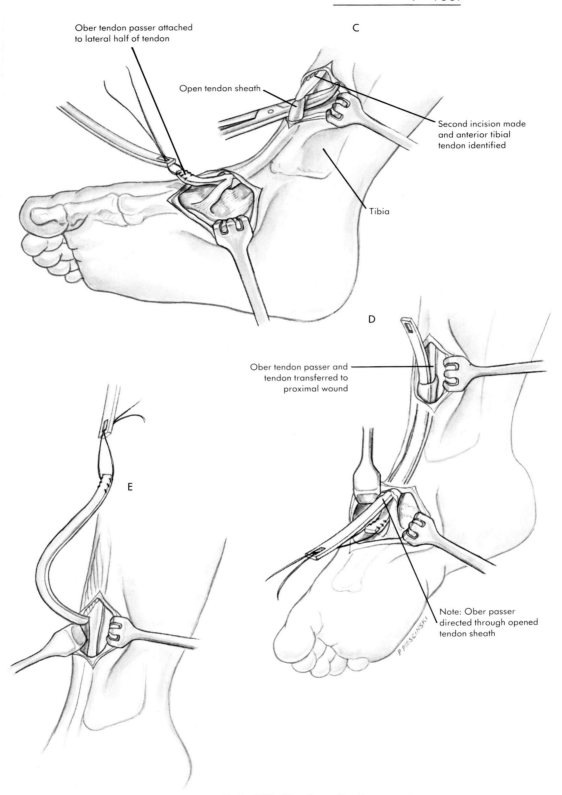

Ober tendon passer attached to lateral half of tendon

C

Open tendon sheath

Second incision made and anterior tibial tendon identified

Tibia

D

Ober tendon passer and tendon transferred to proximal wound

E

Note: Ober passer directed through opened tendon sheath

P. PIESCINSKI

Plate 213. (Continued)

F. and **G.** A third longitudinal incision is made over the dorsolateral aspect of the foot, 5 cm. long, and centered over the cuboid. The lateral half of the anterior tibial tendon is delivered into a third wound subcutaneously deep to the extensor retinaculum with an Ober tendon passer. With an electric drill, two holes are made on the cuboid at converging angles.

H. and **I.** The holes are joined at their depth with a small curet. *Preserve the dorsal roof of the cuboid! Do not fracture it!* The lateral half of the split anterior tibial tendon is passed into the holes and sutured to itself with the ankle in 5 to 10 degrees of dorsiflexion.

If the child's foot is small or the cuboid bone is osteoporotic, a drill hole is made in the cuboid bone, and with two Keith needles the whip suture at the distal end of the split tendon is delivered into the plantar aspect of the foot. The tendon is firmly anchored in the hole in the cuboid bone, and the sutures are tied down firmly over a piece of sterile felt and a button with the foot in 5 degrees of dorsiflexion. (This technique is not illustrated in this drawing.) The tourniquet is released, and, after complete hemostasis, the wounds are closed in the usual fashion and a below-knee cast is applied.

Postoperative Care. Four weeks postoperatively, the cast is removed and active and passive exercises are performed to develop motor function over the anterior tibial muscle. A plastic splint is made to be worn at night, holding the ankle in 5 degrees of dorsiflexion or neutral position and the forefoot in 10 to 15 degrees of pronation.

REFERENCES

Hoffer, M. M., Barakat, G., and Koffman, M.: 10-year follow-up of split anterior tibial tendon transfer in cerebral palsied patients with spastic equinovarus deformity. J. Pediatr. Orthop., 5:432, 1985.

Hoffer, M. M., Reiswig, J. A., Garrett, A. M., and Perry, J.: The split anterior tibial tendon transfer in the treatment of spastic varus hindfoot of childhood. Orthop. Clin. North Am., 5:31, 1974.

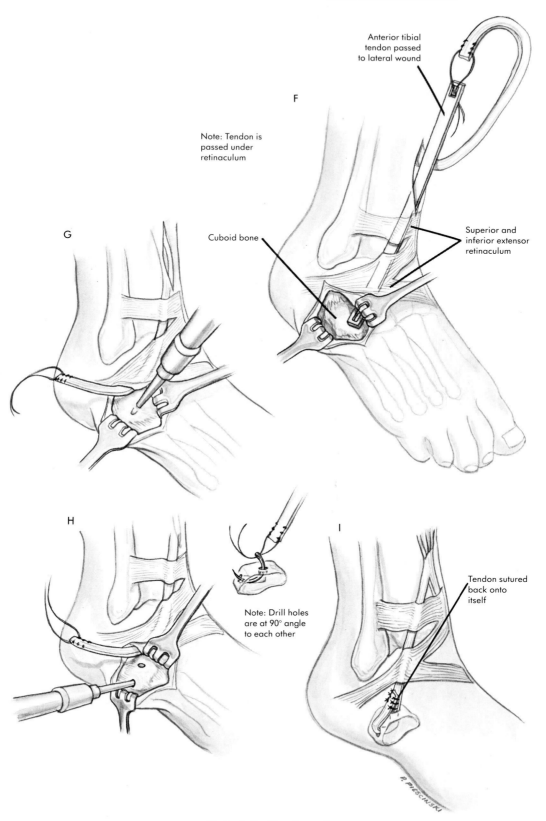

Anterior tibial tendon passed to lateral wound

F

Note: Tendon is passed under retinaculum

Superior and inferior extensor retinaculum

Cuboid bone

G

H

Note: Drill holes are at 90° angle to each other

I

Tendon sutured back onto itself

R. PIESCINSKI

Plate 213. (Continued)

PLATE 214   ## Reverse Evans Operation for Lengthening of the Lateral Column of the Foot for Correction of Calcaneal Valgus Deformity

Indications. Calcaneovalgus deformity of the foot with lateral subluxation of the calcaneocuboid and talonavicular joints. This procedure is recommended for correction of midfoot valgus deformity with lateral subluxation of the navicular on the head of the talus and lateral tilting of the calcaneocuboid joint. The lateral border of the foot is concave. The lateral column of the foot is short in relation to the medial column of the foot.

Radiographic Control. Image intensifier.

Patient Position. Supine.

Operative Technique

A. A 5-cm.-long incision is made over the lateral aspect of the calcaneus and cuboid bones, parallel with and immediately dorsal to the peroneal tendons. Subcutaneous tissue is divided in line with the skin incision.

B. and C. The skin margins are undermined and retracted. Avoid inadvertent division of the sural nerve. The deep fascia and cruciate ligament are incised, and the tendons of the peroneus longus and brevis are identified and retracted plantarward. The calcaneocuboid joint is exposed by elevating and reflecting the extensor digitorum brevis muscle distally and medially from the anterolateral part of the os calcis. The calcaneocuboid joint is identified with a Keith needle. If in doubt, make radiograms for accurate identification. Do not divide the capsule and open the calcaneocuboid joint!

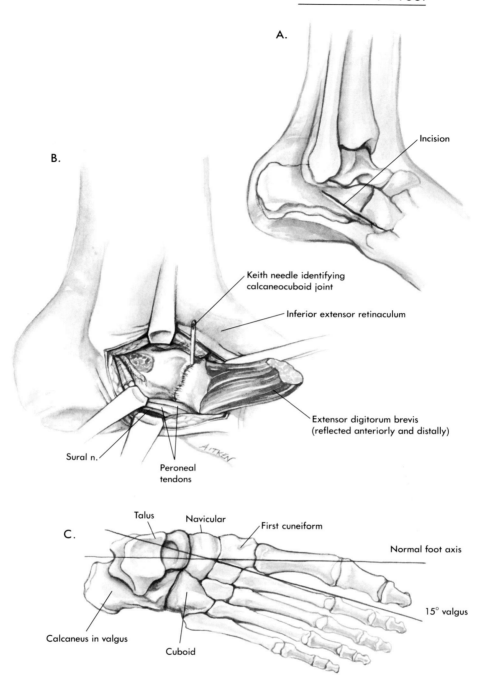

Plate 214. A.–F., Reverse Evans operation for lengthening of the lateral column of the foot for correction of calcaneal valgus deformity.

D. The anterior part of the calcaneus is subperiosteally exposed. With a straight, sharp osteotome, the anterior end of the calcaneus is sectioned in front of the peroneal tubercle. The line of osteotomy is parallel with and 1.5 cm. behind the calcaneocuboid joint.

E. and **F.** The osteotomized segments are pried apart with an osteotome, then a large Cobb periosteal elevator, and then a spreader.

Insert broad, straight osteotomes of various sizes (1.25 to 3.0 cm. or more) into the osteotomy site to determine the optimum width of the bone graft to be used. The foot is inspected clinically, and radiograms are made to ensure that the desired degree of correction is obtained.

Next, a bone graft of appropriate size and thickness is taken from the ilium with both cortices intact. The graft is inserted between the calcaneal fragments. The spreader is removed, and the degree of correction is again ascertained by radiograms. The forepart of the foot should be adducted, and the heel slightly inverted. The graft is fixed to the calcaneus with two criss-cross threaded Steinmann pins. The tourniquet is deflated, and, after complete hemostasis, the wound is closed in the usual fashion. A below-knee cast is applied for immobilization.

Postoperative Care. The cast is changed in four weeks. Radiograms are made to assess bone healing. The pins are removed, a new below-knee cast is applied, and weight-bearing is allowed. The total period of cast immobilization is two months for solid consolidation of the graft. (Evans recommended that the plaster cast be retained for about four months; this author finds two months to be adequate.)

REFERENCES

Evans, D.: Calcaneo-valgus deformity. J. Bone Joint Surg, 57-B:270, 1975.

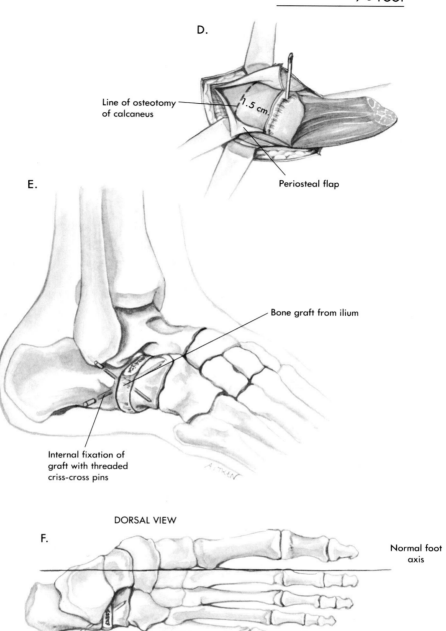

D.

Line of osteotomy of calcaneus

1.5 cm

Periosteal flap

E.

Bone graft from ilium

Internal fixation of graft with threaded criss-cross pins

DORSAL VIEW

F.

Normal foot axis

Corrected calcaneus

Plate 214. (Continued)

PLATE 215 **Correction of Flexible Pes Planovalgus Due to Plantar Sag of the Naviculocuneiform Joint and Medial Sag of the Talonavicular Joint (Giannestras Technique)**

Indications. Painful flat foot due to plantar sag of the naviculocuneiform joint with minimal to moderate degree of medial sag of the talonavicular joint.

Age. Patient near skeletal maturity.

Radiographic Control. Image intensifier.

Patient Position. Supine.

Operative Technique

A. A slightly dorsally curved incision is made on the medial aspect of the foot; it begins immediately posterior to the medial malleolus, extends anteriorly to the navicular tubercle, and ends at the middle of the midshaft of the first metatarsal. The subcutaneous tissue is divided in line with the skin incision, and the wound margins are undermined, elevated, and gently retracted. Avoid a short and inadequate incision.

B. The abductor hallucis muscle is detached and elevated from the medial and plantar surfaces of the medial cuneiform, navicular, plantar calcaneonavicular (spring), and laciniate ligaments. Take care not to injure the muscle's nerve supply.

C. Next, the posterior tibial tendon is identified. In the posterior part of the wound immediately behind the posterior tibial tendon are the flexor digitorum longus tendon and medial plantar branch of the tibial nerve; they are retracted posteriorly and plantarward. Over a blunt elevator, the sheath of the posterior tibial tendon is split longitudinally from the medial malleolus to its insertion at the tuberosity of the navicular.

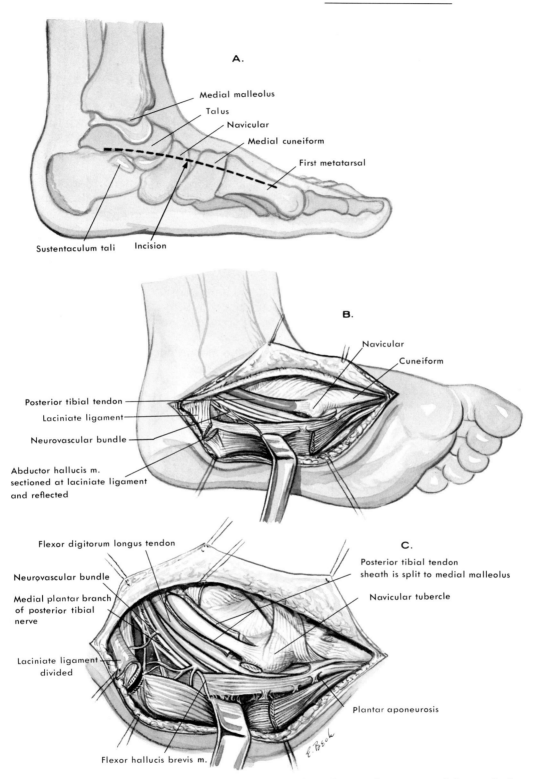

A.

Medial malleolus

Talus

Navicular

Medial cuneiform

First metatarsal

Sustentaculum tali   Incision

B.

Navicular

Cuneiform

Posterior tibial tendon

Laciniate ligament

Neurovascular bundle

Abductor hallucis m.
sectioned at laciniate ligament
and reflected

Flexor digitorum longus tendon

Neurovascular bundle

Medial plantar branch
of posterior tibial
nerve

Laciniate ligament
divided

C.

Posterior tibial tendon
sheath is split to medial malleolus

Navicular tubercle

Plantar aponeurosis

Flexor hallucis brevis m.

E. Beck

Plate 215. A.–P., Correction of flexible pes planovalgus due to plantar sag of the naviculo-cuneiform joint and medial sag of the talonavicular joint (Giannestras technique).

D. The posterior tibial tendon is sectioned from its insertion to the navicular tubercle, and a 00 Mersilene or Tycron whip suture is passed through the distal end of the tendon for traction and later reattachment.

Caution! It is imperative to leave a moderate amount of stump of posterior tibial tendon covering the navicular tuberosity.

E. The anterior tibial tendon is identified in the dorsal and anterior part of the wound. The inferior extensor retinaculum is sectioned, and the sheath of the anterior tibial tendon is split longitudinally. The tendon is divided at its insertion to the base of the first metatarsal, and a 00 Mersilene or Tycron suture is passed through its distal end.

F. The talonavicular, naviculocuneiform, and cuneiform–first metatarsal joints are identified; this should not be difficult, but, if in doubt, can be verified by making a radiogram with a Keith needle marking the first metatarsocuneiform joint. Next, on the medial aspect of the foot, 1.5 cm. apart, two parallel incisions are made down to underlying bone, dividing the capsule and ligamentous tissues; the two incisions extend from the distal end of the medial cuneiform to the neck of the talus adjacent to the sustentaculum tali. Do not divide the flexor digitorum longus tendon or the neurovascular bundle in the posterior part of the wound. The capsule of the first metatarsocuneiform joint is sectioned between the two parallel incisions, and, with a sharp, thin osteotome, an osteocartilaginous flap is elevated. The flap begins at the distal end of the medial cuneiform and extends proximally to include a thin cortical layer of the medial cuneiform and the navicular.

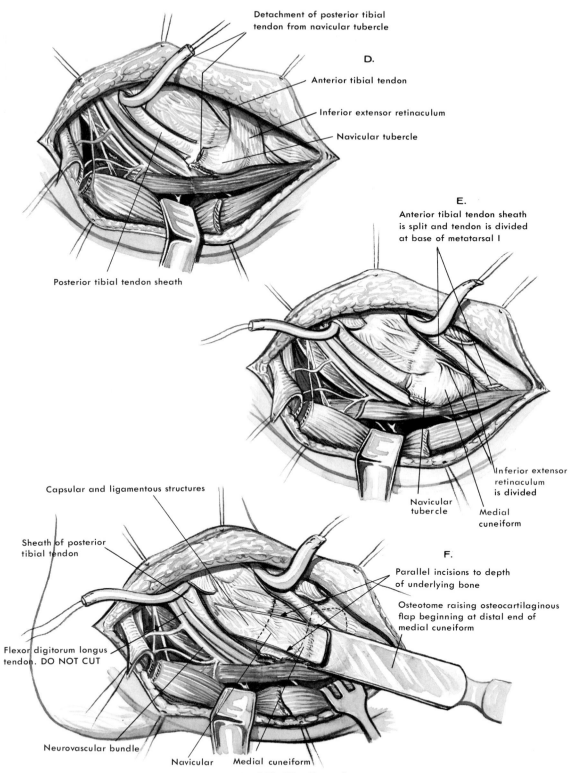

Detachment of posterior tibial tendon from navicular tubercle

D.

Anterior tibial tendon

Inferior extensor retinaculum

Navicular tubercle

Posterior tibial tendon sheath

E.

Anterior tibial tendon sheath is split and tendon is divided at base of metatarsal I

Inferior extensor retinaculum is divided

Navicular tubercle

Medial cuneiform

Capsular and ligamentous structures

Sheath of posterior tibial tendon

F.

Parallel incisions to depth of underlying bone

Osteotome raising osteocartilaginous flap beginning at distal end of medial cuneiform

Flexor digitorum longus tendon. DO NOT CUT

Neurovascular bundle

Navicular

Medial cuneiform

Plate 215. (Continued)

G. The osteocartilaginous flap and the capsular and ligamentous tissues are reflected. Care is taken not to tear the thin ligamentous structure between the navicular and cuneiform. The hyaline articular cartilage of the talonavicular joint should not be disturbed.

H. The plantar calcaneonavicular (or spring) ligament is identified and divided from its attachment to the navicular. It is dissected free and lifted back to its origin from the sustentaculum tali.

I. The ligamentous and capsular structures are gently dissected and elevated to expose the dorsal, medial, and plantar surfaces of the navicular and medial cuneiform bones.

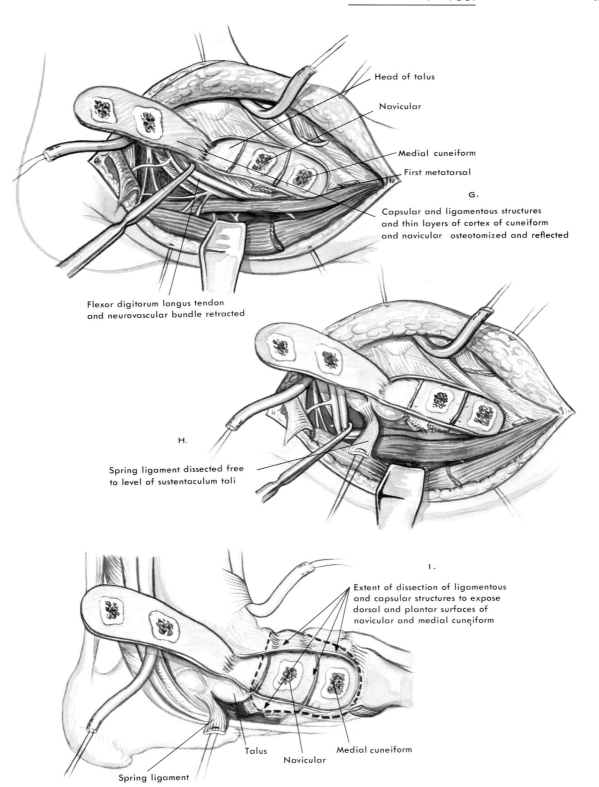

Head of talus

Navicular

Medial cuneiform

First metatarsal

G.

Capsular and ligamentous structures
and thin layers of cortex of cuneiform
and navicular osteotomized and reflected

Flexor digitorum longus tendon
and neurovascular bundle retracted

H.

Spring ligament dissected free
to level of sustentaculum tali

I.

Extent of dissection of ligamentous
and capsular structures to expose
dorsal and plantar surfaces of
navicular and medial cuneiform

Talus

Navicular

Medial cuneiform

Spring ligament

Plate 215. (Continued)

J. The plantar aspect of the navicular is denuded of soft tissue, and the cortex is roughened with a sharp curet or rasp.

K. With a thin, sharp osteotome, a wedge of bone is excised from the proximal surface of the medial cuneiform. The base of the wedge, directed plantarward, is about 2 to 3 mm. in width. The opposing distal articular cartilage of the navicular is excised, exposing the subjacent cortical bone.

L. The adequacy of correction of the plantar sag of the naviculocuneiform joint is checked by pronation and plantar flexion of the forepart of the foot. There should be close apposition of the bone surfaces between the medial cuneiform and navicular. Then a drill hole $5/16$ inch in diameter is made in the navicular, beginning on its plantar surface; it is directed dorsally and distally to exit at the center of the denuded distal articular surface of the navicular. A second drill hole, $5/16$ inch in diameter, is made in the medial cuneiform; it begins on the plantar surface, extends dorsally and proximally, and exits on the proximal denuded joint surface immediately below the dorsal cortex. An adequate amount of cortex should be left in both bones so that the suture does not tear out of the cancellous bone.

M. Giannestras does not recommend the use of staples or Kirschner wires across the naviculocuneiform joint for internal fixation. A double No. 2 chromic suture is passed through the holes from the plantar surface of the navicular into the dorsal holes in the navicular and medial cuneiform, exiting on the plantar aspect of the cuneiform. The forefoot is held in plantar flexion and pronation, and the suture is tied. This author recommends the use of a small-fragment cancellous screw or two threaded Kirschner wires for transfixing the naviculocuneiform joint.

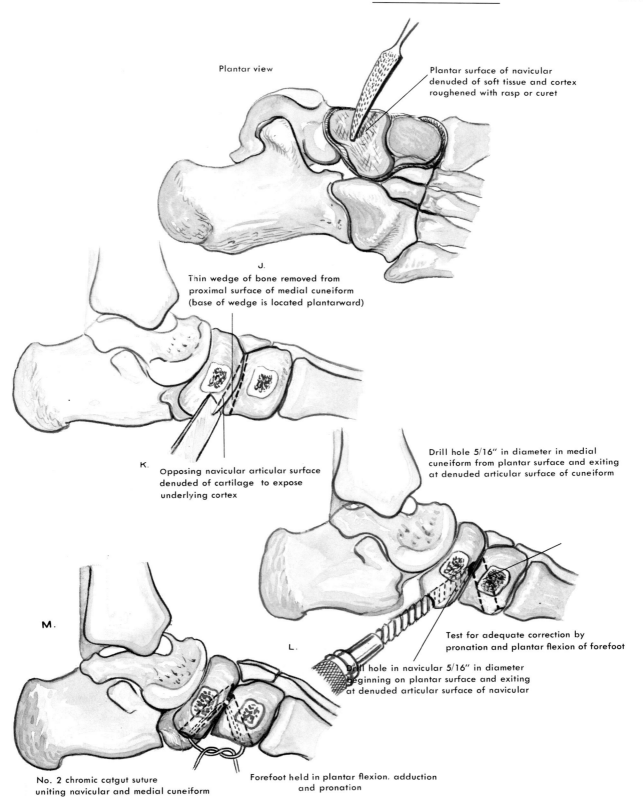

Plantar view

Plantar surface of navicular denuded of soft tissue and cortex roughened with rasp or curet

J.

Thin wedge of bone removed from proximal surface of medial cuneiform (base of wedge is located plantarward)

K.

Opposing navicular articular surface denuded of cartilage to expose underlying cortex

Drill hole 5/16" in diameter in medial cuneiform from plantar surface and exiting at denuded articular surface of cuneiform

M.

Test for adequate correction by pronation and plantar flexion of forefoot

L.

Drill hole in navicular 5/16" in diameter beginning on plantar surface and exiting at denuded articular surface of navicular

No. 2 chromic catgut suture uniting navicular and medial cuneiform

Forefoot held in plantar flexion, adduction and pronation

Plate 215. (Continued)

N. With the foot held in maximally corrected position—the forepart of the foot plantar-flexed and adducted—the osteocartilaginous flap is pulled distally with a Kocher clamp to cover the denuded surfaces of the navicular and cuneiform bones. The distal end is anchored securely to the base of the first metatarsal with 00 Mersilene or Tycron suture. The flap should be taut, forming a bowstring on the medial and plantar aspects of the foot. With a fine, small cutting needle, the dorsal and plantar margins of the flap are anchored to adjacent capsular structures with interrupted sutures. Any distal redundant portion of the flap is excised. The spring ligament is tautly resutured to the navicular. The security of fixation and degree of correction are checked with the foot released.

O. A drill hole 7/64 inch in diameter is made in the navicular from the dorsal to the plantar surface, approximately 1.5 to 2.0 cm. lateral to the medial edge of the navicular tubercle. The plantar surface of the navicular is denuded of all fibrous tissue and roughened with a sharp curet, exposing raw cancellous bone.

P. The ends of the tibialis anterior and tibialis posterior tendons are sutured together with 00 Mersilene or Tycron suture, which is passed in a figure-of-eight fashion. The two ends of the suture are loose, one coming out of the end of the tibialis anterior and the other through the end of the tibialis posterior, similar to Bunnell's suture but without the pull-out wire. Then the two suture ends are threaded through a large, slightly curved needle and passed through the plantar drill hole and up through the dorsal drill hole. The suture ends are then separated, and each one is threaded through a sharp cutting needle and passed separately through the overlying capsular and ligamentous soft tissues. Next, with a forceps the two tendons are pulled and held down snugly under the plantar aspect of the navicular and the sutures are tied. The tendons are against the plantar aspect of the navicular but are not pulled up through the drill hole; only the sutures pass up through the drill hole. Additional sutures are applied through the two tendons to the overlying spring ligament.

The tourniquet is deflated, and complete hemostasis obtained. It is best to insert a closed-suction Hemovac unit. The subcutaneous tissues are closed with interrupted sutures, and the skin is closed with a subcuticular suture.

A below-knee cast is applied for immobilization. Avoid an overcorrected position. The purpose of the cast is to retain the correction achieved surgically. Giannestras recommends that the cast be applied in two sections. The heel should be slightly varus, the plaster under the newly formed longitudinal arch well molded, and the forefoot in maximal pronation.

Before the patient leaves the operating room, anteroposterior and lateral radiograms of the foot are made to determine the position of the talonavicular and naviculocuneiform joints.

Postoperative Care. Immobilization in the cast is maintained for eight weeks. The cast is changed as necessary. Radiograms of the foot are made to ascertain the fusion of the naviculocuneiform joint. If union is delayed or does not take place, a below-knee walking cast is applied for another four weeks. Persistence of non-union is ignored, however, as it usually does not cause any symptoms.

On removal of the cast, the foot may appear overcorrected; parents should be reassured that it will return to normal position after two to three weeks of walking. In the beginning, a three-point or four-point crutch gait is used to protect the limb. Active exercises are performed to strengthen the triceps surae, toe extensors, tibialis posterior, and tibialis anterior muscles.

Initially, the tendency is to walk on the lateral aspect of the foot. Proper heel-toe gait should be taught by the physical therapist. The child is fitted with simple Oxford shoes with a rigid shank. No arch supports of any type in the shoe are required.

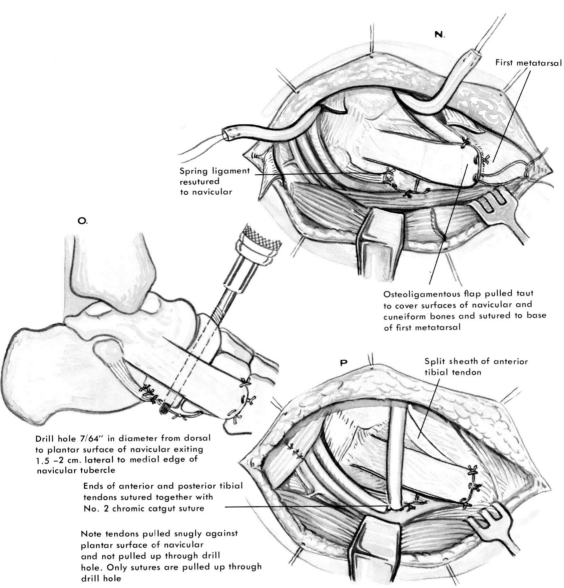

N.

First metatarsal

Spring ligament
resutured
to navicular

Osteoligamentous flap pulled taut
to cover surfaces of navicular and
cuneiform bones and sutured to base
of first metatarsal

O.

Drill hole 7/64" in diameter from dorsal
to plantar surface of navicular exiting
1.5 –2 cm. lateral to medial edge of
navicular tubercle

Ends of anterior and posterior tibial
tendons sutured together with
No. 2 chromic catgut suture

Note tendons pulled snugly against
plantar surface of navicular
and not pulled up through drill
hole. Only sutures are pulled up through
drill hole

P

Split sheath of anterior
tibial tendon

Plate 215. (Continued)

REFERENCES

Butte, F. L.: Navicular-cuneiform arthrodesis for flatfoot. J. Bone Joint Surg., 19:496, 1937.

Caldwell, G. D.: Surgical correction of relaxed flatfoot by the Durham flatfootplasty. Clin. Orthop., 2:221, 1953.

Crego, C. H., Jr., and Ford, L. T.: An end-result study of various operative procedures for correcting flat feet in children. J. Bone Joint Surg., 34-A:183, 1952.

Giannestras, N. J.: Static foot problems in the pre-adolescent and adolescent stages. In: Foot Disorders. Medical and Surgical Management. Philadelphia, Lea & Febiger, 1967, pp. 119–155.

Giannestras, N. J.: Flexible valgus flatfoot resulting from naviculocuneiform and talonavicular sag. Surgical correction in the adolescent. In: Bateman, J. E. (ed.): Foot Science. Philadelphia, W. B. Saunders Co., 1976, pp. 67–105.

Hoke, M.: An operation for the correction of extremely relaxed flat feet. J. Bone Joint Surg., 13:773, 1931.

Jack, E. A.: Naviculocuneiform fusion in the treatment of flat foot. J. Bone Joint Surg., 35-B:279, 1953.

Miller, O. L.: A plastic flat foot operation. J. Bone Joint Surg., 9:84, 1927.

Seymour, N.: The late results of naviculo-cuneiform fusion. J. Bone Joint Surg., 49-B:558, 1967.

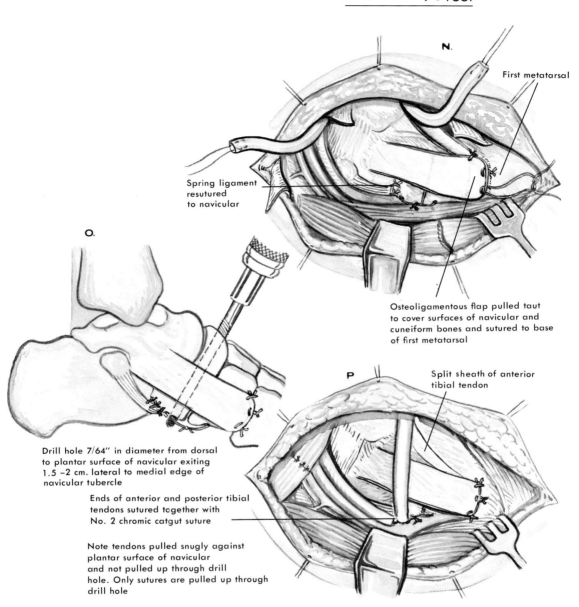

N.

First metatarsal

Spring ligament
resutured
to navicular

Osteoligamentous flap pulled taut
to cover surfaces of navicular and
cuneiform bones and sutured to base
of first metatarsal

O.

Drill hole 7/64" in diameter from dorsal
to plantar surface of navicular exiting
1.5 –2 cm. lateral to medial edge of
navicular tubercle

Ends of anterior and posterior tibial
tendons sutured together with
No. 2 chromic catgut suture

Note tendons pulled snugly against
plantar surface of navicular
and not pulled up through drill
hole. Only sutures are pulled up through
drill hole

P

Split sheath of anterior
tibial tendon

Plate 215. (Continued)

PLATE 216 — Vertical Osteotomy of the Medial Cuneiform with Wedge of Bone Graft Based on the Plantar Aspect with Transfer of the Anterior Tibial Tendon to the Dorsum of the Medial Cuneiform

Indications. Cavovarus deformity of the foot in which the hindfoot is flexible and there is satisfactory extrinsic muscle balance.

Radiographic Control. Image intensifier.

Patient Position. Supine, with the knee flexed and the hip laterally rotated.

Operative Technique

A. The medial and plantar aspects of the midfoot are approached through a 5-cm.-long medial incision, beginning at the head of the talus and extending distally to the juncture of the proximal one fourth of the first metatarsal. The subcutaneous tissue is divided in line with the skin incision. The veins crossing the field are clamped and coagulated. The wound flaps are undermined and retracted dorsally and plantarward.

First, the anterior tibial tendon is exposed and traced distally to its insertion on the plantar aspect of the foot.

B. The medial cuneiform bone is identified; with a small drill bit, its center is marked and confirmed by radiography.

Chandler retractors are inserted on the plantar and dorsal surfaces of the medial cuneiform, and with an electric saw a vertical osteotomy of the medial cuneiform is performed. Its dorsal cortex is left intact.

C. A wedge of bone of the appropriate size is taken from the crest of the ilium in routine fashion. With the help of a bone spreader, the osteotomy is opened up and the wedge of bone is inserted on the plantar aspect of the opened-up medial cuneiform and impacted in place. This will elevate the middle ray of the foot from equinus to normal position. If there is rigid contracture of the soft tissues, the incision is extended posteriorly and a plantar release is performed as described in Plate 206.

D. Drill holes are made in the distal segment of the medial cuneiform, and the anterior tibial is detached from the plantar aspect of the base of the first metatarsal and transferred to the dorsum of the medial cuneiform. The anterior tibial tendon should be firmly anchored to bone with nonabsorbable sutures. The bone graft and the osteotomized medial cuneiform are fixed internally with one or two threaded Steinmann pins.

The tourniquet is released, and completed hemostasis is achieved. The wound is closed in the usual fashion, and a below-knee cast is applied.

Postoperative Care. Weight-bearing is not permitted until the pin is removed four weeks postoperatively. Following pin removal, another below-knee cast is applied for an additional two weeks and the patient is allowed partial to full weight-bearing.

REFERENCES

Legg, A. T.: The treatment of congenital flatfoot by tendon transplantation. Am. J. Orthop. Surg., 10:584, 1912–1913.

Muller, E.: Ueber die Resultate der Ernst Muller'schen Plattfussoperation. Beitr. Klin. Chir., 75:424, 1913.

Young, C. S.: Operative treatment of pes planus. Surg. Gynecol. Obstet., 68:1099, 1939.

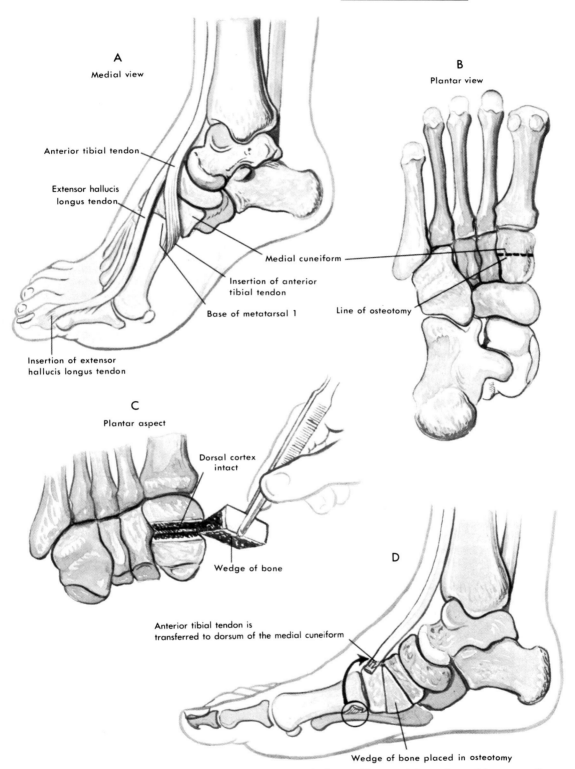

A
Medial view

Anterior tibial tendon

Extensor hallucis longus tendon

Insertion of extensor hallucis longus tendon

Insertion of anterior tibial tendon

Base of metatarsal 1

Medial cuneiform

B
Plantar view

Line of osteotomy

C
Plantar aspect

Dorsal cortex intact

Wedge of bone

D

Anterior tibial tendon is transferred to dorsum of the medial cuneiform

Wedge of bone placed in osteotomy

Plate 216. A.–D., Vertical osteotomy of the medial cuneiform with wedge of bone graft based on the plantar aspect with transfer of the anterior tibial tendon to the dorsum of the medial cuneiform.

PLATE 217 — Vertical Dorsal Wedge Osteotomy of the Base of the First Metatarsal to Correct a Fixed Equinus Deformity of the Medial Ray in Pes Cavus

Indications. Fixed equinus deformity of the first metatarsal in pes cavus.

Radiographic Control. Yes.

Patient Position. The patient is placed in supine position with the knee flexed and the hip rotated laterally.

Operative Technique

A. A 5-cm.-long incision is made over the medial aspect of the foot centered over the base of the first metatarsal. The subcutaneous tissue is divided in line with the skin incision. The wound margins are elevated and retracted.

B. Identify the anterior tibial tendon with its sheath and carefully dissect to its insertion into the medial plantar aspect of the first metatarsal.

C. Retract the anterior tibial tendon posteriorly and identify the cuneiform–first metatarsal joint, but do not section the capsule. Immediately distal to the insertion of the anterior tibial tendon, perform a vertical osteotomy of the first metatarsal, leaving its dorsal cortex intact. Do not injure the growth plate of the first metatarsal. Use radiographic control.

D. and **E.** A wedge of bone of appropriate size is taken in routine fashion from the ilium. The first metatarsal is elevated, and the wedge of bone is inserted into the open-up wedge osteotomy. It is transfixed with two criss-cross pins.

The tourniquet is released, and complete hemostasis is achieved. The wound is closed in the usual fashion, and a below-knee cast is applied.

Postoperative Care. Weight-bearing is not permitted until the pin is removed four weeks postoperatively. Following pin removal, another below-knee cast is applied for an additional two weeks and the patient is allowed partial to full weight-bearing.

REFERENCES

Fowler, B., Brooks, A. L., and Parris, T. F.: The cavo-varus foot. J. Bone Joint Surg., 41-A:757, 1959.

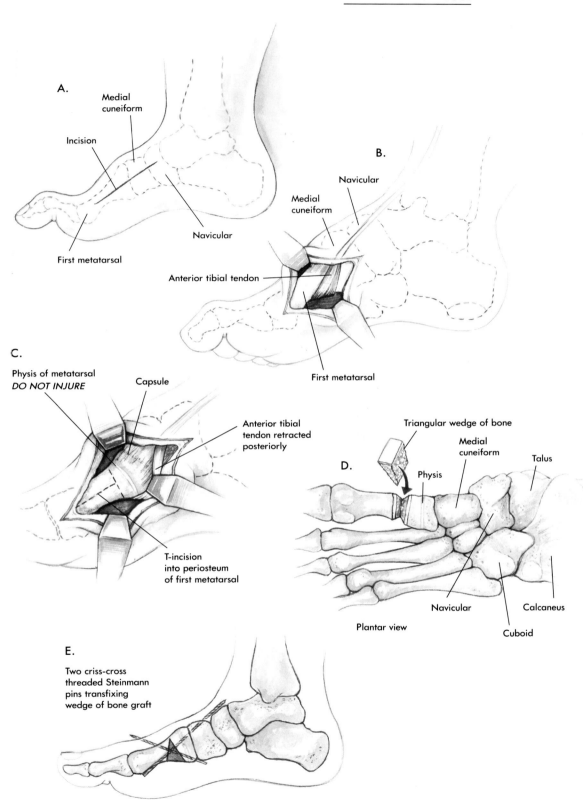

A.

Medial cuneiform

Incision

First metatarsal

Navicular

B.

Navicular

Medial cuneiform

Anterior tibial tendon

First metatarsal

C.

Physis of metatarsal
DO NOT INJURE

Capsule

Anterior tibial tendon retracted posteriorly

T-incision into periosteum of first metatarsal

D.

Triangular wedge of bone

Medial cuneiform

Physis

Talus

Navicular

Calcaneus

Cuboid

Plantar view

E.

Two criss-cross threaded Steinmann pins transfixing wedge of bone graft

Plate 217. A.–E., Vertical dorsal wedge osteotomy of the base of the first metatarsal to correct a fixed equinus deformity of the medial ray in pes cavus.

PLATE 218   Transfer of the Long Toe Extensors of the Metatarsal Heads

Indications. In corrected cavovarus deformity of the foot, on active dorsiflexion of the foot, the toes hyperextend but the metatarsal heads do not elevate and remain in equinus posture.

Objective. To increase the power of dorsiflexion of the forefoot and elevate the metatarsal heads, providing a dynamic force against forefoot equinus deformity.

Requisites. A flexible foot. A release of the contracted soft tissues on the plantar aspect of the foot should always be carried out first.

Operative Technique

A. A longitudinal incision is made on the dorsomedial aspect of the first metatarsal, extending from the base of the proximal phalanx to the proximal one fourth of the metatarsal shaft. The incision should be placed medial to the extensor hallucis longus tendon, toward the second metatarsal. The subcutaneous tissue is divided, and the wound flaps are retracted with 0 silk sutures. The digital nerves and vessels should not be injured.

B. The extensor hallucis longus and brevis tendons are identified and sectioned at the base of the proximal phalanx. An alternate technique is to leave the insertion of the extensor hallucis brevis tendon intact; the stump of the extensor hallucis longus tendon is sutured to the intact brevis tendon. (This latter method is faster and is utilized by the author when the long toe extensors of all five toes are to be transferred to the heads of the metatarsals.)

C. Silk whip sutures (00) are inserted in the ends of the long and short toe extensors. The long toe extensor is dissected free, and with a sharp scalpel its sheath is thoroughly excised as far proximally as possible.

D. The epiphyseal plate of the first metatarsal is proximal, whereas that of the lateral four metatarsals is distal in location. The extensor hallucis longus tendon is transferred to the head of the first metatarsal. The long toe extensors of the lesser toes are transferred to the distal one third of the metatarsal shafts, with care taken not to disturb the growth plate. When the patient is over the age of 10 to 12 years, the tendons are transferred to the heads of the metatarsals, as, by then, growth of the foot is almost complete.

With small Chandler elevator retractors, the soft tissues are retracted. The periosteum is not stripped. Through a stab wound in the periosteum, a hole is drilled in the center of the first metatarsal head and is enlarged to receive the tendon. The extensor hallucis longus tendon is passed through the hole in the first metatarsal in a medial to lateral direction and sutured to itself, with the forefoot in maximal dorsiflexion.

E. The extensor hallucis brevis tendon is then sutured to the stump of the long toe extensor, with the toe held in neutral extension or in 10 degrees of dorsiflexion.

A similar technique is employed to transfer the long extensor tendons of the lesser toes. Longitudinal incisions are made between the second and third metatarsals and between the fourth and fifth metatarsals. The extensor brevis tendon of the little toe is either absent or not of adequate size to transfer to the stump of the longus.

The tourniquet is released, and complete hemostasis is obtained. The wounds are closed with interrupted sutures.

Postoperative Care. A below-knee walking cast is applied, to be worn for four to six weeks. A sturdy, well-padded toe plate is made in the cast. The plantar aspect of the metatarsals should be well padded.

Special muscle training for the transferred tendons is not required, as the transfer is in phase.

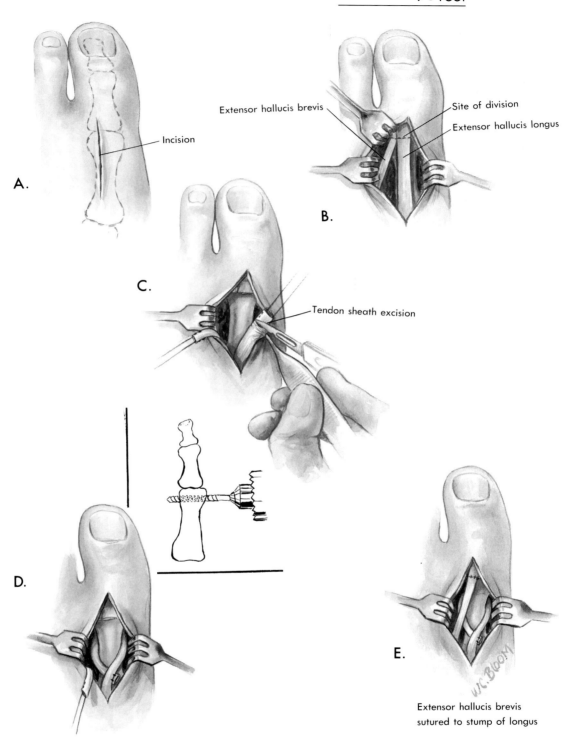

A.

B.

Extensor hallucis brevis — Site of division

Extensor hallucis longus

— Incision

C.

Tendon sheath excision

D.

E.

Extensor hallucis brevis
sutured to stump of longus

Extensor hallucis longus passed through
hole in metatarsal head and sutured to itself

Plate 218. A.–E., Transfer of the long toe extensors of the metatarsal heads.

REFERENCES

Chuinard, E. G., and Baskin, M.: Claw-foot deformity. Treatment by transferring the long extensors into the metatarsals and fusion of the interphalangeal joints. J. Bone Joint Surg., 55-A:351, 1973.

Frank, G. R., and Johnson, W. M.: The extensor shift procedure in the correction of clawtoe deformities in children. South. Med. J., 59:889, 1966.

Jones, R.: The soldier's foot and the treatment of common deformities of the foot. Part II: Claw-foot. Br. Med. J., 1:749, 1968.

Sherman, H. M.: The operative treatment of pes cavus. Am. J. Orthop. Surg., 2:374, 1904–1905.

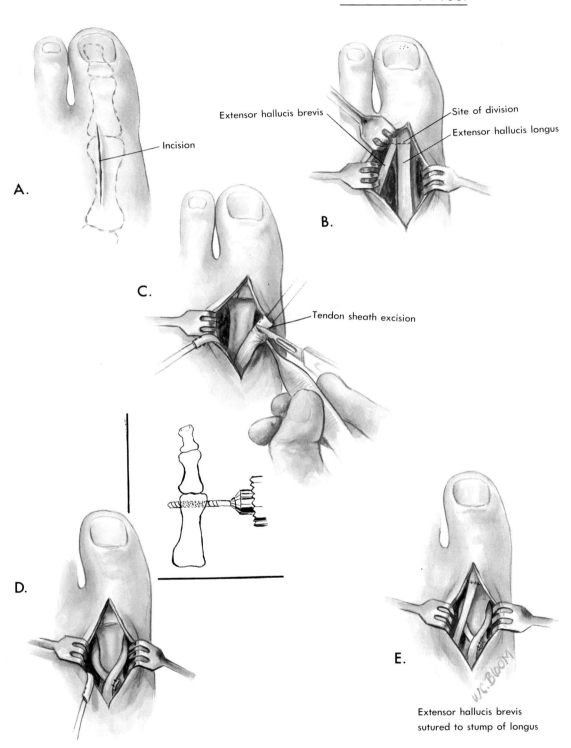

A.

Incision

B.

Extensor hallucis brevis

Site of division

Extensor hallucis longus

C.

Tendon sheath excision

D.

Extensor hallucis longus passed through
hole in metatarsal head and sutured to itself

E.

Extensor hallucis brevis
sutured to stump of longus

Plate 218. (Continued)

PLATE 219   Resection of Entire Ray of Foot

Indications. Macrodactyly.

Radiographic Control. Yes.

Patient Position. Supine.

Operative Technique

A. Make a dorsal, longitudinal, racquet-shaped incision beginning 1 to 2 cm. proximal to the tarsometatarsal joint of the ray to be resected. Extend the incision distally along the metatarsal shaft. At the head of the metatarsal, curve it medially and laterally plantarward across the crease of the metatarsophalangeal joint of the toe. Extend the incision proximally to join the point of its origin. In the case of macrodactyly, an appropriate-sized width of skin and subcutaneous tissue is excised on the plantar aspect of the foot. The subcutaneous tissue is divided in line with the skin incision, and the superficial fascia is incised.

B. The digital nerves of the ray to be ablated (which are usually hypertrophic) are excised. The vessels are clamped and coagulated.

C. The extensor longus and brevis tendons are pulled distally and divided.

D. With sharp and dull dissection, the involved metatarsal is exposed and sectioned at its base with an oscillating power saw or sharp osteotome.

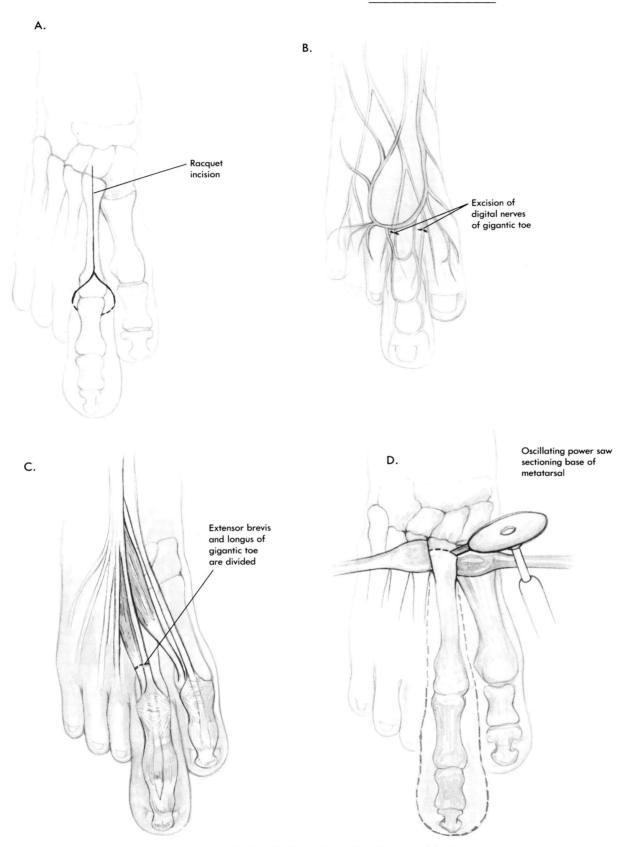

A.

Racquet
incision

B.

Excision of
digital nerves
of gigantic toe

C.

Extensor brevis
and longus of
gigantic toe
are divided

D.

Oscillating power saw
sectioning base of
metatarsal

Plate 219. A.–G., Resection of entire ray of foot.

E. The entire ray is removed extraperiosteally. Next, the flexor tendons on the plantar aspect of the foot are pulled distally and resected. The plantar digital nerves of the ablated ray are dissected and excised. The vessels are clamped and coagulated.

F. The adjoining metatarsal heads are approximated and sutured tautly with interrupted, nonabsorbable sutures such as 0 Tycron. The tourniquet is released. Complete hemostasis is achieved, and a Hemovac suction drain is placed.

G. The subcutaneous tissue is closed with 00 Vicryl interrupted sutures, and the skin with 00 subcuticular nylon.

Postoperative Care. A below-knee cast is applied, compressing the metatarsal heads together. The cast is removed three weeks after surgery. Weight-bearing is allowed as tolerated.

REFERENCES

Barsky, A. J.: Macrodactyly. J. Bone Joint Surg., 49-A:1255, 1967.

Dennyson, W. G., Bear, J. N., and Bhoola, K. D.: Macrodactyly in the foot. J. Bone Joint Surg., 59-B:355, 977.

Herring, J. A., and Tolo, V. T.: Macrodactyly. J. Pediatr. Orthop., 4:503, 1984.

Kumar, K., Kumar, D., Gadegone, W. M., and Kapahtia, N. K.: Macrodactyly of the hand and foot. Int. Orthop., 9:259, 1985.

E.

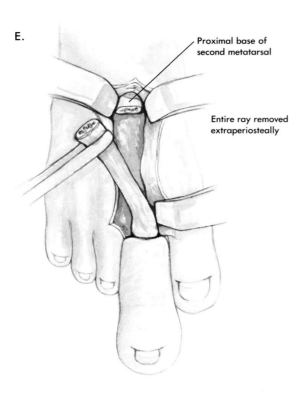

Proximal base of
second metatarsal

Entire ray removed
extraperiosteally

F.

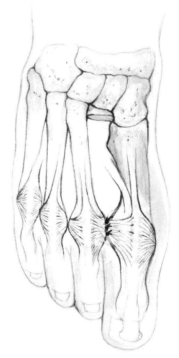

Interosseous ligaments
sutured

G.

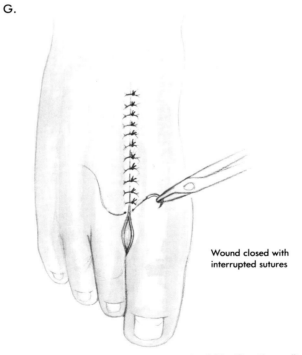

Wound closed with
interrupted sutures

Plate 219. (Continued)

PLATE 220

Mobilization of the Tarsometatarsal and Intermetatarsal Joints by Capsulotomy and Ligamentous Release for Resistant Varus Deformity of the Forefoot (Heyman, Herdon, and Strong Methods)

Indications. Rigid metatarsus varus deformity in a child between the ages of 3 and 7 years not responding to conservative management by manipulation and cast, especially when skew foot is being produced by failure to correct the forefoot varus.

Disadvantage. The popularity of this procedure has waned; it is seldom performed because of the resultant arthritis of the tarsometatarsal joint with a bony prominence and pain. This author prefers simple soft-tissue medial release with capsulotomy of the first metatarsal cuneiform joint. The varus deformity of the lateral metatarsals (two to five) is corrected by osteotomy at their bases. Osteotomy does not disturb growth and does not cause arthritis.

Patient Position. Supine.

Operative Technique

A. A curved transverse skin incision is made, extending from the base of the first metatarsal to the lateral border of the cuboid bone. It runs obliquely across the dorsum of the forepart of the foot just distal to the tarsometatarsal joints.

An alternative method of exposure of the tarsometatarsal joints is to make three longitudinal incisions on the dorsum of the foot—the first overlies the first ray, the second is between the second and third rays, and the third overlies the fourth ray. In the young child, two instead of three linear skin incisions may be made—one between the first and second rays and the other overlying the fourth ray.

B. The subcutaneous tissue and deep fascia are divided. The skin flaps are mobilized and retracted with 00 silk sutures. By meticulous linear dissection, the tendons of the extensor digitorum longus, extensor hallucis longus, anterior tibial, and peroneus brevis are exposed and freed. The dorsalis pedis vessels are identified. Meticulous care is taken not to injure the neurovascular structures.

C. The anterior tibial tendon is retracted medially, and the extensor hallucis longus tendon with the dorsalis pedis vessels is retracted laterally. The intermetatarsal space between the first and second metatarsals is identified with a small hemostat, and the intermetatarsal ligament is divided, beginning distally and progressing proximally. By this method, the first metatarsocuneiform joint is located. The epiphyseal plate of the first metatarsal is proximally located; it should not be damaged. The medial and dorsal capsules are divided. The plantar capsule is not sectioned at this time. The anterior tibial tendon should be carefully protected in order to prevent its inadvertent sectioning. The articular cartilage should not be injured.

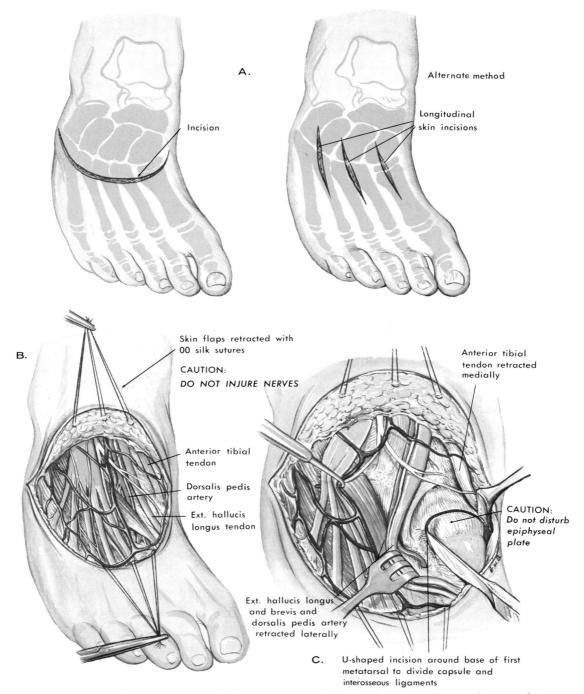

A.

Alternate method

Incision

Longitudinal
skin incisions

B.

Skin flaps retracted with
00 silk sutures

CAUTION:
DO NOT INJURE NERVES

Anterior tibial
tendon

Dorsalis pedis
artery

Ext. hallucis
longus tendon

Anterior tibial
tendon retracted
medially

CAUTION:
*Do not disturb
epiphyseal
plate*

Ext. hallucis longus
and brevis and
dorsalis pedis artery
retracted laterally

C. U-shaped incision around base of first
metatarsal to divide capsule and
interosseous ligaments

Plate 220. A.–G., Mobilization of the tarsometarsal and intermetatarsal joints by capsulotomy and ligamentous release for resistant varus deformity of the forefoot (Heyman, Herdon, and Strong methods).

D. Next, the second metatarsocuneiform joint is exposed; it is located slightly proximal to the first metatarsocuneiform joint. The intermetatarsal ligaments and dorsal capsule are divided. Then longitudinal dissection is carried out in a plane overlying the third ray, taking care to protect the neurovascular structures and the extensor tendons. Again, with a small hemostat, the intermetatarsal space between the second and third metatarsals is identified, and the intermetatarsal ligaments are sectioned. Dorsal capsulotomy of the second and third metatarsocuneiform joints is completed. The fourth metatarsotarsal joint is essentially at the same level as the second and third; the articulation is readily identified after division of the intermetatarsal ligaments. Dorsal capsulotomy is similarly carried out.

At the fifth metatarsocuboid joint, the attachment of the peroneus brevis is protected and the lateral capsule is not disturbed; the latter will serve as a hinge that prevents lateral displacement of the fifth metatarsal as the foot is manipulated.

E. Attention is then directed to the plantar capsule and the plantar ligaments. The metatarsotarsal joints are opened by plantar flexion of the forefoot and distal traction on the individual metatarsals. The medial two thirds of the plantar capsule and ligaments at each joint are divided, leaving the lateral one third intact. This will provide sufficient stability to prevent displacement of the metatarsals while the forefoot is manipulated out of adduction. The intermetatarsal ligaments must be divided completely to permit gliding of the metatarsals as the deformity is corrected.

F. and **G.** The forefoot is manipulated into abduction and eversion. After correction is achieved, there will be considerable incongruity of the articular surfaces. If there is marked instability of the tarsometatarsal joints, Kirschner wires may be inserted to fix the first metatarsal to the first cuneiform and the fifth to the cuboid. The author, however, has not found routine use of Kirschner wires to be necessary.

The tourniquet is released, and complete hemostasis is secured. The wound is closed with interrupted sutures, and a well-molded, above-knee cast is applied, holding the foot in the corrected position.

Postoperative Care. For the first few days after surgery, the leg should be elevated to prevent excessive swelling. In ten to 14 days, when the reactive swelling has subsided, the cast is changed and a new snug, well-molded one is applied. It is best to carry this out with the patient under general anesthesia and the foot manipulated into the corrected position prior to application of the cast. The skin sutures should not be removed at this time, as the wound edges will separate.

Three weeks later (about four to five weeks after surgery), the cast and sutures are removed and a carefully molded below-knee walking cast is applied. Immobilization in the cast is continued for a minimum of three to four months; this is important to allow adequate time for remodeling of articular surfaces. The casts are changed every three to four weeks (depending on how robust the child is, as walking is encouraged). Each time, the foot is manipulated into the corrected position.

REFERENCES

Heyman, C. H., Herndon, C. H., and Strong, J. M.: Mobilization of the tarsometatarsal and intermetatarsal joints for the correction of resistant adduction of the forepart of the foot in congenital clubfoot or congenital metatarsus varus. J. Bone Joint Surg., 40-A:299, 1958.

Kendrick, R. E., Sharman, N. K., Hassler, W. L., and Herndon, C. H.: Tarsometatarsal mobilization for resistant adduction of the forepart of the foot. J. Bone Joint Surg., 52-A:61, 1970.

Stark, J. G., Johanson, J. E., and Winter, R. B.: The Heyman-Herndon tarsometatarsal capsulotomy for metatarsus adductus: Results in 48 feet. J. Pediatr. Orthop., 7:305, 1987.

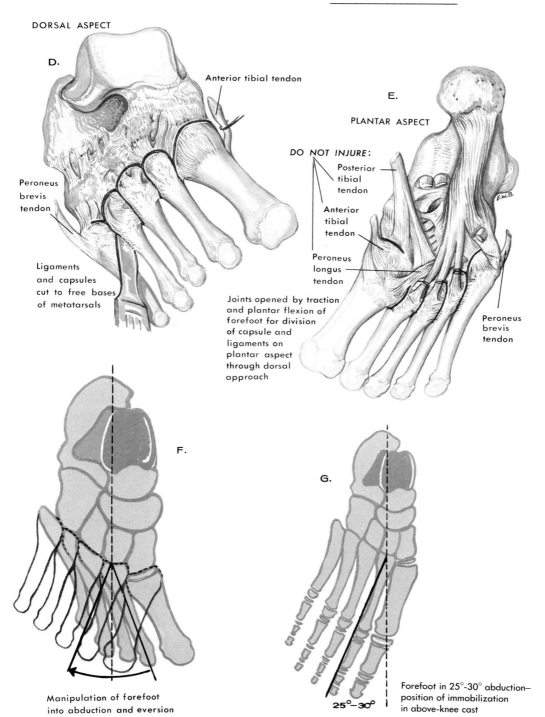

DORSAL ASPECT

D.

Anterior tibial tendon

Peroneus
brevis
tendon

Ligaments
and capsules
cut to free bases
of metatarsals

E.

PLANTAR ASPECT

DO NOT INJURE:

Posterior
tibial
tendon

Anterior
tibial
tendon

Peroneus
longus
tendon

Peroneus
brevis
tendon

E.W.B.

Joints opened by traction
and plantar flexion of
forefoot for division
of capsule and
ligaments on
plantar aspect
through dorsal
approach

F.

Manipulation of forefoot
into abduction and eversion

G.

25°–30°

Forefoot in 25°-30° abduction—
position of immobilization
in above-knee cast

Plate 220. (Continued)

PLATE 221 **Osteotomy of Bases of Metatarsals for Correction of Varus Deformity of Forepart of Foot**

Indications. Fixed, rigid varus deformity of the forefoot in a child eight years of age or older, especially if it is causing the hindfoot to go into valgus deviation and resulting in a skew foot.

Patient Position. Supine.

Operative Technique

A. The bases of all five metatarsals are exposed by three longitudinal skin incisions, all approximately 5 cm. long—the first on the medial side of the first metatarsal; the second in the interval between the second and third rays; and the third between the fourth and fifth rays. The subcutaneous tissue and fascia are divided in line with the skin incisions. The dorsal cutaneous nerves and the dorsalis pedis and metatarsal vessels should be protected from injury. The epiphyseal plate of the first metatarsal, in contrast to the lateral four metatarsals, is proximal in location and should not be damaged. By appropriate retraction of the extensor tendons and the anterior tibial tendon, the bases of all metatarsals are exposed.

B. The lines of osteotomy may be marked with a small starter and drill holes. The osteotomies are dome-shaped, with their apices directed posteriorly. In the first four metatarsals, the medial limb is longer than the lateral limb; in the fifth metatarsal, the lateral (fibular) limb is longer than the medial one in order to prevent lateral displacement of the distal fragment when the forefoot is manipulated into abduction. In moderate varus deformity, osteotomy of the fifth metatarsal is not necessary. Often a laterally based wedge is excised from the lateral half of the base of the first metatarsal. The osteotomy is completed with a sharp dental osteotome or a small oscillating electric saw.

C. A heavy threaded Kirschner wire is inserted across the distal one fourth of the metatarsal shafts. The wound is closed and the foot is manipulated, swinging the forepart into abduction. An alternate method is internal fixation of the osteotomized fragments with two Kirschner wires—one inserted across the first metatarsal to the medial cuneiform and the other across the fifth metatarsal to the cuboid. A well-molded, above-knee or below-knee cast is applied, holding the forepart of the foot in 5 to 10 degrees of abduction. The heel should be in neutral position. Weight-bearing is not allowed.

Radiograms are made in the operating room with the patient under anesthesia to ensure that the desired degree of correction is achieved and that the osteotomized bone fragments are in satisfactory apposition.

Postoperative Care. At three to four weeks, the cast, Kirschner wires, and sutures are removed. A below-knee walking cast is applied while the foot is held in the corrected position. Immobilization in the cast is continued for an additional two to three weeks.

REFERENCES

Berman, A., and Gartland, J. J.: Metatarsal osteotomy for the correction of adduction of the forepart of the foot in children. J. Bone Joint Surg., 53-A:498, 1971.
Coleman, S. S.: Complex Foot Deformities in Children. Philadelphia, Lea & Febiger, 1983, pp. 267–290.
DalMonte, A., Manes, E., Soncini, G., Bandini, E., and Andrisano, A.: Surgical treatment of metatarsus varus during the growth period. Ital. J. Orthop. Traumatol., 8:390, 1982.
Holden, D., Siff, S., Butler, J., and Cain, T.: Shortening of the first metatarsal as a complication of metatarsal osteotomies. J. Bone Joint Surg., 66-B:582, 1984.

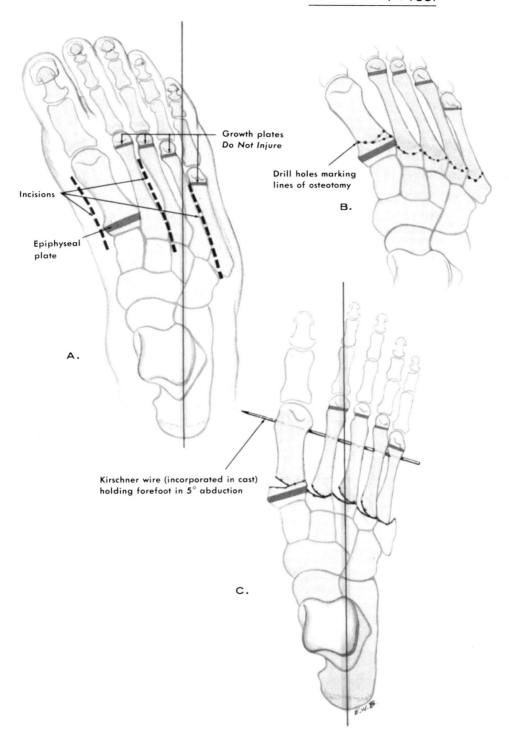

Growth plates
Do Not Injure

Incisions

Epiphyseal
plate

Drill holes marking
lines of osteotomy

B.

A.

Kirschner wire (incorporated in cast)
holding forefoot in 5° abduction

C.

Plate 221. **A.–C.,** Osteotomy of bases of metatarsals for correction of varus deformity of forepart of foot.

PLATE 222 **Treatment of Dorsal Bunion by "Open-Up" Plantarflexion Osteotomy of Base of First Metatarsal and Transfer of Flexor Hallucis Longus Tendon to Head of First Metatarsal**

Indications. Fixed dorsiflexion deformity of the first metatarsal with plantarflexion contracture of the great toe caused by muscle imbalance between a poor peroneus longus and a strong anterior tibial.

Requisites. Good motor strength of flexor hallucis longus and flexor hallucis brevis muscles.

Radiographic Control. Yes.

Patient Position. Supine.

Operative Technique

A. A longitudinal incision is made over the dorsomedial aspect of the foot, starting at the first cuneiform bone and extending distally to the first metatarsal head, where it is curved plantarward.

B. The base of the first metatarsal is exposed. A dorsal capsulotomy of the tarsometatarsal and navicular-cuneiform joint may be necessary to bring the first metatarsal bone into plantar flexion. Do not perform capsulotomy of the medial cuneiform–first metatarsal joint because after osteotomy the proximal metatarsal fragment will be unstable and difficult to fix.

With a starter and drill, the line of open-up osteotomy on the dorsal aspect of the base of the first metatarsal is marked. The plantar cortex should be left intact. Next, with a scalpel, a U-shaped flap of capsule is raised from the dorsum of the metatarsophalangeal joint with its base attached to the proximal phalanx. If necessary, any abnormally prominent bone on the metatarsal head is excised. If the flexion contracture of the great toe is not corrected by manipulation, capsulotomy of the plantar aspect of the first metatarsophalangeal joint is performed. Next, the flexor hallucis longus tendon is divided near its insertion and delivered into the proximal part of the wound. A tunnel is drilled in the head of the first metatarsal from its dorsal to its plantar aspect.

C. The osteotomy of the dorsal, medial, and lateral parts of the base of the first metatarsal is completed. The distal part of the metatarsal is manipulated into plantar flexion, taking due care not to break the plantar cortex. A wedge of autogenous bone graft from the ilium is obtained and inserted at the osteotomy site, correcting the dorsiflexion deformity of the first metatarsal. The flexor hallucis longus tendon, with a whip suture in its distal end, is brought from the plantar to the dorsal aspect through the tunnel in the first metatarsal head and sutured to itself; this makes the flexor hallucis longus muscle a plantar flexor of the first metatarsal instead of the great toe.

D. The dorsal U-flap of the capsule is sutured to the flexor hallucis longus tendon on the dorsum of the metatarsal head, holding the great toe in neutral position. The wound is closed in the usual fashion. A below-knee, well-molded walking cast with a toe plate is applied and is worn for five to six weeks.

Postoperative Care. The cast is removed in five to six weeks. Radiograms are made to determine the consolidation of the bone graft and osteotomy. Active and passive exercises are performed to develop plantarflexion of the first ray.

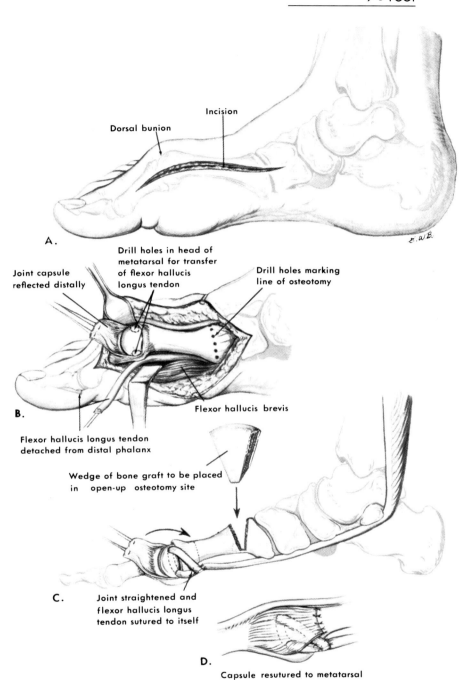

Incision

Dorsal bunion

A.

Drill holes in head of metatarsal for transfer of flexor hallucis longus tendon

Joint capsule reflected distally

Drill holes marking line of osteotomy

B.

Flexor hallucis brevis

Flexor hallucis longus tendon detached from distal phalanx

Wedge of bone graft to be placed in open-up osteotomy site

C.   Joint straightened and flexor hallucis longus tendon sutured to itself

D.

Capsule resutured to metatarsal

Plate 222. A.–D., Treatment of dorsal bunion by "open-up" plantarflexion osteotomy of base of first metatarsal and transfer of flexor hallucis longus tendon to head of first metatarsal.

PLATE 223   ## McKay's Technique for Correction of Dorsal Bunion

Indications. Dorsal bunion deformity of the great toe with no fixed structural deformity. It can be passively corrected by manipulation.

Patient Position. Supine.

Operative Technique

In this procedure, the tendinous insertions of the flexor hallucis brevis and the abductor and adductor hallucis are transferred to the neck of the first metatarsal.

A. Make a longitudinal incision on the medial aspect of the foot, extending from the base of the first metatarsal to the interphalangeal joint of the great toe. The subcutaneous tissue and superficial fascia are divided in line with the skin incision.

B. Identify the abductor hallucis and medial part of the flexor hallucis brevis and detach them from their insertion. Dissect and mobilize the distal half of these muscles, preserving their tendons as much as possible.

C. Through a separate dorsolateral longitudinal incision, if necessary, the lateral tendon of the flexor hallucis brevis and the tendon of adductor hallucis are sectioned from their origin and dissected free.

If there is any associated hallux valgus, leave the insertion of the abductor hallucis intact; if hallux varus is present, leave the adductor hallucis attached to its insertion.

A.

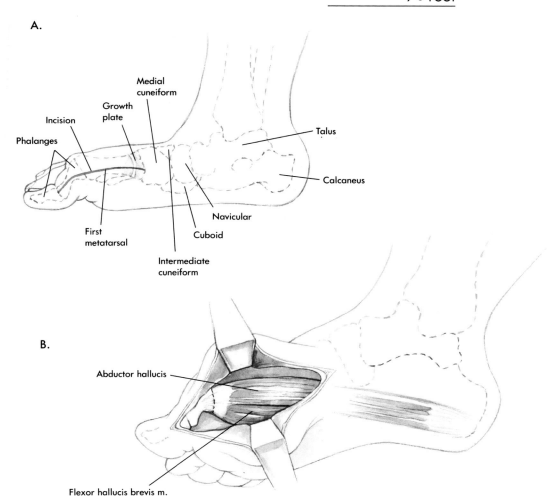

B.

C.

PLANTAR VIEW

Plate 223. **A.–E.,** McKay's technique for correction of dorsal bunion.

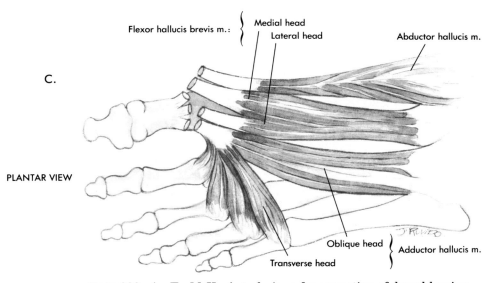

D. and **E.** Remove the sesamoid bones of the tendinous part of the flexor hallucis brevis. Next, make a circumferential incision in the periosteum of the first metatarsal at its neck and elevate it proximally for a distance of 1 cm.

The tendons of the abductor hallucis and medial part of the flexor hallucis brevis are transferred on the dorsal aspect of the first metatarsal neck; the adductor hallucis and lateral part of the flexor hallucis brevis are transferred dorsally between the first and second metatarsals.

All four tendons are sutured together and to the adjoining capsule and periosteum, creating a myotendinous ring around the neck of the first metatarsal. The collar of the periosteum is sutured to the tendons. Next, the interphalangeal joint of the great toe is stabilized by a standard arthrodesis (fixed internally with a cannulated AO screw) or by tenodesis in the skeletally immature child.

The wounds are closed in the usual fashion. A below-knee walking cast is applied.

Postoperative Care. The cast is removed in three to four weeks. Active exercises are performed to strengthen the motor power of the muscles.

REFERENCE

McKay, D. W.: Dorsal bunions in children. J. Bone Joint Surg., 65-A:975, 1983.

D.

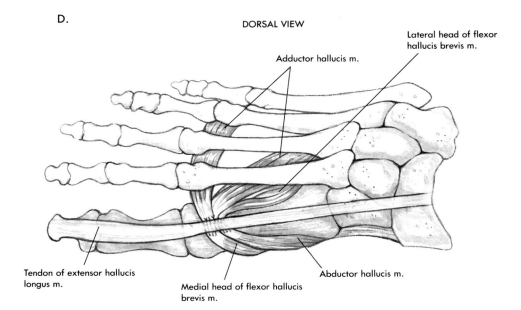

DORSAL VIEW

Lateral head of flexor
hallucis brevis m.

Adductor hallucis m.

Tendon of extensor hallucis
longus m.

Medial head of flexor hallucis
brevis m.

Abductor hallucis m.

E.

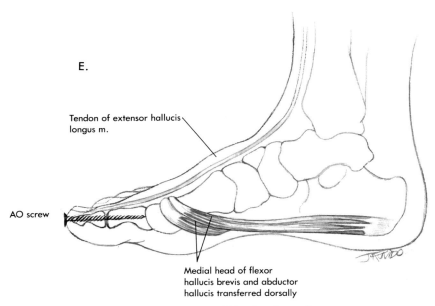

Tendon of extensor hallucis
longus m.

AO screw

Medial head of flexor
hallucis brevis and abductor
hallucis transferred dorsally

Plate 223. (Continued)

PLATE 224　**Correction of Hallux Valgus and Metatarsus Primus Varus**

Indications. Severe deformity with pain over the prominent first metatarsal head "bunion" and difficulty with shoe wear and walking.

Choice of Operative Procedures. In the preoperative assessment, congruity of the metatarsophalangeal (MP) joint of the hallux should be determined. When the MP joint is noncongruous (i.e., the base of the proximal phalanx is deviated and subluxated medially), realignment of the MP joint by soft tissue reconstruction combined with a proximal osteotomy to decrease the angle between the first and second metatarsals is performed.

When the MP joint is congruous (i.e., the corresponding metatarsal and phalangeal articular surfaces have concentric apposition), realignment of the joint should not be performed because it will result in articular malalignment with pain, stiffness, and arthritis. When the MP joint is congruous—a rare occurrence in the juvenile or adolescent bunion—the deformity is corrected by extra-articular repair, primarily distal metatarsal osteotomy and/or proximal phalangeal osteotomy.

When there is marked splaying of the forefoot due to ligamentous hyperlaxity with obliquity of the first metatarsocuneiform joint of greater than 30 degrees, arthrodesis of the metatarsal cuneiform–first metatarsal (MCF1) joint is indicated in the adolescent with a skeletally mature foot. When the first metatarsal is significantly longer than the second metatarsal, it can be performed in the skeletally immature foot. Motion at the MCF1 joint is eliminated by the fusion, but ordinarily its absence is not missed functionally by the patient.

In the anteroposterior radiograms of the weight-bearing foot, the site of varus angulation of the first metatarsal is determined—is it at the MCF1 joint or in the first metatarsal? When the medial inclination of the MCF1 joint exceeds 20 degrees and the angle between the first and second metatarsals is abnormally high, an open-up osteotomy of the medial cuneiform with a wedge of iliac bone graft is performed to correct the varus inclination of the first metatarsal. Otherwise, an open-up osteotomy of the first metatarsal base with bone graft taken from the excised prominent metatarsal head is carried out.

Patient Position. Supine.

Radiographic Control. Image intensifier.

Operative Technique

A. The incision is made on the dorsomedial aspect of the first metatarsal and hallux. It begins at the middle of the proximal phalanx of the great toe and extends in a curvilinear fashion proximally and medially on the dorsomedial border of the first metatarsal and terminates at the MCF1 joint. When osteotomy of the medial cuneiform is to be performed, the incision extends farther proximally to end at the tuberosity of the navicular.

B. Subcutaneous tissue is divided in line with the skin incision. The skin margins are retracted with skin hooks. The wound flaps are undermined, elevated, and retracted. The digital vessels and nerves are identified and kept out of harm's way. Exercise caution, particularly at the proximal part of the wound, where the neurovascular bundle is at risk under the scalpel of the inexperienced surgeon. Identify the MCF1 joint and the metatarsophalangeal joint of the great toe. The growth plate of the first metatarsal is at its base; do not disturb it. With Metzenbaum (or dull) scissors, dissect and mobilize the distal half of the abductor hallucis muscle; do not detach it from its insertion. At the end of the operation, the abductor hallucis muscle will be transferred from its plantar medial location to straight medial.

Make a U-shaped incision in the capsule of the metatarsophalangeal joint of the great toe. Leave the capsule attached to the base of the proximal phalanx of

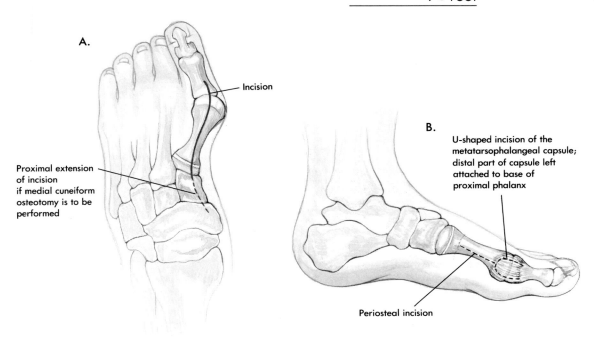

A.

Incision

Proximal extension
of incision
if medial cuneiform
osteotomy is to be
performed

B.

U-shaped incision of the
metatarsophalangeal capsule;
distal part of capsule left
attached to base of
proximal phalanx

Periosteal incision

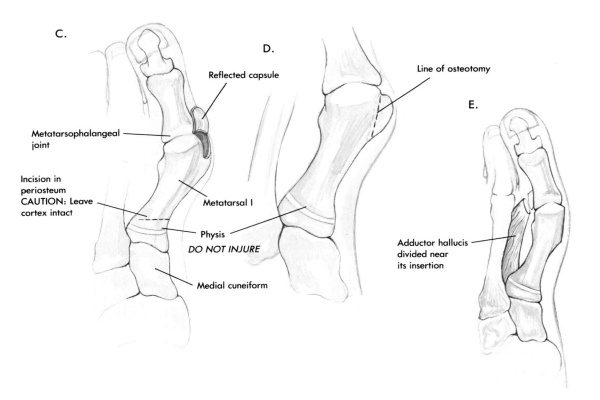

C.

Reflected capsule

Metatarsophalangeal
joint

Incision in
periosteum
CAUTION: Leave
cortex intact

Metatarsal I

Physis
DO NOT INJURE

Medial cuneiform

D.

Line of osteotomy

E.

Adductor hallucis
divided near
its insertion

Plate 224. A.–N., Correction of hallux valgus and metatarsus primus varus.

the hallux. A longitudinal incision is made in the periosteum on the medial aspect of the first metatarsal. The periosteal incision extends from the neck of the first metatarsal to its base. Proximally, a transverse incision is made in the periosteum immediately distal and parallel to the physis of the first metatarsal. Avoid injury to the growth plate. Do not divide the capsule at the MCF1 joint.

C. The incised capsule is elevated by sharp and dull dissection and reflected distally. The metatarsal head is exposed on its dorsal, medial, and plantar aspects. With a Freer elevator, the periosteum is elevated, exposing the dorsal, medial, and plantar aspects of the first metatarsal shaft.

A groove separates the prominent exposed part of the metatarsal head (the "bunion") from the articulating cartilaginous part of the metatarsal head. A pair of whip sutures are placed in the U-shaped, detached-reflected capsule—one over the dorsal margin and the other on the plantar margin. With a sharp AO thin osteotome, delineate the boundaries of the bunion to be excised.

Caution! Do not weaken the first metatarsal shaft by taking an excess amount of bone from its neck.

D. With sharp, thin osteotomes, the prominent nonarticular portion of the metatarsal head is resected in one piece and kept sterile in a moist sponge for later use as a bone graft.

E. The big toe is laterally displaced, and with sharp tenotomy scissors the lateral capsule of the metatarsophalangeal joint and the tendon of the adductor hallucis are divided. This author has not found it necessary to transfer the adductor hallucis to the head of the first metatarsal.

Occasionally, one may have to make a separate short dorsolateral incision and section the adductor hallucis tendon under direct incision.

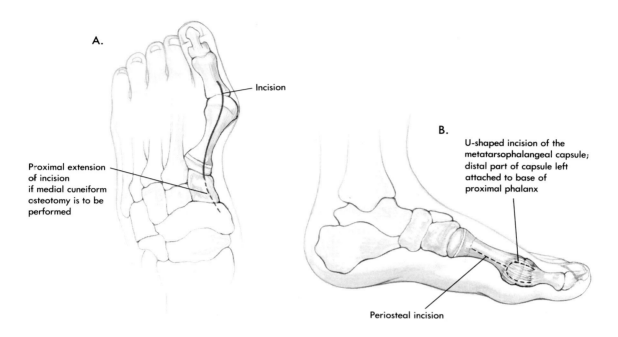

A.

Incision

Proximal extension
of incision
if medial cuneiform
osteotomy is to be
performed

B.

U-shaped incision of the
metatarsophalangeal capsule;
distal part of capsule left
attached to base of
proximal phalanx

Periosteal incision

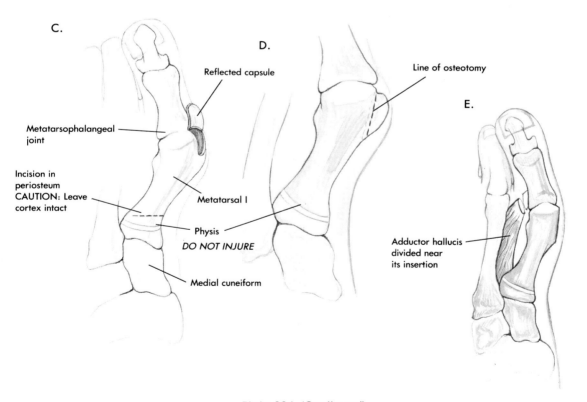

C.

Reflected capsule

D.

Line of osteotomy

E.

Metatarsophalangeal
joint

Incision in
periosteum
CAUTION: Leave
cortex intact

Metatarsal I

Physis
DO NOT INJURE

Medial cuneiform

Adductor hallucis
divided near
its insertion

Plate 224. (Continued)

F. When medial divergence of the first metatarsal is only moderate, an open-up osteotomy of the first metatarsal is performed. Make drill holes at the base of the first metatarsal 0.5 mm. distal to its growth plate. The lateral cortex is left intact. The bone is divided transversely with a thin osteotome. The osteotome is directed dorsoplantarward, not mediolaterally.

G. The osteotomy cleft is spread open with periosteal elevators, leaving the lateral cortex intact. The bone previously removed from the metatarsal head is shaped into a wedge and driven into the osteotomized fragments, with care taken that the lateral cortex not be broken. Precautions should be taken to avoid elevating or depressing the first metatarsal unless this is indicated.

H. If the metatarsus varus deformity is severe, perform a modified dome-shaped osteotomy with a medial buttress on the proximal segment; this effectively corrects the deformity. The line of osteotomy is drawn, and holes are made with a power drill. The osteotomy is completed with sharp, thin osteotomes.

I. The first metatarsal is abducted and primus varus deformity is fully corrected.

J. The alignment of the osteotomized fragments is maintained by internal fixation with a heavy threaded Steinmann pin, which is inserted obliquely from the medial aspect of the distal one third of the first metatarsal into the lateral metatarsals. The pin protrudes on the lateral aspect of the foot for ease of removal when the osteotomy is healed.

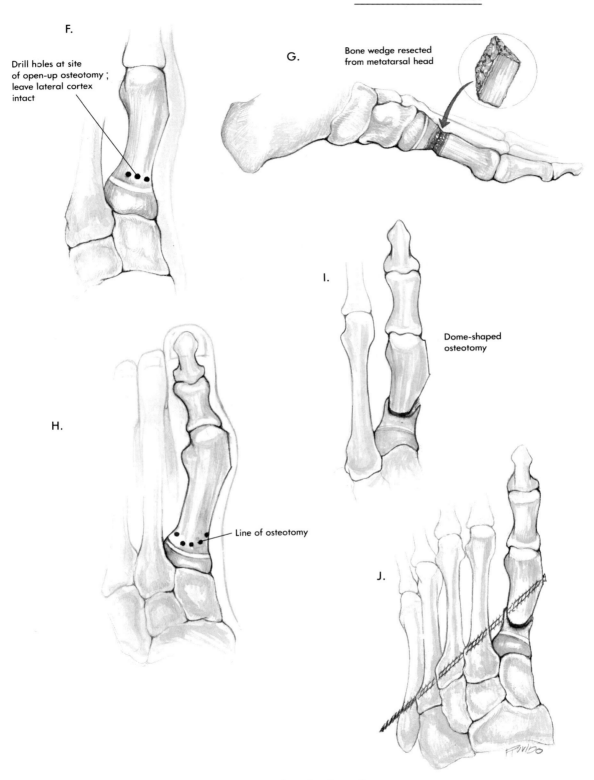

F.

Drill holes at site of open-up osteotomy ; leave lateral cortex intact

G.

Bone wedge resected from metatarsal head

I.

Dome-shaped osteotomy

H.

Line of osteotomy

J.

Plate 224. (Continued)

K. When medial deviation of the first metatarsal takes place at the MCF1 joint and the varus deformity exceeds 20 degrees, an open-up osteotomy of the medial cuneiform is performed as follows: Extend the skin incision to the tuberosity of the navicular. Divide the subcutaneous tissue and fascia in line with the skin incision and identify the MCF1 and naviculomedial cuneiform joints. Do not divide their capsules.

Under image intensifier, exactly determine the level of the osteotomy in the center of the medial cuneiform. With the help of an electric saw, perform an osteotomy of the medial cuneiform.

L. With osteotomes, pry open the site of the osteotomy in the medial cuneiform and insert a wedge of appropriate-sized bone graft taken from the iliac crest into the osteotomy cleft. A large, long piece of bone graft is required; the size of the resected medial prominence of the first metatarsal head is not adequate. Two threaded Kirschner wires are inserted criss-crossed for internal fixation.

M. The Tycron whip (or other nonabsorbable) sutures inserted into the proximal end of the capsule are attached firmly to the distal shaft of the first metatarsal through drill holes made in the first metatarsal shaft, with the hallux held in neutral extension and abduction-adduction.

N. If the abductor hallucis tendon is displaced plantarward, it is transfixed to a more dorsal site on the medial aspect of the base of the proximal phalanx.

The tourniquet is released, and complete hemostasis is achieved. A small Hemovac suction tube is inserted for drainage. The wound is closed in the usual fashion, and a non–weight-bearing, below-knee cast is applied with the ankle and foot in neutral position and with a toe cap.

Postoperative Care. Ordinarily, the osteotomy will heal in six weeks; however, the pins are removed three to four weeks postoperatively, and a new below-knee walking cast is applied. Full weight-bearing is allowed. When the cast is removed, passive exercises of the first metatarsophalangeal joint and tiptoe rising active exercises are performed several times a day until full range of motion is obtained; this may take six to nine months.

REFERENCES

Bonney, G., and Macnab, I.: Hallux valgus and hallux rigidus. A critical survey of operative results. J. Bone Joint Surg., 34-B:366, 1952.

Coughlin, M. J.: The pathophysiology and treatment of the juvenile bunion. Chapter 36. In: Gould, J. S. (ed.): Surgery of the Foot. Philadelphia, W. B. Saunders Co., 1993.

DuVries, H.: Static deformities of the forefoot. In: DuVries, H. L. (ed.): Surgery of the Foot, 2nd ed. St. Louis, C. V. Mosby, 1965.

Giannestras, N. J.: The Giannestras modification of the Lapidus operation. In: Giannestras, N. J. (ed.): Foot Disorders, Medical and Surgical Management. Philadelphia, Lea & Febiger, 1973.

Goldner, J. L., and Gaines, R. W.: Adult and juvenile hallux valgus: Analysis and treatment. Orthop. Clin. North Am., 7:863, 1976.

Hart, J. A. L., and Bentley, G.: Metatarsal osteotomy in the treatment of hallux valgus. J. Bone Joint Surg., 58-B:261, 1976.

Kelikian, H.: Hallux Valgus, Allied Deformities of the Forefoot and Metatarsalgia. Philadelphia, W. B. Saunders Co., 1965.

Lapidus, P. W.: Operative correction of the metatarsus varus primus in hallux valgus. Surg. Gynecol. Obstet., 58:183, 1934.

Mann, R. A., and Coughlin, M. J.: Hallus valgus—etiology, anatomy, treatment and surgical considerations. Clin. Orthop., 157:31, 1981.

McBride, E. D.: A conservative operation for bunions. J. Bone Joint Surg., 10:735, 1928.

McBride, E. D.: Hallux valgus, bunion deformity: Its treatment in mild, moderate and severe stages. J. Int. Coll. Surg., 21:99, 1954.

McBride, E. D.: The McBride bunion hallux valgus operation. Refinements in the successive surgical steps of the operation. J. Bone Joint Surg., 42-A:965, 1960.

Scranton, P. E., Jr.: Principles in bunion surgery. J. Bone Joint Surg., 65-A:1026, 1983.

Scranton, P. E., Jr., and Zuckerman, J. D.: Bunion surgery in adolescents: Results of surgical treatment. J. Pediatr. Orthop., 4:39, 1984.

Silver, D.: The operative treatment of hallux valgus. J. Bone Joint Surg., 5:225, 1923.

Young, J. D.: A new operation for adolescent hallux valgus. Univ. Penn. Med. Bull., 23:439, 1910.

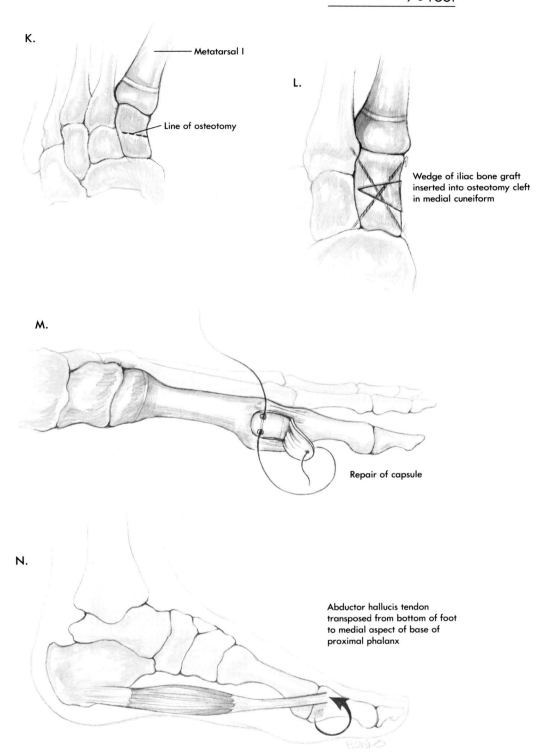

K.

Metatarsal I

Line of osteotomy

L.

Wedge of iliac bone graft inserted into osteotomy cleft in medial cuneiform

M.

Repair of capsule

N.

Abductor hallucis tendon transposed from bottom of foot to medial aspect of base of proximal phalanx

Plate 224. (Continued)

PLATE 225   **Instantaneous Elongation of Short First Metatarsal with Bone Grafting and Intramedullary Pin Fixation**

Indications. Severe or marked shortening of the first metatarsal with callosities under the second and third metatarsal heads. Ordinarily, it is a congenital anomaly associated with hallux varus; occasionally, it is an isolated deformity. Short first metatarsal may be caused by premature closure of its growth plate, which is either post-traumatic or iatrogenically caused by inappropriate surgery.

Requisites. Adequate size of foot: child six years of age or older.

Special Instrumentation. Mini-Orthofix.

Radiographic Control. Image intensifier.

Patient Position. Supine.

Operative Technique

A. On the dorsomedial aspect of the first metatarsal, a longitudinal incision is made; it begins at the interphalangeal joint of the big toe and terminates at the naviculocuneiform joint. Subcutaneous tissue is divided in line with the skin incision. The wound flaps are elevated and retracted. Digital vessels and nerves are identified and kept out of harm's way.

B. Identify the extensor hallucis longus and brevis tendons and retract them laterally. On the medial aspect of the foot, the abductor hallucis muscle is identified; it is detached from its insertion to the base of the proximal phalanx of the great toe, reflected proximally, and partially excised. Do not section the flexor hallucis brevis muscle. With a Keith needle, the growth plate of the first metatarsal is located and verified by image intensifier radiographic control.

C. With a power drill, mini-Orthofix pins are inserted mediolaterally in a transverse plane; the first is inserted into the medial cuneiform, and a second is inserted into the proximal diaphysis of the first metatarsal immediately distal to the growth plate. The pin in the first metatarsal is drilled farther laterally into the second metatarsal for secure fixation.

Distally, drill a set of two pins to transfix the metatarsophalangeal joint of the big toe—one pin into the head of the first metatarsal and the other pin into the middle of the proximal phalanx, avoiding its growth plate. The position of the pins is double checked by image intensifier radiography; the pins should engage in both cortices. The mini-Orthofix lengthener is adjusted appropriately and applied to the pins.

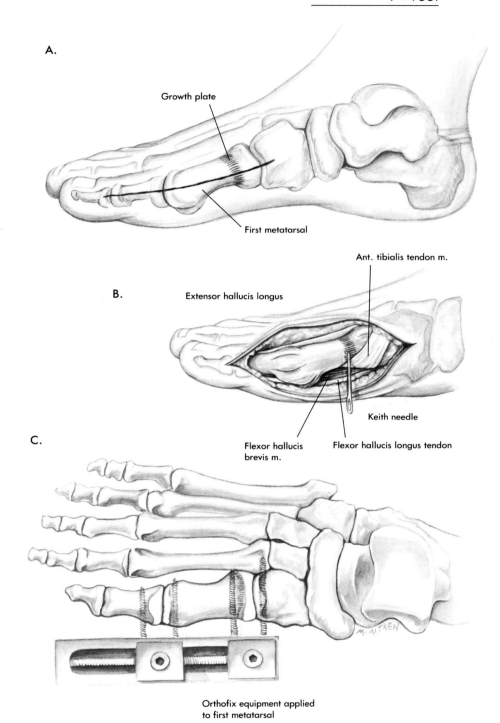

A.

Growth plate

First metatarsal

B.

Ant. tibialis tendon m.

Extensor hallucis longus

Keith needle

Flexor hallucis longus tendon

Flexor hallucis
brevis m.

C.

M. AITKEN

Orthofix equipment applied
to first metatarsal

Plate 225. A.–H., Instantaneous elongation of short first metatarsal with bone grafting and intramedullary pin fixation.

D. With drills and sharp AO osteotomes, the first metatarsal is divided in its middle.

E. The metatarsal is slowly elongated to the desired length. During lengthening, the pneumatic tourniquet is deflated in order to assess circulation.

A Z-lengthening of the extensor hallucis longus and/or flexor hallucis longus may be indicated if the tendons become very taut.

F. After the desired amount of lengthening is achieved, a thick, double cortical bone graft is obtained from the ilium and placed in the elongated gap of the first metatarsal. (Iliac bone graft is performed over fibular graft because it heals faster and does not produce ankle valgus due to short fibula.)

G. The divided metatarsal bones are compressed, and the Orthofix pins are removed.

H. Under image intensifier radiographic control, carefully insert an intramedullary smooth Steinmann pin of appropriate diameter from the tip of the great toe into the first metatarsal, across the graft, into the proximal segment of the first metatarsal, and into the medial cuneiform. The tip of the pin at the great toe is bent in order to prevent pin migration. The wound is closed, and a below-knee cast is applied with a toe cap over the great toe.

Postoperative Care. Weight-bearing is not allowed. Periodic radiograms are made to check the position of the pins and bone healing. Ordinarily, the cast is changed and the pin is removed six weeks postoperatively. Another below-knee cast is applied for an additional three to four weeks. Weight-bearing is permitted in the second cast. Adequate incorporation of the graft and bone healing usually require eight to 12 weeks.

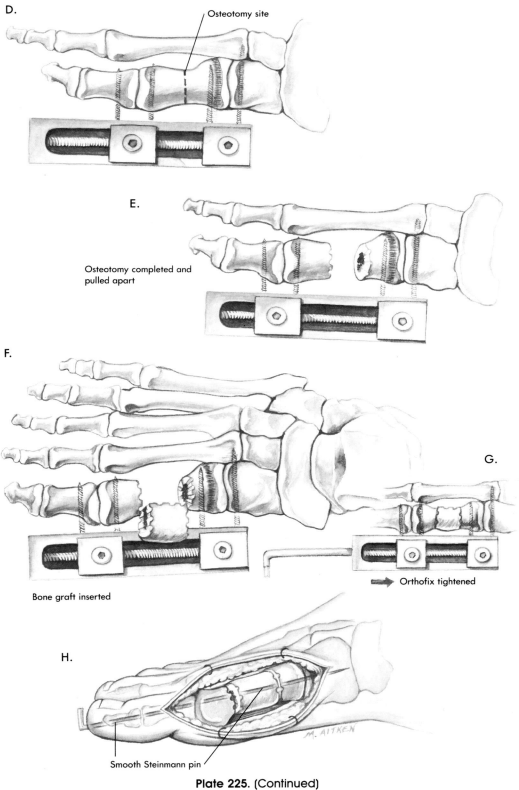

D.

Osteotomy site

E.

Osteotomy completed and
pulled apart

F.

G.

Bone graft inserted

Orthofix tightened

H.

Smooth Steinmann pin

M. AITKEN

Plate 225. (Continued)

PLATE 226   Farmer's Operation for Correction of Congenital Hallux Varus

Indications. Presence of deformity with difficulty wearing shoes.

Age. Between the ages of six and 12 months.

Surgical Procedure. First, provide a fatty skin flap on the medial side of the forefoot in order to permit lengthening of the soft tissues. The taut, contracted structures at the level of the metatarsophalangeal joint are sectioned. The skin flap is obtained from the adjoining sides of the hallux and second toe, where there is an abundant amount of skin. The flap is taken from the plantar surface and rotated to cover the medial side of the forefoot. If there is any tautness of the skin on the lateral side, a free, full-thickness skin graft is used to fill in the defect. This author recommends internal fixation.

Patient Position. Supine.

Operative Technique

With Duplication of the Hallux

A. and **B.** Draw the outline of the flap on the plantar aspect of the foot. The incision begins at the web interspace between the second toe and the duplicated hallux and extends proximally to the middle one third of the first and second metatarsals.

Next, make the incision for excision of the duplicated hallux dorsally. It begins between the two nails of the duplicated hallux and extends proximally to the neck of the first metatarsal, where it is extended medially and transversely to a point 1 cm. proximal to the plantar skin flap.

C. Subcutaneous tissue is divided in line with the skin incision. Digital vessels and nerves are identified and retracted. The contracted abductor hallucis muscle is sectioned. The capsule of the first metatarsophalangeal joint is sectioned transversely, and the duplicated hallux on the medial side is excised. The skin web between the second toe and the hallux is excised for surgical syndactyly of the second toe to the great toe following the technique of McFarland and Kelikian (see Plate 230).

D. The hallux is sutured to the second toe and webbed, and the skin flap on the plantar surface is elevated and retracted proximally.

E. The skin flap on the plantar aspect of the foot is trimmed to fit into the defect and sutured in place with interrupted sutures.

F. and **G.** The incision on the dorsal aspect of the foot is lengthened as necessary, and the skin flap from the plantar-medial aspect of the foot is sutured to the dorsum of the foot.

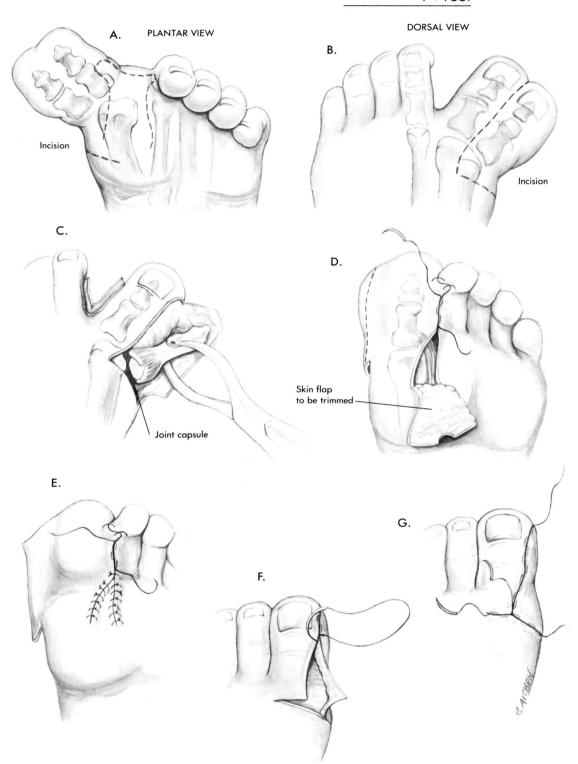

A. PLANTAR VIEW

Incision

B. DORSAL VIEW

Incision

C.

Joint capsule

D.

Skin flap
to be trimmed

E.

F.

G.

Plate 226. A.–O., Farmer's operation for correction of congenital hallux varus.

Without Duplication of the Hallux

H. An incision is made on the plantar surface of the foot in the web interspace between the big toe and the second toe and extended proximally toward the distal one third of the hallux. Subcutaneous tissue is divided in line with the skin incision. Tendons and nerves are retracted out of harm's way.

I. and J. The abductor hallucis tendon is sectioned, and all contracted fibrous tissue on the medial aspect of the metatarsophalangeal joint of the big toe is sectioned. The capsule of the first metatarsophalangeal joint is divided.

K. The big toe and the second toe are surgically syndactylized following the technique of McFarland and Kelikian.

H.

First
metatarsal

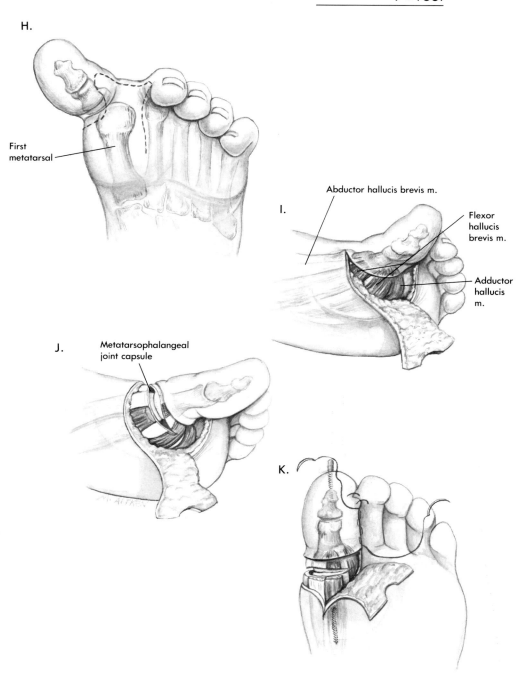

I.

Abductor hallucis brevis m.

Flexor
hallucis
brevis m.

Adductor
hallucis
m.

J.

Metatarsophalangeal
joint capsule

K.

Plate 226. (Continued)

L.–N. The flap of skin on the plantar aspect of the foot is rotated medially and dorsally and sutured to the dorsum of the forefoot with interrupted sutures.

O. The defect left on the plantar aspect of the foot is covered with a full-thickness skin graft taken from the lower abdomen above the groin.

In both techniques, the metatarsophalangeal joint is fixed with one threaded Steinmann pin to maintain alignment of the big toe.

Postoperative Care. A below-knee cast is applied, and the patient is allowed weight-bearing for a period of three weeks. The sutures and pin are removed, and another below-knee cast is applied for an additional week or ten days. The patient is then allowed to be ambulatory.

REFERENCES

Farmer, A. W.: Congenital hallux varus. Am. J. Surg., 95:274, 1958.
Johnson, K. A., and Spiegel, P. V.: Extensor hallucis longus transfer for hallux varus deformity. J. Bone Joint Surg., 66-A:681, 1984.
Kelikian, H.: The hallux. In: Jahss, M. H. (ed.): Disorders of the Foot. Philadelphia, W. B. Saunders Co., 1982, pp. 616–618.
Kelikian, H., Clayton, L., and Loseff, H.: Surgical syndactylism of the toes. Clin. Orthop., 19:208, 1961.
McElvenny, R. T.: Hallux varus. Q. Bull. Northwest. Med. School, 15:277, 1941.

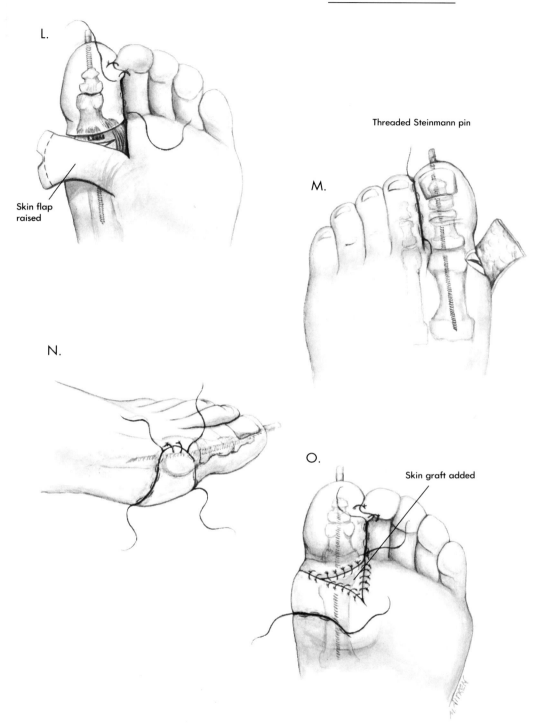

L.

Skin flap
raised

Threaded Steinmann pin

M.

N.

O.

Skin graft added

Plate 226. (Continued)

PLATE 227   **Correction of Hallux Valgus Interphalangeus**

Indications. Moderate or severe valgus deformity at the interphalangeal joint of the great toe with irritation of the skin, adventitious bursa, blisters, and pain due to shoe pressure. This operation is performed in the skeletally immature foot of the child.

Patient Position. Supine.

Operative Technique

    A. A 4-cm., slightly oblique longitudinal incision is made on the dorsolateral aspect of the deformed great toe. The incision begins in the middle of the distal phalanx immediately proximal to the nail bed, curves medially at the interphalangeal joint, and terminates on the dorsomedial aspect of the base of the proximal phalanx. The subcutaneous tissue is divided in line with the skin incision.

    B. The digital vessels and nerves and the tendon of the extensor hallucis longus are identified and retracted laterally with a blunt retractor. Then, Homan or Davies retractors are inserted on the medial and lateral aspects of the plantar surface of the proximal phalanx. With an electric saw and/or AO osteotome, resect a wedge of bone based medially. The medial base of the resected wedge should be wide enough so that when the bone fragments are aligned, the deformed big toe will be straight.

    C. The bone fragments are manipulated, anatomically aligned, and internally fixed with a Kirschner wire or Steinmann pin. The tip of the pin is bent to prevent pin migration. Be sure that there is no rotational malalignment.

    The wound is closed, and a below-knee walking cast is applied with a cap over the great toe.

Postoperative Care. The cast is changed three to four weeks postoperatively. The pin is removed, and another below-knee cast is applied for an additional two to three weeks.

Correction of Hallux Valgus Interphalangeus in the Skeletally Mature Foot by Wedge Resection and Fusion of the Interphalangeal Joint

    D. The incision and surgical exposure are similar to those described in **A.** The capsule is divided, and the interphalangeal joint is resected, removing a wedge based medially with excision of the prominent, hypertrophied, medial portion of the base of the epiphysis of the distal phalanx.

    E. The cancellous surfaces of the phalanges of the great toe are anatomically aligned and fixed internally with an AO cannulated screw of appropriate diameter and length. The tip of the screw extends to the base of the proximal phalanx. The interphalangeal joint is fused in neutral extension or 2 to 3 degrees of flexion, but not in hyperextension.

Postoperative Care. The foot is immobilized in a below-knee cast for three to four weeks and then supported in a shoe with a rigid shank-toe portion. The screw is removed six to 12 months after surgery.

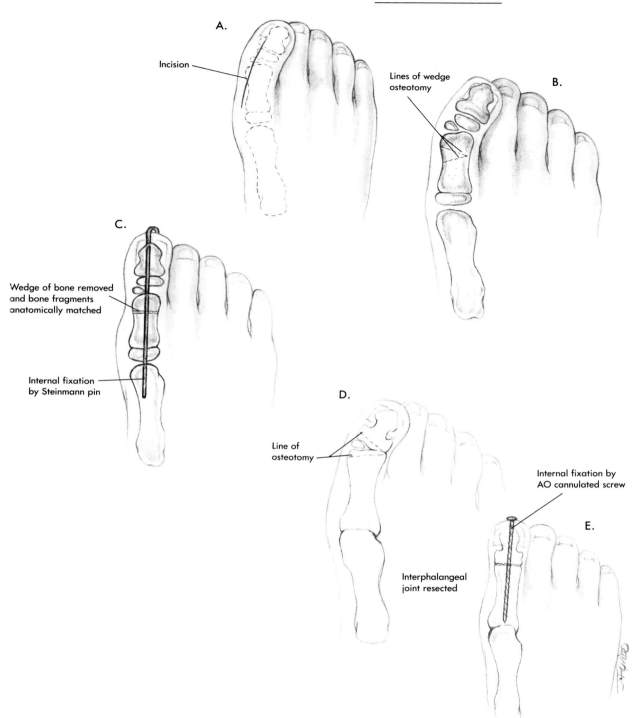

Plate 227. A.–E., Correction of hallux valgus interphalangeus.

PLATE 228 Correction of Hammer Toe by Resection and Arthrodesis of the Proximal Interphalangeal Joint

Indications. Severe deformity with painful calluses over the dorsum of the flexed interphalangeal joint.

Radiographic Control. Yes.

Patient Position. Supine.

Operative Technique

A. A 3- to 4-cm. longitudinal incision is made over the dorsal aspect of the proximal interphalangeal joint parallel to and at the lateral border of the extensor digitorum longus tendon. The subcutaneous tissue is divided, and the skin flaps are retracted.

B. The long extensor tendon is split and retracted to expose the capsule of the proximal interphalangeal joint. The digital vessels and nerves are protected from injury. A transverse incision is made in the capsule, and the joint surfaces are widely exposed.

C. and **D.** With a rongeur, wedges of bone based dorsally are resected from the head of the proximal phalanx and the base of the middle phalanx. Enough bone should be removed to allow correction of deformity.

E. and **F.** The proximal and middle phalanges are held together by internal fixation with a Kirschner wire that is inserted retrograde. The Kirschner wire should not cross the metatarsophalangeal joint. The cancellous bony surfaces of the middle and proximal phalanges should be apposed, and the rotational alignment should be correct. The capsule is resutured tightly by reefing. The wound is closed in routine manner. With a pair of long nose pliers, the end of the Kirschner wire is bent 90 degrees and cut, leaving 0.5 cm. protruding through the skin.

Postoperative Care. A below-knee walking cast is applied with a band of plaster of Paris protecting the toe. The wire and cast are removed in six weeks, when the radiograms show fusion of the interphalangeal joint.

REFERENCES

Jones, R.: Notes on Military Orthopaedics. New York, P. B. Hoeber, 1917, pp. 38–57.
Soule, R. E.: Operation for the cure of hammertoe. N. Y. Med. J., 91:649, 1910.

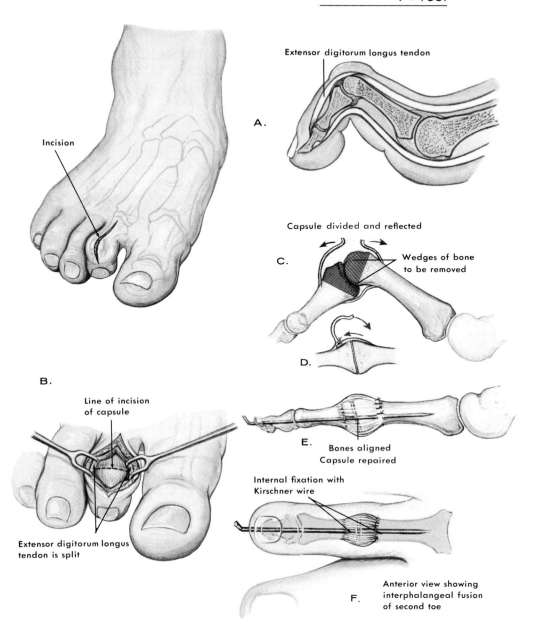

Incision

Extensor digitorum longus tendon

A.

Capsule divided and reflected

C.

Wedges of bone to be removed

D.

B.

Line of incision of capsule

Extensor digitorum longus tendon is split

E.

Bones aligned
Capsule repaired

Internal fixation with Kirschner wire

Anterior view showing interphalangeal fusion of second toe

F.

Plate 228. A.–F., Correction of hammer toe by resection and arthrodesis of the proximal interphalangeal joint.

PLATE 229 **Correction of Underriding of the Second Toe by Transfer of Long Flexor to Dorsolateral Aspect of Second Toe; Fenestrated Distal Surgical Syndactyly of the Second and Third Toes**

Indications. Underriding of a toe under the neighboring one with pain and discomfort while walking. There is a combination of flexion deformity, varus deviation, and lateral rotation of one or both interphalangeal joints of a toe. When the metatarsophalangeal joint of the affected toe is flexed and the deformities of the proximal interphalangeal and/or distal interphalangeal joints can be fully corrected by passive manipulation, a simple open tenotomy of the flexor tendons is performed.

Patient Position. Supine.

Operative Technique

Tenotomy of Flexor Tendons

A. Make a transverse incision proximal to the proximal plantar crease of the affected toe. Divide the subcutaneous tissue in line with the skin incision. With a blunt scissors, spread the skin flaps apart and keep the digital neurovascular bundle out of harm's way.

B. and C. Make a longitudinal incision in the flexor sheath. Identify the three flexor tendons—the flexor longus in the center and the flexor brevis on each side of the longus—and withdraw these tendons from the wound over a fine dissecting forceps. Section the tendons with a sharp scalpel. With a small hemostat, explore the wound to ensure that all of the slips of tendons are sectioned.

Manipulate the toes. If the natural resting posture of the toe is neutral, the wound is closed with 00 or 000 fine absorbable sutures. If the toe is still curly after division of the tendons and manipulation of the toe, it is best to use an intramedullary pin inserted from the tip of the affected toe to the base of the proximal phalanx for internal fixation. If no pin is inserted for internal fixation, a simple dressing is applied. If pins are used, it is best to apply a below-knee cast for a period of ten to 14 days.

Alternative Method of Management: Flexor-to-Extensor Tenodesis

D. A 3-cm. longitudinal incision is made on the dorsolateral aspect of the deformed toe. The subcutaneous tissue is divided, and the digital nerve and long toe extensor tendon are pulled medially with a blunt retractor.

E. The affected toe is acutely flexed, and on its plantar aspect the long toe flexor tendon is identified. A longitudinal incision is made in the flexor tendon sheath; the tendon is pulled dorsally with a small, blunt hook, and two sutures are passed through the tendon. The tendon is sectioned distal to the suture site.

F. and G. Transfer the long toe flexor to the dorsolateral aspect of the proximal phalanx of the affected toe.

The long toe flexor is sutured to the extensor expansion with the interphalangeal joints of the toe in full extension and with the metatarsophalangeal joint in flexion. The tourniquet is released, and the wound is closed in the usual manner. Alignment of the affected toe is maintained by a smooth Kirschner wire drilled from the distal end of the toe into the base of the proximal phalanx.

Postoperative Care. A below-knee walking cast is applied. The cast and wire are removed three to four weeks after surgery.

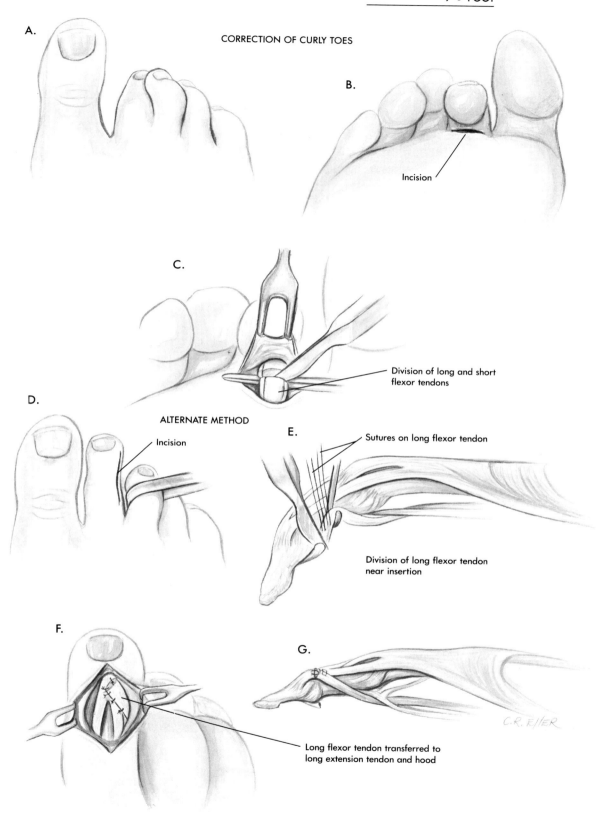

A.

CORRECTION OF CURLY TOES

B.

Incision

C.

Division of long and short flexor tendons

D.

ALTERNATE METHOD

Incision

E.

Sutures on long flexor tendon

Division of long flexor tendon near insertion

F.

G.

C.R. Eller

Long flexor tendon transferred to long extension tendon and hood

Plate 229. A.–G., Correction of underriding of the second toe by transfer of the long flexor to the dorsolateral aspect of the second toe. Fenestrated distal surgical syndactyly of the second and third toes.

REFERENCES

Kelikian, H.: Hallux Valgus, Allied Deformities of the Forefoot, and Metatarsalgia. Philadelphia, W. B. Saunders Co., 1965, p. 330.

Pollard, J. P., and Morrison, P. J. M.: Flexor tenotomy in the treatment of curly toes. Proc. R. Soc. Med., 68:480, 1975.

Ross, E. R., and Menelaus, M. B.: Open flexor tenotomy for hammer toes and curly toes in childhood. J. Bone Joint Surg., 66-B: 770, 1984.

Sharrard, W. J. W.: The surgery of deformed toes in children. Br. J. Clin. Pract., 17:263, 1963.

Sharrard, W. J. W.: Congenital varus (curly) toes. In: Paediatric Orthopaedics and Fractures and Developmental Abnormalities of the Foot and Toes. Oxford, Blackwell, 1971, pp. 295–299.

Sweetnam, R.: Congenital curly toes: An investigation into the value of treatment. Lancet, 2:398, 1958.

Watson, H. K., and Boyes, J. H.: Congenital angular deformities of the digits. J. Bone Joint Surg., 49-A:333, 1967.

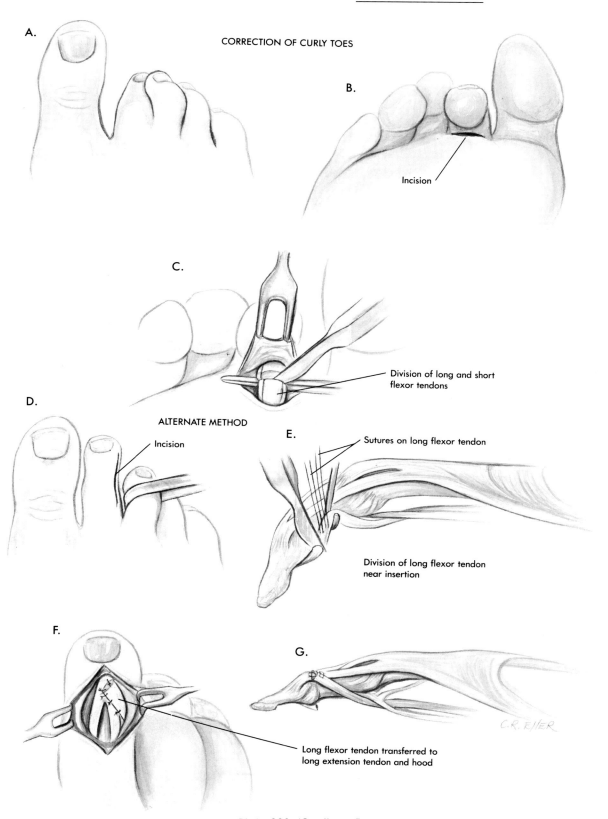

A.

CORRECTION OF CURLY TOES

B.

Incision

C.

Division of long and short
flexor tendons

D.

ALTERNATE METHOD

Incision

E.

Sutures on long flexor tendon

Division of long flexor tendon
near insertion

F.

G.

C.R. EJIER

Long flexor tendon transferred to
long extension tendon and hood

Plate 229. (Continued)

PLATE 230   Correction of Digitorum Minimus Varus (McFarland and Kelikian Technique)

Indications. The presence of a painful hard callus over the dorsum of the fifth toe caused by irritation from a shoe in an adolescent or adult.

Patient Position. Supine.

Operative Technique

A. First, a 00 nylon whip suture is passed through the pulps of the fourth and fifth toes. The suture ends are clamped with hemostats, and the toes are pulled apart, bringing the web space into full view.

B. Three sets of incisions are made:

1. A web-bisecting incision starts on the dorsum of the forefoot in the groove between the metatarsal heads, extends distally to bisect the web, and then passes plantarward to terminate at about the same point posteriorly on the plantar aspect of the forefoot as it does on the dorsum.

2. Two *paradigital incisions,* one for each toe, begin at the point where the web-bisecting incision begins to dip plantarward and extend lengthwise along the adjacent side of each toe. The paradigital incision for the little toe ends on the side of the distal phalanx at a point plantar and just proximal to the base of the nail, whereas the incision for the fourth toe is the same length as that for the fifth. The paradigital incisions are placed slightly toward the plantar border of the toe to give a semblance of an interdigital groove after surgical syndactylism.

3. Two connecting oblique incisions extend from the terminal point of the paradigital incision on each side to the proximal end of the web-bisecting incision on the plantar aspect.

C. The triangular patches of skin between the paradigital and oblique connecting incisions are excised. In dissection of subcutaneous tissue in this area, care is taken not to injure the plexus of veins. The skin flaps are mobilized and retracted to their respective sides. The digital nerves and vessels should be identified and protected from injury.

D. and E. The long extensor tendon of the fifth toe is divided at its insertion; a 00 Tycron whip suture is applied to its distal end. (This end is later transferred to the fifth metatarsal head according to the technique for the Jones procedure described in Plate 218.) Next, the long flexor of the fifth toe is dissected free of the proximal phalanx. Small retractors are placed on the dorsal and plantar aspects of the bone to protect the soft tissues. The capsules of the metatarsophalangeal and proximal interphalangeal joints of the little toe are divided, and the proximal phalanx is excised. The long fifth toe extensor is transferred to the fifth metatarsal head. The wound is packed with moist gauze, the pneumatic tourniquet is deflated, and bleeding vessels are clamped and coagulated.

F. The terminal points of the paradigital incisions are sutured together with 0000 nylon, bringing the toes together. The alignment of the toes is inspected. Care is taken to avoid eversion or inversion of the toes; if necessary, the terminal suture is removed and reapplied. The dorsal wound is closed with 0000 nylon, and the plantar skin edges with 0000 Vicryl.

Postoperative Care. A below-knee walking cast is applied. Three to four weeks following surgery, the cast and sutures are removed. The patient is allowed to bear weight and resume normal activities.

REFERENCES

Kelikian, H.: Hallux Valgus, Allied Deformities of the Forefoot, and Metatarsalgia. Philadelphia, W. B. Saunders Co., 1965.
McFarland, B.: Congenital deformities of the spine and limbs. In: Platt, H. (ed.): Modern Trends in Orthopedics. New York, P. B. Hoeber, 1950, p. 107.

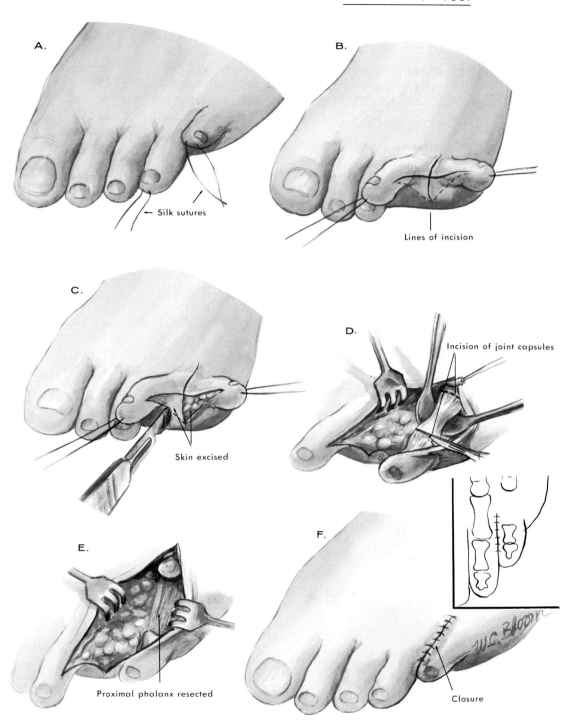

Plate 230. A.–F., Correction of digitorum minimus varus (McFarland and Kelikian technique).

PLATE 231   Butler's Operation for Correction of Overriding Fifth Toe

Indications. Presence of a painful hard callus over the dorsum of the fifth toe caused by irritation from a shoe in an adolescent or adult with marked contracture of the skin and soft tissues on the dorsum of the fifth ray and toe.

Patient Position. Supine.

Operative Technique

A. and **B.** A racquet incision is made on the dorsal aspect of the little toe; then, add a second handle to the racquet on the plantar aspect of the little toe and fifth metatarsal. The plantar handle is inclined toward the fibula (laterally) and is longer than the dorsal handle. The subcutaneous tissue is divided. The wound flaps are undermined and elevated.

C. The contracted extensor tendon of the fifth toe is exposed.

D. Digital vessels and nerves are identified and carefully kept out of harm's way. Avoid excessive traction on the neurovascular bundle and circulatory embarrassment.

E. The long extensor tendon to the little toe and the dorsomedial capsule of the metatarsophalangeal joint are sectioned. The little toe can now be manipulated freely plantarward and laterally into the correct anatomic alignment.

A.

B.

Line of incision

C.

Neurovascular bundle

Extensor digitorum longus tendon

D.

Flexor digitorum longus tendon

Neurovascular bundle

E.

Sectioning of metatarsophalangeal joint

Extensor digitorum longus tendon

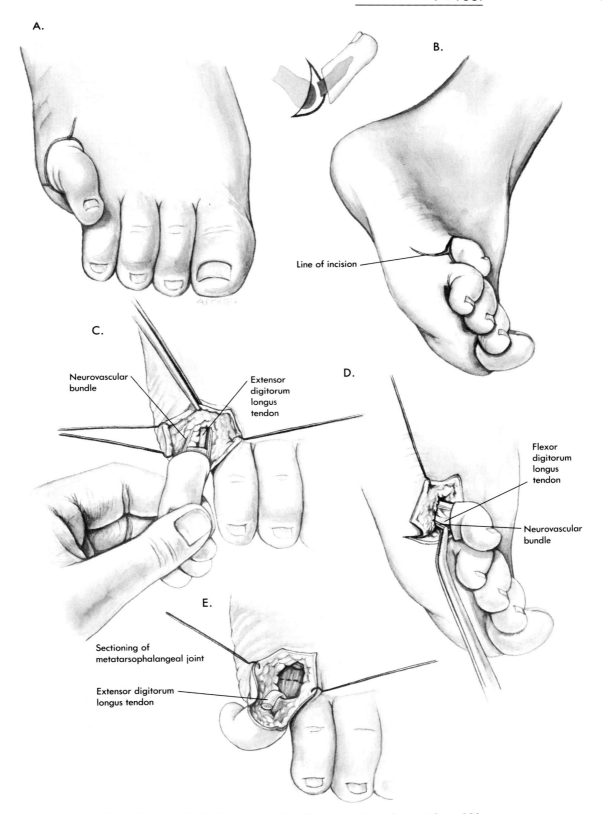

Plate 231. A.–J., Butler's operation for correction of overriding fifth toe.

F. and **G.** In severe deformity, the plantar capsular adhesions may prevent correction of deformity. In such an instance, the capsular adhesions are freed from the metatarsal head by blunt dissection with a Freer elevator.

H. Now the toe is manipulated into the plantar handle of the wound; it should dangle in normal alignment without any soft-tissue tension.

I. and **J.** The pneumatic tourniquet is released, and complete hemostasis is achieved. Close the wound, holding the little toe in normal anatomic position. Subcutaneous tissue is closed with 000 Vicryl interrupted sutures, and the skin is closed with 000 or 0000 nylon interrupted sutures.

The mechanics of the operation are illustrated in the diagrams.

Postoperative Care. A single dressing with an Ace bandage is applied. In an uncooperative child, a below-knee cast is applied to keep the little toe and wound out of reach of the child's hand.

REFERENCE

Cockin, J.: Butler's operation for an overriding fifth toe. J. Bone Joint Surg., 50-B:78, 1968.

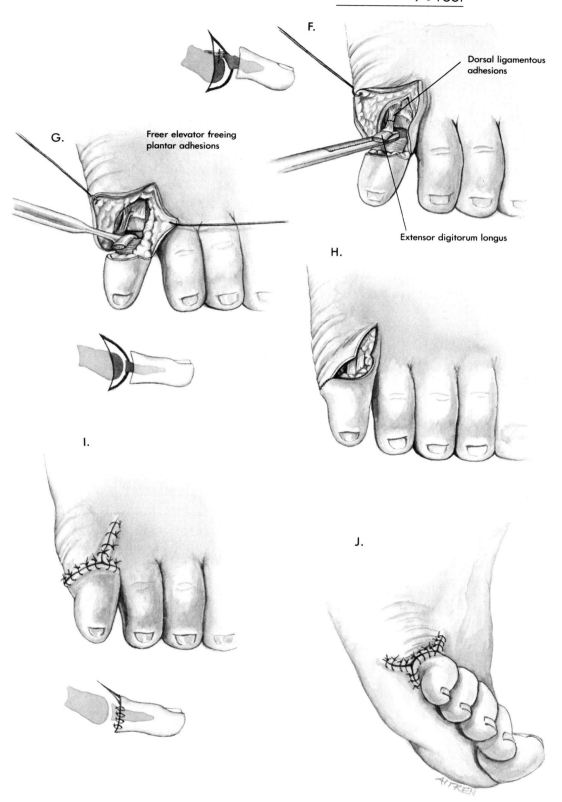

F. Dorsal ligamentous adhesions

Extensor digitorum longus

G. Freer elevator freeing plantar adhesions

H.

I.

J.

AITKEN

Plate 231. (Continued)

PLATE 232 **Sliding Osteotomy of the Fifth Metatarsal Neck for Correction of Tailor's Bunion (Bunionette) (Sponsel-Hansson Technique)**

Indications. Painful prominence of the fifth metatarsal head causing disabling pain and difficulty wearing shoes.

Patient Position. Supine.

Operative Technique

A. A dorsal incision is made, extending from the middle of the fifth metatarsal shaft to the fifth metatarsophalangeal joint. The subcutaneous tissue is divided in line with the skin incision. The long toe extensor tendon of the fifth toe is retracted medially. The periosteum is incised, and the neck and distal third of the metatarsal shaft are subperiosteally exposed.

B. Insert Homan or small Chandler retractors subperiosteally to protect the soft tissues. With a sharp AO osteotome, mark the line of oblique osteotomy; it begins laterally and distally immediately proximal to the metatarsal head and extends proximally on the metatarsal shaft at a 45-degree oblique angle. The osteotomy is completed with a reciprocating saw.

C. With a rongeur, excise the lateral distal corner of the distal metatarsal shaft.

D. Displace the metatarsal head medially and proximally to bring the prominent lateral surface of the metatarsal head to the level of the lateral surface of the distal end of the metatarsal shaft.

Hansson maintains the position with absorbable sutures.

E. This author recommends internal fixation with two threaded Steinmann pins inserted from the lateral surface of the metatarsal shaft and directed medially and distally to engage the cortex of the displaced metatarsal head. Radiograms in the anteroposterior and lateral planes are made to determine the adequacy of correction of the deformity and the position of the pins. The wound is closed in the usual fashion. A below-knee cast is applied.

Postoperative Care. The cast is changed, and the pins are removed three to four weeks after surgery. Another below-knee cast is applied. Partial weight-bearing is allowed. The total period of cast immobilization is about six weeks.

REFERENCES

Hansson, G.: Sliding osteotomy for tailor's bunion: Brief report. J. Bone Joint Surg., 71-B:324, 1989.
Sponsel, K. H.: Bunionette correction by metatarsal osteotomy. Orthop. Clin. North Am., 7:809, 1976.

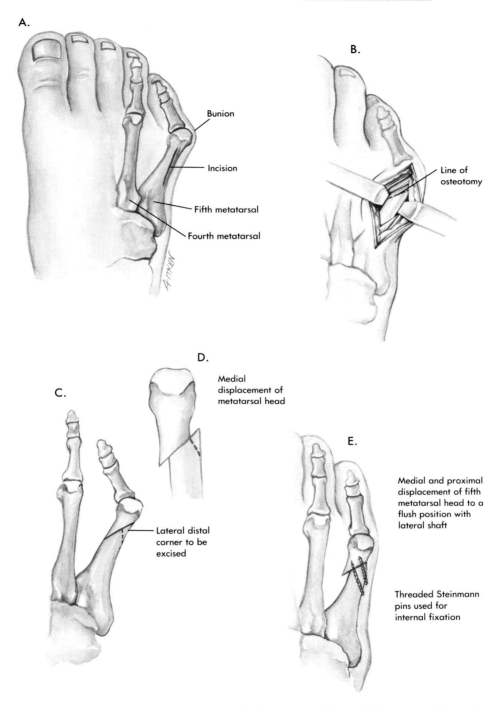

A.

Bunion

Incision

Fifth metatarsal

Fourth metatarsal

B.

Line of osteotomy

D.

Medial displacement of metatarsal head

C.

Lateral distal corner to be excised

E.

Medial and proximal displacement of fifth metatarsal head to a flush position with lateral shaft

Threaded Steinmann pins used for internal fixation

Plate 232. **A.–E.,** Surgical correction of a bunionette (Sponsel-Hansson technique).

PLATE 233 **Arthrodesis of the Metatarsophalangeal Joint of the Great Toe**

Indications. Painful and disabling hallux rigidus in the skeletally mature foot.

Radiographic Control. Yes.

Patient Position. Supine.

Operative Technique

   A. A dorsal longitudinal incision is made to expose the metatarsophalangeal joint. It begins at the distal interphalangeal joint of the great toe, immediately lateral to the extensor hallucis longus tendon, and extends proximally to terminate at the distal one third of the first metatarsal. Subcutaneous tissue and superficial fascia are divided in line with the skin incision. Do not injure the digital vessels and nerves.

   B. The extensor hallucis longus and brevis tendons are exposed, mobilized, and retracted laterally. The capsule of the metatarsophalangeal joint is divided first by a transverse incision, which is then converted to a "T" by a longitudinal incision on the center of the first metatarsal. Small Homan or Davies retractors are placed medially and laterally under the first metatarsal head.

   C. With sharp AO osteotomes, small rongeurs, and curets, the articular cartilage of the base of the proximal phalanx is completely removed.

   Next, the joint cartilage from the first metatarsal head is excised with an oscillating saw or sharp AO osteotome. The angle and wedge of bone excised from the base of the proximal phalanx and first metatarsal head should be such that when the denuded raw bony surfaces are apposed, the position of the arthrodesis is optimum (i.e., it should be in 10 to 15 degrees of valgus; in the male, in 10 to 15 degrees of dorsiflexion; and, in the female, in 15 to 20 degrees of dorsiflexion).

   D.–F. The first metatarsal head and base of the proximal phalanx are snugly held in the desired position and internally fixed with a cannulated screw (AO or Herbert). The guide pin and then the drill are directed proximally and slightly plantar through the base of the proximal phalanx, emerging on the side of the first metatarsal. The screw is inserted and countersunk, lying against the flare of the base of the proximal phalanx. Bony spurs are excised so that the medial and dorsal surfaces of the first metatarsal head are smooth.

   The tourniquet is released. Complete hemostasis is achieved. A small Hemovac drain is inserted, and the wound is closed in the usual fashion. The foot and leg are immobilized in a below-knee walking cast.

Postoperative Care. The cast is changed two to three weeks postoperatively. The sutures are removed. Radiograms are made. Another walking cast is applied for an additional three weeks. The screw is removed six to 12 months later.

REFERENCES

Fitzgerald, J. A. W.: Review of long-term results in arthrodesis of the first metatarsophalangeal joint. J. Bone Joint Surg., 51-B:488, 1969.
Harrison, M.: Hallux limitus. J. Bone Joint Surg., 53-B:772, 1971.
Kelikian, H.: Hallux Valgus, Allied Deformities of the Forefoot, and Metatarsalgia. Philadelphia, W. B. Saunders Co., 1965, p. 273.
Kelikian, H.: The hallux. In: Jahss, M. H. (ed.): Disorders of the Foot. Philadelphia, W. B. Saunders Co., 1983, pp. 608–613.

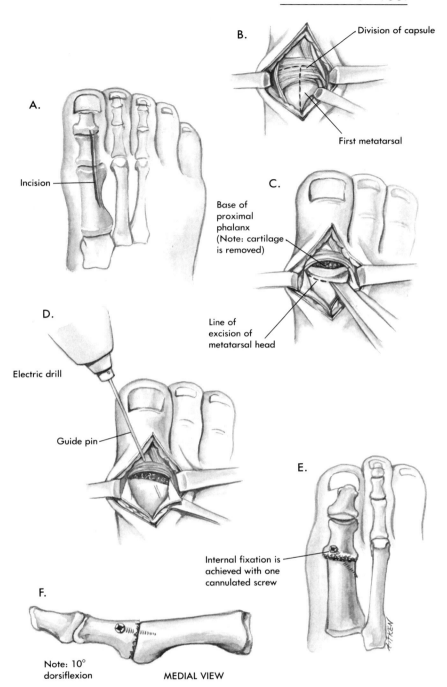

A.

Incision

B.

Division of capsule

First metatarsal

C.

Base of
proximal
phalanx
(Note: cartilage
is removed)

Line of
excision of
metatarsal head

D.

Electric drill

Guide pin

E.

Internal fixation is
achieved with one
cannulated screw

F.

Note: 10°
dorsiflexion

MEDIAL VIEW

Plate 233. A.–F., Arthrodesis of the metatarsophalangeal joint of the great toe.

PLATE 234

Cuneiform Osteotomy of the Head-Neck of the First Metatarsal with Dorsally Based Wedge (Waterman Technique)

Indications. Symptomatic and disabling hallux rigidus in the growing foot (the physis of the proximal phalanx is open).

Patient Position. Supine.

Operative Technique

A. Make a dorsomedial longitudinal incision, beginning at the middle of the first metatarsal and extending distally across to the metatarsophalangeal joint to terminate at the interphalangeal joint of the great toe. The subcutaneous and superficial fascia are divided in line with the skin incision. The extensor hallucis longus and brevis tendons with digital vessels and nerves are mobilized and retracted laterally. The dorsal capsule is elevated distally; expose the head of the first metatarsal.

B. and **C.** If the metatarsophalangeal (MP) joint of the great toe cannot be dorsiflexed to neutral position, perform a plantar capsulotomy of the first MP joint and, if necessary, release of the flexor hallucis brevis at its insertion on the base of the proximal phalanx. Do not divide the flexor hallucis longus.

D. Next, with an oscillating saw and sharp AO osteotome, a cuneiform osteotomy with a wedge of bone directed distally and including the hypertrophic spurs is removed from the proximal part of the metatarsal head-neck.

E. and **F.** The bone fragments are anatomically apposed, and the osteotomy is transfixed with two threaded Steinmann pins inserted through the distal metatarsal shaft and drilled obliquely and distally into the metatarsal head across the joint and into the proximal phalanx. Anteroposterior and lateral radiograms are made to determine the degree of correction of the deformity and the position of the pins.

The tourniquet is released, and complete hemostasis is achieved. The wound is closed in the usual fashion.

A below-knee cast is applied. Weight-bearing is not allowed.

Postoperative Care. The pins are removed four weeks post surgery. A new below-knee walking cast is applied for an additional two to three weeks.

REFERENCES

Kelikian, H.: Hallux Valgus, Allied Deformities of the Forefoot and Metatarsalgia. Philadelphia, W. B. Saunders Co., 1965, p. 273.
Watermann, H.: Die Arthritis deformans Grosszehengrundgelenkes. Z. Orthop. Chir., 48:346, 1927.

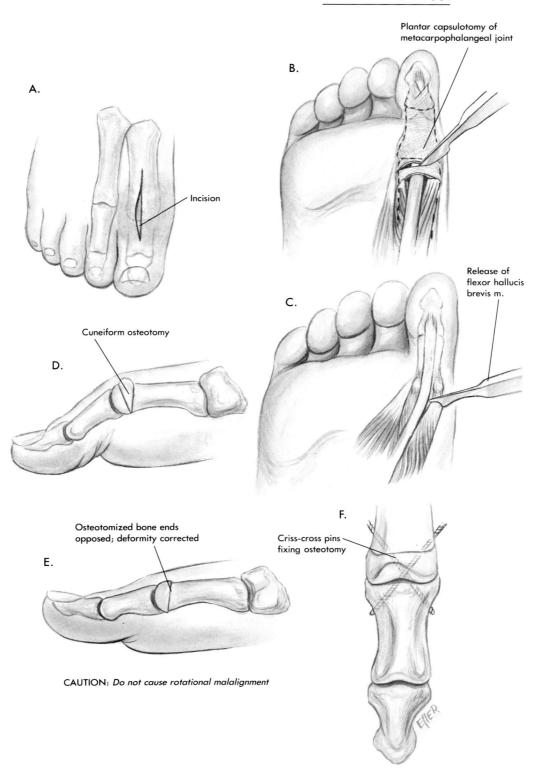

A.

B.

Plantar capsulotomy of
metacarpophalangeal joint

Incision

Release of
flexor hallucis
brevis m.

C.

Cuneiform osteotomy

D.

Osteotomized bone ends
opposed; deformity corrected

E.

F.

Criss-cross pins
fixing osteotomy

CAUTION: *Do not cause rotational malalignment*

Plate 234. A.–F., Cuneiform dorsiflexion wedge osteotomy of the first metatarsal head-neck
for treatment of hallux rigidus (Waterman technique).

PLATE 235 — Extension Osteotomy of the Base of the Proximal Phalanx of the Great Toe for Treatment of Hallux Rigidus

Indications. The adolescent or adult patient with persisting pain at the metatarsophalangeal joint of the great toe with disability in the form of limping and difficulty with shoe fitting. Failure of conservative measures to relieve symptoms, i.e.:

1. Stiffening of the sole of the shoe between the shank and toe portions medially under the first metatarsal head.

2. Wearing a slightly larger shoe with its leather softened dorsally over the first metatarsophalangeal joint.

3. Passive manipulative exercises performed several times a day to increase the range of dorsiflexion of the great toe.

Radiographic Control. Image intensifier.

Patient Position. Supine.

Operative Technique

A. A curved dorsal incision about 4 cm. long is made, centering over the base of the proximal phalanx. The subcutaneous tissue is divided. The extensor hallucis longus tendon and digital nerves are retracted to one side to expose the proximal phalanx and metatarsophalangeal joint of the great toe with a sharp AO osteotome. The capsule of the metatarsophalangeal joint is not disturbed.

B. The proximal and distal lines of osteotomy, with its base dorsally, are delineated. Under image intensifier radiographic control through the tip of the great toe, two threaded Kirschner wires are inserted obliquely with a power drill, stopping short of the distal level of osteotomy. The interphalangeal joint of the hallux is in marked extension. This preliminary step will assist in criss-cross pinning of the osteotomy.

C. With a power saw and small osteotomes, a wedge of bone with a dorsal base of predetermined width is resected from the phalanx as far proximally as possible. Leave the cortex and periosteum on the plantar aspect intact. It is best to use drill holes to mark and control the extent of osteotomy. The phalanx is angulated dorsally, and the gap is closed.

D. and E. The two Kirschner wires are drilled, advancing them proximally into the metatarsal head-neck, holding the osteotomized fragments firmly together. The wound is closed, and a below-knee walking cast with a sturdy toe plate is applied. The great toe should be held in extension by appropriate padding underneath.

Postoperative Care. The pins are removed in three to four weeks, and a new below-knee cast is applied; weight-bearing is allowed. Ordinarily, the osteotomy will heal in six weeks.

REFERENCE

Kessel, L., and Bonney, G.: Hallux rigidus in the adolescent. J. Bone Joint Surg., 40-B:668, 1958.

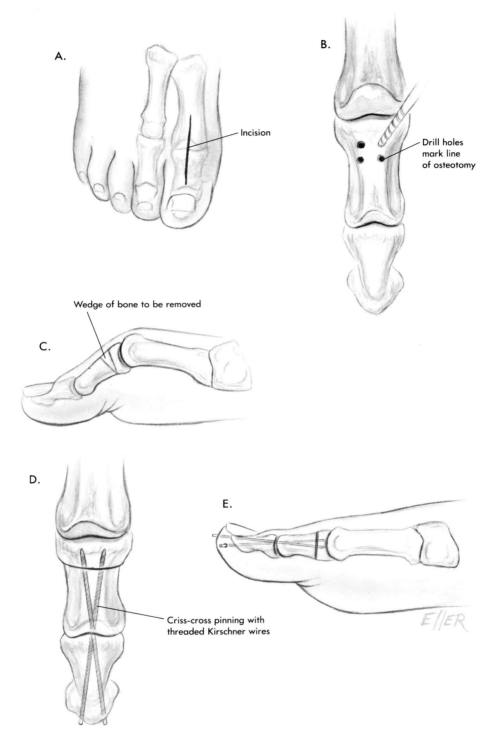

A.

Incision

B.

Drill holes
mark line
of osteotomy

Wedge of bone to be removed

C.

D.

E.

Criss-cross pinning with
threaded Kirschner wires

ELLER

Plate 235. **A.–E.,** Extension osteotomy of the base of the proximal phalanx of the great toe
for treatment of hallux rigidus.

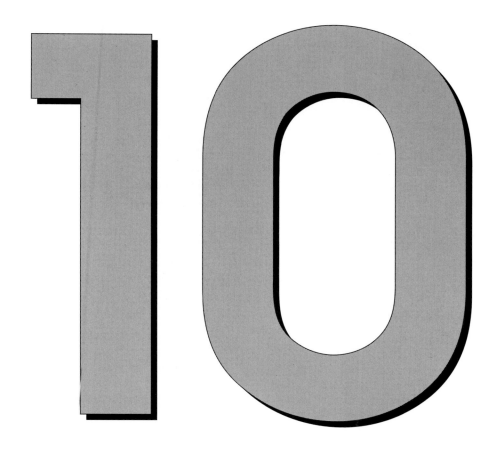

Spine

PLATE 236 **Cervical Spine Fusion for Absence or Hypoplasia of Odontoid Process (Atlantoaxial Instability) (Gallie Technique)**

Indications

1. Atlantoaxial instability (atlas-dens interval) greater than 5 mm. in children (3 mm. in adults) anteriorly or posteriorly. The atlas-dens interval (ADI) is greater in the child than in the adult because part of the odontoid process is cartilaginous and is not completely ossified. The causes of instability may be (a) congenital owing to aplasia or hypoplasia of the odontoid process; (b) developmental bone dysplasia, such as in Morquio's disease; (c) ligamentous hyperlaxity, such as in Down syndrome and rheumatoid arthritis; or (d) post-traumatic, such as in fracture-dislocation.

2. Neurologic deficit caused by spinal cord or spinal nerve compression owing to atlantoaxial instability.

3. Persistent neck pain and muscle spasm with failure to respond to conservative measures of management, such as traction and/or support in a cervical orthosis.

Preoperative Assessment

1. A thorough neurologic examination. Obtain neurologic or neurosurgical consultation.

2. Cervical spine radiograms with (a) open mouth views, (b) lateral-neutral, flexion, and extension views, and (c) tomograms.

3. Computed tomography (CT) scan in flexion and extension and three-dimensional CT reconstruction.

4. Magnetic resonance imaging (MRI) of the cervical spine and spinal cord, particularly if a neurologic deficit is detected.

Cineradiography and myelography are ordinarily not performed.
The following determinations should be made:

1. *Atlas-dens interval.* This interval is the space between the anterior aspect of the dens and the posterior aspect of the anterior ring of the atlas, as measured in the lateral projection. The distance is often greatest in flexion views. In children, the ADI should be 4 mm. or less; in adults, the interval should be 3 mm. or less. In trauma, an increase in ADI in the neutral position indicates an avulsion or tear of the transverse atlantal ligament; in such an instance, flexion views should not be obtained because it would be dangerous to do so.

2. *Space available for the spinal cord (SAC).* The SAC is the distance between the posterior aspect of the odontoid process or axis and the nearest posterior structures, that is, the posterior ring of the atlas or the foramen magnum. When this space is narrowed, as shown on routine radiograms, it is vital to obtain an MR image.

3. *Anatomic reduction of the atlantoaxial joint.* If the atlantoaxial joint is subluxated, apply skull traction for one or two weeks to obtain reduction.

4. *Integrity of the posterior arch of C-1.* The C-1 posterior arch may be hypoplastic—a rare anomaly but not uncommon in patients with os odontoideum. In patients with poor development of the posterior arch of C-1, the fusion should be extended to the occiput.

Radiographic Control. Image intensifier.

Blood for Transfusion. Yes.

Patient Position. The patient is placed in a prone position, and the neck, shoulder, and posterior iliac graft area are prepared and draped sterile in the usual orthopedic fashion.

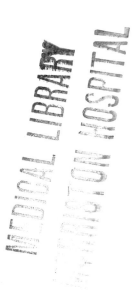

Operative Technique

In this book, the Gallie technique for posterior atlantoaxial arthrodesis is described and illustrated. It is preferred by this author.

A. The surgeon should be familiar with the anatomic structures of the upper cervical spine, specifically, the occiput, atlas, axis, vertebral arteries, articular capsules, lateral alar ligament, cruciform ligament (vertical and horizontal limbs), and tectorial membrane.

B. In patients with marked atlantoaxial instability and risk of neurologic damage, a halo vest or cast is applied preoperatively. Lateral radiograms of the cervical spine are made to confirm an anatomic reduction of the atlantoaxial joint.

C. An intradermal injection of 1:500,000 solution of epinephrine minimizes bleeding. Make a midline posterior incision from the protuberance of the base of the skull to the spinous process of C-4. The subcutaneous tissue and fascia are divided in line with the skin incision. Keep the dissection within the relatively avascular midline.

Use palpation to locate the spinous process of C-2. Mark the process with a small towel clip, and document it with a lateral radiogram of the spine.

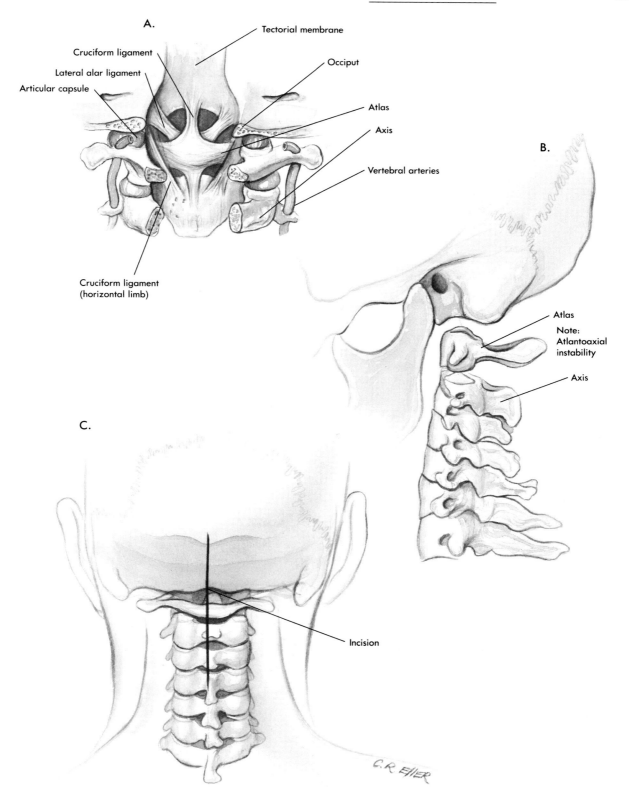

A.

Tectorial membrane

Cruciform ligament

Lateral alar ligament

Articular capsule

Occiput

Atlas

Axis

Vertebral arteries

Cruciform ligament
(horizontal limb)

B.

Atlas

Note:
Atlantoaxial
instability

Axis

C.

Incision

C.R. EILER

Plate 236. **A.–G.,** Cervical spine fusion for absence or hypoplasia of the odontoid process (atlantoaxial instability) (Gallie technique).

D. Divide the intermuscular septum and the ligamentum nuchae, and subperiosteally expose only the area to be fused—C-1, C-2. In children, exposure of the base of the skull or vertebrae distal to C-2, C-3 results in spontaneous extension of the fusion. With a periosteal elevator, expose the spinous process and lamina of C-1, C-2 and denude them of all muscular and fibrous tissues.

Caution! Do not injure the vertebral arteries and veins on the posterolateral aspect of the ring of C-1.

The superior aspect of C-1 should not be dissected more than 1 cm. laterally in children and 1.5 cm. from the midline in adolescents. Do not decorticate the posterior ring of C-1. Elevate the periosteum from the anterior surface of the arch of C-1 by a small angulated neural elevator. Usually, it is not necessary to decorticate the exposed lamina of C-1, C-2. In the adolescent and young adult, however, it may be done with a dental burr.

E. Pass a loop of wire inferosuperiorly under the arch of C-1. Stainless steel wire, 22 to 18 gauge depending on the age of the patient and the size of the spinal canal, is used to hold the iliac bone graft in place against the posterior arches of the atlas and the axis. In children younger than six years of age, internal fixation with wire is not necessary.

F. A corticocancellous autogenous bone graft is harvested from the ilium and trimmed to fit over the lamina of C-1 and C-2. The graft is positioned in place.

G. The loop of wire is bent inferiorly and passed around the spinous process of C-2. The two loose ends of the wire that protrude from the inferior surface of the atlas are brought over the posterior surface of the graft. The wire is twisted, locking the graft in place.

Lateral radiograms of the cervical spine are made to determine the position of the graft and the wires and anatomic reduction of the atlantoaxial joint.

A medium-sized Hemovac suction tube is placed. The wound is closed in layers in the usual fashion.

Postoperative Care. A patient who is in a halo vest or cast continues to wear the appliance for six weeks and then is placed in a cervical orthosis for a total period of immobilization of about 12 weeks.

REFERENCES

Fielding, J. W., Hawkins, R. J., and Ratzan, S. A.: Spinal fusion for atlantoaxial instability. J. Bone Joint Surg., 58-A:400, 1976.
Gallie, W. E.: Fractures and dislocations of the cervical spine. Am. J. Surg., 46:495, 1939.

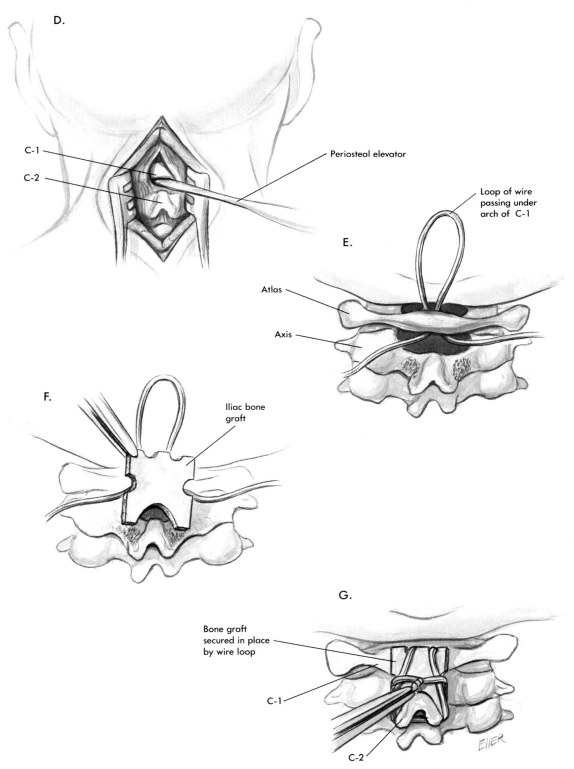

D.

C-1

C-2

Periosteal elevator

Loop of wire
passing under
arch of C-1

E.

Atlas

Axis

F.

Iliac bone
graft

G.

Bone graft
secured in place
by wire loop

C-1

C-2

ELIER

Plate 236. (Continued)

PLATE 237   Posterolateral Lumbosacral in Situ Fusion for Stabilization at L-5, S-1 Spondylolisthesis

Indications. Operative intervention is indicated in the following circumstances:

1. When there is persistent back pain and marked disability interfering with activities of daily living despite conservative management, such as temporary support to the spine, activity restriction, and physical therapy for six months to a year.

2. In severe slip (greater than 50 per cent) with severe tautness of the hamstrings, postural deformity, and abnormal gait unresponsive to aggressive physical therapy.

3. When there is progression of the slip beyond 25 to 50 per cent owing to marked instability at the defect.

4. In the presence of neurologic deficit that does not improve with conservative management and may or may not progress.

5. When persistent sciatic scoliosis is unresponsive to rest, physical therapy, and support of the spine.

When spondylolisthesis is 50 per cent or more and the slip angle is more than 50 degrees in a growing child or adolescent, the period of conservative management should not be prolonged if the symptoms and disability persist. Results of surgical stabilization are excellent; the parents and patient should be informed of the psychosocial importance of normal physical activity for an adolescent.

Objectives. The goals of surgery are (1) to stabilize the unstable spondylolytic segment; (2) to prevent further slip; (3) to relieve any nerve root irritation and prevent further neurologic deficit; and (4) to correct hamstring tautness, poor posture, and abnormality of gait.

The posterolateral alar transverse processes (all the way to their tips) and fusion of facets extends from the midsacrum to the fifth or fourth lumbar vertebra. The arthrodesis should extend to L-4 when the transverse process of L-5 is small, the degree of listhesis is 50 per cent or more, and the slip angle is more than 50 degrees. The dorsal aspects of the transverse process, the pars articularis, and the articular facets in the posterolateral lower lumbar spine and sacrum provide an adequate bone surface for bridging the vertebrae with bone grafts. Additional advantages of posterolateral fusion are the position of the grafts near the center of the anteroposterior motion of the vertebral column and the healthy soft-tissue environment provided by the surrounding muscles.

Preoperative Assessment. When *neurologic deficit* is present (motor and sensory) owing to nerve root involvement, perform MRI or CT scanning, with or without metrizamide myelography. The cause of nerve root irritation is not a loose lamina. When the fifth lumbar nerve root is involved, the offending agent is the upper part of the pars interarticularis or the hypertrophied fibrocartilaginous mass at the site of the defect; when the sacral nerve roots are affected, the nerve irritation is caused by a prominent portion of the body of the first sacral vertebra.

Decompression alone, without fusion, has no place in the treatment of spondylolisthesis in children and adolescents; it causes increased instability, progression of deformity, and greater lumbar kyphosis and deformity.

In the operative plate, only in situ fusion is described and illustrated.

Blood for Transfusion. Yes.

Radiographic Control. Yes.

Patient Position. Under general endotracheal anesthesia, the patient is placed in prone position on the Hall frame. Properly position and pad the upper and lower limbs to prevent pressure sores and nerve palsy.

Operative Technique

A. A longitudinal midline incision is made beginning at the midsacrum and extending proximally to the level of the fourth lumbar spinous process (when only L-5 to the midsacrum is the extent of arthrodesis) and to the spinous process of the third lumbar vertebra when the fusion is to extend to L-4. Subcutaneous tissue is divided in line with the skin incision.

B. The wound flaps are undermined and retracted to either side, exposing the lateral border of each paravertebral muscle. The lumbosacral fascia is divided by two incisions that curve toward the midline like hockey sticks.

C. The paraspinal muscle is split, and blunt dissection with the index finger is used to separate the muscle mass down to the sacrum. Expose the space between the transverse process of the fifth lumbar vertebra and the ala of the sacrum and the articular processes of the fifth lumbar and first sacral vertebrae.

Caution! Split the sacrospinal muscle only enough to expose the vertebrae to be fused. When only L-5, S-1 fusion is planned, do not expose the fourth lumbar vertebra; when L-4, S-1 fusion is to be carried out, do not expose the third lumbar vertebra. The natural tendency is to dissect too far cephalad.

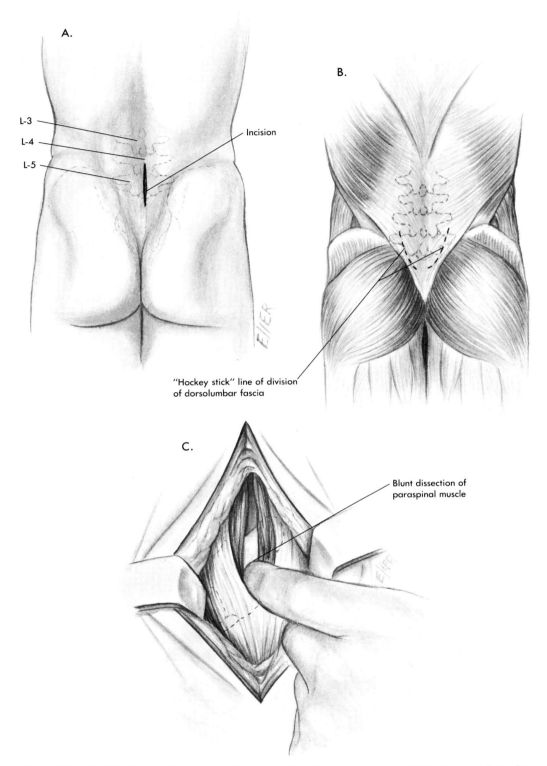

A.

L-3
L-4
L-5

Incision

"Hockey stick" line of division
of dorsolumbar fascia

B.

C.

Blunt dissection of
paraspinal muscle

Plate 237. A.–K., Posterolateral lumbosacral in situ fusion for stabilization at L-5, S-1 spondylolisthesis.

D. Deep right-angle retractors are used to retract the muscles. Expose the ala of the top of the sacrum and the laminae of the vertebrae to be fused to the base of their spinous processes. Denude their dorsal surfaces of all soft tissue.

E. Denude the transverse process of L-5 (or L-4 and L-5 if fusion is to extend to L-4) of soft tissues on the dorsal surface and superior and inferior borders.

Caution! Do not carry the soft-tissue dissection anteriorly, which might injure the spinal nerves that traverse in front of the transverse processes.

F. Denude the lateral surface of the superior articular process of L-5 (if L-5 sacrum fusion) and L-4 (if L-4 sacrum fusion) of all soft tissue. Do not damage the adjacent joint, and do not expose the vertebrae immediately above the fusion.

Denude the lateral surface of the pars interarticularis of all soft tissue and the dorsal surface of the lamina as far medially as the base of the spinous process.

Do not expose the spinous processes, and preserve the ligamentous attachments.

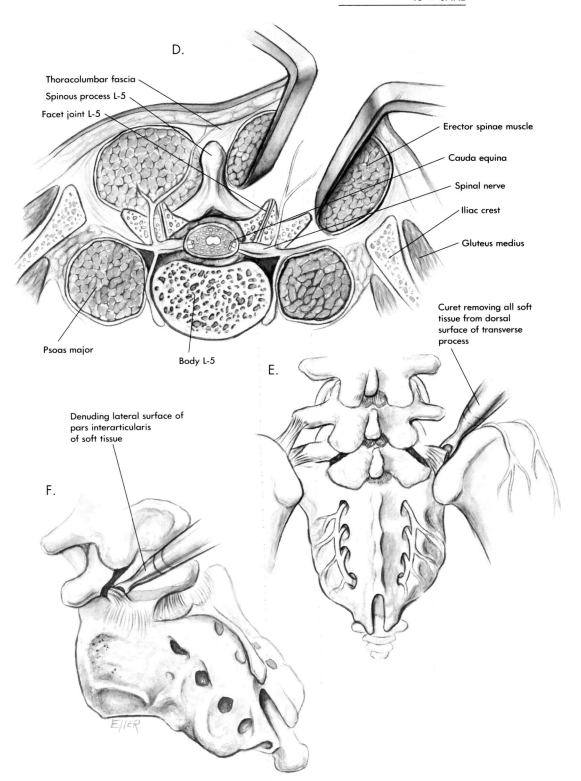

D.

Thoracolumbar fascia

Spinous process L-5

Facet joint L-5

Erector spinae muscle

Cauda equina

Spinal nerve

Iliac crest

Gluteus medius

Curet removing all soft
tissue from dorsal
surface of transverse
process

Psoas major

Body L-5

E.

Denuding lateral surface of
pars interarticularis
of soft tissue

F.

Plate 237. (Continued)

G. and **H.** Decompression of the nerve roots, if indicated, may be carried out through the posterolateral approach. When the L-5 nerve root is irritated, only the superior half of the lamina of the affected side is removed and the nerve is traced laterally and completely decompressed.

G.

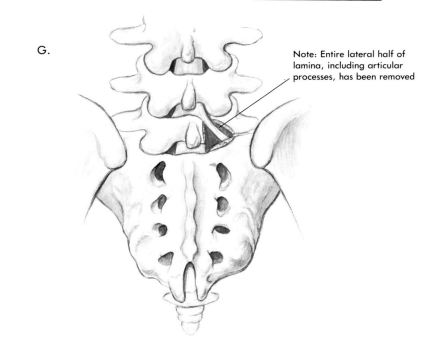

Note: Entire lateral half of
lamina, including articular
processes, has been removed

H.

L-4   L-5   Sacrum

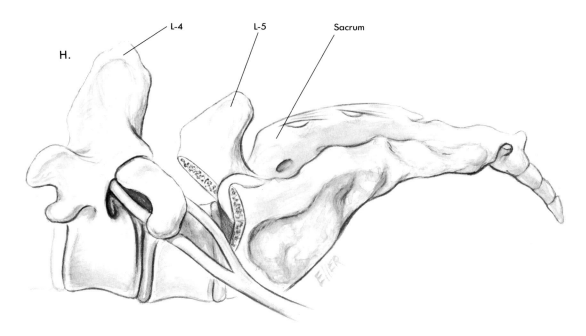

Decompression of nerve root

Plate 237. (Continued)

I. and J. The procedure continues with the following steps:

1. The articular facets of L-5, S-1 (and L-4, L-5 if fusion is extended to L-4) are completely excised with osteotomes.

2. With a curet, all remaining articular cartilage is thoroughly removed from each facet joint.

3. A flap of bone is then raised from the transverse process and turned into the joint.

4. From the ala of the sacrum, multiple flaps of bone, based anteriorly, are also raised and turned forward and cephalad to form a bridge to the transverse process of the fifth lumbar vertebra (when fusion is extended only to L-5).

5. Flaps of bone are excised from the dorsal surface of each lamina and turned down laterally.

K. Abundant iliac bone grafts are harvested from one or both iliac crests through the ipsilateral wounds. Usually, adequate bone graft may be obtained from one iliac crest.

The ipsilateral iliac crest is exposed through an incision in the fascia over the posterior and superior iliac crest. Do not extend the incision laterally more than one hand's width to avoid injury to the cluneal nerves and the hypogastric and ilioinguinal nerves. Obtain bone graft from the outer wall of the ilium, leaving the inner cortex intact.

Cancellous bone strips are laid across the fusion area, followed by cancellous and cortical bone.

The wound is closed in the usual fashion with suction drainage tubes.

Postoperative Care. Postoperative care depends on the degree of listhesis. When in situ fusion is performed for first- and second-degree slip without decompression, spine support in the form of a thoracolumbosacral orthosis (TLSO) is usually adequate. For slips greater than 50 per cent, it is best to immobilize the spine in a pantaloon (including the hips and thighs) body cast for two or three months, then provide support in a TLSO for an additional three months.

REFERENCES

Watkins, M. B.: Posterolateral fusion in pseudarthrosis and posterior element defects of the lumbosacral spine. Clin. Orthop., 35:80, 1964.
Wiltse, L. L., Bateman, J. G., Hutchinson, R. H., and Nelson, W. E.: The paraspinal sacrospinalis–splitting approach to the lumbar spine. J. Bone Joint Surg., 50-A:919, 1968.

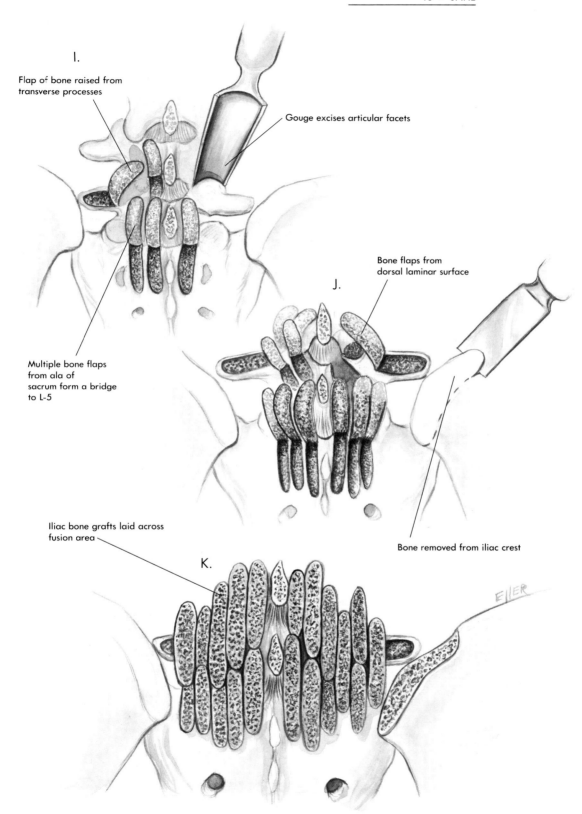

I.

Flap of bone raised from transverse processes

Gouge excises articular facets

Multiple bone flaps from ala of sacrum form a bridge to L-5

J.

Bone flaps from dorsal laminar surface

Bone removed from iliac crest

Iliac bone grafts laid across fusion area

K.

Plate 237. (Continued)

PLATE 238 Posterior Spinal Fusion for Scoliosis

Indication. Idiopathic structural scoliosis, progressive and greater than 35 to 40 degrees, with decompensation of the spine.

Blood for Transfusion. The availability of blood should be double-checked before the operation is started. To replace blood adequately throughout the procedure, the use of two large-gauge intravenous needles is mandatory. A red blood cell saver may be used.

Radiographic Control. Yes.

Patient Position. Surgery is performed under general endotracheal anesthesia. The operating surgeon should supervise the proper positioning of the patient. This is important to minimize blood loss and to adequately expose the surgical field. The patient is turned in the prone position and placed on a four-poster or Relton-Hall frame. The abdomen should remain completely free—minimizing abdominal pressure decreases venous bleeding. There should be no pressure on the axillae. The upper pads should rest on the upper chest–manubrium, clavicles, and acromion. Shoulder abduction should be less than 90 degrees; elbows are flexed and placed over soft pads. Proper positioning of the upper limbs is vital; there should be no stretch on the brachial plexus or pressure on the ulnar nerves.

The entire back is prepared and draped. The spinous process of the seventh cervical vertebra and the ilium on both sides should be in the sterile field. The use of a large self-adhering povidone-iodine (Betadine) drape is of great value in ensuring asepsis.

Operative Technique

A. The incision is made from above downward, initially through the dermis only from a level one vertebra superior to the proposed fusion area to a level one vertebra inferior to it.

B. To minimize bleeding, the intradermal and subcutaneous tissues are infiltrated with an epinephrine solution (1:500,000). The direction of the skin incision is planned so that when the curve is maximally corrected by spinal instrumentation, the operative scar will be straight. This technique improves the appearance of the back and draws less attention to any residual curve.

C. The superficial and deep fasciae are divided in a straight line over the spinous processes to be fused. Three or four Wheatlander retractors are placed to spread the wound under tension.

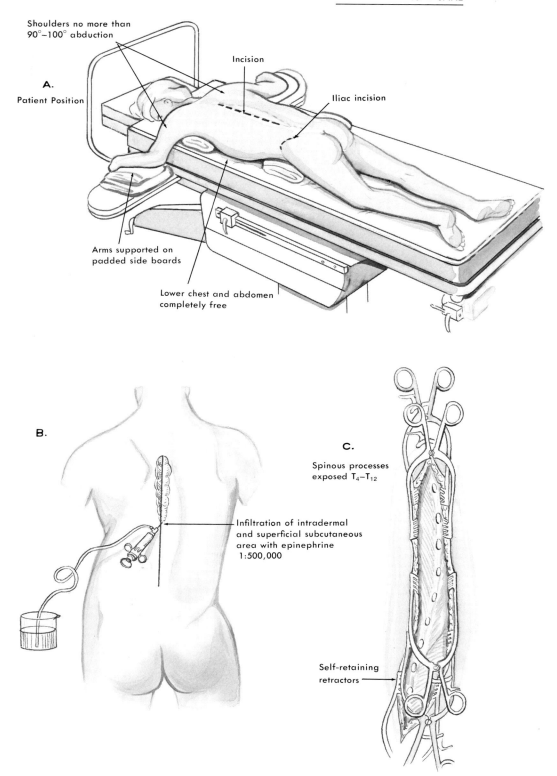

A. Patient Position

Shoulders no more than 90°–100° abduction

Incision

Iliac incision

Arms supported on padded side boards

Lower chest and abdomen completely free

B.

Infiltration of intradermal and superficial subcutaneous area with epinephrine 1:500,000

C.

Spinous processes exposed T₄–T₁₂

Self-retaining retractors

Plate 238. A.–Q., Posterior spinal fusion for scoliosis.

D. The median raphe is incised, exposing the tips of the spinous processes. Starting at the proximal end, the assistant presses down over the spinous process with a Kelly clamp, and the surgeon, with a scalpel or a Bovie knife, splits the cartilaginous tip of the spinous process longitudinally in the midline down to bone. Dissection in this avascular plane minimizes blood loss.

E. Next, with Cobb periosteal elevators, the spine is subperiosteally exposed as far laterally as the transverse process in the thoracic area and beyond the articular facets in the lumbar area. In the thoracic area, begin dissection distally and proceed proximally—the inferosuperior dissection facilitates the subperiosteal elevation of the oblique attachments of short rotator muscles and ligaments from the lamina. Subperiosteal stripping of muscle and soft tissues from the spinous process, lamina, and transverse process should be meticulous. Avoid excessive force and muscle tearing. Use sharp dissection with a scalpel to detach tendons and ligaments, particularly the superior margin of the lamina.

F. As the subperiosteal dissection is carried out, each level is packed firmly with gauze to minimize bleeding.

Dissect laterally with caution! A branch of segmented vessel lies immediately lateral to the facet joint—do not injure it! Be gentle—do not tear muscles laterally!

G. When this dissection is completed, the packing is removed and Wheatlander retractors or laminectomy spreader retractors, or both, are placed deeply to spread the soft tissues out of the field. Next, with the scalpel, rongeurs, and curets, the interspinous ligaments and all remaining soft tissue tags are removed from the spinous processes, laminae, facet joints, and transverse processes. The soft-tissue clean-up should be thorough. Any bleeding, which may be vigorous in the intertransverse process spaces, is controlled with electrocautery. At this stage, radiopaque markers are placed in the spinous processes of the superior and inferior vertebrae and radiograms are made to double-check and confirm the correct level of fusion.

D.

Incision of periosteum over spinous processes to bony tip

Interspinous ligament

E.

Cobb periosteal elevator reflecting cartilaginous caps to expose spinous processes on both sides

T₁₂

NOTE: Subperiosteal stripping to facet joints begins at T_{12} and proceeds to T_4

F.

Hemostasis facilitated by subperiosteal sponge packing

G.

T₄

Transverse processes exposed

CAUTION:

DO NOT DAMAGE COSTOTRANSVERSE ARTICULATION

DO NOT TEAR LIGAMENTS AND MUSCLES ALONG INFERIOR MARGINS OF LAMINAE. USE SCALPEL

Metal markers on spinous process of T_{12}

NOTE: X-ray is taken at this step to confirm correct level of exposure

Plate 238. (Continued)

H–L. *Facet joint fusion* is performed by thoroughly excising the cartilaginous material from the articular facet and firmly packing cancellous bone within the remaining space. Facet joint excision and grafting should be performed regardless of the type of spinal instrumentation. A variety of techniques of facet joint fusion have been described.

In the *Hibbs technique,* in the thoracic area first, intra-articular fusion in the dorsal area is performed as follows. First, the posterior half of the facet joint is removed with a Hibbs or Cobb gouge. Then, with a curet, all of its articular cartilage is removed. Next, flaps of bone from the base of the transverse process are elevated and turned into the joint. The Hibbs technique is advocated by Risser and is simple and relatively quick.

In the *Moe technique* of facet joint fusion, two hinged fragments of bone are elevated from adjacent transverse processes and tilted laterally to the intertransverse area. The facet joint is excised, removing all articular cartilage, and a block of corticocancellous bone is packed in the remaining defect.

First, a cut is made at the base of the lamina of the superior articular process, carried along the transverse processes to its tip. Then the split lamina is elevated, leaving it attached to the tip of the transverse process, and then bent to lie between the transverse process.

Second, the facet joint surface is resected with a separate cut and discarded.

Third, the articular cartilage is thoroughly curetted.

Fourth, a hinged fragment of bone is elevated from the midportion of the inferior transverse process.

Fifth, a corticocancellous bone graft is impacted in the defect of the previously resected facet joint. Moe's technique is time-consuming but achieves excellent facet joint fusion.

H. In the *Hall technique,* the inferior facet joint is sharply cut with a semicircular gouge, removing the bone fragment with underlying articular cartilage in one piece.

I. This exposes the superior facet cartilage, which is removed with a sharp curet.

J.–L. The outer cortex of the superior facet is resected, creating a trough into which cancellous bone from the outer wall of the ilium is layered and impacted.

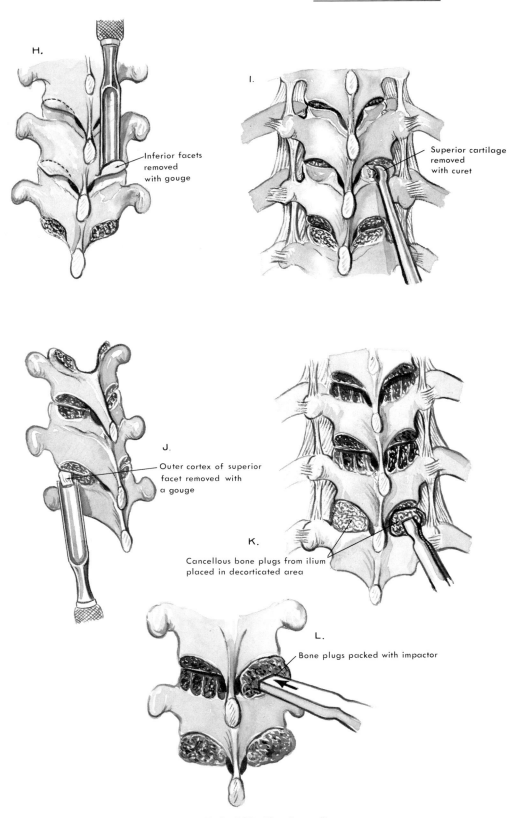

H.
Inferior facets
removed
with gouge

I.
Superior cartilage
removed
with curet

J.
Outer cortex of superior
facet removed with
a gouge

K.
Cancellous bone plugs from ilium
placed in decorticated area

L.
Bone plugs packed with impactor

Plate 238. (Continued)

M. and N. In the lumbar area the articular facet joints are directed sagittally; they are best excised with small, thin osteotomes. A spreader bar is applied between the spinous processes. The articular cartilage is curetted out, and into each joint a block of bone (obtained from the spinous processes or the ilium) is inserted and countersunk. The posterior elements of the spine should be thoroughly cleaned of all soft tissue.

O. The spinous processes are resected with a bone cutter and saved for bone grafting. The spinous processes at the superior and inferior ends are left intact to facilitate secure internal fixation with either the Harrington rod or the L-rod.

P. Next, with a sharp Hibbs or Cobb gouge, multiple flaps of bone, half of its thickness and half of its width, are elevated from the base of the spinous processes and laminae. The assistant, with a suction tube, keeps the edge of the bone gouge free of blood and clearly visible to the surgeon. It is easy to keep the flaps attached at their base by rotating the edge of the sharp gouge. The free end of the flap from the lamina below is turned up and locked under the laterally bent flap of the lamina above. The superior halves of the spinous process of the most cephalic vertebra of the fusion area and the most inferior one are left intact. The facet joints at the extremes of the fusion area (i.e., between the superior vertebra and the one above, and the inferior vertebra and the one below) are not disturbed. Then, the remaining portion of each spinous process is partially divided with a Hibbs bone cutter, broken down, and turned up to bring it in contact with the next spinous process above. Thus, when decortication is completed, there is contact of abundant cancellous bone at the laminae and spinous processes and at the facet joints.

The wound is copiously irrigated with antibiotic solution and is firmly packed with lap pads.

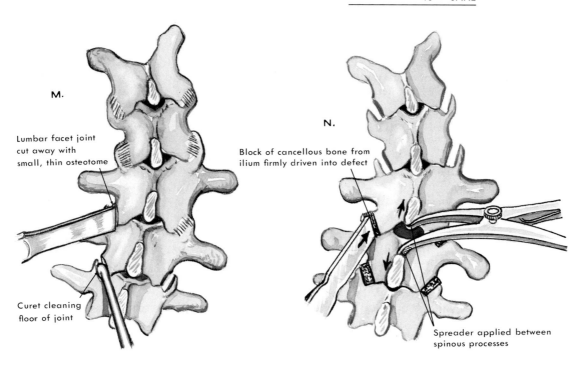

M.

Lumbar facet joint
cut away with
small, thin osteotome

Curet cleaning
floor of joint

N.

Block of cancellous bone from
ilium firmly driven into defect

Spreader applied between
spinous processes

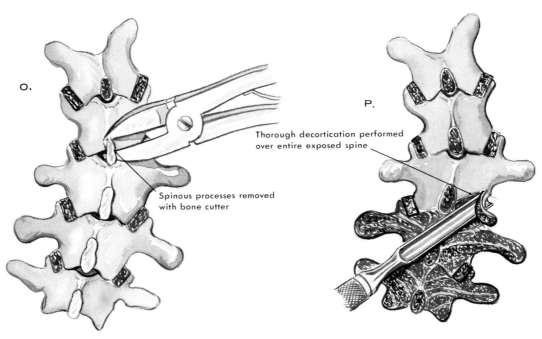

O.

Spinous processes removed
with bone cutter

P.

Thorough decortication performed
over entire exposed spine

Plate 238. (Continued)

Q. *Bone grafting* is done after decortication to ensure surface-cell biologic viability. The bone graft is usually autogenous and is taken from the outer table of the ilium. A separate vertical incision over the iliac crest is made; it is preferred over a curved incision made just distal to the posterior half of the iliac crest, because the operative scar is more pleasing. By sharp and dull dissection, more than half of the posterolateral wall of the ilium is exposed. The most abundant and best quality cancellous bone is adjacent to the upper part of the sciatic notch. By gentle dissection, identify the sciatic notch; avoid injury to the superior gluteal vessels and nerve. With the help of gouges and osteotomes, harvest cancellous cortical strips of bone graft in the usual fashion. Use bone wax for hemostasis. The cancellous and cortical bone grafts are placed over the facet joints and the laminae.

Occasionally, bone graft is taken from the tibia. The graft is divided into two unequal pieces. The longer piece should reach the end vertebra of the fusion area. It is sutured to the base of the intact half of the spinous process of the inferior vertebra and placed snugly on the convex side of the curve. There should be adequate overlap of the two fragments. Fragments of autogenous bone from the tibia are laid down over the facet joint in the intertransverse process spaces and overlap the laminae.

The retractors are removed, and the muscles are allowed to fall into place. The periosteum, with the deep layers of the muscle, is closed with interrupted sutures. The remaining wound is closed in layers in the usual manner. The skin is closed with subcutaneous 00 nylon suture.

Postoperative Care. This depends on the type of internal fixation (see Plates 239 to 242 and Plate 244).

REFERENCES

Hibbs, R. A.: An operation for progressive spinal deformities. A preliminary report of three cases from the service of the Orthopaedic Hospital. N.Y. State J. Med., 93:1013, 1911.

Hibbs, R. A.: A report of fifty-nine cases of scoliosis treated by the fusion operation. J. Bone Joint Surg., 6:3, 1924.

King, H. A., Moe, J. H., Bradford, D. S., and Winter, R. B.: The selection of fusion levels in thoracic idiopathic scoliosis. J. Bone Joint Surg., 65-A:1302, 1983.

Moe, J. H.: A critical analysis of methods of fusion for scoliosis: An evaluation of 276 patients. J. Bone Joint Surg., 40-A:529, 1958.

Winter, R. B.: Posterior spinal fusion in scoliosis: Indications, techniques, and results. Orthop. Clin. North Am., 10:787, 1979.

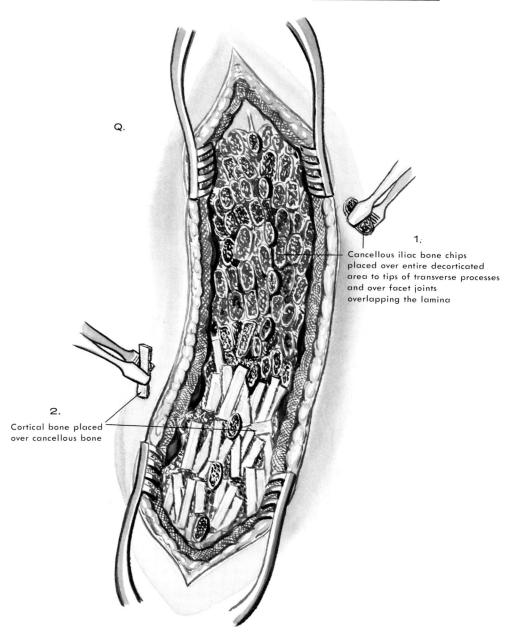

Q.

1.
Cancellous iliac bone chips
placed over entire decorticated
area to tips of transverse processes
and over facet joints
overlapping the lamina

2.
Cortical bone placed
over cancellous bone

Plate 238. (Continued)

PLATE 239   ## Posterior Spinal Instrumentation by the Harrington System

Indication. The Harrington system is rarely used.

Radiographic Control. Yes.

Patient Position. Prone (see Plate 238).

Operative Technique. The posterior spine is exposed as described in Plate 238 for spinal fusion. There should be meticulous subperiosteal exposure out to the tip of the transverse processes. The first stage of Harrington instrumentation is the *placement of the hooks*. To provide a normally aligned spine, it is vital to select the correct level for the purchase site for the superior and inferior distraction hooks: The *superior distraction hook* should be anchored at or one vertebra above the superior end vertebra, whereas the *inferior distraction hook* should be at one or two vertebrae below the inferior end vertebra *within the stable zone*. The inferior distraction hook rarely, if ever, is placed distal to L-4.

A. and **B.** The *superior distraction hook* is seated in a facet joint. The purchase site is prepared as follows: First, all ligamentous and capsular tissue is removed from the lamina. The direction of the facet joint is determined by tapping a narrow periosteal elevator in the facet joint. Next, with a ¼-inch osteotome or a Capener gouge, the inferior facet joint is squared off. The direction of the osteotomy is oblique, with the medial border directed more superiorly than is the lateral margin.

C. A No. 1251 sharp hook is inserted into the facet interspace with the hook tilted anteriorly at a driving angle of 45 degrees; this forward tilting of the hook is important in order to prevent fracturing of the lamina. Once the hook has engaged the pedicle, it is impacted with a mallet.

D. The No. 1251 sharp hook is removed and replaced with a dull No. 1262 flanged hook or a dull No. 1253 unflanged hook. This author prefers a flanged hook because it firmly grips the bone and does not fracture the lamina. It is best to place the medial one third of the hook medial to the facet joint to prevent lateral hook displacement or dislodgment. The hook should be firmly impacted into the pedicle.

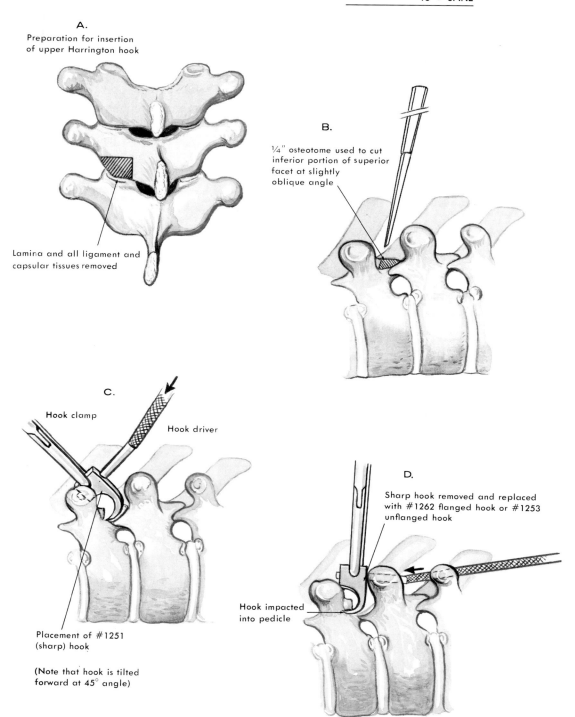

A.
Preparation for insertion
of upper Harrington hook

Lamina and all ligament and
capsular tissues removed

B.
¼″ osteotome used to cut
inferior portion of superior
facet at slightly
oblique angle

C.
Hook clamp

Hook driver

Placement of #1251
(sharp) hook

(Note that hook is tilted
forward at 45° angle)

D.
Sharp hook removed and replaced
with #1262 flanged hook or #1253
unflanged hook

Hook impacted
into pedicle

Plate 239. A.–T., Posterior spinal instrumentation by the Harrington system.

E. The *inferior distraction hook* is seated underneath the superior border of the selected vertebra. First, remove a portion of the lamina and adjacent inferior facet with a Kerrison rongeur, producing a flat margin that extends to the pars interarticularis. To facilitate hook insertion, distract the spinous processes of the adjacent vertebra with a Blount or lamina spreader.

F. Insert a No. 1254 hook under the lamina. The shoe of the hook is in the epidural space.

G. Prior to placing the Harrington outrigger or rod, pack cancellous bone at the lower hook site.

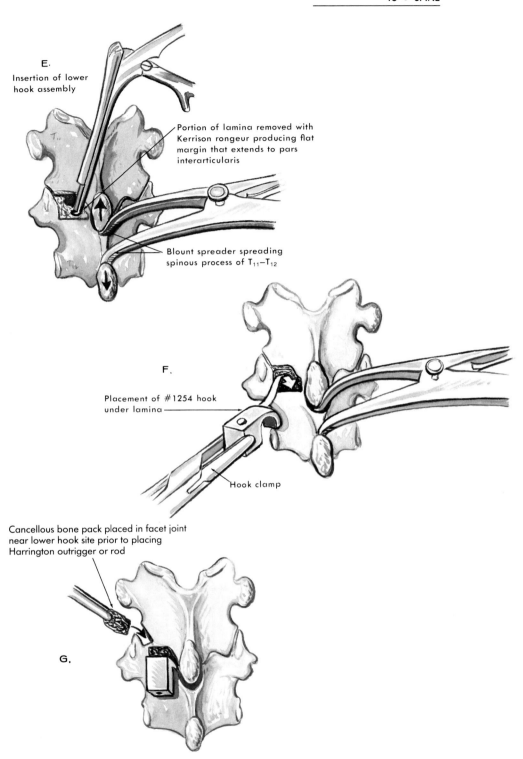

E.
Insertion of lower
hook assembly

Portion of lamina removed with
Kerrison rongeur producing flat
margin that extends to pars
interarticularis

Blount spreader spreading
spinous process of $T_{11}-T_{12}$

F.

Placement of #1254 hook
under lamina

Hook clamp

Cancellous bone pack placed in facet joint
near lower hook site prior to placing
Harrington outrigger or rod

G.

Plate 239. (Continued)

H. and **I.** The Harrington outrigger is then inserted between the superior and the inferior distraction hooks. Passive force is applied to the apex of the convexity of the curve, and the screw device on the outrigger is tightened, distracting and correcting the curve. The use of the Harrington outrigger is optional. It is recommended by this author because it facilitates exposure and correction; with the spine in the corrected position, it is easier to perform decortication and spinal fusion, and assists in choosing a rod of proper length.

J. Next, decortication of the posterior elements of the spine and facet fusion is carried out (see Plate 238). The posterior elements on which the hooks are seated should be left intact.

K. The outrigger is removed, and the distraction rod is placed between the superior and the inferior hooks. Then, using the Harrington spreader, gradual distraction is carried out, stopping short of rod bending or bone disruption. The degree of maximum distraction that can be performed safely depends on the experience of the surgeon. It is best to perform a Stagnara wake-up test and determine neurologic status by asking the patient to actively move the foot, ankle, and knee. If spinal cord and nerve function is intact, anesthesia is deepened and surgery continued. It is best to insert a C-ring or thread an 18-gauge wire around the superior ratchet of the rod immediately inferior to the hook in order to checkrein telescoping of the rod within the hook.

In the lumbar spine, contoured square-end rods should be used to preserve lumbar lordosis. In double major curves, a single distraction rod provides better balance to the spine than do two overlapping distraction rods.

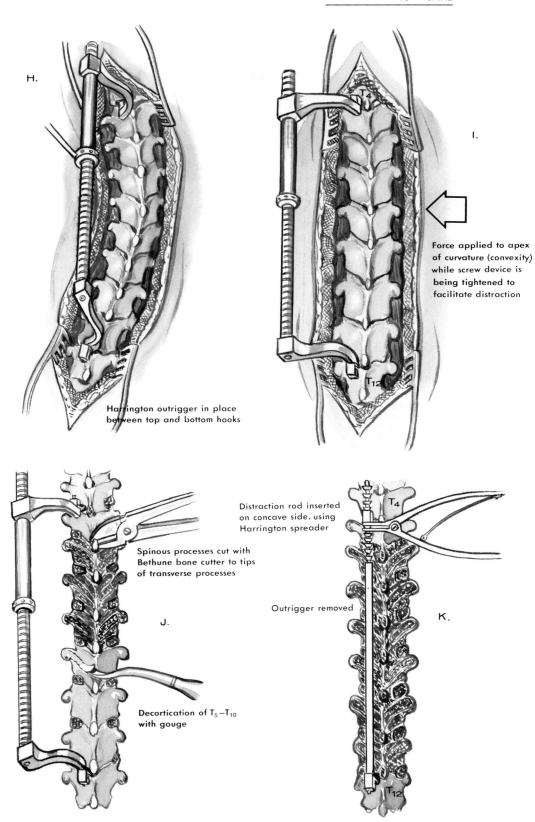

H.

Harrington outrigger in place between top and bottom hooks

I.

T4

Force applied to apex of curvature (convexity) while screw device is being tightened to facilitate distraction

T12

J.

Spinous processes cut with Bethune bone cutter to tips of transverse processes

Decortication of T5–T10 with gouge

K.

T4

Distraction rod inserted on concave side, using Harrington spreader

Outrigger removed

T12

Plate 239. (Continued)

Application of the Harrington Compression Instrumentation on the Convex Side of the Curve

This procedure is used when kyphosis is associated with scoliosis in the thoracic region. Some surgeons prefer to use compression in conjunction with distraction, because it provides more stable fixation and increases the degree of correction (an average of 10 degrees). The use of the compression assembly is contraindicated when the thoracic spine is hypokyphotic.

The compression assembly comes in two sizes: $\frac{1}{8}$ inch and $\frac{5}{11}$ inch. Ordinarily, the smaller size with the No. 1259 hook is used because it is flexible, contouring easily to the dorsal roundback. In the proposed fused area, the lamina and facet joint should be thoroughly cleared of all soft tissue.

L.–N. The upper hooks (usually three in number) are inserted under the selected transverse processes at the junction of the transverse process and the lamina. The shoe of the hook has a sharp edge that sections the costotransverse ligament. It is important that the edge of the hook not cut into the transverse process. Insert the hooks in a horizontal direction. Do not tilt the hook to slide under the transverse process. The upper three hooks are placed temporarily.

O.–Q. The lower hooks (usually three in number) are inserted underneath the lamina as close to the facet joint as possible. This is because the transverse processes of T-11 and those of more inferior vertebrae are not suitable for hook purchase. The laminae of the selected distal vertebrae are prepared for hook placement. With an osteotome or Kerrison rongeur, an adequate amount of bone is resected from the laminae and inferior facet. Next, the two adjacent spinous processes are spread apart with a Blount or laminectomy spreader, and the hook is inserted underneath the lamina in a horizontal fashion.

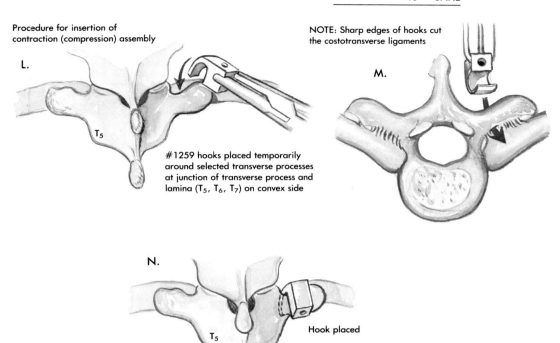

Procedure for insertion of contraction (compression) assembly

L.

T₅

#1259 hooks placed temporarily around selected transverse processes at junction of transverse process and lamina (T₅, T₆, T₇) on convex side

NOTE: Sharp edges of hooks cut the costotransverse ligaments

M.

N.

T₅

Hook placed

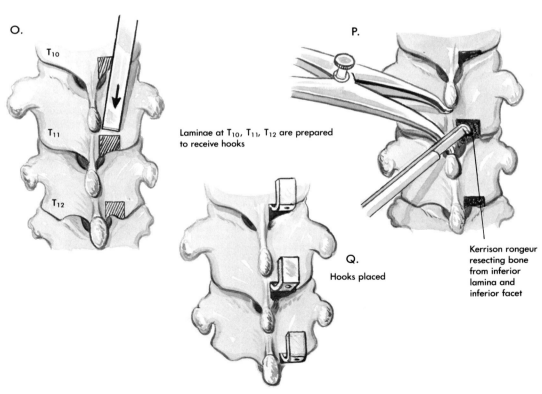

O.

T₁₀

T₁₁

T₁₂

Laminae at T₁₀, T₁₁, T₁₂ are prepared to receive hooks

P.

Kerrison rongeur resecting bone from inferior lamina and inferior facet

Q.

Hooks placed

Plate 239. (Continued)

R. and **S.** Three hooks are placed under the transverse processes of the upper thoracic vertebrae and three hooks under the laminae of the lower thoracic or the upper lumbar vertebrae, or both. Next, a threaded rod with the hooks attached to it is inserted. Cranially directed hooks are inserted first, followed by the caudally directed hooks. Once the hooks are firmly secured in place, the compression assembly is tightened, using wire holders and a Harrington spreader and spinning the nut around the hook using a Penfield dissector. Finally, the nut is tightened with a wrench.

T. Next, the lower three hooks are tightened. After maximal contraction is achieved, the central threads adjacent to the nuts are stripped (damaged) with a clamp as close to the nut as possible to prevent unwinding and loosening.

In kyphosis without scoliosis, two compression rods are used, one on each side.

Postoperative Care. The spine is supported in a plastic TLSO for three months followed by wearing the brace during the day for an additional three months.

REFERENCES

Dickson, J. H.: Twenty year follow-up on patients with idiopathic scoliosis having Harrington instrumentation and fusion. Presented at 19th Annual Meeting, Scoliosis Research Society, Orlando, 1984.

Dickson, J. H., and Harrington, P. R.: The evolution of the Harrington instrumentation technique in scoliosis. J. Bone Joint Surg., 55-A:993, 1973.

Goldstein, L. A.: Treatment of idiopathic scoliosis by Harrington instrumentation and fusion with fresh autogenous iliac bone grafts. J. Bone Joint Surg., 51-A:209, 1969.

Harrington, P. R.: Surgical instrumentation for management of scoliosis. J. Bone Joint Surg., 42-A:1448, 1960.

Harrington, P. R.: Treatment of scoliosis: Correction and internal fixation by spine instrumentation. J. Bone Joint Surg., 44-A:591, 1962.

Harrington, P. R.: The management of scoliosis by spine instrumentation: An evaluation of more than 200 cases. South. Med. J., 56:1367, 1963.

Harrington, P. R.: Technical details in relation to the successful use of instrumentation in scoliosis. Orthop. Clin. North Am., 3:49, 1972.

Moe, J. H.: A critical analysis of methods of fusion for scoliosis: An evaluation of 276 patients. J. Bone Joint Surg., 40-A:529, 1958.

Nachemson, A., and Elfstrom, G.: A force-indicating distractor for Harrington-rod procedure. J. Bone Joint Surg., 51-A:1660, 1969.

Tamborino, J. M., Armbrust, E. N., and Moe, J.: Harrington instrumentation in correction of scoliosis: A comparison with cast correction. J. Bone Joint Surg., 46-A:313, 1964.

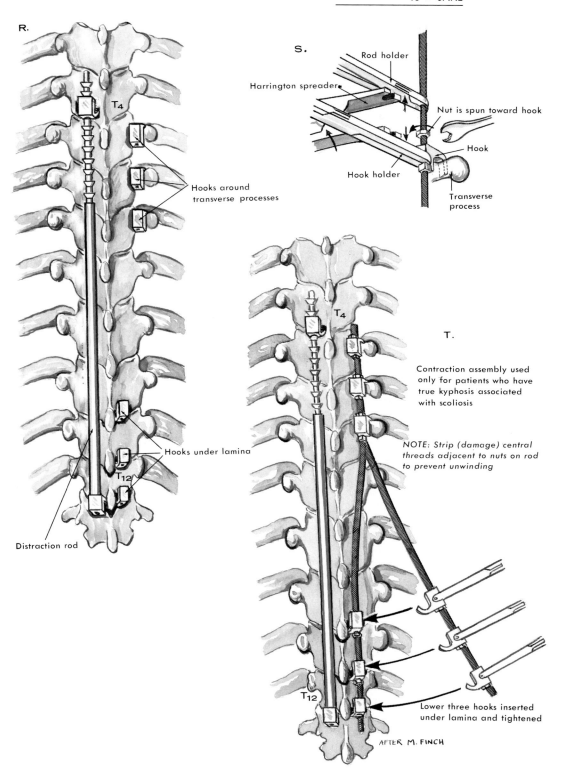

R.

T₄

Hooks around
transverse processes

Hooks under lamina

T₁₂

Distraction rod

S.

Rod holder

Harrington spreader

Nut is spun toward hook

Hook

Hook holder

Transverse
process

T.

Contraction assembly used
only for patients who have
true kyphosis associated
with scoliosis

*NOTE: Strip (damage) central
threads adjacent to nuts on rod
to prevent unwinding*

T₄

T₁₂

Lower three hooks inserted
under lamina and tightened

AFTER M. FINCH

Plate 239. (Continued)

PLATE 240 — Bilateral L-Rod Sublaminar Symmetrical Instrumentation (Luque Procedure)

Indications. Paralytic scoliosis of 35 degrees or greater. This system of internal fixation is preferred by some surgeons because it is much less expensive than the newer instrumentation systems.

Procedure. Two stainless steel rods are contoured with the spine in the maximally corrected position and transfixed to the laminae of both sides of the vertebrae by sublaminar 16- or 18-gauge stainless steel wires. Nickel-chrome (MP-35-N) alloy rods and wires are also available. The rods and wires should be compatible, that is, stainless steel with stainless steel and alloy with alloy. The rods are either $\frac{3}{16}$ inch (4.8 mm.) or $\frac{1}{4}$ inch (6.4 mm.). The wires press through the spinal canal; therefore, the risk of spinal cord or nerve injury is high. The procedure is always combined with facetectomy, decortication, and bone grafting. Proximally, the fusion area and stabilization should extend high—avoid the common pitfall of fusing too short. Inferiorly, the L-rod often has to be fixed to the pelvis by the Galveston technique, because the sacrum is often the distal part of neuromuscular scoliosis.

Radiographic Control. Yes.

Patient Position. Prone on a Hall frame (see Plate 238).

Operative Technique

A1.–A3. Surgical exposure of the thoracolumbar spine is similar to that described in Plate 238 (posterior spinal fusion). After exposure of the spinous processes and laminae, the spine is straightened as much as possible by external manual pressure applied by an assistant, and the rods are bent to closely fit the laminae. The rods are contoured in both the coronal and sagittal planes. An "L" is bent at one end of each rod.

A₁.

A₂.

Contouring
of L-rods

Incision

ANTEROPOSTERIOR VIEW

A₃.

L-rod

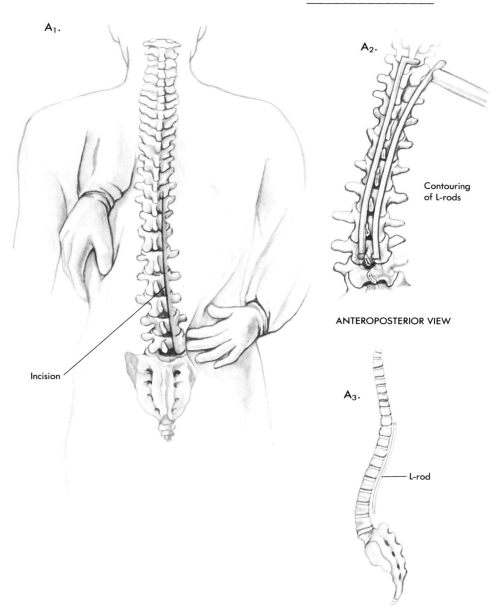

Plate 240. A.–R., Bilateral L-rod sublaminar symmetrical instrumentation (Luque procedure).

B. and **C.** The ligamentum flavum of each vertebra is then exposed. In the thoracic region, the spinous processes slant caudally and overlap the distal spinous process. With a rongeur or bone biter, each spinous process is excised to expose the intervening ligamentum flavum. In the lumbar spine, ordinarily there is adequate space between the lumbar vertebrae; therefore, excision of spinous processes is not usually required.

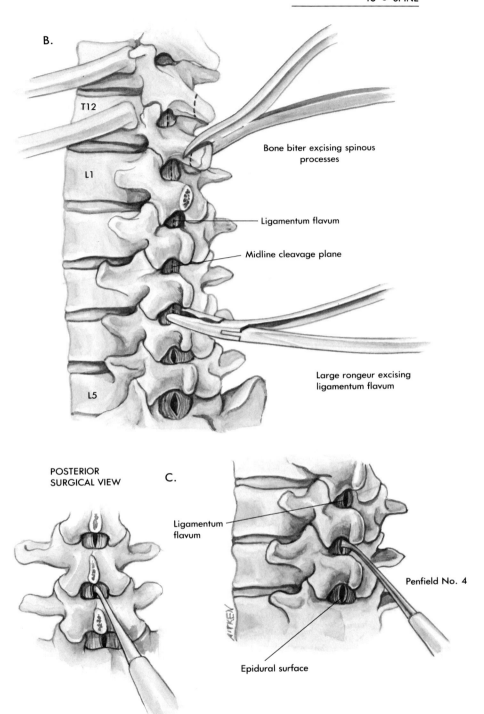

B.

T12

L1

Bone biter excising spinous
processes

Ligamentum flavum

Midline cleavage plane

Large rongeur excising
ligamentum flavum

L5

POSTERIOR
SURGICAL VIEW

C.

Ligamentum
flavum

Penfield No. 4

Epidural surface

Plate 240. (Continued)

D1., **D2.**, and **E.** The ligamentum flavum is thinned by removing small bites until the midline cleavage plane is visualized. With a small dissector (Penfield No. 4), the deep surface of the ligamentum flavum is freed and separated; next, the remainder of the ligamentum flavum is removed with a Kerrison rongeur. Because it is easier to pass the wires on the convex side of the curve, enlarge the opening in the ligamentum flavum more on that side. Make the opening just large enough for the wire to pass through.

Caution! Do not damage the epidural vessels or dura! All the facets in the fusion area are excised as described in Plate 238.

F. Bend a double 16- or 18-gauge wire with the major diameter of the bend slightly larger than the width of the lamina. Do not create a curve with a large radius—the wire will impinge on the spinal cord.

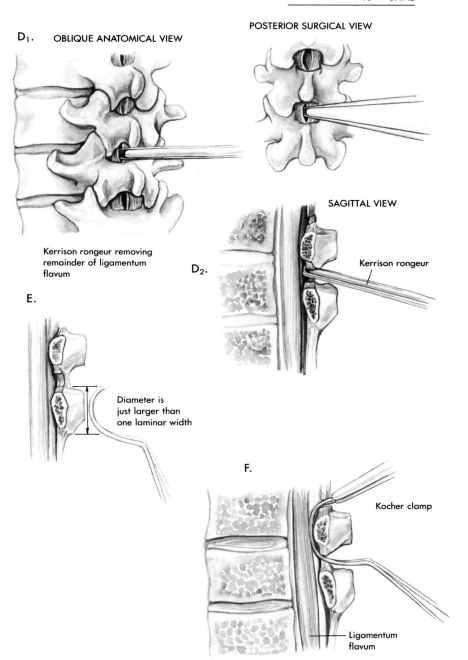

D₁. OBLIQUE ANATOMICAL VIEW

POSTERIOR SURGICAL VIEW

Kerrison rongeur removing
remainder of ligamentum
flavum

SAGITTAL VIEW

D₂.

Kerrison rongeur

E.

Diameter is
just larger than
one laminar width

F.

Kocher clamp

Ligamentum
flavum

Plate 240. (Continued)

G. The wires are passed from below upward (caudad to cephalad direction). Do not use force. Maintain the wires snugly against the undersurface of the lamina. When the tip of the wire is seen on the upper margin of the lamina, grasp it with a needle holder or Kocher clamp and pull it upward until half the length of the wire is pulled through.

H. Cut the tip of the double wire, and position each wire on the right and left sides of the lamina. At the ends of the fixation area, where stress is greatest, pass another double wire because it is best to have double wires on each side of the top and bottom ends of the rods.

Each wire is crimped to prevent accidental protrusion into the spinal canal and consequent spinal cord injury.

An alternate method is to bend each end of the wire over the lamina and then lay it over the margin of the wound.

I. In paralytic scoliosis, first wire the concave rod and then wire the convex rod.

1. With the rod bender, make the final adjustments and ensure that the appropriate degree of lordosis and kyphosis is bent into the rod.

2. Make a hole through the base of the most distal lumbar spinous process to be instrumented.

3. Insert the L-rod on the concave side of the curve, and pass its short limb transversely across the lamina and through the hole at the base of the spinous process of the most caudal vertebra.

4. Tighten the double wire on the concave side of the most distal vertebra, thereby firmly fixing it inferiorly.

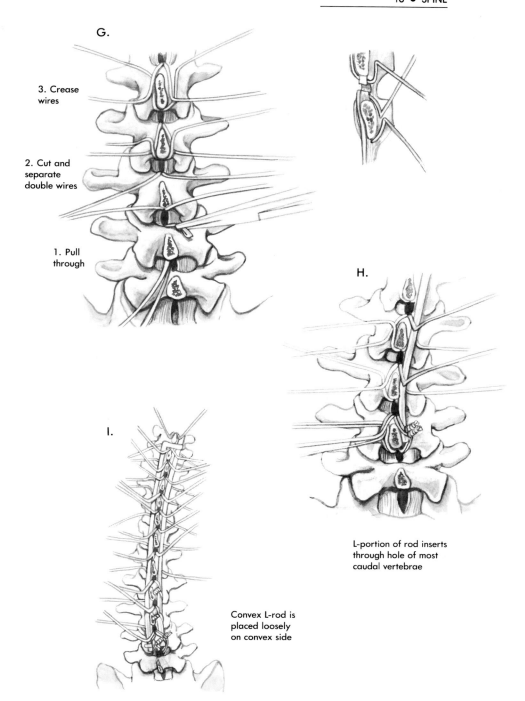

G.

3. Crease wires

2. Cut and separate double wires

1. Pull through

H.

L-portion of rod inserts through hole of most caudal vertebrae

I.

Convex L-rod is placed loosely on convex side

Plate 240. (Continued)

J. Loosely place the second L-rod on the convex side of the curve with its short limb inserted across the lamina of the most cephalad vertebra to be instrumented and under the long limb of the concave rod. Placing the L-rod on the convex side of the curve before tightening the wires on the concave rod makes it simple to insert the short limb of the convex rod under the long limb of the concave rod.

K. The L-rod on the *concave side* is stabilized with a rod holder or pusher, and the spine is straightened by an assistant applying external manual pressure on the trunk.

Caution! Do not use the wires to pull the spine to the rod! With a wire twister, tighten the wires sequentially—on the concave side, begin at each end of the curve and proceed toward its apex. Breakage of the wire is a potentially troublesome problem. Begin tightening the wires with twists at a 45-degree angle to the axis of the wire; as the wires are tightened, the direction of the twists changes to 90 degrees. At this point, stop twisting—the wires are taut enough! As the wires are being tightened, rotation of the L-segment is a problem—prevent it by stabilizing the L-segment with a rod holder.

L. After complete wiring of the concave side, the rod on the convex side is wired—on the convex side. First, tighten the wires on the apex and then proceed sequentially toward the end. Then the Texas Scottish Rite cross-links are inserted to prevent the rods from slipping through the wires.

The convex rod technique is used primarily in the correction and sequential instrumentation of thoracic curves. It is not illustrated because there are much more effective and less risky means of instrumentation of thoracic curves. The rod is placed on the convex side of the curve with its short limb inserted transversely across the lamina "inferior" to the most cephalad vertebra of the curve.

First, the second and third wires on the convex side are tightened. Then the curved spine is straightened maximally toward the rod by an assistant applying external manual pressure; the rod is stabilized by a rod holder; and half of the wires on the convex side are tightened sequentially, proceeding superoinferiorly. Next, the concave rod is applied by insertion of its short L-limb transversely through a hole made in the spinous process of the most distal vertebra. The distal end of the concave rod is secured to the most distal lamina by tightening of the wires. The long segment of the concave L-rod overlies (i.e., it is superficial to) the short leg of the convex rod. Finally, the wires are tightened sequentially—on the convex side proceeding proximally to distally and on the concave side distally to proximally to distally. The wire ends are cut and turned down toward the midline.

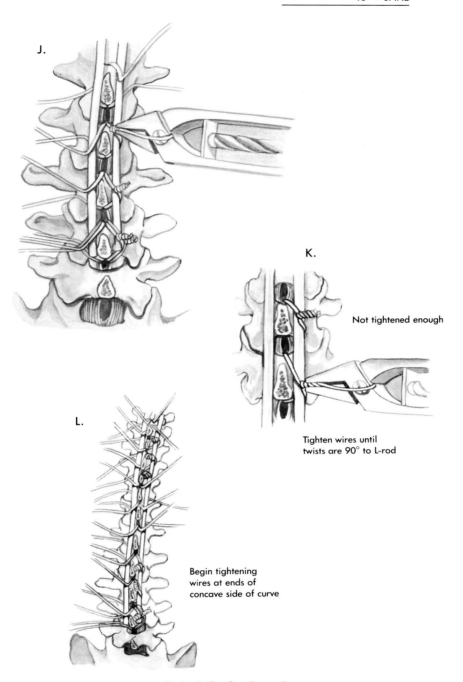

J.

K.

Not tightened enough

Tighten wires until
twists are 90° to L-rod

L.

Begin tightening
wires at ends of
concave side of curve

Plate 240. (Continued)

M. Facet fusion is already performed before the wires are passed underneath the lamina. The rods cover most of the external surface of the lamina, leaving little space exposed. The cortical surface of the laminae and transverse processes is decorticated *gently* as much as possible. Abundant corticocancellous bone is harvested from the posterior ilium, and the bone grafts are laid bilaterally lateral to the rods. Bone bank bone is used if additional bone grafting is required. Bone grafting should be voluminous, and it should extend laterally to the tip of the transverse processes.

Before closure of the wound, a wake-up test is performed to ensure integrity of the spinal cord and spinal nerves.

N. In neuromuscular scoliosis, the curve extends distally to include the sacrum, and pelvic fixation is required in instrumentation of the spine. Fixation is carried out by the Galveston technique (developed by Allen and Ferguson) in which the short limb of the L-rod is passed through the posterior iliac spine.

Both iliac crests are exposed subperiosteally. Beginning at the level of the posterior superior iliac spine, with the use of a power drill, insert a guide pin along the transverse bar of the ilium that is the same diameter as the Luque rod to be used. The depth of the pin into the ilium should be 6 to 9 cm.

O. and **P.** Next, contour the Luque rod in three separate planes. First, bend it to a right angle, with the short limb 12 cm. long, by the use of two sleeve benders. Second, contour the rod to fit the curve of the ilium (i.e., the angle of the ilium to the midsagittal plane of the spine). The angulation of the rod should be 2 cm. lateral to the first bend in the rod, and it is best performed by the use of a pelvic rod-bending clamp and a sleeve bender. Last, contour the rod to fit the lumbar lordosis by the use of a French rod bender. The short limb of the rod should be parallel to the angle of the inferior tilt of the guide pin.

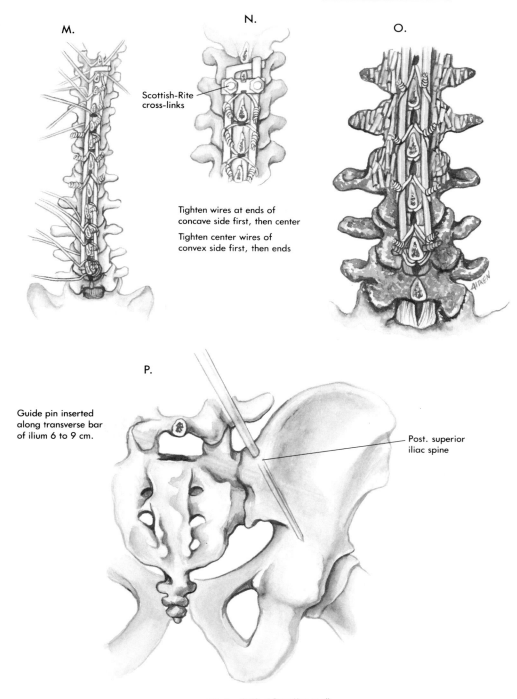

M.

N.

Scottish-Rite
cross-links

Tighten wires at ends of
concave side first, then center

Tighten center wires of
convex side first, then ends

O.

P.

Guide pin inserted
along transverse bar
of ilium 6 to 9 cm.

Post. superior
iliac spine

Plate 240. (Continued)

Q. and **R.** Finally, the iliac portion of the rod is inserted into the holes made by the guide pin and the sublaminar wires are tightened.

The wound is closed in the usual fashion.

Postoperative Care. Postoperative immobilization in cast or spinal orthotics is usually not necessary unless there is osteoporosis of the vertebral column. Patients are allowed to sit with assistance as soon as they are comfortable.

REFERENCES

Allen, B. L., Ferguson, R. L.: The Galveston technique for L rod instrumentation of the scoliotic spine. Spine, 7:276, 1982.

Luque, E. R.: The Luque system. In: Bradford, D. S., and Hensinger, R. M. (eds.): The Pediatric Spine. New York, Thieme, Inc., 1985, pp. 448–471.

Luque, E. R.: Segmental spinal instrumentation for correction of scoliosis. Clin. Orthop., 163:192, 1982.

Luque, E. R.: The anatomic basis and development of segmental spinal instrumentation. Spine, 7:256, 1982.

Luque, E. R.: Anatomy of scoliosis and its correction. Clin. Orthop., 105:198, 1984.

Luque, E. R. (ed.): Segmental Spinal Instrumentation. Thorofare, N.J., Slack, 1984.

Watkins, M. B.: Posterolateral fusion of the lumbar and lumbosacral spine. J. Bone Joint Surg., 35-A: 1014, 1953.

Wilber, G., Thompson, G. H., Shaffer, J. W., Brown, R. H., and Nash, C. L.: Postoperative neurological deficits in segmental spinal instrumentation. J. Bone Joint Surg., 66-A:1178, 1984.

Wiltse, L. L.: The paraspinal sacrospinalis—splitting approach to the lumbar spine. J. Bone Joint Surg., 50-A:919, 1968.

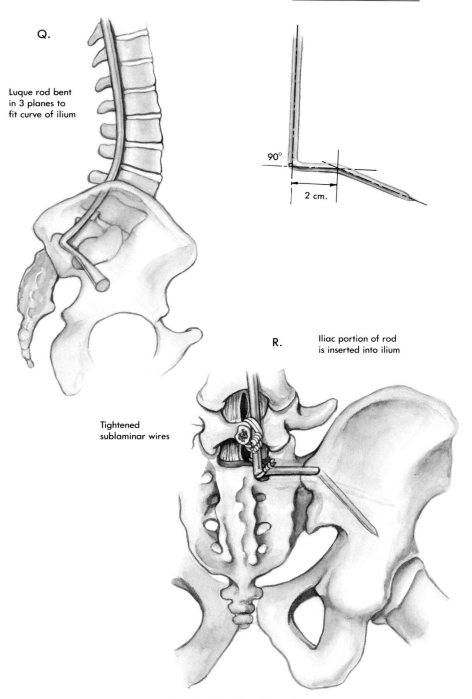

Q.

Luque rod bent
in 3 planes to
fit curve of ilium

90°

2 cm.

R.   Iliac portion of rod
is inserted into ilium

Tightened
sublaminar wires

Plate 240. (Continued)

PLATE 241   ## Harrington Rod Instrumentation with Luque Sublaminar Wiring (the "Harri-Luque" Procedure)

Indications. Thoracic lordoscoliosis. This technique corrects both coronal and sagittal deformities, thereby producing a normal, gentle kyphosis of the thoracic spine and preserving the normal lumbar lordosis. The Harri-Luque procedure is performed by surgeons who choose not to use the Cotrel-Dubousset instrumentation—the latter provides better correction and more secure fixation but is more technically demanding with a steep learning curve.

Special Instrumentation. Harrington and Luque instrumentation. A square-ended rod and a square-holed distal hook are required. The rod is contoured first into the desired configuration; the use of the square-ended rod and square-holed distal hook pulls the deformity into the rod and prevents the rod from rotating into the deformity.

Blood for Transfusion. Yes.

Radiographic Control. Image intensifier.

Patient Position. Prone on a Hall frame.

Operative Technique

A. The vertebrae to be fused are exposed as described in Plate 238. The ligamentum flavum of the vertebrae is excised throughout the upper and lower Harrington hook placement sites. (Follow the technique as described in Luque instrumentation; see Plate 240.)

On the concavity of the curve, the facet joints are excised and bone grafted; however, the laminae should be decorticated extremely lightly, if at all.

B. Next, place a double loop of stainless steel wire under the laminae of each vertebrae to be fused following the technique of Luque instrumentation, as described in Plate 240. Avoid penetration into the spinal canal and neurologic damage. Do not cut the wire loop.

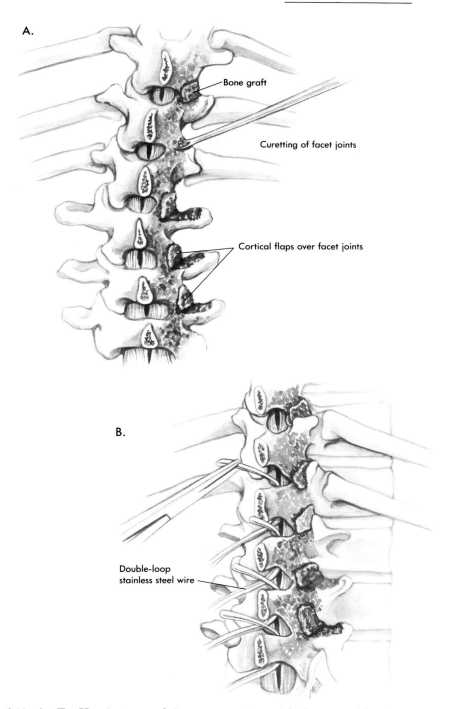

A.

Bone graft

Curetting of facet joints

Cortical flaps over facet joints

B.

Double-loop
stainless steel wire

Plate 241. A.–F., Harrington rod instrumentation with Luque sublaminar wiring (the Harri-Luque procedure).

C. The hooks and the Harrington rod are placed on the concave side of the curve, as described and illustrated in Plate 240. When the lumbar spine is included in the Harrington rod instrumentation, it is vital to preserve the normal lumbar lordosis. Bend the rod to fit the normal sagittal contours of the lumbar spine.

D. Use a square-holed Harrington hook and a square-ended rod to prevent rotation of the rod.

E. After the hook is inserted, wire the spinous processes of the two most distal vertebrae together, that is, the spinous process of the vertebra into which the hook is inserted and the spinous process of the next cephalad vertebra. Wiring of these spinous processes prevents distraction of the two distal vertebrae, and when distraction forces are exerted to correct the scoliosis, the lumbar lordosis is maintained because the convexity of the lordotic curve of the rod lies against the lamina in the concavity of the curve.

F. The Harri-Luque technique is designed to correct thoracic lordoscoliosis or hypokyphosis. The rod is contoured to provide 20 to 25 degrees of gentle, smooth, normal thoracic kyphosis. The distal and proximal 2 to 3 cm. of the rod are flat.

First, distract the rod minimally; symmetrically, slowly tighten the wires several times up and down the spine to correct the thoracic lordosis. Ordinarily, in the flexible adolescent with scoliosis, 3 cm. of space between the laminae and the rod can be readily corrected. In rigid deformities, a preliminary anterior discectomy is performed; the anterior release permits an easy correction of the thoracic lordosis.

Postoperative Care. During the first three months after surgery, the spine is supported in a plastic TLSO full time. The brace is then worn only during the day for an additional three months.

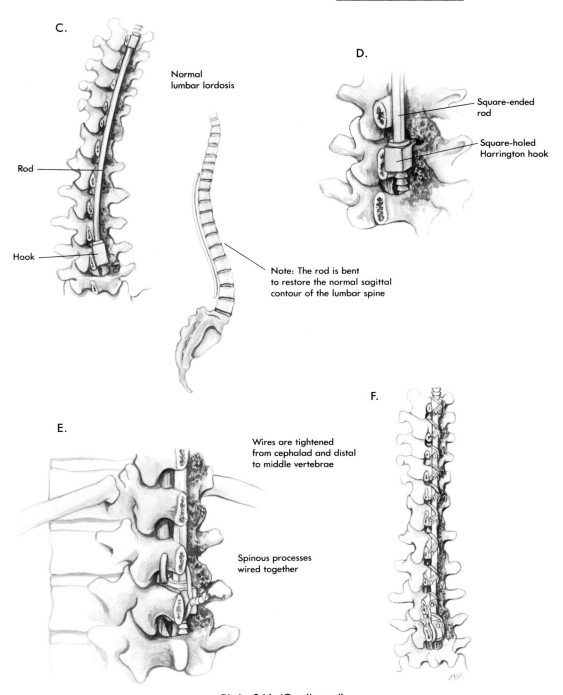

C.

Normal
lumbar lordosis

Rod

Hook

Note: The rod is bent
to restore the normal sagittal
contour of the lumbar spine

D.

Square-ended
rod

Square-holed
Harrington hook

E.

Wires are tightened
from cephalad and distal
to middle vertebrae

Spinous processes
wired together

F.

Plate 241. (Continued)

PLATE 242 ## Wisconsin or Drummond Technique of Segmental Spinal Instrumentation

Principle. In the Wisconsin or Drummond technique, distraction with a Harrington rod on the concavity of the curve is combined with a lateral corrective force provided by a Luque rod on the convexity of the curve. Segmental fixation of the spine is obtained by wires passing through the base of the spinous processes connecting the two rods with each other. The wires do not traverse the spinal canal; therefore, the risk of spinal cord or nerve root injury is minimized. This technique provides secure segmental fixation and lateral corrective force. The forces, however, are purely translational, and sagittal plane deformities of kyphosis and lordosis are not corrected. Rotational deformity may be aggravated by tautening of the wires around the Harrington distraction rod.

In double major curves, a long central distraction Harrington rod is used and two separate Luque rods are placed, one for the convexity of each curve.

Indications. Idiopathic or paralytic scoliosis with minimal exaggeration of lordosis and kyphosis.

Blood for Transfusion. Yes.

Radiographic Control. Yes.

Special Instrumentation

1. Harrington and Luque rods.
2. Drummond (Wisconsin) instrumentation apparatus.
3. Special curved awls.
4. Special button-wire implants.
5. Wire tighteners.

Contraindications. Kyphosis and lordosis.

Patient Position. Prone on a Hall frame.

Operative Technique

A. The spinous processes and the posterior elements of the spine are exposed as described in Plate 238. The level of fusion is determined by following the guidelines set forth by King et al.

The proximal and distal hook sites for the Harrington rod are prepared as described in Plate 239.

B. With a special curved awl, make a hole through the base of the spinous process of each vertebra to be fixed by segmental instrumentation. The holes should be deep, immediately superficial to the ventral cortex of the base of the spinous process. Exercise meticulous care not to enter the spinal canal. Some surgeons prefer to begin to make the holes on each side of the base of the spinous process with a small air-driven burr and then connect the holes by a right-angled clamp.

C. Next, through each hole, two wires are passed, one on each side of the spinous process. These wires have small stainless steel buttons that abut the base of the spinous process to prevent cutting through by the wire. Each button has an additional hole through which the wire from the opposite side passes. Pull the wires tight until the buttons seat firmly against the base of the spinous process.

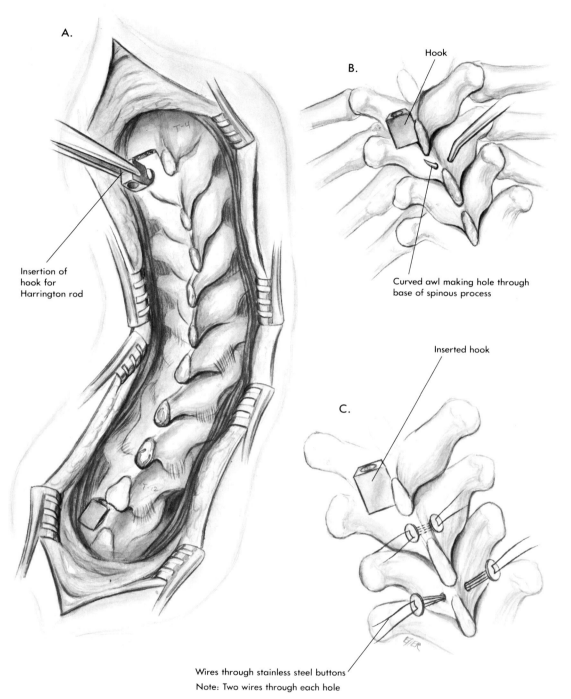

A.

Insertion of
hook for
Harrington rod

B.

Hook

Curved awl making hole through
base of spinous process

Inserted hook

C.

Wires through stainless steel buttons
Note: Two wires through each hole

Plate 242. A.–F., Wisconsin or Drummond technique of segmental spinal instrumentation.

D. Next, the facet joints are excised, and the laminae and transverse processes are decorticated, exposing raw cancellous bone. In the concavity of the curve, insert the proximal and distal hooks of the Harrington rod into the previously made holes. Each button has two wires—lay down the deep wire from the midline toward the side of the patient.

E. The Harrington rod is placed superficial to the deep wires and inserted into the hooks. The rod is then slowly distracted to correct the lateral curvature. Next, the superficial wire is brought over the rod and the wires are tautly twisted down against the rod. Begin twisting at the proximal and distal ends of the curve, and proceed toward the apex of the curve where the rod is farthest away from the spine.

F. Shape the Luque rod to fit on the convex side of the curve. At *both* ends of the extent of the fusion, the rod is contoured to an "L" to seat the rod firmly and keep it from sliding. The Luque rod is contoured to somewhat less curvature than the degree of scoliosis after Harrington distraction. Also, the rod is shaped to fit the kyphosis and lordosis.

Already on the convex side of the curve, the facet joints are incised and the laminae and transverse processes are decorticated. The fusion site on the concave side of the curve is bone grafted. The deep wire on the side of the spinous process is laid out. The Luque rod is placed snugly on the side of the spinous process with the L parts extending across the superior and inferior spinous processes of the fusion site. The superficial wires are placed over the Luque rod and twisted with the deep wires. Then, beginning at the center and proceeding distally and proximally, the wires are tightened. Go back and forth between the concave and convex sides, and gently distract the Harrington distraction rod further.

Final radiograms are made. The protruding ends of the wires are cut and buried deep in soft tissue. Hemovac suction tubes are placed, and the wound is closed in the usual fashion.

Postoperative Care. The patient is immobilized in a TLSO for three or four months.

REFERENCES

Drummond, D. S., Narechania, R., Wenger, D., Corolla, J., and Breed, A.: Wisconsin segmental spinal instrumentation. Orthop. Trans., 1982, 22–23.

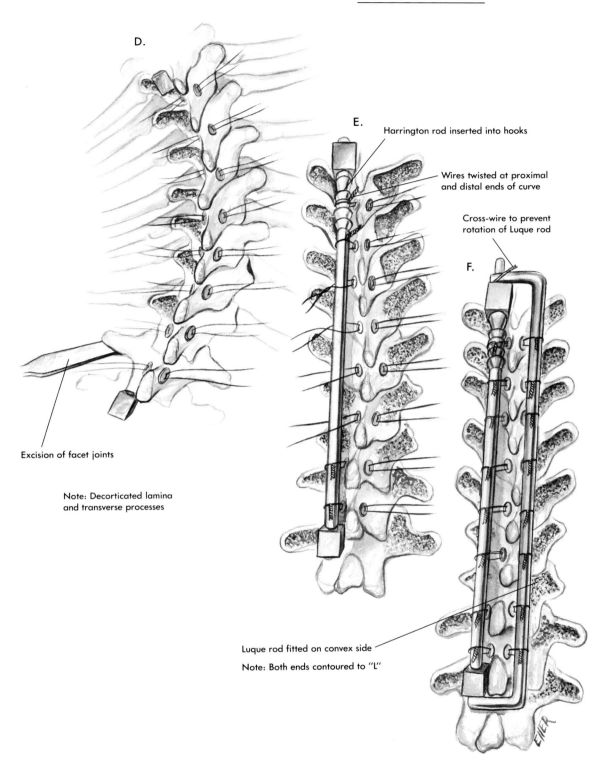

D.

Excision of facet joints

Note: Decorticated lamina
and transverse processes

E.

Harrington rod inserted into hooks

Wires twisted at proximal
and distal ends of curve

Cross-wire to prevent
rotation of Luque rod

F.

Luque rod fitted on convex side

Note: Both ends contoured to "L"

Plate 242. (Continued)

PLATE 243 Harrington Instrumentation Without Fusion (Subcutaneous Rod Technique)

Indications. Progressive scoliosis in young children in whom correction and stabilization of the spine are indicated. In this technique, subperiosteal exposure (except in cases of hook placement) and arthrodesis are not performed; therefore, longitudinal growth of the vertebral column is not disturbed. Postoperatively, the spine is supported in a Milwaukee CTLSO, and the rod is periodically lengthened or replaced as necessary.

Historically, Harrington developed this technique of spinal instrumentation in the treatment of juvenile scoliosis; however, he did expose the spine subperiosteally, which frequently resulted in spontaneous fusion and arrested longitudinal growth of the vertebral column in the skeletally immature child. Marchetti is credited for the concept of periodic lengthening and replacement of the rod and external support of the spine by orthosis. Moe introduced the technique of placing the rod in the soft tissues and not exposing the spine subperiosteally.

Blood for Transfusion. Yes.

Radiographic Control. Image intensifier.

Special Instrumentation

 1. Harrington rod—be sure that pediatric-sized hooks are available.
 2. Moe rod or ratchet rod.

Patient Position. The child is placed prone on a Hall frame, as described in Plate 238 for posterior spinal fusion.

Operative Technique

A. The skin and subcutaneous tissue are incised throughout the extent of the curve to be corrected by instrumentation. Do not make two small incisions at each end of the curve and try to pass the rod subcutaneously. Without exposure of the posterior elements, it is difficult to connect the vertebrae and determine the exact levels of instrumentation. Using radiography, identify and mark the most cephalad and caudad vertebrae at the ends of the planned area of instrumentation.

Subperiosteally, expose the two vertebrae at each end of the curve—one at the top and the other at the bottom of the curvature.

B. Identify and excise the ligamentum flavum; then at each end vertebra, gently insert an appropriate pediatric-sized hook under the laminae into the spinal canal. The facet joints of the end vertebrae are fused next; this measure assists in stabilizing the hook.

C. Next, a special rod designed by Moe is inserted into the hooks. The Moe rod has a 6-mm. unthreaded shank with threads at both ends to allow distraction at both the top and the bottom. If the Moe rod is not available, use a ratchet-type rod. The rod should be long enough to allow periodic lengthening. Ordinarily, one has to incise the deep fascia and partially divide the muscles at the site of the entrance of the rod into the hooks. It is vital to keep the rod superficial to the paravertebral muscles at all of the intervening areas. Great care should be exercised to avoid subperiosteal exposure because it will result in spontaneous fusion owing to the young age of the patient and the immobilization.

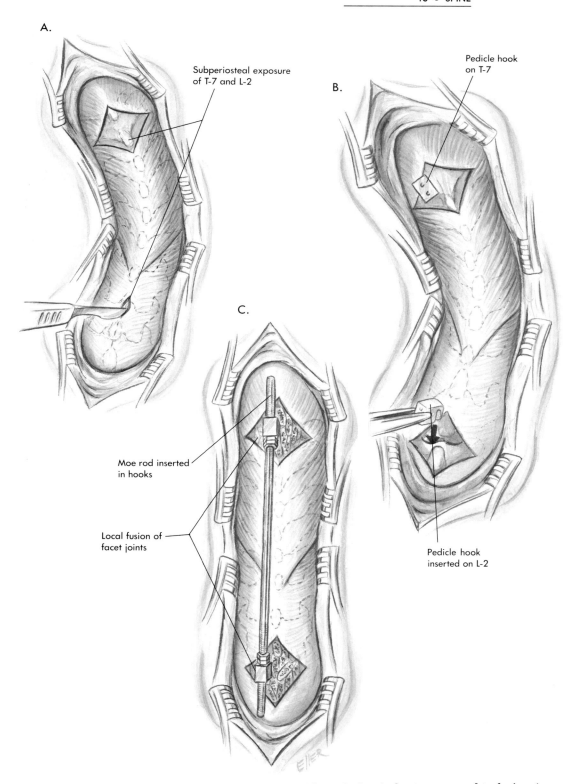

A.

Subperiosteal exposure
of T-7 and L-2

B.

Pedicle hook
on T-7

C.

Moe rod inserted
in hooks

Local fusion of
facet joints

Pedicle hook
inserted on L-2

Eller

Plate 243. A.–G., Harrington instrumentation without fusion (subcutaneous rod technique).

D. In a double structural curve, the rod is inserted in an "S" fashion. To allow the rod to lie deep to the skin and subcutaneous tissue, one often has to excise one or two spinous processes at the level where the rod crosses over them at the junction of the two curves.

E. Insert a C-ring or a wire to checkrein shortening of the rod. The wound is closed in the usual fashion.

Postoperative Care. The spine is supported in a Milwaukee CTLSO that is manufactured preoperatively but adjusted to the elongated trunk of the child with appropriate positioning and tautening of the pads. It is vital to support the spine with a Milwaukee orthosis before ambulation. The use of an underarm spinal orthosis is not recommended because it does not provide adequate support.

F. and **G.** Depending on the longitudinal growth of the spine, the rod is usually lengthened every six to nine months. The technique of lengthening is as follows:

1. Expose only one end of the rod, and clear the ratchet or threads of all soft tissue.
2. Unlock the rod by removing the C-ring or wire.
3. Place a hook holder on the hook and a rod clamp on the rod.
4. With a distractor between the two clamps, gently lengthen, achieving further correction. The amount of lengthening is individualized—there is no fixed rule.
5. Lock the rod in its lengthened position by inserting a new C-ring or wire.

Replacement of the rod is usually required after one or two lengthenings. For rod replacement, the entire extent of the instrumentation of the spine is subcutaneously opened. Only the ends of the curve and the hooks are subperiosteally exposed. Check the position and stability of anchorage of the hooks. Remove the rod and insert a longer one.

When the adolescent growth spurt begins, the longitudinal growth of the vertebral column is so rapid that the subcutaneous rod technique is ineffective in controlling progression of the curvature. At this stage, spinal fusion is performed. The hooks are usually stable and do not require replacement; however, the old rod should be removed, and a new strong rod should be inserted. The technique of spinal fusion and instrumentation is the same as described in Plate 239 for Harrington instrumentation.

REFERENCES

Moe, J. H., Kharrat, K., Winter, R. B., and Cummine, J. L.: Harrington instrumentation without fusion plus external orthotic support for the treatment of difficult curvature problems in young children. Clin. Orthop., 185:35, 1984.

Moe, J. H., Winter, R. B., Bradford, D., and Lonstein, J.: Scoliosis and Other Spinal Deformities, 2nd ed. Philadelphia, W.B. Saunders Co., 1987.

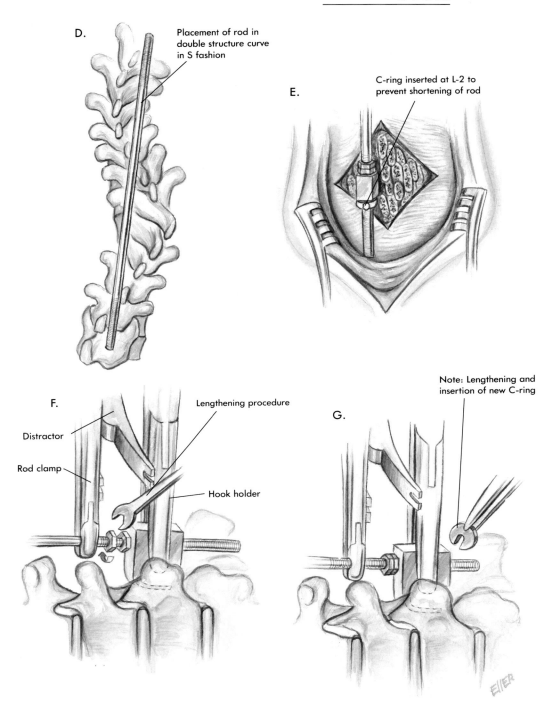

D. Placement of rod in double structure curve in S fashion

E. C-ring inserted at L-2 to prevent shortening of rod

F. Distractor / Rod clamp / Lengthening procedure / Hook holder

G. Note: Lengthening and insertion of new C-ring

Plate 243. (Continued)

PLATE 244 ## Cotrel-Dubousset (C-D) Instrumentation of the Spine for Treatment of Scoliosis

Indication. Idiopathic structural scoliosis, progressive and greater than 35 to 40 degrees, with decompensation of the spine.

Advantages. The C-D instrumentation has the following distinct advantages over other systems:

1. It provides excellent and unequaled correction of the scoliosis and thoracic hypokyphosis and lordosis.

2. The system achieves excellent correction of the rib hump and thoracic prominence and restores the sagittal contour to near normal.

3. When the vertebrae are of good bone quality, the system provides very rigid and strong fixation, obviating the need for postoperative immobilization. The comfort of the absence of a cast or spinal brace following surgery is very pleasing to the patient.

Disadvantages. The C-D system has certain drawbacks:

1. The instrumentation is difficult and technically demanding, and there is a steep learning curve.

2. There is a greater potential risk of nerve or spinal canal injury, particularly in the hands of an inexperienced surgeon.

3. The instruments occupy an extensive surface of laminae; therefore, the total area of bone that is decorticated is less than with other methods of instrumentation; some loss of correction may occur.

4. The cost of C-D instrumentation is much higher than that of other methods of instrumentation.

The C-D Instrumentation System. It consists of two rods placed on either side of the posterior elements of the spine. Multiple hooks anchor the rods to the spine. The two rods are cross-linked by devices for transverse traction (DTTs) into a rectangular configuration, thereby providing a very rigid and strong fixation.

Operative Technique

A. *The C-D rods.* The C-D rod is knurled with toric notches. These rods are very strong. There were no failures of the rods on testing their bending strength with a loading of 26 kiloponds at a frequency of 10 hertz (Hz) up to 1,200,000 cycles. On testing to axial compression with a loading of 20 kiloponds at a frequency of 10 Hz, the C-D rod did not fail at 204,000 cycles; under similar forces of axial compression, the Harrington distraction rod failed at 86,310 cycles. The fixation of the hook to the rod via the screws is very strong; with one screw fixation, it required a load of 1600 N to displace the hook on the rod, and with two-screw fixation, it required 2100 N.

In addition to its great strength, the C-D knurled rod is more flexible and more ductile than the Harrington rod.

The C-D rod comes in two different types: (1) the standard rod, which has enough ductility to allow complex bending of the rod in severe deformities, and (2) a cold-rolled rod that is stiff and provides resistance to bending forces.

B. and **C.** *The hooks.* These are designed for firm purchase of the pedicle, lamina, and transverse process. The hooks are of two basic types: open and closed.

The *pedicle hook* is bifid—it embraces the posterior base of the pedicle, the strongest part of the posterior arch. The bifid ends of the pedicle hook catch the cortices of the pedicle, thereby greatly increasing its rotational strength.

The *laminar hooks.* They come in different sizes: thoracic and lumbar. The *thoracic* laminar hooks are thin, adapted for the thin thoracic laminae; and the *lumbar* laminar hooks for insertion in the thick lumbar lamina. The laminar hooks

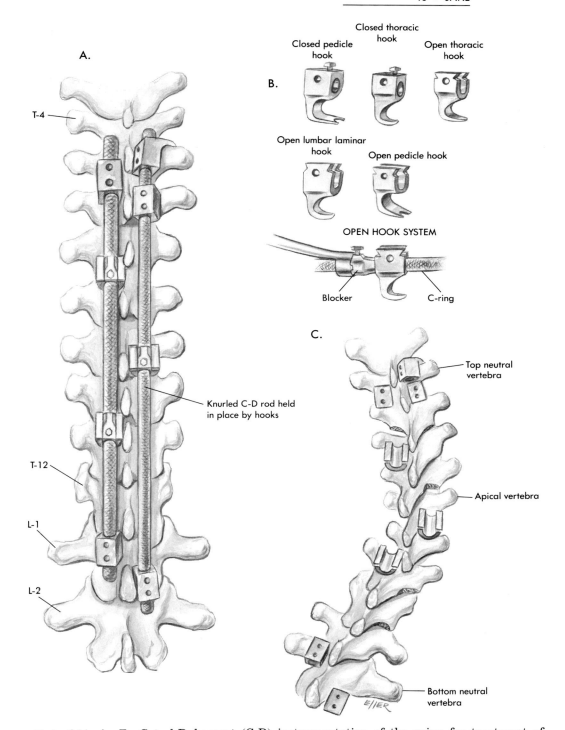

A.

B.

Closed pedicle
hook

Closed thoracic
hook

Open thoracic
hook

Open lumbar laminar
hook

Open pedicle hook

OPEN HOOK SYSTEM

Blocker   C-ring

T-4

Knurled C-D rod held
in place by hooks

T-12

L-1

L-2

C.

Top neutral
vertebra

Apical vertebra

Bottom neutral
vertebra

EILER

Plate 244. A.–Z., Cotrel-Dubousset (C-D) instrumentation of the spine for treatment of scoliosis.

come in various sizes and depth of the blade portion. It is vital to use the appropriate hook to prevent the penetration of the hooks into the spinal canal.

When an open hook is used, it is secured to the rod by a blocker that first slides onto the rod and then is inserted into the opening of the hook. Position the screws on the closed hooks or the blocker (in the open hooks), and lock them to the rod. *C-rings* are inserted next to the hooks; the screws of the C-ring are not tightened initially, thereby allowing them to rotate on the hook while the hook is held in place in distraction.

In C-D instrumentation the hooks provide numerous purchase points on the spine. In contrast with the Harrington system, the C-D instrumentation provides greater security of fixation, thereby obviating the necessity of external support in most patients.

The "claw configuration" consists of a hook for the thoracic transverse process above and a pedicle hook for the pedicle below. The strength of each hook is markedly increased by tightening of these hooks against each other. Sliding of the hooks is prevented by the claw configuration.

Preoperative Planning—Determination of Levels of Instrumentation

Standing and traction radiograms in the anteroposterior and lateral projections are used—the traction films depict the structure of both the major curve and its attendant minor curve. The level of fusion extends stable zone to stable zone as proposed by Harrington and subsequently substantiated by King et al. Basically, the rules are similar to Harrington instrumentation, except the following:

1. C-D achieves greater correction than does Harrington instrumentation; therefore, inferiorly, C-D can stop one level shorter than the Harrington technique.
2. Proximally, the most superior vertebra should extend beyond the hypokyphosis as seen in the lateral radiograms of the spine.

Originally, Cotrel recommended that the fusion area extend from proximal to distal neutral vertebrae; usually, in thoracic curves that are flexible on side-bending, this is quite adequate.

In this text, the basic technique of C-D instrumentation and fusion of a right thoracic curve are presented and illustrated. Four hooks are placed on the concave side and four hooks on the convex side. The type of hooks are as follows:

For the Top (Upper End) Vertebra

1. Closed pedicle hook on the *concave side*.
2. On the opposite *convex side,* a pedicle transverse claw, that is, a closed pedicle hook plus a transverse process hook. (When the procedure is technically difficult, a simple laminar hook in compression may be substituted for the pedicle transverse claw.)

For the Bottom (Lower End) Vertebra

1. A closed lumbar laminar hook on the superior margin of the hemilamina on the *concave side*.
2. A closed lumbar laminar hook on the inferior margin of the hemilamina on the *convex side*.

This hook selection for the lower end vertebra is applied in most cases. The hook on the convex side of the bottom vertebra may dislodge. To prevent this complication, a claw configuration using the transverse process of the adjacent vertebra may be used.

On the Apical Vertebra (with the Convex Vertical Edge)

An open pedicle hook is inserted.

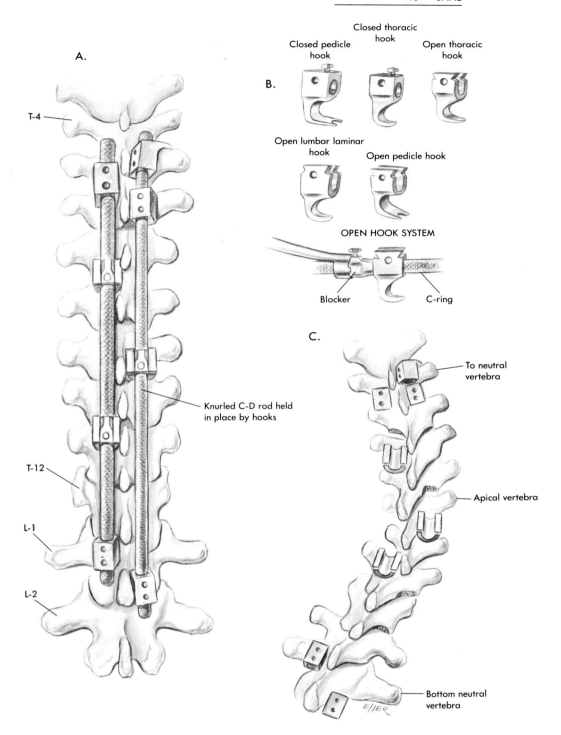

A.

T-4

Knurled C-D rod held
in place by hooks

T-12

L-1

L-2

B.

Closed pedicle
hook

Closed thoracic
hook

Open thoracic
hook

Open lumbar laminar
hook

Open pedicle hook

OPEN HOOK SYSTEM

Blocker   C-ring

C.

To neutral
vertebra

Apical vertebra

Bottom neutral
vertebra

Plate 244. (Continued)

Upper Intermediate Hook

1. Convex—open pedicle hook.
2. Concave—one or two levels inferior to the convex intermediate hook—open pedicle hook.

Lower Intermediate Hooks

Note: The lower intermediate vertebrae are one or two levels below the apical vertebra with the convex vertical edge.

1. Convex—open thoracic laminar hook.
2. Concave—open thoracic laminar hook.

The surgical exposure of the spine is through a routine subperiosteal exposure, as described in Plate 239 for Harrington instrumentation. The transverse process of the upper-end vertebra and the inferior aspect of the lamina of the lower-end vertebra are thoroughly exposed. Pay meticulous attention to hemostasis.

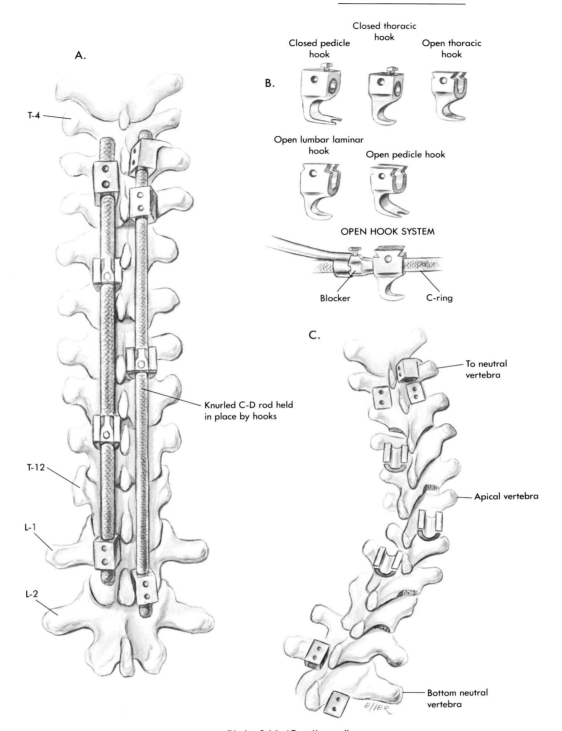

A.

T-4

Closed pedicle
hook

Closed thoracic
hook

Open thoracic
hook

B.

Open lumbar laminar
hook

Open pedicle hook

OPEN HOOK SYSTEM

Blocker   C-ring

Knurled C-D rod held
in place by hooks

C.

To neutral
vertebra

Apical vertebra

T-12

L-1

L-2

Bottom neutral
vertebra

Plate 244. (Continued)

D1. and **D2.** *Insertion of the pedicle hook.* In the thoracic spine (T-1 to T-9 and, in some cases, down to T-11), pedicle hooks are inserted.

First, part of the inferior facet is removed with a *vertical cut* made at the junction between the convexity of the superior facet and the concavity at its junction with the spinous process, and a *horizontal cut* is made 4 to 5 mm. distal to the inferior transverse process line. For apical purchase of the pedicle hook, the horizontal cut should be perpendicular to the line of instrumentation and the proposed path of the rod.

Excise a sufficient amount of the lamina. Partial excision of the inferior facet is required for placing the hook directly in front of the pedicle and for having the bifid part of the blade of the hook against the base of the pedicle while keeping secure contact of the hook against the inferior facet itself.

E. Curet out the cartilage of the superior facet of the vertebra below.

F1. and **F2.** The pedicle and the plane of the facet joint are identified. The pedicle finder is inserted very gently into the space and pushed against the pedicle.

Caution! Do not "plunge" the pedicle finder into the spinal canal, thereby injuring the spinal cord and causing paraplegia.

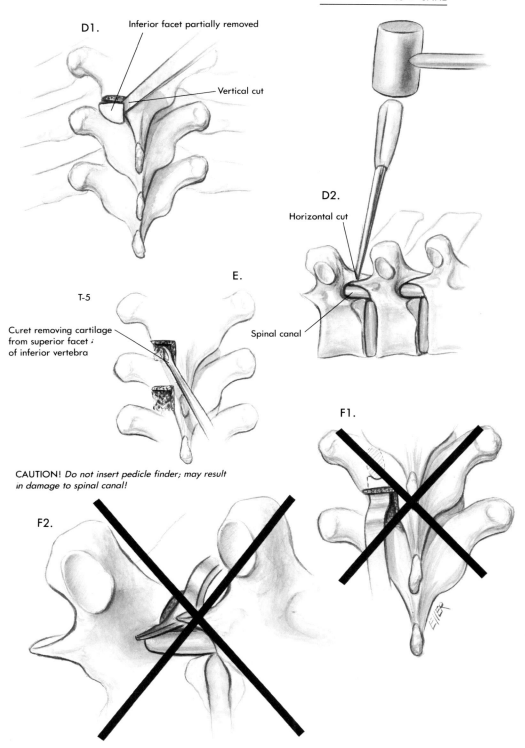

D1.

Inferior facet partially removed

Vertical cut

D2.

Horizontal cut

Spinal canal

E.

T-5

Curet removing cartilage
from superior facet
of inferior vertebra

CAUTION! *Do not insert pedicle finder; may result
in damage to spinal canal!*

F1.

F2.

Plate 244. (Continued)

G1. and **G2.** The pedicle hook, held by a hook holder and directed by an angled hook inserter, is directed cephalad and anteriorly and inserted cautiously into the joint space. If necessary, insertion of the pedicle hook may be facilitated by excising some of the posterior part of the transverse process of the vertebra below with a Leksell rongeur. Both horns of the bifid blade should penetrate in the appropriate plane to engage the pedicle. The pedicle hook should sit on the superior facet from below.

H1.–H3. Avoid these serious pitfalls:

1. Too low an angle of approach to the facet plane with resultant penetration of the inferior facet posterior to the plane of the joint by the horns of the hook. Fracture of the inferior facet may result if one pounds with force.

2. Do not force the pedicle hook anteriorly and injure the spinal canal—this consequence is a problem particularly when the superior facet is relatively short in relation to the inferior facet from below. In such a situation, the pedicle hook may engage only the very tip of the superior part from below and slip forward and damage the spinal cord, if pushed with force.

3. Fracture of the superior facet may be produced during the insertion of the pedicle finder or the hook. Be suspicious of a fracture if a cracking sound is heard. Remove the hook immediately, and rule out superior facet fracture. If the fracture is undisplaced, it may be left intact. If the fracture fragment is displaced, it may be pushed toward the spinal cord. Perform a laminectomy and remove the floating fragment of the superior facet. Do not reinsert a hook at this level. Choose another site.

The following pedicle hooks are inserted:

1. One closed pedicle hook on the concave side of the upper-end vertebra.
2. One closed pedicle hook on the convex side of the upper-end vertebra.
3. One open pedicle hook on the apical vertebra on the convex side.
4. One open pedicular hook (the upper intermediate concave hook) on the concave side one or two levels above the apical vertebra.

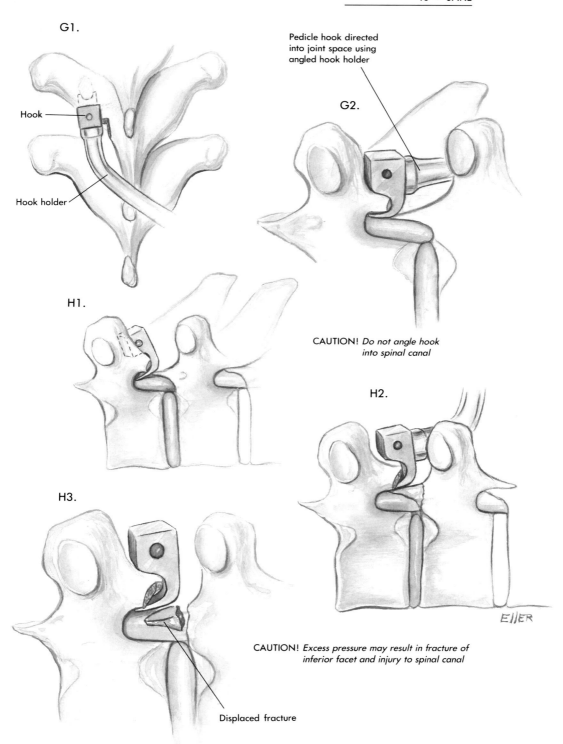

G1.

Hook

Hook holder

G2.

Pedicle hook directed
into joint space using
angled hook holder

CAUTION! *Do not angle hook
into spinal canal*

H1.

H2.

H3.

EllER

CAUTION! *Excess pressure may result in fracture of
inferior facet and injury to spinal canal*

Displaced fracture

Plate 244. (Continued)

I. Insert the laminar hook in the supralaminar position. During this procedure, there is definite risk of injury to the spinal cord because the spinal canal is relatively taut and the hooks are in the spinal canal. Pay diligent attention to details of technique.

First, remove the spinous process. Second, perform a laminotomy of the superior margin of the lamina. Keep the size of laminotomy for hook insertion as small as possible. Displacement of the hook into the spinal canal is a serious complication. With a small aperture in the interlaminar space, the cephalad end of the hook locks against the lamina above and checkreins its protrusion into the spinal canal. The bone of the upper end of the lamina should be strong and thick for good purchase, and its axis should be at right angles to the anticipated rod axis.

Insert the hook with a hook holder. Keep a vigilant eye on the position of the laminar hooks during rod insertion and during facet fusion.

In the simple right thoracic curve, the two lower concave hooks are laminar.

J.–L. Insert the infralaminar hook. The thick lamina may have to be trimmed down with a rongeur; however, it is important to maintain the strength of the bone on the medial aspect of the inferior lamina. First, perform a small laminotomy of the inferior part of the lamina of the vertebra to provide a horizontal purchase for the hook. Preserve the adjacent capsule as much as possible.

With a hook holder, manually insert the laminar hook gently, and then push it with a hook inserter into the plane between the anterior aspect of the lamina and the ligamentum flavum attached to it. This hook is inserted on the lower-end vertebra on the convex side on the inferior surface of the lamina.

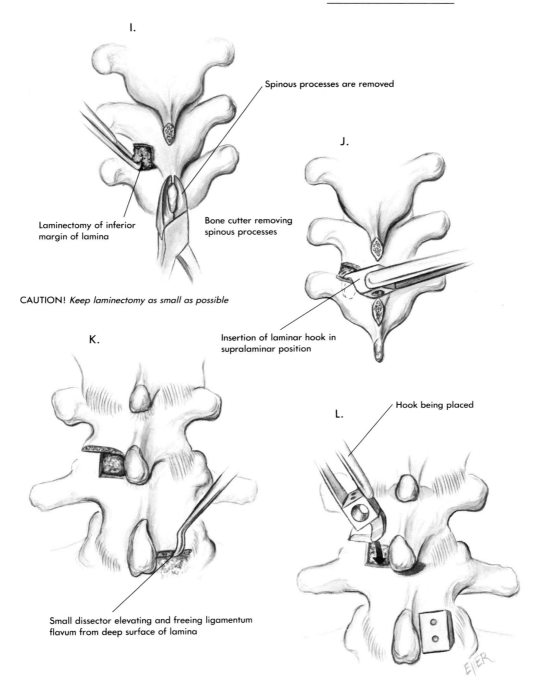

I.

Spinous processes are removed

J.

Laminectomy of inferior
margin of lamina

Bone cutter removing
spinous processes

CAUTION! *Keep laminectomy as small as possible*

Insertion of laminar hook in
supralaminar position

K.

L.

Hook being placed

Small dissector elevating and freeing ligamentum
flavum from deep surface of lamina

Plate 244. (Continued)

M., N1., and **N2.** Insert the transverse process hook. The hook usually used is a closed lumbar laminar hook. It is much simpler when the transverse process hook is inserted before insertion of the pedicle hook with which it forms a claw.

Prepare the space for the hook with a transverse process elevator by inserting it on the superior aspect of the base of the transverse process and then rotating it; some of the ligaments between the rib and the transverse process are sectioned without damage to the joint.

The closed lumbar hook is held with a hook holder and inserted onto the transverse process following the path created by the transverse process elevator.

Next, check the position and purchase of all the hooks. During decortication and facet fusion, it may be safer to remove all the hooks during chiseling and pounding of the bone because those actions may cause risky displacement of the hooks against the spinal cord.

O. and **P.** Perform facet fusion and meticulous decortication of the transverse spinous process and the medial laminar process, as described in Plate 238.

Caution! Do not compromise hook purchase.

Autogenous bone grafts taken from the ilium are placed beneath the rods. Replace all of the hooks. As a rule, concave facet fusion is performed first and then the concave rod is inserted. Next, the convex facet fusion is performed. Finally, the convex rod is inserted.

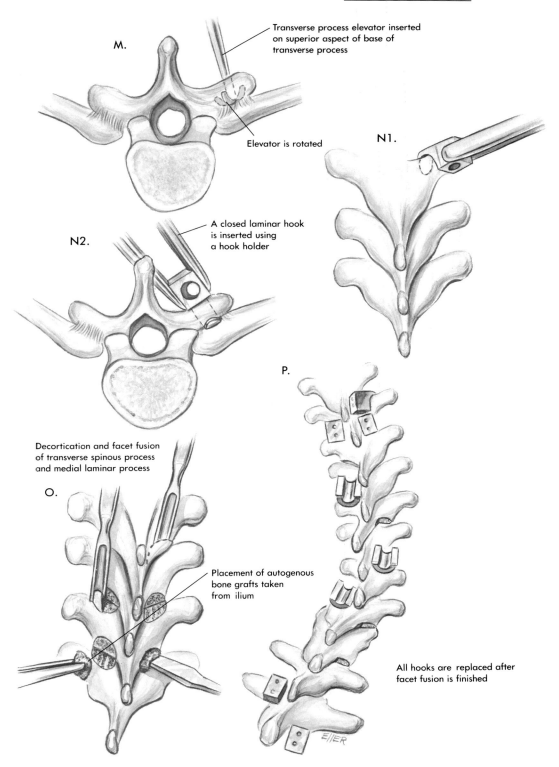

M.

Transverse process elevator inserted on superior aspect of base of transverse process

Elevator is rotated

N1.

N2.

A closed laminar hook is inserted using a hook holder

Decortication and facet fusion of transverse spinous process and medial laminar process

O.

P.

Placement of autogenous bone grafts taken from ilium

All hooks are replaced after facet fusion is finished

Plate 244. (Continued)

Concave Rod Contouring

Q. and **R.** The objectives of the concave rod are (1) to *distract* the concavity of the scoliotic curve, with its greatest effect within the short structural apical segment; (2) to provide normal sagittal *contours* by posteriorly pulling the apex of the thoracic lordosis or hypokyphosis; and (3) to *derotate* as a result of pulling the concavity backward and pushing the convexity forward.

The initial rod shape (at the time of insertion) and the final rod shape (after it has rotated 90 degrees) should be more or less similar; otherwise, tremendous forces will be exerted on the hooks and cause fracture of the laminae during rod rotation.

Contour the rod on the concave side to the shape of the scoliosis and to the shape of the anticipated sagittal contour of the normal thoracic kyphosis and lumbar lordosis.

LATERAL VIEW

ANTEROPOSTERIOR VIEW

Q.

Contouring rod to fit normal thoracic spinal curve

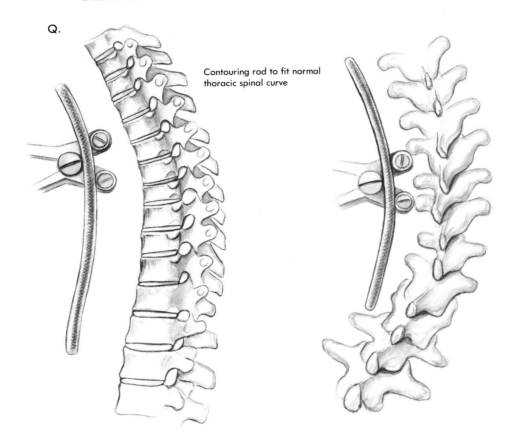

R.

C-D rods

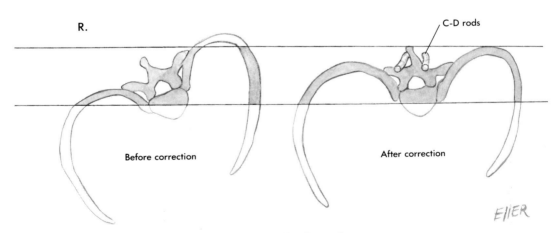

Before correction

After correction

EllER

Plate 244. (Continued)

S., T1., and T2. The rod is passed through the upper pedicle hook and is then pulled inferiorly. Next, introduce two blockers (back to back) on the lower end of the rod. Gently tighten the hex bolts, locking the blockers in the midpart of the rods and preventing their upward displacement during rod insertion. The blockers, because of the midposition, are kept away from the open hooks as the rod is pushed into the holes. Finally, insert the rod into the bottom closed hook.

With proper contouring, the rod can be easily positioned into the open box of the open upper and lower intermediate hooks. Occasionally, the positioning may be difficult, requiring the use of a rod introducer.

Place the rod into the opening of the open hook, unlock the blocker, and with a hook holder pointing the hook down to the blocker, push the blocker into the hook box. Blocker manipulation is facilitated by the use of a hook driver (which has lateral flanges for rotational control) and hook and block pushers.

S.

T1.

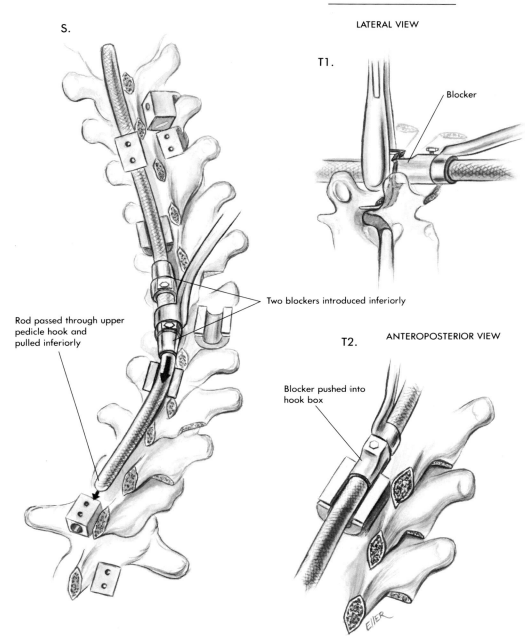

Blocker

Two blockers introduced inferiorly

Rod passed through upper
pedicle hook and
pulled inferiorly

T2.   ANTEROPOSTERIOR VIEW

Blocker pushed into
hook box

Eller

Plate 244. (Continued)

U., V1., and **V2.** Place the *C-rings* over the rod between the intermediate hooks, and apply distraction between a rod holder and the C-rings on either side. The C-rings hold the hooks securely in place, permitting distraction of the apical vertebra without blocking rotation.

Next, seat the intermediate hooks under some distraction and tighten the set screw of the C-ring. Double check the position of the upper and lower hooks.

W. With two large rod holders, slowly rotate the rod 90 degrees from its scoliotic configuration to a kyphotic configuration. Carefully inspect the hooks; occasionally, under great stress, the lamina (particularly the one purchased by the top concave hook) may fracture and spinal cord injury may result.

Another problem is lateral displacement of the upper intermediate hook—when this movement takes place, the hook should be repositioned in place immediately.

With rotation of the rod, the spine straightens. The degree of straightening depends on the flexibility of the spine. Correct placement of the hooks and contouring of the rod are also important.

Following complete derotation, tighten the set screws on the hooks and blockers, and remove the C-rings.

U.

V1.

Distraction is applied

C-rings placed over rod
between intermediate hooks

Derotation of rod

W.

C-rings tightened

V2.

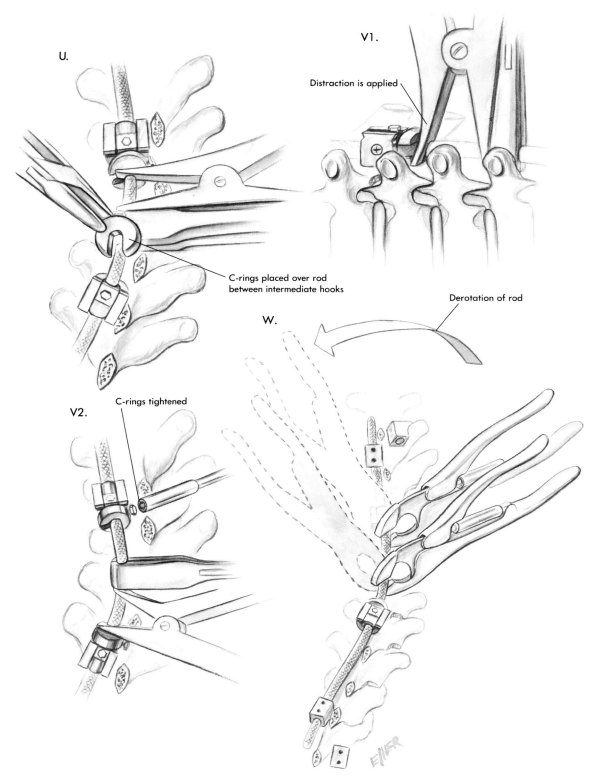

Plate 244. (Continued)

X. and **Y.** Contour and insert the convex rod. The purpose of the convex rod is to provide further rigidity of fixation by compression and the construction of a rigid frame. The rod on the convex side is undercontoured to the kyphosis; that is, it is flat in its middle section. On rotation of the rod, the flat segment is forced against the rotated vertebrae and some further correction can be obtained. The lower part of the rod on the concave side is contoured for some lordosis.

The technique for inserting the rod on the convex side is similar to that for the concave side. First, pass the rod through the upper claw, then push it through the apical open hook. Move the blocker upward into the apical hook. Slip the rod into the lower hook.

Z. Tauten the upper claw, and compress the convex apical hook against the upper claw. With a hook compressor, compress the lower hook segment against a rod gripper.

The remaining parts of the posterior arches are decorticated, and any remaining bone graft is added to the wound.

One device for transverse traction (DTT) is inserted just below the upper hook, and a second DTT is inserted above the lower hooks. The Texas Scottish Rite system of cross-linking is very superior to other systems. These cross-links provide a rectangular configuration, making the spinal instrumentation very strong.

Spinal cord monitoring is checked, and a formal wake-up test is performed. When the patient moves the lower limbs and toes, he or she is reawakened.

The C-rings are removed, and all the set screws are tightened until they break off. Hex screws are inserted and sheared on all the closed hooks.

The wound is drained and closed in the routine fashion.

Postoperative Care. Spinal orthotics or casts are not required for immobilization when the degree of scoliosis corrected is moderate and the instrumentation is satisfactory, with strong normal bone quality of the vertebrae. However, if the scoliosis is severe, the vertebral bones are osteoporotic, and the security of instrumentation is under par, it is best to support the spine full time in a TLSO for six months.

REFERENCES

Bradford, D. S.: Spinal fusion with Cotrel-Dubousset instrumentation for correction of scoliosis. Strategies in Orthopaedic Surgery, Vol. 7, No. 1, 1988.

Cotrel, Y., and Dubousset, J.: New segmental posterior instrumentation of the spine. Orthop. Trans., 9:118, 1985.

Denis, F.: Cotrel-Dubousset instrumentation in the treatment of idiopathic scoliosis. Orthop. Clin. North Am., 19:291, 1988.

Nash, C. L., Jr., Schatzinger, L., and Lorig, R.: Intraoperative monitoring of spinal cord function in scoliosis undergoing correction. J. Bone Joint Surg., 56-A:1765, 1974.

Nash, C. L., Jr., Gregg, E. C., Brown, R. H., and Pillai, N. S.: Risk of exposure to x-rays in patients undergoing long-term treatment for scoliosis. J. Bone Joint Surg., 61-A:371, 1979.

Nash, C. L., Jr., Lorig, R. A., Schatzinger, L. A., and Brown, R. H.: Spinal cord monitoring during operative treatment of the spine. Clin. Orthop., 126:100, 1977.

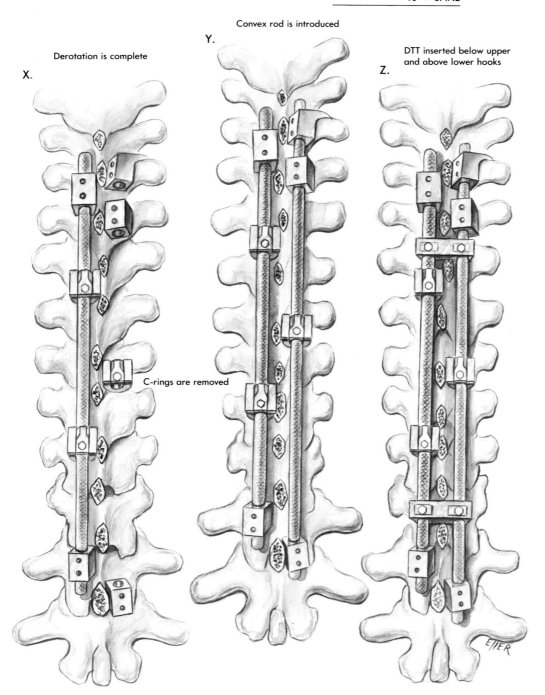

Convex rod is introduced

Y.

Derotation is complete

X.

DTT inserted below upper
and above lower hooks

Z.

C-rings are removed

Plate 244. (Continued)

PLATE 245 **Anterior Instrumentation of the Spine (Thoracoabdominal Approach) (Zielke Technique)**

Indications. Anterior spine fusion is performed in the pediatric spine for three specific purposes:

1. *To remove the discs and ligaments in order to provide increased curve correctability.* An example is the child with a severe cerebral palsy scoliosis with a marked pelvic obliquity. The achievement of a level pelvis is most important for long-term sitting balance. Without the anterior release and fusion, adequate correction would not be possible.

2. *To bone graft the spine anteriorly if solid arthrodesis is unlikely by posterior fusion alone.* An example is the child with a significant kyphosis problem, such as a congenital or neurofibromatosis diagnosis. Solid arthrodesis cannot be achieved without anterior and posterior fusion.

3. *To eradicate the anterior convex growth plates to prevent late bending of the fused area.* An example is the child with severe juvenile idiopathic scoliosis in which a posterior fusion alone would result in deformity increase as a result of the "crankshaft" effect.

Patient Position. The patient is placed in the lateral decubitus position with the convex side of the curve upward. The upper arm is flexed forward and abducted to rotate the scapula away from the vertebral column. At the apex of the curve, the table is elevated to facilitate excision of the intervertebral discs.

Operative Technique

A. and **B.** It is necessary to remove a rib for exposure of the spine; the rib that is removed is the one immediately superior to the most cephalic vertebral body to be exposed; for example, for exposure from T-5 or T-6 to T-11, the fifth rib is removed. Removal of the tenth rib allows exposure of the spine from T-10 to the sacrum. The costal cartilage of the tenth rib is split longitudinally for exposure of the retroperitoneal plane and diaphragm. The attachments of the diaphragm to the rib cage are sectioned. In this plate, the thoracoabdominal approach for exposure of the lower thoracic and lumbar spine is described.

Skin Incision

The incision begins at the spinous process of T-10 (or T-9) and extends along the course of the tenth rib to the costocartilaginous junction, across the upper abdomen to the lateral edge of the rectus abdominis. At this point, the incision is carried distally toward the symphysis pubis. This single incision allows exposure of the spine all the way to the sacrum.

A.

Incision
(along path of 10th rib)

Spinous process of T$_{10}$

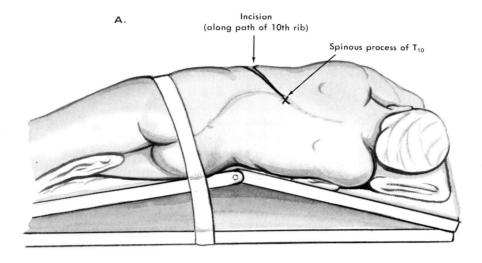

B.

Incision

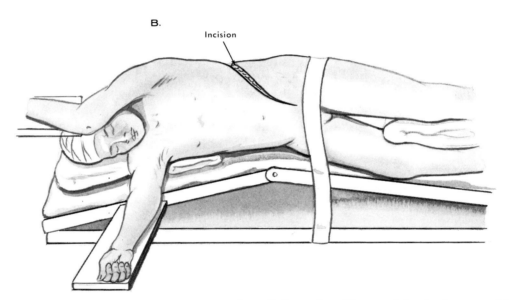

Plate 245. A.–Q., Anterior instrumentation of the spine (thoracoabdominal approach) (Zielke technique).

C. The tenth rib is freed by sharp and dull dissection, divided at its costocartilaginous junction, and excised. Removal of the rib permits a larger working aperture, and also the rib is used as autogenous bone graft.

D. and **E.** The costal cartilage of the tenth rib is split longitudinally with a scalpel. It is best to place stay sutures on either side of the costal cartilage so that the tissue plane is easily identifiable for later closure.

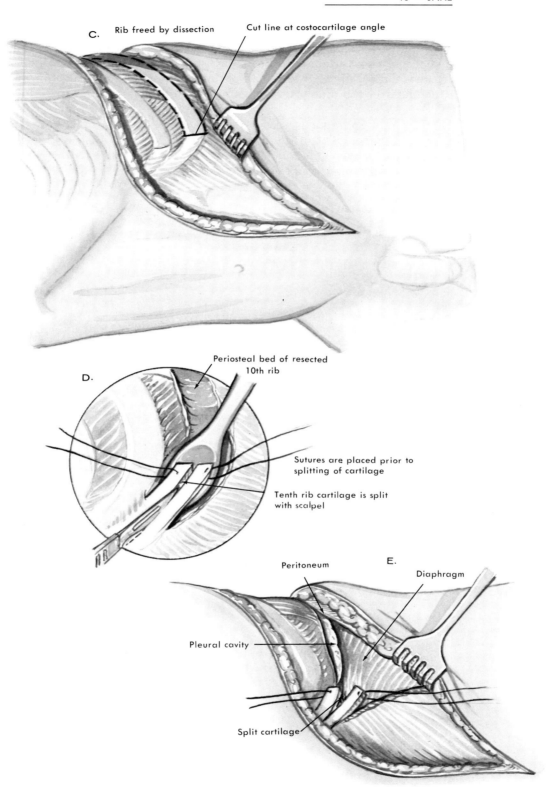

C. Rib freed by dissection   Cut line at costocartilage angle

D.

Periosteal bed of resected
10th rib

Sutures are placed prior to
splitting of cartilage

Tenth rib cartilage is split
with scalpel

Peritoneum   E.   Diaphragm

Pleural cavity

Split cartilage

Plate 245. (Continued)

F. By blunt dissection, the peritoneum is gently peeled off from the underside of the diaphragm. Upon freeing of the peritoneum, the viscera will fall anteriorly away from the vertebral bodies. Stay sutures are placed on either side of the intended line of division of the diaphragm, which is ½ to ¾ inch from the site of attachment of the diaphragm. This will facilitate closure of the diaphragm later on.

G. The diaphragm is sectioned from its costal attachments. An alternative method of detachment of the diaphragm is to carry it out from the thoracic side along its costal attachment using a Bovie knife (not illustrated). By this technique, bleeding is minimized and the problem of postoperative atelectasis is less common.

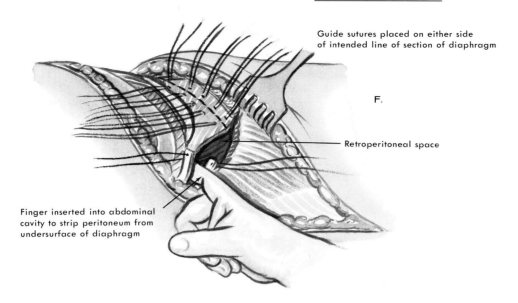

Guide sutures placed on either side
of intended line of section of diaphragm

F.

— Retroperitoneal space

Finger inserted into abdominal
cavity to strip peritoneum from
undersurface of diaphragm

Diaphragm (free from peritoneum on undersurface)
is divided circumferentially 1.5 cm. from its costal attachment

G.

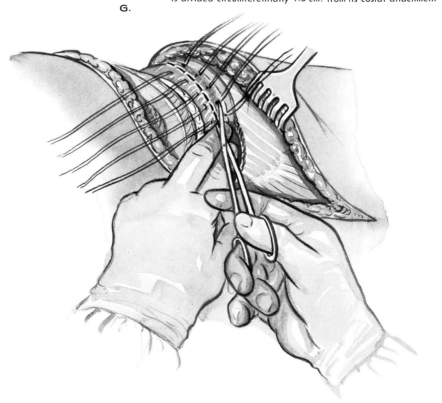

Plate 245. (Continued)

H. Next, the parietal pleura is incised along the vertebral bodies throughout the extent of the vertebrae to be exposed.

I. In the lumbar region, the psoas muscle is gently elevated off the vertebral bodies and intervertebral discs. The segmented vessels are ligated either close to their origin from the aorta or in the middle of the vertebral body; therefore, the vital vascular anastomosis near the intervertebral foramen is avoided and potential vascular infarct of the cord is obviated.

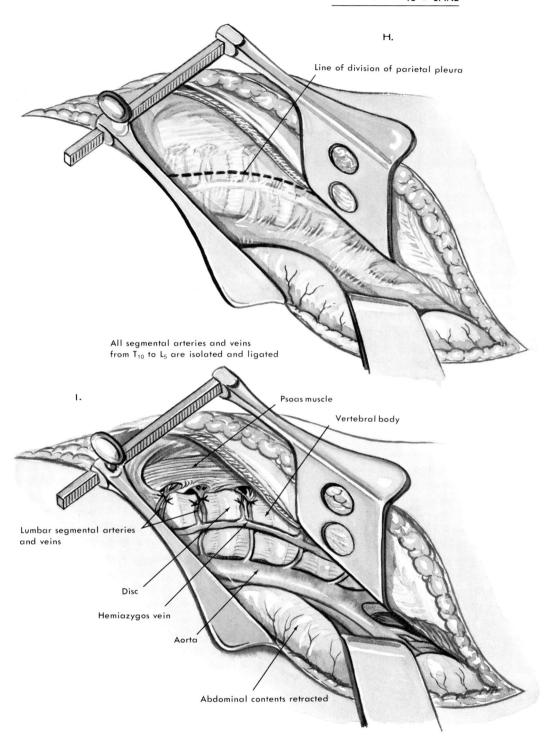

H.

Line of division of parietal pleura

All segmental arteries and veins
from T₁₀ to L₅ are isolated and ligated

I.

Psoas muscle

Vertebral body

Lumbar segmental arteries
and veins

Disc

Hemiazygos vein

Aorta

Abdominal contents retracted

Plate 245. (Continued)

Interbody Fusion

J. and **K.** The annulus is exposed anteriorly from the margin of one intervertebral foramen to the contralateral foramina. The aorta and vena cava are protected, and the anterior longitudinal ligament is incised with a sharp scalpel. Next, with a duck-bill rongeur, the discs are excised. Once the discs are excised, the posterior annulus and posterior longitudinal ligaments are visualized.

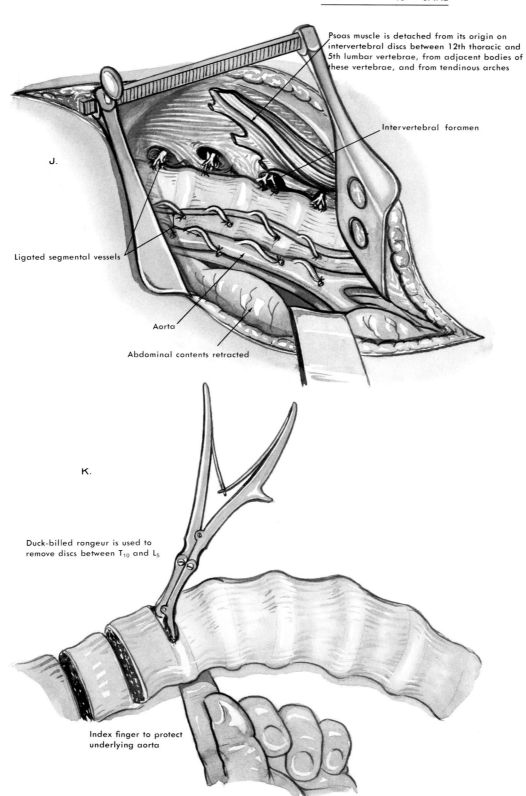

Psoas muscle is detached from its origin on intervertebral discs between 12th thoracic and 5th lumbar vertebrae, from adjacent bodies of these vertebrae, and from tendinous arches

Intervertebral foramen

J.

Ligated segmental vessels

Aorta

Abdominal contents retracted

K.

Duck-billed rongeur is used to remove discs between T_{10} and L_5

Index finger to protect underlying aorta

Plate 245. (Continued)

L. The aorta and vena cava are protected with Chandler or other appropriate elevator retractors. With a sharp osteotome and mallet, the vertebral end-plates are removed.

M. With a curet, any retained disc and vertebral end-plates are removed. In correction of kyphosis, all annular ligamentous tissue down to the posterior longitudinal ligament is removed; in scoliosis, however, the outer annular fibers on the concave side are preferably left intact. For hemostasis, the excised disc interspaces are packed with Gelfoam soaked in thrombin solution.

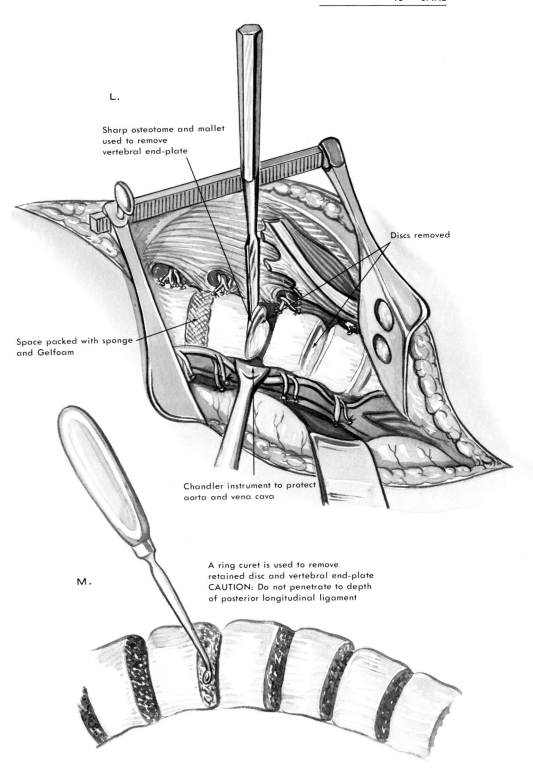

L.

Sharp osteotome and mallet
used to remove
vertebral end-plate

Discs removed

Space packed with sponge
and Gelfoam

Chandler instrument to protect
aorta and vena cava

M.

A ring curet is used to remove
retained disc and vertebral end-plate
CAUTION: Do not penetrate to depth
of posterior longitudinal ligament

Plate 245. (Continued)

Zielke Instrumentation—Ventral Derotation Spondylodesis

N. The anterior aspect of the vertebrae is exposed, and the discs are excised as described previously. The outer annular fibers on the concave side are left intact. Intraoperative radiograms of the spine are made with radiopaque markers to ensure that the exposed vertebrae correspond to the proposed level and extent of fusion. Begin instrumentation with the most cephalic vertebra.

First, measure the diameter of the vertebral body with a caliper. The length of the screw should be such that its tip perforates the opposite vertebral cortex. The thickness of the washers and angle plates should be taken into consideration; therefore, the selected screw will be 5 to 9 mm. longer than the diameter of the vertebral body as measured by caliper. It is vital to have bicortical fixation.

The threads of the Zielke screws are broad and self-cutting for firm anchoring in cancellous bone. The pressure force of the screws is distributed by angle plates and washers. Double-bladed angle plate (similar to Dwyer staples) is used for the end vertebrae, whereas washers are used for the intervening vertebrae. The screw heads have either lateral or upper slits, through which the compression rod is passed. The notches (slits) of the most cephalic and caudal screws are side-opening, whereas the intervening screws are top-opening.

Make a borehole for the screw with an awl; then insert the Zielke screw of appropriate length with an attached blade or washer across the center of the vertebral body. At the end vertebrae, the flanges of the staples should be in the vertebral body only; they should not penetrate the normal intervertebral disc. The screws should not penetrate the intraspinal canal. The screw in the apical vertebrae should now be posterolateral, with the most proximal and distal screws being 1 cm. anterior to the apical screws. From the lateral projection, the line drawn between the screw heads should form a gentle C-curve. When the spine derotates and straightens, the rod will be straight.

O. Next, insert a flexible stainless steel threaded rod of appropriate length into the notches of each screw head. The compression mechanism of ventral derotation spondylodesis (VDS) is similar to the Harrington compression rod; it is transmitted by similar hex nuts that have a central threaded hole fitting the threads of the compression rod. The cylindrical process of the nuts is received by bilateral cuttings of the screw heads. The nuts are advanced into screw heads manually. The terminal screws are fitted with two hex nuts, one facing the other, for locking. The intervening screws are fitted with only one locking nut, facing the apex of the scoliosis. With appropriate fitting of the hex nuts into the screw heads, the threaded compression rod is tautly anchored in the screw head, checkreining it from slipping out.

Next, the derotation bar is installed by fitting its shoes on the ends of the compression rod. Using the handle bar, the convexity of the curve is gently pulled anteriorly. Simultaneously, the force on the tension screw is adjusted. Avoid sudden maneuvers because they may rupture the vertebral body or fracture the pedicle. Normal lordosis is produced by derotating the spine.

P. and Q. After desired derotation is achieved, the intervertebral spaces are packed with autogenous bone obtained from the resected rib and ilium. Bone graft wedges of 1 to 2 cm. are placed anteriorly; small pieces of bone graft are placed posteriorly. It is vital to have complete bone-to-bone contact to ensure solid fusion. Next, the hex nuts are tightened to achieve compression correction of the scoliotic deformity. After the desired degree of correction is achieved, the screws at the end of the system are firmly locked. The threads of the proximal and distal parts of the compression rod are destroyed by a mallet and impactor; this step ensures that the lock nuts do not unwind. Chest tubes are inserted and the wound is closed in the usual fashion.

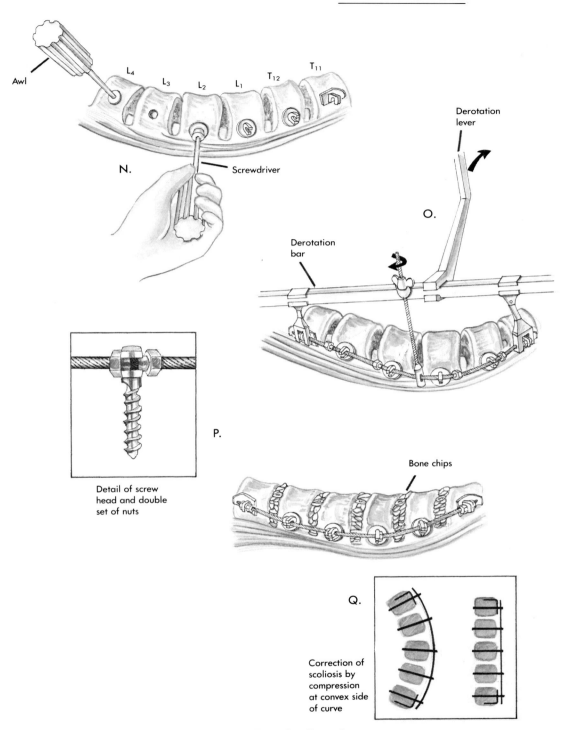

N.

Awl

Screwdriver

L_4 L_3 L_2 L_1 T_{12} T_{11}

O.

Derotation lever

Derotation bar

P.

Detail of screw
head and double
set of nuts

Bone chips

Q.

Correction of
scoliosis by
compression
at convex side
of curve

Plate 245. (Continued)

Postoperative Care. After routine care in the intensive care unit, removal of the chest tube, and the return of bowel and bladder function, a plaster-of-Paris body jacket is applied. Cast immobilization is usually for four months; this is followed by support of the spine in a TLSO for an additional six months. Solid interbody fusion should be documented by tomography before orthotic support to the spine is discontinued.

REFERENCES

Giehl, J. P., Zielke, K., and Hack, H. P.: Zielke ventral derotation spondylodesis. Orthopade, 18:101, 1989.

Hack, H. P., Zielke, K., and Harms, J.: Spinal instrumentation and monitoring. In: Bradford, D. S., and Hensinger, R. M. (eds.): The Pediatric Spine. New York, Thieme, Inc., 1985, p. 491.

Moe, J. H., Purcell, G. A., and Bradford, D. S.: Zielke instrumentation (VDS) for the correction of spinal curvature. Analysis of results in 66 patients. Clin. Orthop., 180:133, 1983.

Zielke, K.: Ventrale Derotationsspondylodese, Behandlungsergebnisse bei idiopathischen Lumbalskoliosen. Z. Orthop., 120:320, 1982.

Zielke, K., and Berthet, A.: Ventrale Derotationsspondylodese—vorlaufiger Bericht uber 58 Falle. Beit. Orthop. Traumatol., 25:85, 1978.

Zielke, K., and Pellin, B.: Ventrale Derotationsspondylodese. Symposium on Kyphosis and Scoliosis, Belgrade, 1975.

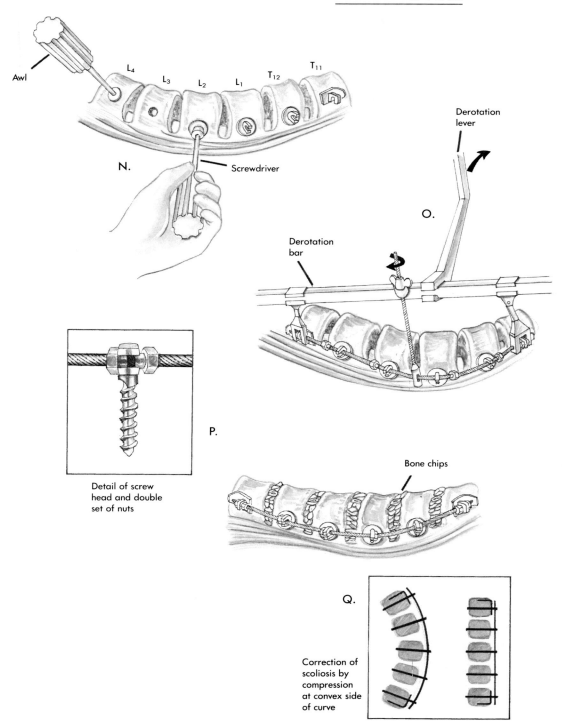

Awl

L₄ L₃ L₂ L₁ T₁₂ T₁₁

N.

Screwdriver

Detail of screw
head and double
set of nuts

P.

Derotation
lever

O.

Derotation
bar

Bone chips

Q.

Correction of
scoliosis by
compression
at convex side
of curve

Plate 245. (Continued)

Appendix

PLATE 246 **Trapezius Transfer for Shoulder Abduction**

Indications. Paralysis of deltoid and scapulocostal muscles when shoulder fusion cannot be performed to provide shoulder abduction.

Blood for Transfusion. Yes.

Radiographic Control. Yes.

Patient Position. Supine with the shoulder supported on a hand table.

Operative Technique

A. Make an incision beginning 5 cm. proximal to the center of the acromion, midway between the clavicle and the spine of the scapula. The excision extends distally to the acromion and the upper one quarter of the arm. Divide subcutaneous tissue and superficial fascia in line with the skin incision.

B. The trapezius muscle is isolated and completely detached from its attachments to the clavicle, acromion, and the spine of the scapula.

C. The trapezius muscle is undermined, elevated, and reflected proximally. Place three or four 0 Tycron sutures at the anterior, medial, and posterior ends of the trapezius. The deltoid muscle is split in its anterior one quarter. By sharp and dull dissection, the long head of the biceps brachii tendon is exposed.

D. The bicipital groove is subperiosteally exposed, and three or four drill holes are made. The 0 Tycron sutures are passed through the drill holes, and the center is laterally rotated and abducted 120 degrees. The trapezius tendon is transfixed to the upper humeral metaphysis lateral to the bicipital groove.

E. When the subscapularis and pectoralis major and minor muscles are functional and there is a medial rotation–lateral rotation muscle imbalance, the latissimus dorsi muscle is detached from its insertion and transferred to the rotator cuff at its insertion (see Plate 10, p. 64). When the anterior deltoid is good in motor strength and the middle and posterior deltoids are paralyzed, the anterior deltoid may be transferred posteriorly.

Close the wound in the routine fashion. The shoulder and operated upper limb are immobilized in a shoulder spica cast, with the shoulder in 120 degrees of abduction and neutral rotation.

Postoperative Care. Six weeks after surgery, the cast is removed and active-assisted and gentle passive exercises are performed to increase motor strength of the transferred muscle and range of motion of the shoulder.

REFERENCES

Gilbert, A.: Obstetrical brachial plexus palsy. In: Tubiana, R. (Ed.), The Hand. Philadelphia, W.B. Saunders Co., 1991, pp. 595–597.

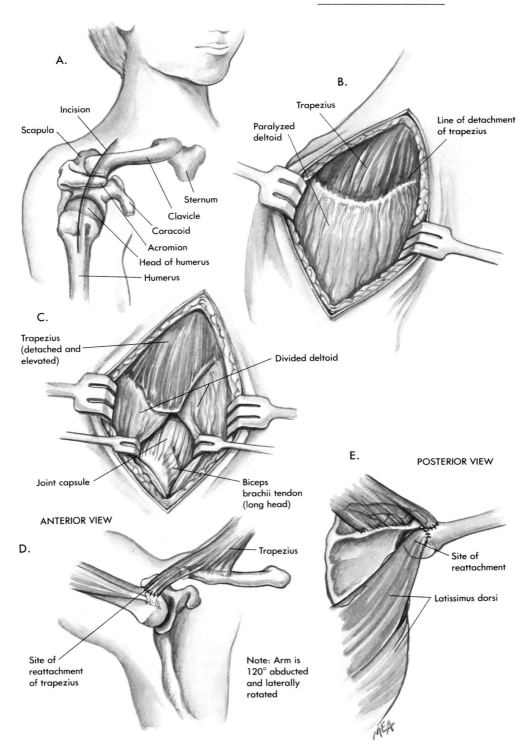

A.

Incision

Scapula

Sternum

Clavicle

Coracoid

Acromion

Head of humerus

Humerus

B.

Trapezius

Paralyzed deltoid

Line of detachment of trapezius

C.

Trapezius (detached and elevated)

Divided deltoid

Joint capsule

Biceps brachii tendon (long head)

ANTERIOR VIEW

D.

Trapezius

Site of reattachment of trapezius

Note: Arm is 120° abducted and laterally rotated

E.

POSTERIOR VIEW

Site of reattachment

Latissimus dorsi

Plate 246. A.–E., Trapezius transfer for shoulder abduction.

PLATE 247 **Surgical Exposure and Epiphyseodesis of Triradiate Cartilage of the Acetabulum (Steel Technique)**

Indications

1. Biopsy or excision of tumors of the acetabular region, such as osteoid osteoma.

2. Epiphyseodesis of the triradiate cartilage of the acetabulum to checkrein progression of intrapelvic protrusion (Otto pelvis) such as in Marfan's syndrome.

Blood for Transfusion. Yes.

Radiographic Control. Image intensifier.

Patient Position. Supine.

Operative Technique

A. The incision begins at the juncture of the middle and distal one third of the iliac crest, extending toward the anterior superior iliac spine and curving anteriorly and medially toward the symphysis pubis. Subcutaneous tissue is divided in line with the skin incision. Superficial fascia is incised, and the cartilaginous apophysis of the iliac crest is exposed.

B. The cartilaginous apophysis is split and retracted medially and laterally, exposing the iliac crest. The inguinal ligament is sectioned to the anterior superior iliac spine.

C. The cartilaginous iliac apophysis is transversely divided at one or two levels for release of tension and facilitation of medial retraction of the iliacus muscle. The inner wall of the ilium and anterior inferior iliac spine and superior ramus of the pubis are subperiosteally exposed.

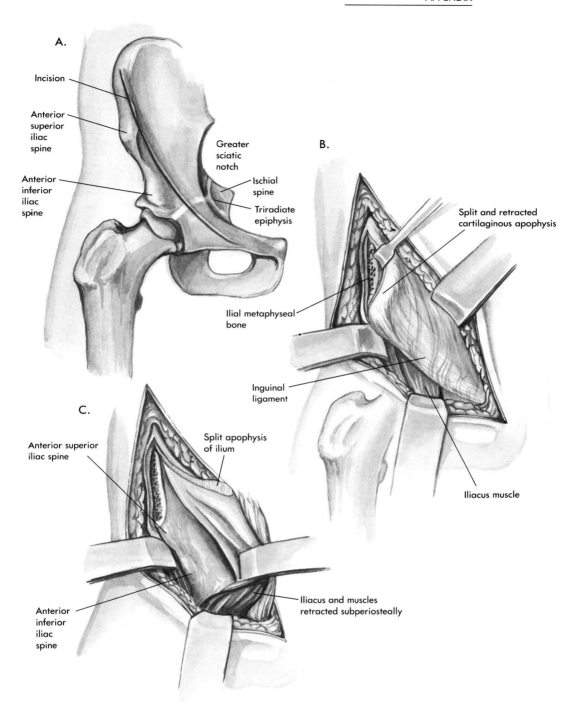

A.

Incision

Anterior superior iliac spine

Anterior inferior iliac spine

Greater sciatic notch

Ischial spine

Triradiate epiphysis

Ilial metaphyseal bone

B.

Split and retracted cartilaginous apophysis

Inguinal ligament

Iliacus muscle

C.

Anterior superior iliac spine

Split apophysis of ilium

Anterior inferior iliac spine

Iliacus and muscles retracted subperiosteally

Plate 247. **A.–I.,** Surgical exposure and epiphyseodesis of triradiate cartilage of the acetabulum (Steel technique).

D. The hip is abducted, flexed, and laterally rotated, and a Chandler retractor is inserted into the greater sciatic notch. A blunt right angle retractor is used for medially retracting the iliopsoas muscle. The triradiate cartilage is exposed.

Caution! Do not injure the obturator vessels or the femoral nerve and vessels medially.

E. and **F.** Under image intensifier radiographic control and with the help of a K-wire, determine the exact site and extent of the triradiate cartilage and then drill it with a burr.

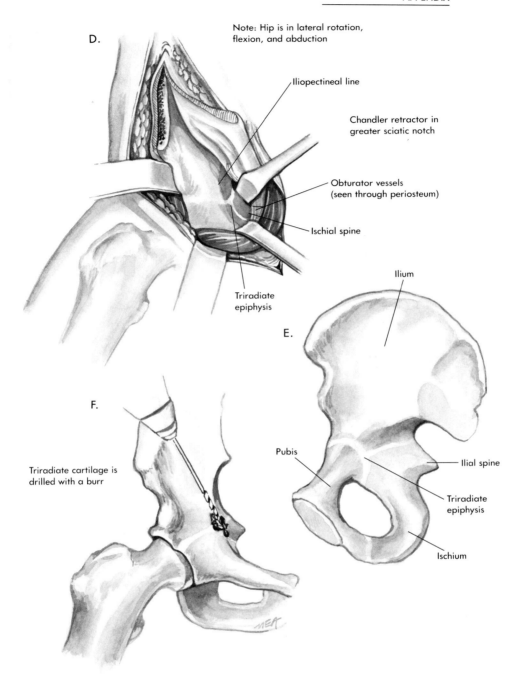

D.

Note: Hip is in lateral rotation, flexion, and abduction

Iliopectineal line

Chandler retractor in greater sciatic notch

Obturator vessels (seen through periosteum)

Ischial spine

Triradiate epiphysis

E.

Ilium

Pubis

Ilial spine

Triradiate epiphysis

Ischium

F.

Triradiate cartilage is drilled with a burr

Plate 247. (Continued)

G. and **H.** With the help of curved sharp osteotomes, remove a rectangular piece of the inner plate of the acetabulum. Do not enter the hip joint. Harvest an autogenous bone graft of appropriate size and shape from the inner wall of the ilium, and firmly insert it into the rectangular defect on the inner wall of the acetabulum. Note the thinness of the acetabular floor. *Do not penetrate the hip joint!*

I. The inguinal ligament is reattached to the anterior superior iliac spine, and the split cartilaginous iliac apophysis is firmly sutured. Close the wound in the usual fashion.

Postoperative Care. Immobilization in a hip spica cast is not ordinarily required. Place the patient in counterpoised, bilateral, split Russell's traction for comfort. Range of motion exercises are performed several times a day, and the patient is allowed to ambulate with a three-point crutch gait protecting the operated lower limb for a period of six weeks until the graft has solidified.

REFERENCE

Steel, H. H.: Personal communication, 1993.

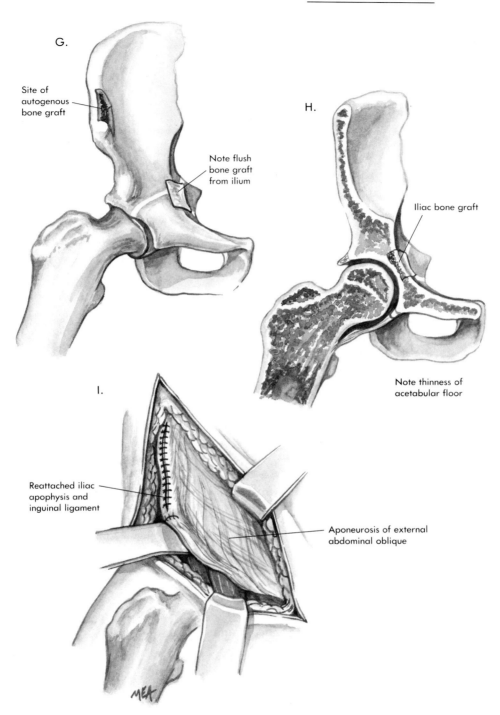

G.

Site of
autogenous
bone graft

Note flush
bone graft
from ilium

H.

Iliac bone graft

Note thinness of
acetabular floor

I.

Reattached iliac
apophysis and
inguinal ligament

Aponeurosis of external
abdominal oblique

MEA

Plate 247. (Continued)

PLATE 248   ### Arthrodiatasis of the Hip Using the Orthofix Articulated Body

Arthrodiatasis is a procedure developed by surgeons in Verona, Italy. In this procedure, the hip joint is distracted by the use of the Orthofix articulating body, which crosses the hip joint. The contracted muscles, ligamentous tissues, and capsule are stretched, distracting the femoral head from the acetabulum. An external hinge, located laterally and parallel to the center of the axis of the hip joint, allows hip motion in the sagittal plane. The creation of a space between the bony surfaces, with reduction of mechanical stress and the preservation or restoration of movement, attempts to improve the synovial circulation and encourage fibrous repair of the articular cartilage without the formation of adhesions. Open surgery to release soft-tissue contractures or to improve joint congruity (through limited arthroplasty) may be required to facilitate movement; it may be combined with osteotomy.

Indications

1. Marked stiffness of the hip joint.
2. Contractural deformity due to chondrolysis.
3. Avascular necrosis.
4. Incongruity of the hip caused by collapse of the femoral head secondary to avascular necrosis, fracture dislocation, and rheumatoid arthritis.

Other Indications. The apparatus can be used as a means of external fixation for pathologic fractures of the femur, such as through a unicameral bone cyst. The technique and apparatus can also be used for hip fusion. In this case, an articulated body is not used.

Special Equipment

1. Orthofix Dynamic Axial Fixator, Model 10.000.
2. One T-clamp, Model 10.007.
3. One articulated body, Model 10.022.
4. Four cortical screws, 6/5 mm. in diameter. Determine the overall screw length and thread length preoperatively using the patient's x-ray films and the Orthofix overlay screw template. For thread length, approximately 5 mm. of screw thread should remain outside the entry cortex and 2 mm. should project beyond the second cortex.
5. Guide template for the articulated body, Model 11.136.
6. Standard instrumentation together with the guide template, Model 11.101 for the standard fixator, Model 10.000, applied fully closed.
7. One 2-mm. diameter Kirschner wire.

Note. When applying the standard fixator, with the body fully closed and using the T-clamp and articulated body, make sure that the minimum distance between the outer screws is 22.6 cm.

Preoperative Measures. Anteroposterior and lateral radiograms of the hip and proximal femur are made, including a computed tomography (CT) scan of the hip joint and a magnetic resonance imaging (MRI) study, if available. These studies are performed to assess the congruence of the hip joint, the quality and structural strength of the ilium, and the length and position of screws to be inserted.

Blood for Transfusion. Yes.

Radiographic Control. Image intensifier.

Patient Position. Supine on a fracture table.

Operative Technique. Using general anesthesia, test the range of motion of the hip. If the hip joint is fixed with marked contracture of the soft tissues, an open soft-tissue release is indicated.

A. Place the patient on a fracture table with the hip in 10 degrees of abduction, if possible. Place the knee in neutral position to visualize the ilium, head of the femur, and proximal femoral shaft in the anteroposterior (AP) projection. If functional exploration of the bone or core decompression is contemplated, obtain a lateral image of the head and neck of the femur. The pelvis, hip, and thigh are then prepared and draped.

B. Under image intensifier radiographic control, determine the axis of flexion-extension of the hip by inserting a 2-mm. Kirschner wire from the greater trochanter into the center of the femoral head perpendicular to the longitudinal axis of the femur.

C. Align the hinge of the articulated body with the axis of flexion-extension of the hip. Slide the hole in the center of the guide template for the articulated body over the Kirschner wire.

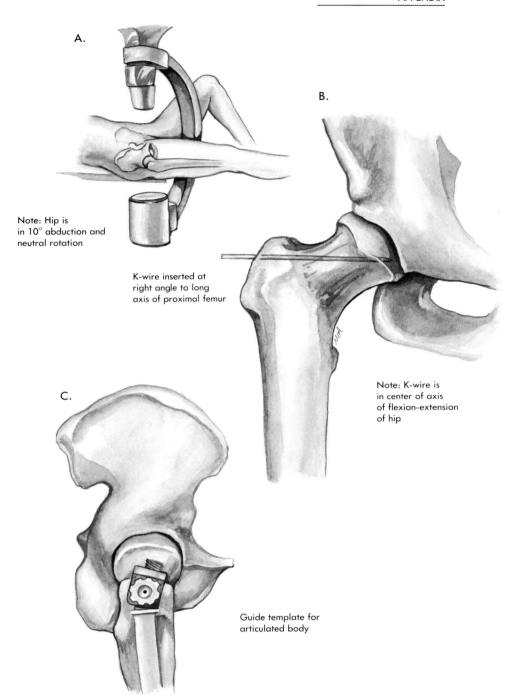

A.

Note: Hip is
in 10° abduction and
neutral rotation

K-wire inserted at
right angle to long
axis of proximal femur

B.

Note: K-wire is
in center of axis
of flexion-extension
of hip

C.

Guide template for
articulated body

Plate 248. **A.–Q.**, Arthrodiatasis of the hip using the Orthofix articulated body.

D. and **E.** Select and mark the sites of insertion of the pelvic and femoral screws. This is guided by the use of template clamps—a T-clamp template for the pelvis and a straight clamp template for the femur.

First, insert the pelvic screws. The site of insertion should be immediately superior to the acetabulum, where the bone is thick, thus providing more secure fixation. It is vital that the pelvic screws be placed correctly in order to prevent loosening of the screws and removal of the Orthofix apparatus, which would result in discontinuation of treatment. In adolescents and adults, with a large ilium screw, use seats 1, 2, and 4 or 2, 4, and 5. In children with a small pelvis and inadequate space for three screws, insert two screws. It is crucial to use image intensifier radiographic control in the AP, oblique, and lateral projections.

Mark the sites of the femoral screws with a straight clamp template. These sites should be as far distal as possible. Three screws provide more stable fixation.

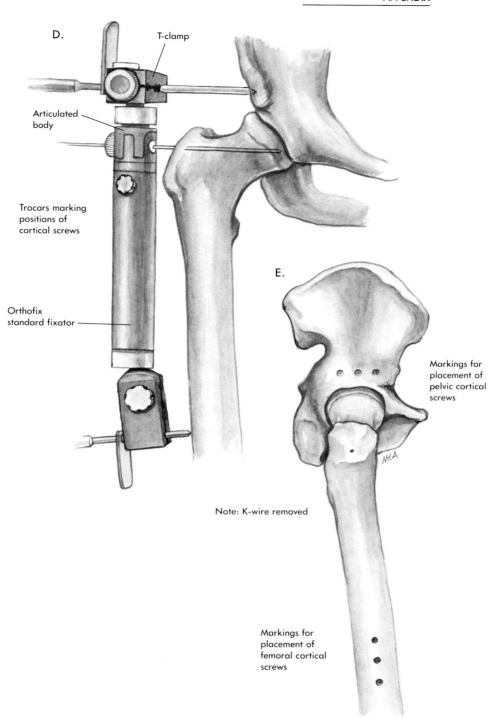

D.

T-clamp

Articulated body

Trocars marking positions of cortical screws

Orthofix standard fixator

E.

Markings for placement of pelvic cortical screws

Note: K-wire removed

Markings for placement of femoral cortical screws

Plate 248. (Continued)

F. and **G.** After selecting and marking the screw sites for the pelvis and femur, insert the pelvic screws first. With a sharp scalpel, make a 6- to 10-mm. longitudinal incision in the skin at the most anterior pin site. With sharp tenotomy and dull Metzenbaum scissors, spread the soft tissues down to the outer wall of the ilium medially.

A 100-mm.-long screw guide and trocar are inserted medially under image intensifier radiographic control through the incision and wound to touch the outer wall of the ilium. The trocar and screw guide tend to slip posteriorly as a result of the obliquity of the pelvic wall. Double-check the position of the trocar by use of image intensifier radiography. Remove the trocar. With a hammer, tap the screw guide so that its teeth engage the lateral cortex of the ilium.

Next, insert an 80-mm.-long, 4.8-mm. drill guide in the screw guide. Then insert a long (240-mm.) drill bit into the drill guide, and drill both the outer and inner table of the ilium.

The resistance of the cortical bone will be felt during penetration of the outer and inner walls of the iliac bone. Image intensifier radiographic control and the use of a drill stop prevent overpenetration of the inner table of the ilium.

Remove the drill bit and the drill guide, and insert a long cortical screw using a T-wrench. Once the resistance of the inner cortical wall of the ilium is felt, check its position by image intensifier radiogram and give the T-wrench six half-turns.

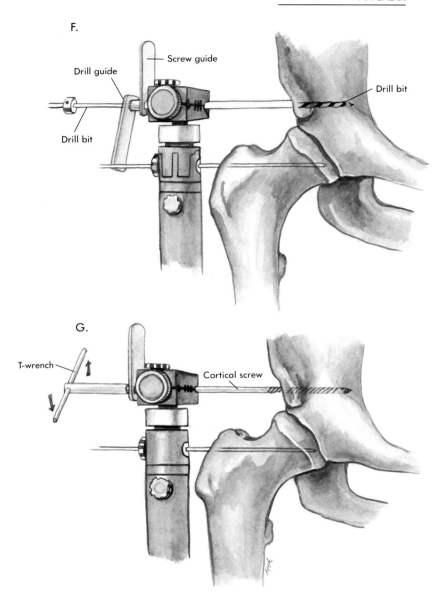

F.

Drill guide

Screw guide

Drill bit

Drill bit

G.

T-wrench

Cortical screw

Plate 248. (Continued)

H. Insert the second and third screws in the pubis in the same manner as the first screw.

I. Next, with the pelvic screw in place, fully close the template and determine the site of the distal three femoral screws. As stated previously, use a straight template clamp for the femoral screws. The steps and technique of insertion of femoral screws are similar to those for the pelvic screws. The site of insertion for the femoral screws must be as distal as possible in the mid diaphysis. Insert the femoral screws through screw seats 1, 3, and 5 of the straight clamp template in a plane 15 degrees anterior to the lateral plane. Two or three threads of the tip of the screw should protrude from the medial cortex of the femur, and three or four threads of the screw should remain outside the lateral cortex. Verify the proper position and length of the cortical screws by image intensifier radiography.

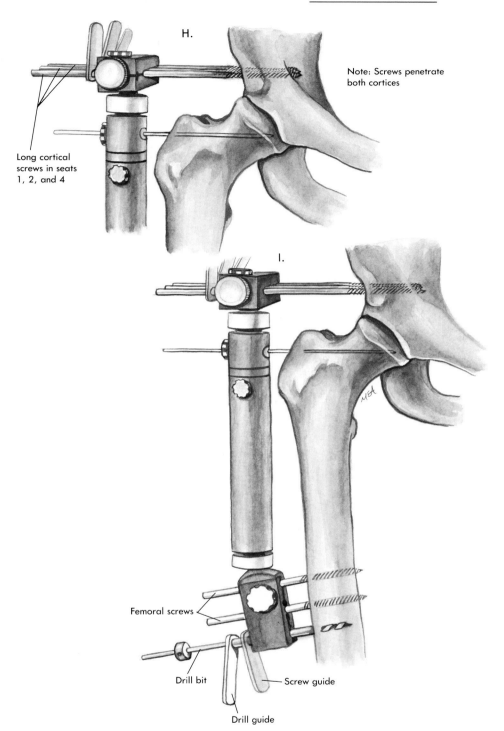

H.

Note: Screws penetrate
both cortices

Long cortical
screws in seats
1, 2, and 4

I.

Femoral screws

Drill bit

Screw guide

Drill guide

Plate 248. (Continued)

J. Remove the template and the Kirschner wire. Apply the permanent Orthofix articulating body apparatus through the pelvic and femoral screws.

K. To provide more stability and secure fixation of the pelvic component, drill and insert two cortical screws through the iliac crest into the ilium and attach them to the protruding ends of the pelvic screws.

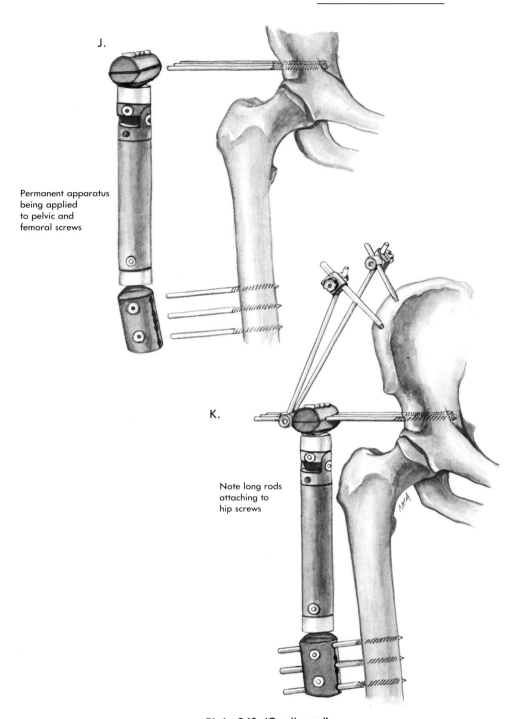

J.

Permanent apparatus
being applied
to pelvic and
femoral screws

K.

Note long rods
attaching to
hip screws

Plate 248. (Continued)

L. and **L1.** Tighten the screw clamps and ball-joint cams with an Allen wrench. Next, with a pre-set torque wrench, lock the cams.

M. Then apply the compression-distraction device with one of its legs in the cam hole of the distal female body and its other leg in the hole of the articulating body, distal to the hinge so that the articulating body is free to move.

Distract the compression-distraction unit 15 full turns with an Allen wrench. This will result in 15 mm. of distraction, which will separate the subchondral bones of the femoral head and acetabulum (hip joint space) 5 mm.

Flex the hip and knee 90 degrees, and check whether there is tension on the skin and puckering of the soft tissues at the screw sites. Perform further soft-tissue release as necessary.

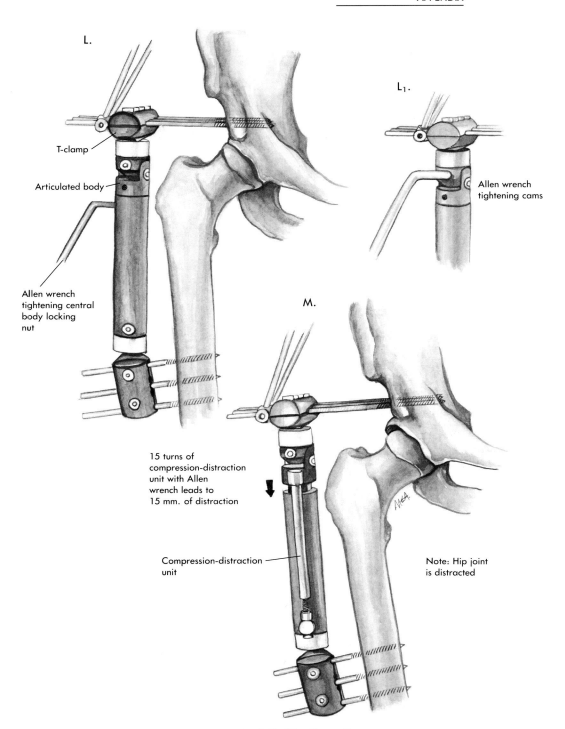

L.

T-clamp

Articulated body

Allen wrench
tightening central
body locking
nut

L₁.

Allen wrench
tightening cams

M.

15 turns of
compression-distraction
unit with Allen
wrench leads to
15 mm. of distraction

Compression-distraction
unit

Note: Hip joint
is distracted

Plate 248. (Continued)

N. Determine the range of motion of the hip. When passive range of hip motion is adequate, the central body locking unit is tightened and the compression-distraction device is removed, making the apparatus lighter and less cumbersome.

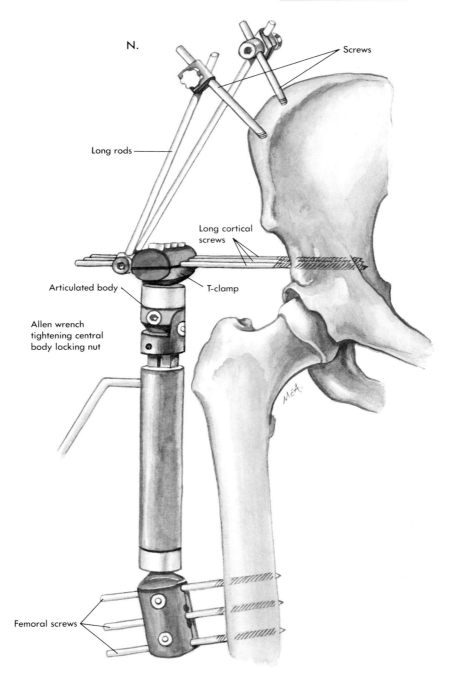

N.

Screws

Long rods

Long cortical
screws

Articulated body

T-clamp

Allen wrench
tightening central
body locking nut

Femoral screws

Plate 248. (Continued)

O1. and **O2.** Do not mistake movement between the lumbar spine and pelvis with that occurring at the hip joint. Perform a Thomas test, and inspect for motion at the hip. If the lower limb moves but the articulated body does not, the motion is taking place between the pelvis and lumbar spine, not at the hip. Obtain radiograms of the hip to determine the position and proper placement of the hinge.

Restricted range of hip motion may be due to tension of muscle and soft tissues under distraction, improper position of the hinge, or incongruity of the hip joint. First, decrease the distraction force and test the range of hip motion. If it improves, perform appropriate soft-tissue release while the patient is still under general anesthesia.

If the range does not improve after reduction of distraction, make radiograms of the hips to determine the position of the hinge; it should be in the center of the axis of flexion-extension of the hip. If the placement of the hinge is incorrect and cannot be corrected, remove the fixator and re-start the whole procedure from the beginning. When bony incongruity of the hip is the cause of poor motion, perform osteoplasty of the femoral head and/or of the acetabulum by open surgery.

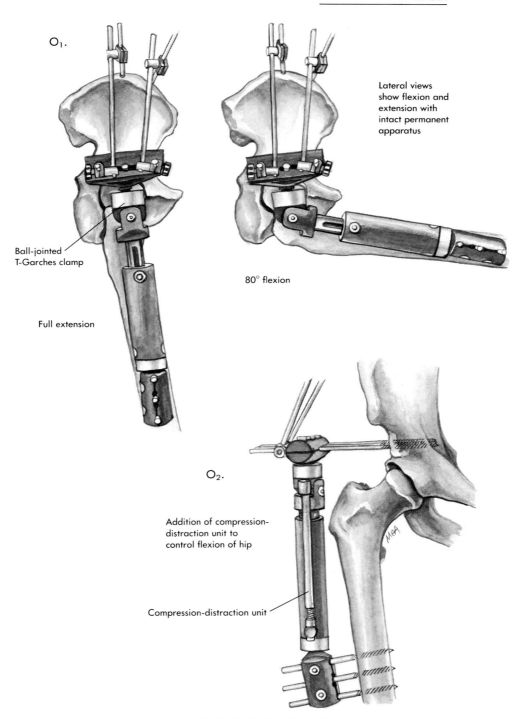

O₁.

Ball-jointed
T-Garches clamp

Full extension

Lateral views
show flexion and
extension with
intact permanent
apparatus

80° flexion

O₂.

Addition of compression-
distraction unit to
control flexion of hip

Compression-distraction unit

Plate 248. (Continued)

O3. and **O4.** When flexion of the hip is a problem and control is required, reattach the compression-distraction device across the articulating body by inserting the legs of the device into the holes in the proximal and distal cams with the fixator in a straight line.

Postoperative Care

Hip Motion. The goal of treatment is to restore and maintain maximum range of hip motion. To achieve this, it is crucial to control postoperative pain and voluntary or involuntary protective muscle spasm. Therefore, during the first two to four postsurgical days, use epidural or patient-controlled analgesia to control pain.

Immediately after surgery, place the patient in a continuous passive motion (CPM) machine. The machine flexes and extends the hip in an arc of motion more or less similar to that obtained at the end of the surgical procedure. When the range of motion is lost or poor because of tension of muscles and soft tissues, reduce the degree of hip distraction until satisfactory range of hip motion is obtained. Afterward, the hip is gradually distracted at the rate of 0.5 mm. per day by the distraction-compression apparatus until 5 mm. of distraction is achieved, as demonstrated by radiograms made with the hip in neutral extension.

Malposition of the hinge (i.e., not in the center of the axis of hip flexion-extension) and anatomic incongruency of the hip are other causes of poor range of hip motion. These causes should have been detected previously in the operating room and rectified by proper placement of the hinge and open surgery of the hip.

Physical Therapy. Intensive therapy (active-assisted and passive range of hip motion and muscle strengthening exercises) are performed several hours a day.

Weight Bearing. Weight bearing is not allowed because it causes loosening of the pelvic screws. The fixator is not dynamized throughout the postoperative course.

Pin Site Care. Instruct the patient and parents (if the patient is a child) to clean the pin sites once or twice a day. With sterile water and sterile cotton swabs, the pin sites are meticulously cleansed and a dry absorbent dressing with a gauze pad is applied around the pins next to the skin. Some serous drainage from the screw sites, particularly around the pelvic region, is common; it should not be mistaken for infection. This drainage is caused by soft-tissue mobility of the skin and soft tissues around the screws. Such serous drainage usually responds to a decrease in patient mobility and meticulous pin site care.

If inflammation develops, with red and warm screw sites draining purulent material, perform bacteriologic studies and administer appropriate antibiotics for 7 to 14 days. If screw site infection does not respond to such outpatient measures, admit the patient to the hospital and give intravenous antibiotic therapy with local débridement of the wound. Removal of the screw or screws and even removal of the fixator may be required. The pelvic screws are ordinarily the site of infection.

Removal of the Fixator. Hip distraction and passive and active movement of the hip are required for six to ten weeks. During this period, the patient should not bear weight on the affected lower limb.

Remove the fixator and screws using general anesthesia on an outpatient basis. I often recommend wound revision at the screw sites in order to provide a hairline scar. The patient is allowed to bear partial weight with crutches. Crutch protection is continued for three to six months after removal of the fixator. Intensive physical therapy is continued. It takes one to two months to change the hip motion from simple hinge to ball-and-socket. I recommend the continuous, around-the-world passive hip motion machine.

REFERENCE

Trivella, G., and Saleh, M.: Operative Technique. Arthrodiatasis. EBI Medical Systems, Parsippany, N.J.

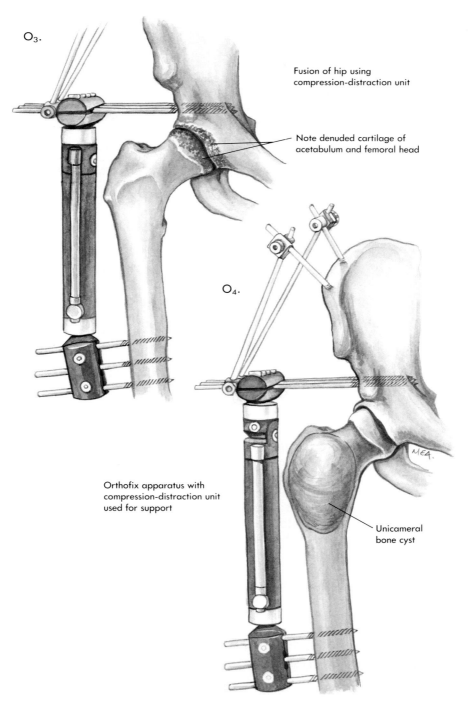

O₃.

Fusion of hip using
compression-distraction unit

Note denuded cartilage of
acetabulum and femoral head

O₄.

Orthofix apparatus with
compression-distraction unit
used for support

Unicameral
bone cyst

Plate 248. (Continued)

PLATE 249   **Proximal Resection of the Femur and Modified Van Nes Rotation-Plasty for Limb Salvage (Carroll Technique)**

Indications. Malignant bone tumors, such as osteosarcomas involving the proximal femur.

Staging with a bone scan using technetium 99m (^{99m}Tc) CT scan, and MRI should be performed prior to surgery. There should be no pulmonary or other metastases and no involvement of the neurovascular structures. The distal third of the femur should be tumor-free and normal.

Preoperative chemotherapy with agents such as methotrexate and citrovarum factor is given by the oncologist.

Blood for Transfusion. Yes.

Radiographic Control. Yes.

Patient Position. Prone, lateral, and supine. Insert a Foley catheter into the bladder. Seal the genitalia and anus with impervious drapes. Initially, the patient is placed in the lateral decubitus position. The entire lower limb, pelvis, abdomen, and thorax, to the nipple level from midline anterior to midline posterior, are prepared. The draping should be meticulous; one should be able to roll the patient from the initial prone position to supine position later on during the procedure.

Operative Technique

Step I

The patient is in the semi-prone position. A sterile pneumatic tourniquet is applied on the proximal thigh, as high as possible. The lower limb is elevated (but not exsanguinated because of the tumor) and the pneumatic tourniquet is inflated to 250 or 300 mm. Hg.

A. Make a midline longitudinal incision beginning at the posterior knee crease and extending proximally as far as the inferior margin of the tourniquet. Later on, the tourniquet will be removed and the longitudinal incision will extend to the subnatal crease and then laterally to make an inverted "L" for exposure of the insertion of the gluteus maximus. Divide the subcutaneous tissue and superficial fascia in line with the skin incision.

B. and **C.** Identify and free the sciatic nerve from the surrounding tissue, and free its common peroneal and tibial branches. Identify and distally section the biceps femoris and medial hamstrings—the gracilis, the semitendinosus, and the semimembranosus. Leave enough length of a stump of the tendons; tag them with 0 Tycron (or other nonabsorbable) suture; later they will be reattached to the iliopsoas tendon.

By blunt and sharp dissection, free the popliteal artery and vein as far proximally as possible to the adductor hiatus and Hunter's canal. Identify and ligate the vascular branches of the thigh musculature.

Pack the wound with moist lap sponges, and apply a compression dressing with an Ace bandage. Release the tourniquet, and obtain complete hemostasis.

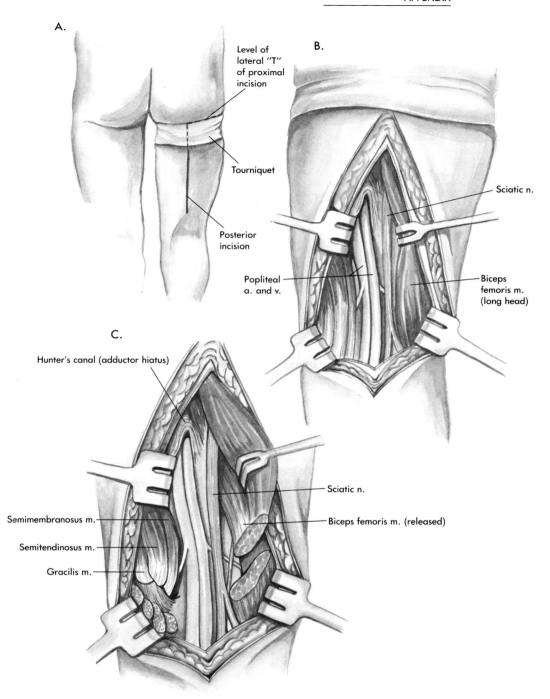

A.

Level of
lateral "T"
of proximal
incision

Tourniquet

Posterior
incision

B.

Sciatic n.

Popliteal
a. and v.

Biceps
femoris m.
(long head)

C.

Hunter's canal (adductor hiatus)

Sciatic n.

Biceps femoris m. (released)

Semimembranosus m.

Semitendinosus m.

Gracilis m.

Plate 249. **A.–Y.**, Proximal resection of the femur and modified Van Nes rotation-plasty for limb salvage.

D. Extend the midline longitudinal incision to the subnatal crease where it curves laterally to the lateral upper thigh. The subcutaneous tissue and superficial fascia are divided in line with the skin incision, and the wound flaps are undermined, elevated, and retracted to their respective sides.

E. Identify the gluteus maximus tendon, and section it near its insertion to the femur. At this time, perform a biopsy and frozen section of the gluteus maximus tendon near its insertion to ensure that it is tumor-free. By dull dissection, elevate and proximally retract the gluteus maximus. Identify the origin of the hamstring muscles at the ischial tuberosity and the sciatic nerve and superior and inferior gluteal vessels as they exit at the greater sciatic notch.

Step II

At this point, the patient is turned over into the complete supine position.

F. The anterior skin incision begins 3 to 4 cm. proximal to the anterior superior iliac spine; it then extends distally and medially 2 to 3 cm. inferior to the iliac crest and inguinal ligament across the femoral triangle to a point where the pulsations of the femoral artery are palpable. The skin incision is extended distally and medially along the course of the femoral artery to join the posterior incision at the Hunter's canal. Excise the biopsy incision with the tumor-involved ablated segment of the proximal femur; make appropriate modification of the skin incision to incorporate it and the wound area employed for biopsy.

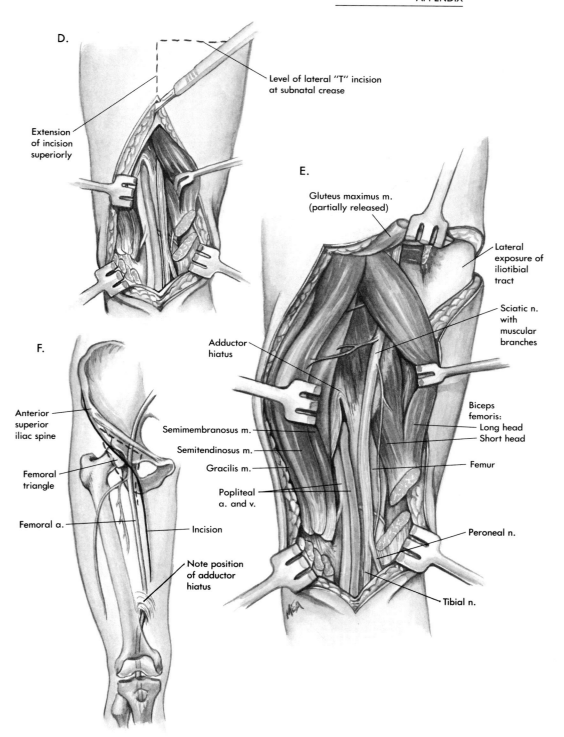

D.

Level of lateral "T" incision at subnatal crease

Extension of incision superiorly

E.

Gluteus maximus m. (partially released)

Lateral exposure of iliotibial tract

Sciatic n. with muscular branches

Adductor hiatus

F.

Anterior superior iliac spine

Femoral triangle

Femoral a.

Semimembranosus m.

Semitendinosus m.

Gracilis m.

Popliteal a. and v.

Incision

Note position of adductor hiatus

Biceps femoris:
Long head
Short head

Femur

Peroneal n.

Tibial n.

Plate 249. (Continued)

G. and **H.** The sartorius muscle is identified, mobilized, and retracted laterally. Medial to the sartorius muscle are the femoral nerve and vessels.

The profundus femoris vessels, as they branch off from the femoral artery and vein and the femoral circumflex vessels, are identified, clamped, and ligated. All of the muscular branches of the femoral artery and veins are freed, clamped, and ligated.

Next, the femoral artery and vein are completely freed and mobilized from the pelvic rim, through Hunter's canal to the popliteal fossa. The femoral nerve is identified and retracted laterally.

Then the hip is flexed, abducted, and laterally rotated. The adductor longus, adductor brevis, pectineus, and gracilis muscles are divided with electrocautery near their origin. The obturator nerve and vessels with their anterior and posterior branches are identified and retracted out of harm's way. Next, the adductor magnus is sectioned with electrocautery near its origin at the proximal level of the anterior skin incision.

I. Connect the anterior and posterior incisions by posterolaterally extending the anterior incision and anteromedially extending the posterior incision. The subcutaneous tissue and superficial fascia are divided in line with the skin incision. The proximal wound flap is undermined, elevated, and retracted superiorly.

Identify the sartorius muscle, and detach it distally; preserve it proximally (at least 10 cm. of length) with its origin and neurovascular supply intact.

Identify the femoral nerve at the pelvic brim. Pull it distally, and pass a suture around the proximal segment of the nerve to prevent bleeding from its vessels. Then section it sharply with a new scalpel.

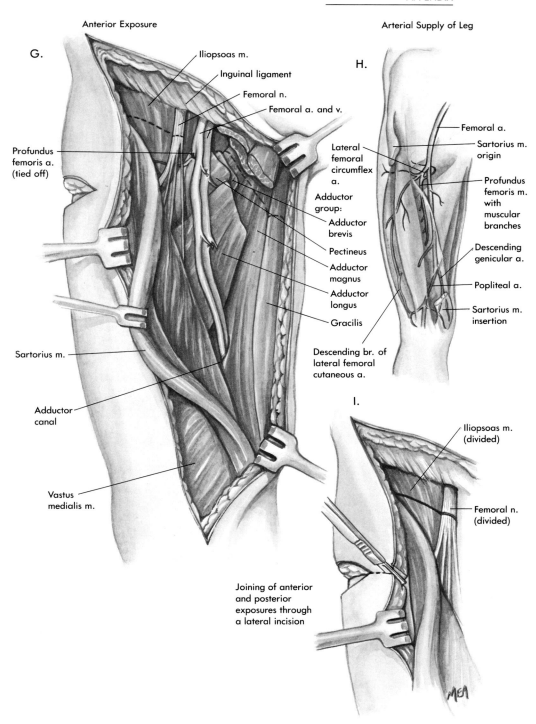

Anterior Exposure

Arterial Supply of Leg

G.

Iliopsoas m.

Inguinal ligament

Femoral n.

Femoral a. and v.

Profundus femoris a. (tied off)

Lateral femoral circumflex a.

Adductor group:

Adductor brevis

Pectineus

Adductor magnus

Adductor longus

Gracilis

Descending br. of lateral femoral cutaneous a.

Sartorius m.

Adductor canal

Vastus medialis m.

H.

Femoral a.

Sartorius m. origin

Profundus femoris m. with muscular branches

Descending genicular a.

Popliteal a.

Sartorius m. insertion

I.

Iliopsoas m. (divided)

Femoral n. (divided)

Joining of anterior and posterior exposures through a lateral incision

Plate 249. (Continued)

J. and **K.** The iliopsoas tendon is identified and traced to its insertion to the lesser trochanter. Tag the tendon with 0 Tycron (or other nonabsorbable) suture, and section the tendon near its insertion. Obtain a biopsy specimen of the distal end of the iliopsoas tendon, and study it by frozen section for tumor cells at the margin.

Identify and section both straight and indirect heads of origin of the rectus femoris.

Flex, abduct, and laterally rotate the hip. In the anteromedial aspect of the wound, identify the obturator vessels and nerve—their anterior and posterior branches. Tie off the vessels, and sharply divide the nerves.

L. With an electrocautery knife, section the gluteus medius and minimus off the greater trochanter, and divide the tensor fasciae latae and vastus lateralis. Elevate these muscles as a soft-tissue flap with the posterolateral skin flap.

M. In the posterior wound, identify and leave the sciatic nerve and its branches intact.

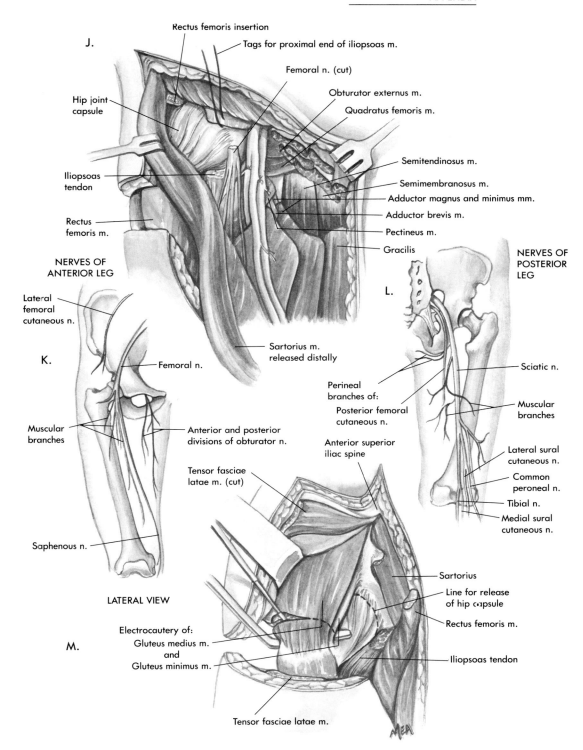

J.

Rectus femoris insertion

Tags for proximal end of iliopsoas m.

Femoral n. (cut)

Obturator externus m.

Quadratus femoris m.

Hip joint capsule

Iliopsoas tendon

Rectus femoris m.

Semitendinosus m.

Semimembranosus m.

Adductor magnus and minimus mm.

Adductor brevis m.

Pectineus m.

Gracilis

Sartorius m. released distally

NERVES OF ANTERIOR LEG

NERVES OF POSTERIOR LEG

Lateral femoral cutaneous n.

K.

Femoral n.

Muscular branches

Anterior and posterior divisions of obturator n.

Saphenous n.

LATERAL VIEW

L.

Perineal branches of:

Posterior femoral cutaneous n.

Sciatic n.

Muscular branches

Lateral sural cutaneous n.

Common peroneal n.

Tibial n.

Medial sural cutaneous n.

Anterior superior iliac spine

Tensor fasciae latae m. (cut)

M.

Electrocautery of: Gluteus medius m. and Gluteus minimus m.

Tensor fasciae latae m.

Sartorius

Line for release of hip capsule

Rectus femoris m.

Iliopsoas tendon

Plate 249. (Continued)

N. Palpate the hip joint capsule, and divide it along the acetabular rim medially, anteriorly, and as far posterolaterally as possible.

Caution! Do not injure the sciatic nerve.

O. Rotate the hip joint medially, and divide the short lateral rotators with electrocautery—the piriformis, superior gemellus, obturator internus, inferior gemellus, and quadratus femoris. Protect the sciatic nerve.

Caution! Do not inadvertently divide the neurovascular structures.

P. Rotate the hip laterally, and identify and section the ligamentum teres.

Next, dislocate the hip and section the remaining posterior capsule and inferior capsule of the hip joint.

Obtain a biopsy specimen of the capsule of the hip joint and ligamentum teres. Perform frozen section and histologic studies to ensure that the margins are free of tumor.

During manipulation and dislocation of the hip, it is vital to keep the tension off the femoral vessels and not to twist them. Monitor the distal pulses with a sterile Doppler flow detector. Intermittently drip warm saline solution with 1 per cent lidocaine without epinephrine onto the vessel to prevent vessel spasm.

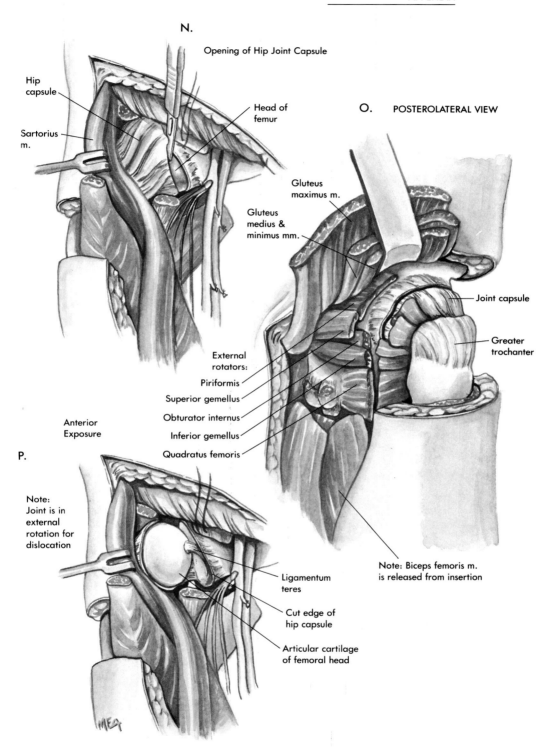

N.

Opening of Hip Joint Capsule

Hip capsule

Sartorius m.

Head of femur

O.   POSTEROLATERAL VIEW

Gluteus maximus m.

Gluteus medius & minimus mm.

External rotators:

Piriformis

Superior gemellus

Obturator internus

Inferior gemellus

Quadratus femoris

Anterior Exposure

Joint capsule

Greater trochanter

P.

Note: Joint is in external rotation for dislocation

Ligamentum teres

Cut edge of hip capsule

Articular cartilage of femoral head

Note: Biceps femoris m. is released from insertion

Plate 249. (Continued)

Q. Measure the level of osteotomy of the distal femur from the knee joint line, which allows adequate tumor-free distal margin. Ordinarily, it is necessary to preserve only 5 to 7 cm. of the distal femur.

Make a circumferential incision through the skin, subcutaneous tissue, and superficial fascia.

R. Identify the rectus femoris tendon, and tag it with 0 Tycron suture for later repair. Then, beginning medially, divide the vastus medialis, rectus femoris, vastus intermedius, and vastus lateralis muscles. Protect and do not injure the neurovascular structures.

Next, divide the periosteum at the intended level of the section of the femur and strip the periosteum distally for 1 cm. With an oscillating power saw (or a Gigli saw), cut the distal femoral shaft.

At this time, obtain a biopsy specimen of the bone marrow proximally and also the distal femoral stump histologically. Study the samples with frozen section to be sure that they are tumor-free.

With the hip dislocated and the femur osteotomized distally, completely remove the upper four fifths of the femoral segment from the wound, with the hip adductors, quadriceps femoris, and hamstring muscles all attached to it.

With the proximal femoral resection completed, left behind are the femoral vessels and the sciatic nerve running from the pelvis to the distal stump. Gently bring the distal femoral stump with the attached knee and leg close to the pelvis to take the tension off the femoral vessels.

S. Expose the acetabulum, and with the help of gouges and curets, remove all articular cartilage from the acetabulum, exposing cancellous bone.

T. Protect the sciatic nerve and femoral vessels, and gently rotate the lower limb externally. Check the fit of the lateral femoral condyle into the acetabulum. Check circulation of the leg and foot with a sterile Doppler flow detector.

Make a step-cut of the remaining distal femoral shaft. Decorticate the lateral wall of the ilium above the acetabulum. With a gouge, prepare a bed on the anterolateral aspect of the ilium to receive the "tailored step-cut" distal femoral stump. The lateral femoral condyle is denuded of articular cartilage and placed into the prepared bed of the acetabulum. The step of the distal femoral metaphysis is placed against the lateral wall of the ilium and transfixed with three cancellous screws.

The patella may be excised extraperiosteally and denuded of all cartilage and soft tissue, cut into small pieces, and used as bone graft to fill any gaps between the 180-degree rotated distal femur and acetabulum. Autogenous bone can be harvested from the ilium as an alternate source of bone graft.

Radiograms are made to determine the position of the screws and the fit of the distal femoral stump into the acetabulum.

The femoral vessels are now anterior and have excessive length with shortening of the femur. The sciatic nerve is brought anteriorly with 180 degrees of lateral rotation of the leg.

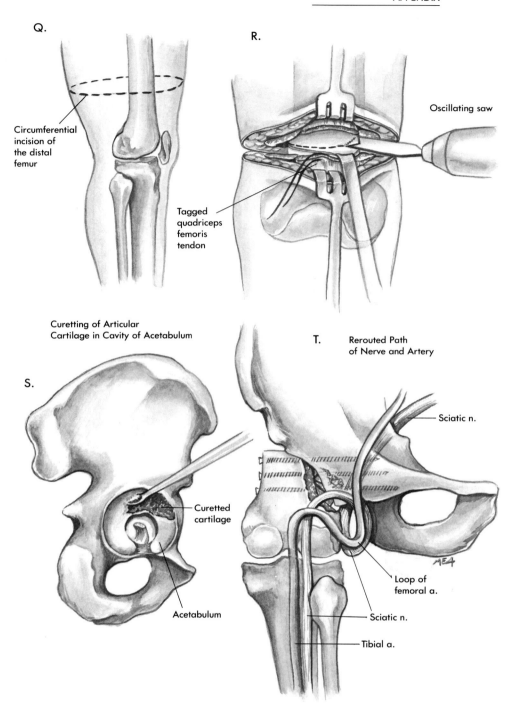

Q.

Circumferential
incision of
the distal
femur

R.

Oscillating saw

Tagged
quadriceps
femoris
tendon

Curetting of Articular
Cartilage in Cavity of Acetabulum

S.

Curetted
cartilage

Acetabulum

T.   Rerouted Path
of Nerve and Artery

Sciatic n.

Loop of
femoral a.

Sciatic n.

Tibial a.

Plate 249. (Continued)

U. The gluteus maximus is sutured to the rectus femoris tendon, which is now located posteriorly to act as a "hip" extensor.

V. The *iliopsoas tendon* is now sutured to the *biceps femoris* and *semimembranosus tendon* (which are now located anteriorly) to provide *flexion* of the "hip." The distal end of the sartorius is sutured to its origin to act as a sling to hold the excess length of the femoral vessels.

W. and **X.** Adductor muscles are debulked, and Z-plasty of skin is performed as necessary; otherwise, the wound is closed in layers and Hemovac suction is inserted in the usual fashion.

Postoperative Care. Apply a one-and-one-half hip spica cast, with the previous knee joint (now the "hip joint") flexed 30 degrees to take the tension off the iliopsoas hamstring tendon repair, the femoral vessels, and the anteriorly transposed sciatic nerve.

Doppler studies are made after application of the hip spica cast to assess the adequacy of circulation. The opposite hip is in 10 to 15 degrees of abduction and 20 degrees of flexion. The patient is allowed to bear weight on the opposite limb. The cast is removed in six weeks, when the distal femoral stump is fused to the acetabulum.

Following removal of the cast, the patient is fitted with a prosthesis. Active exercises are performed to develop motor strength of the "hip" extension and flexion and "knee" (the previous ankle) extension and flexion. Ordinarily, the patient is able to walk without support four months after surgery.

REFERENCES

Shih, C. H., and Carroll, N. C.: Modified Van Nes rotation plasty for the treatment of proximal femoral osteosarcoma in a child. J. Orthop. Surg. Tech., 1:81, 1985.

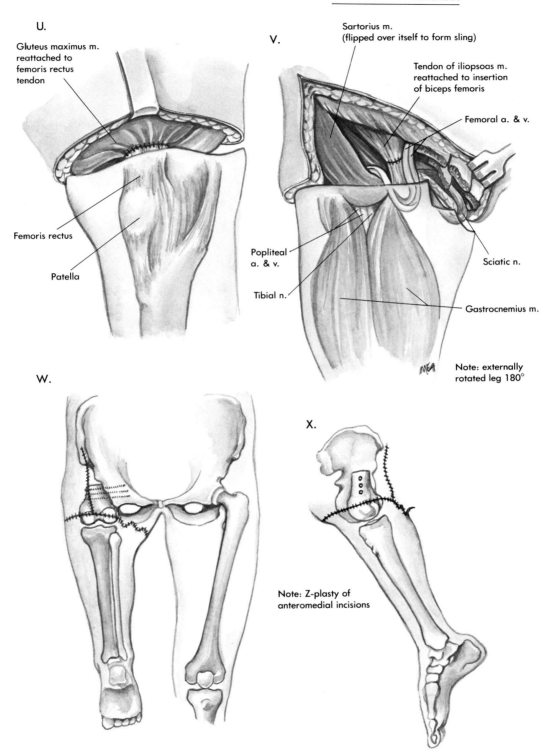

U.

Gluteus maximus m. reattached to femoris rectus tendon

Femoris rectus

Patella

V.

Sartorius m. (flipped over itself to form sling)

Tendon of iliopsoas m. reattached to insertion of biceps femoris

Femoral a. & v.

Sciatic n.

Gastrocnemius m.

Popliteal a. & v.

Tibial n.

Note: externally rotated leg 180°

W.

X.

Note: Z-plasty of anteromedial incisions

Plate 249. (Continued)

PLATE 250   ## Ilizarov Apparatus and Basic Technique

APPARATUS

The Ilizarov apparatus consists of a circular rigid internal fixator constructed of rings with flat surfaces and with multiple holes; the rings are connected to each other and transfixed to the long bones of the limb by smooth wires under tension. The wires pass through bone and soft tissues from one side of the limb to the other. They are placed at multiple levels in several planes and orientations, providing firm circumferential stability against the forces of bending, torsion, compression, shear, and translational displacement. Cyclic axial dynamization stimulates bone regeneration and remodeling. The Ilizarov external fixator is often referred to as the *compression-distraction apparatus* because it distracts and simultaneously compresses the divided ends of bone segments.

The system is very versatile and flexible; it can lengthen, shorten, and transport bone segments and can simultaneously correct any existing angulatory, rotational, or torsional deformity. The drawback of the Ilizarov method is its complexity and the steep learning curve required to master the technique.

The information given in this atlas is intended to serve only as a general guide; the surgeon should study the Ilizarov technique at special workshops and, most importantly, by taking a fellowship in centers where the Ilizarov system is widely used.

The Ilizarov system consists of the following components, which are made of high-quality stainless steel alloys.

Rings

Half-Rings

A. Half-rings are ordinarily joined together to form a full 360-degree ring (**A1.** and **A2.**). The rings have flat surfaces, but their ends are ledges that permit the half-rings to be connected so that their surfaces are on an even plane; *this is crucial!* The half-rings are attached to each other with nuts and bolts or rods. The half-rings are perforated by smooth holes through which bolts are inserted for fixation of the Ilizarov wires. The inner diameter of the holes is 8 mm. The distance between two holes is 4 mm.

The half-rings are available in 12 sizes: 80, 100, 110, 120, 130, 140, 150, 160, 180, 200, 220, and 240 (inner diameter). The half-rings can be extended by short plates and assembled in a multitude of configurations to correct an existing deformity.

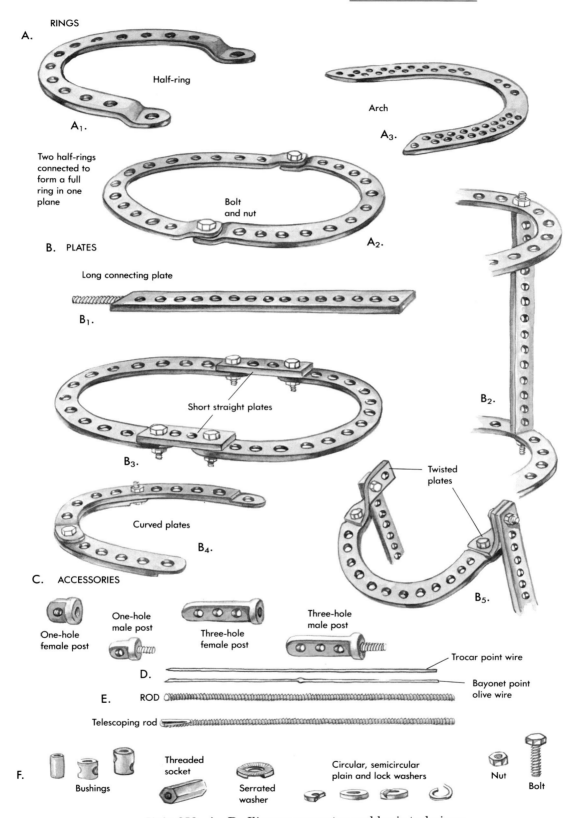

A. RINGS

A₁. Half-ring

A₃. Arch

Two half-rings connected to form a full ring in one plane

Bolt and nut

A₂.

B. PLATES

Long connecting plate

B₁.

B₂.

Short straight plates

B₃.

Twisted plates

Curved plates

B₄.

B₅.

C. ACCESSORIES

One-hole female post

One-hole male post

Three-hole female post

Three-hole male post

D.

Trocar point wire

Bayonet point olive wire

E. ROD

Telescoping rod

F.

Bushings

Threaded socket

Serrated washer

Circular, semicircular plain and lock washers

Nut

Bolt

Plate 250. A.–P., Ilizarov apparatus and basic technique.

Five-eighths (⅝) Rings. These restrict joint motion less than do full rings. They are primarily used at the knee, where wires are to be inserted in the tibial condyles, or at the elbow, for humeral epicondylar wire transfixation. Because the ⅝ rings are not very strong, they are used in combination with full rings.

Arches. Arches are elongated half-rings with staggered holes that allow two rows of fixation points (**A3.**).

Plates

B. The plates are flat and rectangular (5 mm. thick and 14 mm. wide) and perforated with holes (7 mm. in diameter) throughout their length. They are primarily used to connect and reinforce parts of the Ilizarov system and sometimes used to extend the main frame construction. The plates are available in various types.

Long Plates

B1. and **B2.** The long plates are secured to the circular rings and reinforce larger frames, particularly during bone segment transport. These plates are also used as an extension of the frame to serve as auxiliary supports for attachment of wires.

Such modification of the system permits pivoting or translational movement and ready access to the wound when there is soft-tissue damage, such as wound slough or infection. Lengths of the long plates vary from 155 mm. with eight holes, to 235 mm. with 12 holes, to 355 mm. with 17 holes. Connection plates are available with a threaded end.

Short Straight Plates

B3.–B5. The short straight plates are utilized primarily for joining rings (**B3.**), curved plates for lengthening or widening half-rings (**B4.**) and twisted plates (ends rotated 90 degrees to each other) for connecting components that are perpendicular to each other (**B5.**).

Accessories

Posts

C. In essence, a post is a short plate with one or more smooth holes. It can be manufactured as a male or female type. In the *male* post is a threaded rod at one end, which serves as a connection to other components. In the *female* post, one end is tapered into a threaded hole 10 mm. deep (it has no protruding end). The hole in the female post is used to connect bolts or rods.

Posts are available with one, two, three, or four holes. They are used for fixing wires, rods, or plates to the main supports. Posts can be assembled to serve as hinges.

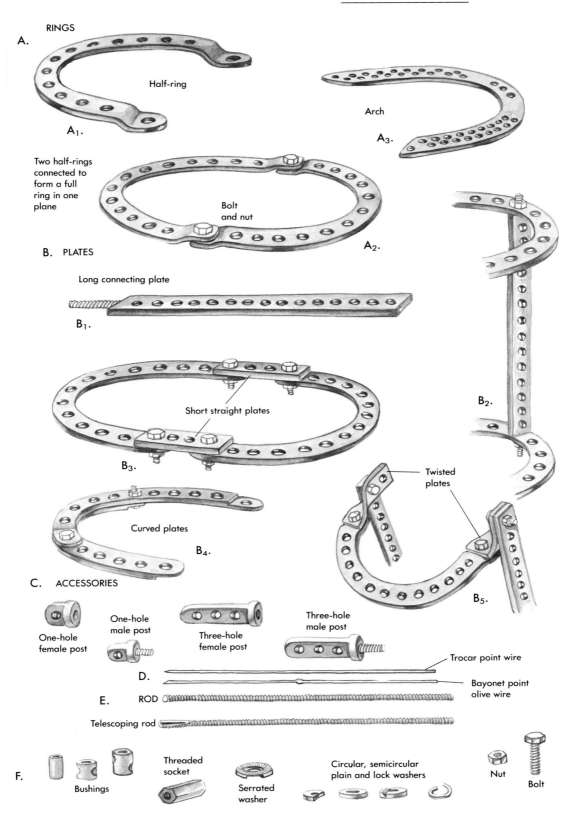

RINGS

A.

Half-ring

A₁.

Arch

A₃.

Two half-rings connected to form a full ring in one plane

Bolt and nut

A₂.

B. PLATES

Long connecting plate

B₁.

Short straight plates

B₃.

B₂.

Twisted plates

Curved plates

B₄.

B₅.

C. ACCESSORIES

One-hole female post

One-hole male post

Three-hole female post

Three-hole male post

Trocar point wire

D.

Bayonet point olive wire

E. ROD

Telescoping rod

F.

Bushings

Threaded socket

Serrated washer

Circular, semicircular plain and lock washers

Nut

Bolt

Plate 250. (Continued)

Wires

D. Ilizarov wires, smooth and round in cross section, pass through bone and soft tissues from one side of the limb to the other. A cyclic, elastic, and axial micromotion and axial dynamization are allowed by the wires which stimulate bone regeneration and remodeling.

Ilizarov wires vary in shape of point, diameter, and length and can be "beaded" or not. The choice of wire depends on the size of the bone and limbs and on the stability of fixation required. In the long bones, wires of 1.5 mm. (for children) and 1.8 mm. (for adults) are used. In very large and heavy patients, 2.0-mm. diameter wires are available. Length varies (300 mm., 370 mm., 400 mm.). In the metacarpals, metatarsals, and phalanges, wires of 0.5 or 1.0 mm. in diameter are used. The wire may be *bayonet point* (cortical), used in diaphyseal dense bones, or *trocar point,* used in cancellous bone.

The wire may have an attached bead or "olive" (referred to as "olive wire"). Olive wires provide interfragmentary compression and increase the stability of fixation. They are available in two sizes: 1.5 mm. × 300 mm. and 1.8 mm. × 400 mm. These wires are resilient and are manufactured from stainless steel.

Rods

E. Rods connect the supporting rings and plates to each other and act as traction devices for the gradual transport of wires or supports. They may be "telescoped" or "threaded."

Threaded rods are constructed of stainless steel and are only 6 mm. in diameter. Their mechanical strength to bending forces is not very strong; therefore, it is recommended that four rods be used to connect two rings. The distance between the threads of the rod is 1 mm.; as a result, one full turn of the lock nut gives a 1-mm. change of distance (distraction or compression) between the two rings. Threaded rods are available in lengths of 60, 80, 100, 120, 150, 200, 250, 300, 350, and 400 mm.

Additional Accessories

F. Other devices used to connect the parts are bushings, threaded sockets, serrated washers, circular and semicircular plain washers, lock washers, regular nuts, and nylon nuts.

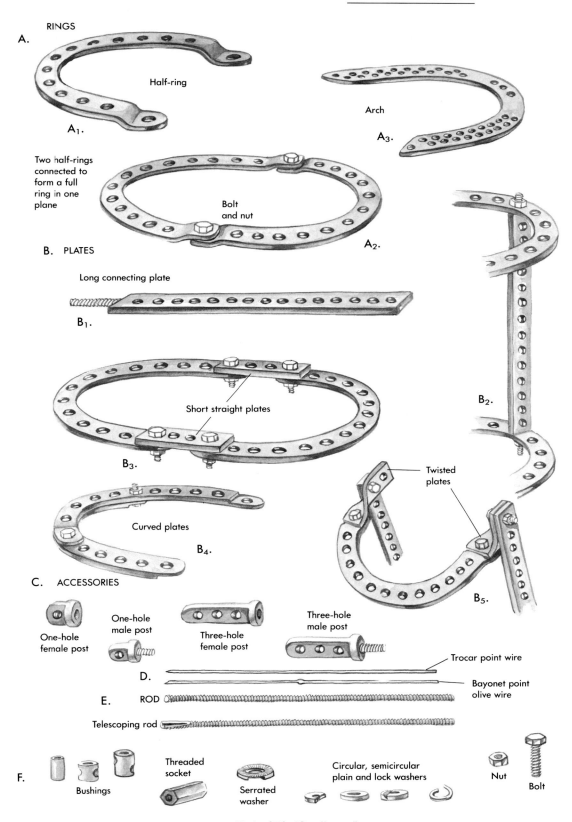

A.   RINGS

Half-ring

A₁.

Arch

A₃.

Two half-rings connected to form a full ring in one plane

Bolt and nut

A₂.

B.   PLATES

Long connecting plate

B₁.

B₂.

Short straight plates

B₃.

Twisted plates

Curved plates

B₄.

B₅.

C.   ACCESSORIES

One-hole female post

One-hole male post

Three-hole female post

Three-hole male post

D.

Trocar point wire

Bayonet point olive wire

E.   ROD

Telescoping rod

F.

Bushings

Threaded socket

Serrated washer

Circular, semicircular plain and lock washers

Nut

Bolt

Plate 250. (Continued)

Wire Fixators

G.–I. Wire fixators consist of either buckles (clamps) or bolts. The buckles are transfixed to the flat surfaces of the ring (not to the holes) with nuts and bolts. They may be an *open frame* (**G.**) wire fixator buckle or a *closed frame* clamp (**H.**). There are two types of wire *fixator bolts* (**I.**), cannulated and slotted; these bolts allow placement of the wire into a hole or slot and fixation of the wire between the ring wall and bolt head.

G.　Open-frame wire fixation buckle (clamp)

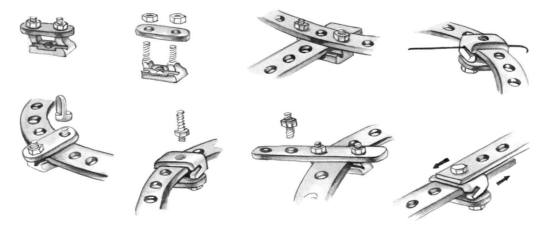

H.　Solid-wire fixation buckle (clamp)

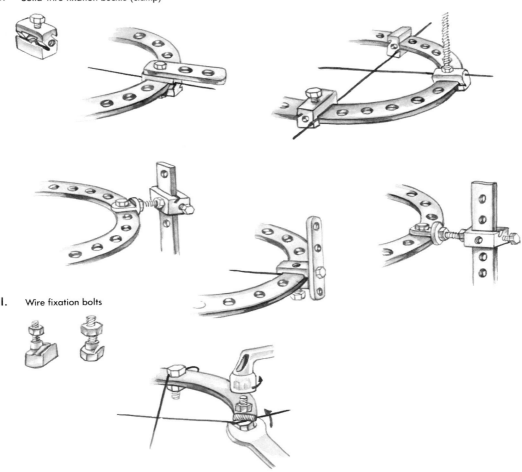

I.　Wire fixation bolts

Plate 250. (Continued)

Graduated Telescoping Rod

J. The graduated telescoping rod consists of a cylindrical tube that is fully threaded inside. The rod is fastened to one ring (usually the distal one) by tightening the bolt. The graduated threaded rod inside is connected by a bolt to the opposing ring (the proximal one). The rod has a square head that is easily adjusted by hand. The square head also has an automatic locking device; depression of a small lever on its side releases the lock. After one fourth of a turn (0.25 mm. distraction or compression), the lever will "pop up" with an audible click (hence the name "the clicker"). On the flat surface, the square-headed clicker (numbered 1, 2, 3, 4) and indented dots are displayed; they moderate the amount of turn in one-quarter increments. On distraction, the clicker number increases (1 to 4); on compression, it decreases (4 to 1).

The cylinder has a hollow section that shows the graduated rod within. The amount of lengthening (distraction) or shortening (compression) is shown in millimeters on a scale on the graduated rod.

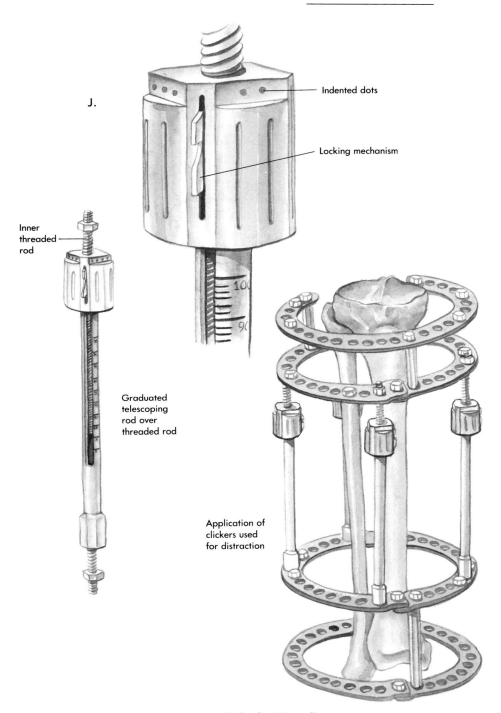

J.

Indented dots

Locking mechanism

Inner threaded rod

Graduated telescoping rod over threaded rod

Application of clickers used for distraction

Plate 250. (Continued)

TECHNIQUE

Wire Insertion

K. Insert the limb through the apparatus, and inspect the orientation of the apparatus on the limb. In children, *the length of the frame must be examined relative to the long bone.* For example, in the tibia, the proximal ring should be immediately distal to the proximal tibial physis and the distal ring should be immediately proximal to the distal tibial physis. There should be a safe distance between the wire and the growth plate. Assess and double-check the position and orientation of the rings by image intensifier radiographic control.

The frame is used as a drill guide for proper insertion of the wires in relation to the long bone. Predetermine the entry and exit sites of the wires. An assistant should point to the site of exit with an instrument. The entry and exit points of the wires must be at least 1.5 to 2.0 cm. away from the major vessels and nerves. The K-wires should be on the same plane on the ring. For example, in the proximal tibia, the wire is inserted horizontally along the distal surface of the proximal ring from the lateral side.

First, poke the wire through the skin down to bone; then drill slowly through the bone with a power drill to avoid burning of tissues. When smooth wires are used, an incision is not required; however, when an olive wire is used, a small stab incision is made after insertion of the wire to allow the olive to pass down to bone. Initially, the drill is chucked close to the skin, and gradually it is chucked back during the drilling.

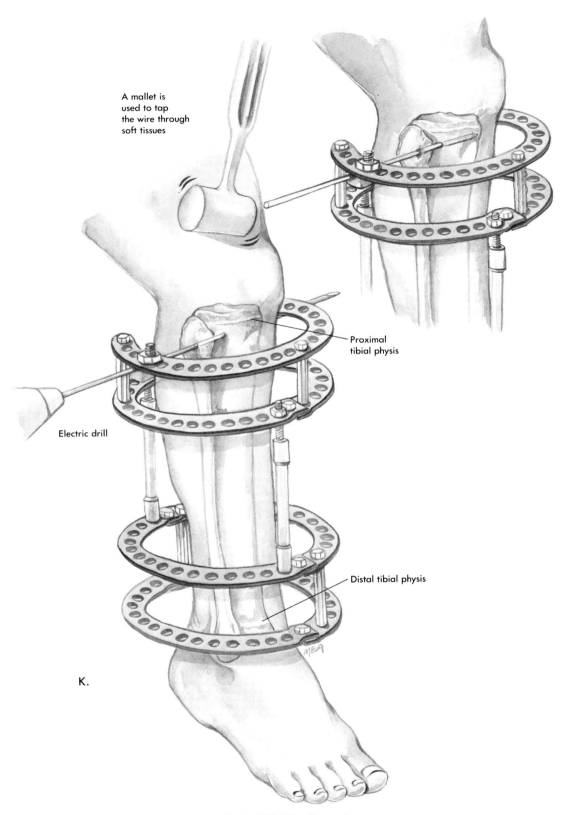

A mallet is
used to tap
the wire through
soft tissues

Proximal
tibial physis

Electric drill

Distal tibial physis

K.

Plate 250. (Continued)

L. At the points of entry and exit, the skin should be held steady with the surgeon's fingers. When limb elongation is to be performed, the skin is pushed toward the site of corticotomy. When compression is planned for treatment of non-union, the skin should be pushed away from the site of the pseudarthrosis. When the ring is to be immobile, the skin is held fixed between two fingers and pushed firmly against underlying hard tissues.

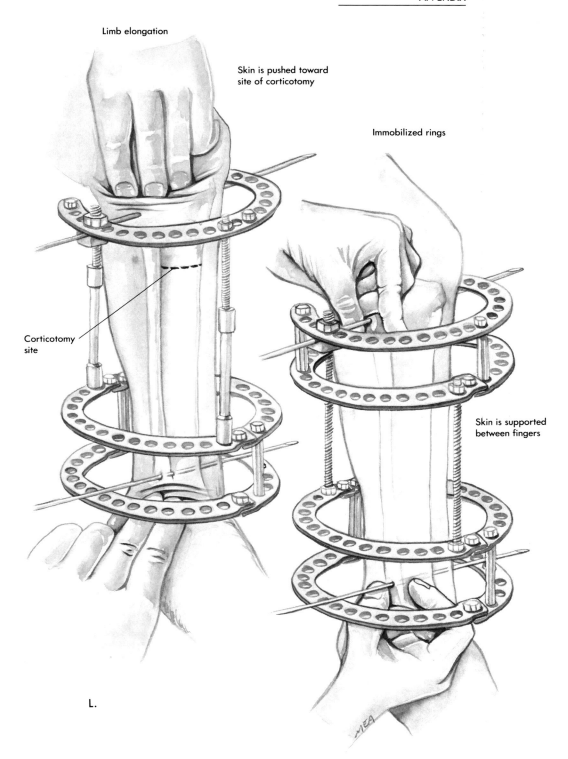

Limb elongation

Skin is pushed toward
site of corticotomy

Immobilized rings

Corticotomy
site

Skin is supported
between fingers

L.

Plate 250. (Continued)

M. In regard to the position of the joint in relation to the wires and the rings, *it is vital to prevent contractural deformity of the joints by providing maximal functional length of the transfixed muscle.* For example, when a wire is inserted through the anterior compartment of the distal tibia, the ankle joint should be maximally plantarflexed (**M1.**); when a wire is inserted through the posterior compartment, the ankle should be maximally dorsiflexed and the knee placed in some flexion to relax the gastrocnemius (**M2.**).

Since the wire will pass through the anterior compartment muscles, the ankle and toes are plantarflexed before insertion to minimize entrapment. This is particularly important in limb lengthening, since the increasing stretch on the muscles is accommodated by transfixing the muscles in their lengthened state. As the wire exits the bone to enter into the posterior compartment, the ankle and toes are dorsiflexed and the wire advanced by tapping it in with a mallet rather than drilling across soft tissues (see **K.**). The latter maneuver minimizes the chance of injury to vessels and nerves because a non-rotating wire pushes such structures out of harm's way rather than perforating them. The wires protruding at each side of the limb should be approximately equal in length.

A cardinal rule is "one wire, one hole." *Insert the wire correctly on the first attempt!* Avoid multiple holes.

First, poke the wire through the skin and soft tissues until it touches cortical bone. Inspect its site through image intensifier radiographic control. Move the tip of the wire anteriorly and posteriorly to ensure that it is in the center of the bone to prevent sliding on the bone slope. Once the correct cortical bone entry point has been determined, grasp the wire with a wet sponge to prevent it from bending while drilling and drill slowly through both cortices under image intensifier radiographic control. Pull the wire backward at this point. If it is easily removable, change the direction of drilling.

N. Fix the wire to the ring by open frame wire fixation buckle clamps, solid frame wire fixation buckle clamps, or wire fixation bolts, either slotted or cannulated, depending on the situation. Never manipulate the position of the wire to facilitate fixation to the ring.

1. If the wire is in the middle of the hole, fix it with a cannulated bolt.
2. If the position of the wire is to the edge of the hole, use a slotted bolt.
3. If the wire position is between two holes, use a buckle clamp.

Minimizing entrapment

M_1.

M_2.

Wire is
inserted
through
anterior
compartment

Wire is
inserted
through
posterior
compartment

Plantarflexed

Dorsiflexed

N.   Fixation of
non-olive wire

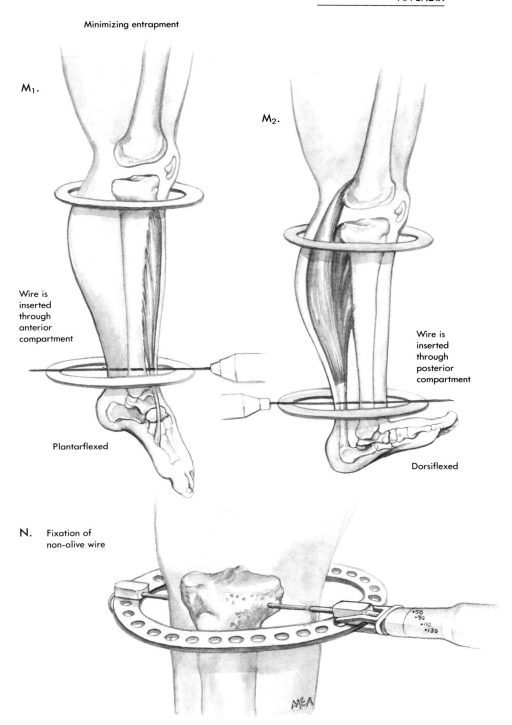

Plate 250. (Continued)

Wire Tensioning

O. A calibrated wire tensioning device is used. Insert the wire into the cannulation in the tensioner, and turn the handle clockwise to tension the wire within the range marked 50 to 130 kg. Non-olive wires should first be fixed to the ring at one side and tensioned from the other side. The olive wires can also be tensioned this way, fixing the olive end to the ring and tensioning from the other side. Use two tensioners and tension the olive wires simultaneously from both ends to ensure even forces across both sides of the olive to decrease the incidence of pressure necrosis of bone from the olive. The tension applied should be between 90 and 130 kg. It is safer to use only 90 kg., since the lengthening process itself generates approximately 30 to 40 kg. of stress on the wires, thereby minimizing the risk of wire breakage.

After tensioning and fixing the wire, cut off only the sharp tip and leave the wire long. The protruding portion is then bent in a smooth arc around the ring to be available to retensioning if necessary.

Mark the ends of the wires with the olives by bending one end in a different manner; this measure prevents accidental pulling of the wire in the wrong direction. Secure the wires to the rings so that they need not be displaced in order to fix them. If a wire lies several millimeters off the ring, use spacer washers on the wire fixation bolt to fix the wire in situ. In this manner, there is no pre-stress on the wire when it is tensioned. Any pre-stress can lead to either displacement of bone fragments or lysis of the bone around the pin with increased risk of pin tract infection.

O.

Olive wire
fixation

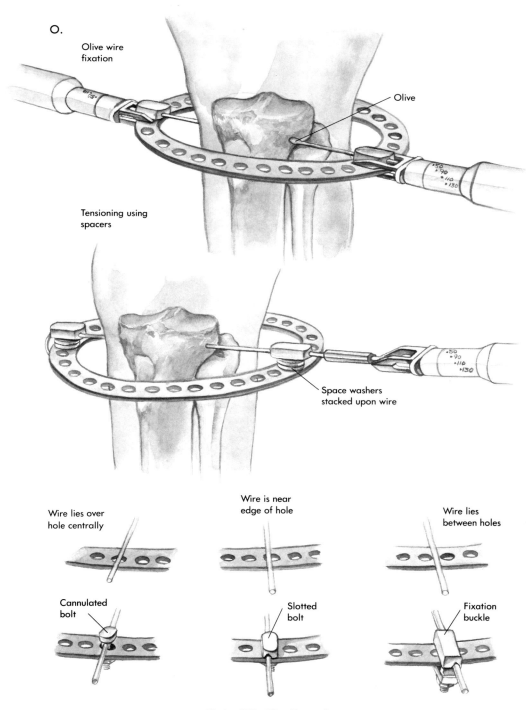

Olive

Tensioning using
spacers

Space washers
stacked upon wire

Wire lies over
hole centrally

Wire is near
edge of hole

Wire lies
between holes

Cannulated
bolt

Slotted
bolt

Fixation
buckle

Plate 250. (Continued)

Corticotomy

P1. Make a 1-cm.-long longitudinal incision over the anterior crest of the tibia. The periosteum is incised and elevated medially and laterally.

P2. Insert a 1-cm.-wide sharp osteotome, and divide the anterior cortex of the tibia.

P3. and **P4.** Insert a 5-mm.-wide sharp osteotome under the protection of the periosteum. Section the medial cortex and then the lateral cortex of the tibia in a similar manner.

P5. and **P6.** Take a wrench, and turn the 5-mm. osteotome 90 degrees. Spread apart the divided posteromedial and, following similar technique, the posterolateral cortices of the tibia. This maneuver, mimicking a laminar spread, cracks open the posterior wall of the cortex.

P7. Perform a rotational osteoclasis. Twist the distal block *laterally*. Under image intensifier radiography, confirm the completeness of corticotomy.

P8. Another method for sectioning the posterior cortex is to use a Gigli saw.

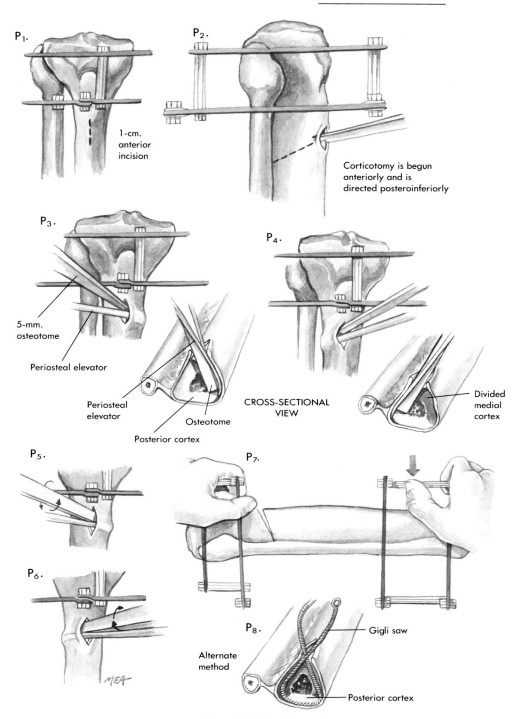

P₁.

1-cm. anterior incision

P₂.

Corticotomy is begun anteriorly and is directed posteroinferiorly

P₃.

5-mm. osteotome

Periosteal elevator

Periosteal elevator

Osteotome

Posterior cortex

CROSS-SECTIONAL VIEW

P₄.

Divided medial cortex

P₅.

P₆.

P₇.

P₈.

Alternate method

Gigli saw

Posterior cortex

MEA

Plate 250. (Continued)

PLATE 251 **Mechanical Axis Deviation**

DEFINITIONS

A. The *mechanical axis* is the line of weight-bearing force from the center of the ankle to the center of the hip joint. Normally in the frontal plane, the mechanical axis of the lower limb passes just medial to the center of the knee near the medial tibial spine.

The mechanical axis of the *tibia* is the line of weight-bearing force from the center of the ankle to the center of the knee. The *anatomic axis* of the tibia and the mechanical axis of the tibia are identical.

The mechanical axis of the *femur* is the line of weight-bearing force from the center of the hip to the center of the knee. The anatomic axis of the femur is the line that traverses from the piriformis fossa to the center of the knee. The mechanical axis of the femur ordinarily subtends an angle of 5 to 7 degrees to the anatomic axis of the femur.

The *orientation line* of each joint is determined next. The orientation line of the *ankle* is the transverse line drawn across the tibial plafond; normally, it is perpendicular to the mechanical axis of the tibia. The joint orientation line of the *distal femur* is the horizontal line drawn between the subchondral bony plates of the medial and lateral femoral condyles; usually, it is in slight valgus of 3 degrees. The mechanical axis of the *tibia* in relation to the knee joint orientation line is in slight varus, about 3 degrees.

The orientation line of the *hip joint* is the line drawn between the tip of the greater trochanter and the center of the femoral head. Normally, this line is perpendicular (90 degrees ±6 degrees) to the mechanical axis of the femur. It alters slightly with rotation of the hip.

B. In the *sagittal plane,* the normal mechanical axis of the *center of gravity* passes from the second sacral vertebra (S-2) to the center of the femoral head, anterior to the center of the knee to a point anterior to the center of the ankle. Normally, the head and neck of the femur are anteverted 15 degrees.

The tibial plateau normally has a posterior tilt of 10 degrees (±2 degrees). When the knee is in neutral extension, the anterior cortex of the distal femur and the anterior cortex of the tibial diaphysis are colinear. The posterior slope of the tibial plateau checkreins recurvatum of the knee and anterior roll of the femoral condyles on the tibia. Normally, the tibial plafond has 5 to 7 degrees of anterior tilt. A sagittal line drawn along the anterior cortex of the diaphysis of the tibia is parallel to the sagittal line projected from the center of the ankle to the center of the knee, whereas the sagittal line from the center of the femoral condyles to the center of the femoral head slopes slightly posterior to the anterior femoral cortex.

Mechanical axis deviation (MAD) may be located in the femur, tibia, or joint, that is, the knees and/or ankle. It may be in the frontal or sagittal plane; it may be uniapical or multiapical. The angular deformity may be only in the femur with a normal tibia, only in the tibia with a normal femur, or in both the femur and tibia. The bony deformity in the femur or tibia may be in the diaphysis, metaphysis, or epiphysis. The knee joint laxity may be the cause of MAD of the lower limb. Bony deformity will cause malalignment of the joints above and below the deformity. In the preoperative planning of surgical correction of malalignment of the lower limb, it is vital to perform the malalignment test and to determine the site of the apex and degree of the angular deformity.

The following text and illustrations are modified from Paley and Tetsworth's description of the malalignment test.

NORMAL MECHANICAL AXIS

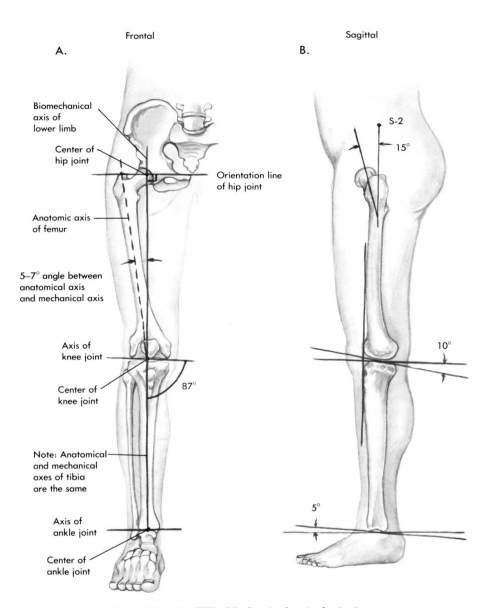

Frontal

A.

Sagittal

B.

Biomechanical axis of lower limb

Center of hip joint

Orientation line of hip joint

Anatomic axis of femur

5–7° angle between anatomical axis and mechanical axis

Axis of knee joint

87°

Center of knee joint

Note: Anatomical and mechanical axes of tibia are the same

Axis of ankle joint

Center of ankle joint

S-2

15°

10°

5°

Plate 251. A.–KK., Mechanical axis deviation.

MALALIGNMENT TEST

Radiology. The first requirement is a standing anteroposterior radiogram of both lower limbs, including the knees and ankles. The knees are in complete extension, and the patellae point straight forward. The most common error by radiology technicians is to make the radiogram with the patient's feet pointing forward. Instruct the radiology technician to orient the patellae, not the feet, straight forward. Look for the position of the patellae in the radiogram; they should be centered between the femoral condyles. When the patellae are malaligned because of patellofemoral joint subluxation or dislocation, use the proximal tibial tuberosity as a landmark. Besides the radiogram, a long transparent ruler, a transparent goniometer, and an x-ray marking pencil are required.

Preoperative Planning

Diaphyseal Varus Deformity of the Tibia with Normal Femur

C. First, draw the mechanical axis line of the lower limb from the center of the femoral head to the center of the ankle.

D. Second, draw joint orientation lines of the ankle (across the tibial plafond) and of the knee (across both the femoral condyles [FC] and tibial plateau [TP]).

E. Third, draw the mechanical axis of the femur from the center of the femoral head to the center of the knee. The lateral angle between the mechanical axis of the femur and the knee joint orientation line is 87 degrees, indicating that the mechanical axis of the femur is normal.

Fourth, extend the normal mechanical axis of the femur distally into the leg toward the ankle. This represents the mechanical axis of the tibia proximal to the apex of the deformity. After the angular deformity is connected, the center of the ankle should be on this line.

Fifth, draw a line from the center of the ankle perpendicular to the ankle joint orientation line; extend it proximally parallel to the distal tibial diaphysis. Because the mechanical and anatomic axes of the tibia are similar, this line represents the mechanical axis of the distal tibia inferior to the apex of the deformity.

The level of intersection of these two mechanical axis lines represents the apex of varus deformity. Measure the angle between the two lines; this is the degree of angular correction required to restore the normal mechanical axis of the lower limb.

Alternate Convex Cortical Line Method. Draw a line downward along the convex cortex of the diaphysis of the tibia proximal to the apex of the deformity. Draw another line upward along the convex cortex of the tibial diaphysis distal to the apex of the deformity. The level of intersection of the convex cortical lines is about the same as that of the mechanical axis lines. The angle formed by these two lines is the angle of correction required to restore normal alignment of the tibial diaphysis.

Proximal Juxta-articular Varus Deformity of the Tibia with Normal Femur. This type of tibia vara deformity frequently occurs in Blount's disease.

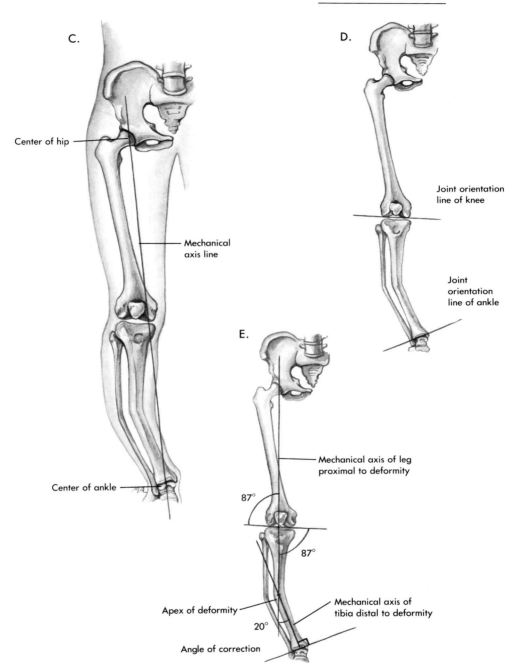

C.

Center of hip

Mechanical
axis line

Center of ankle

D.

Joint orientation
line of knee

Joint
orientation
line of ankle

E.

Mechanical axis of leg
proximal to deformity

87°

87°

Apex of deformity

Mechanical axis of
tibia distal to deformity

20°

Angle of correction

Plate 251. (Continued)

F. First, draw the mechanical axis line from the center of the femoral head to the center of the ankle.

G. Second, draw the joint orientation line of the knee and ankle. At the knee, draw lines across the distal femoral condyles (FC) and the tibial plateau (TP) to rule out lateral ligamentous joint laxity as an additional factor of the varus deformity. If the FC and TP lines are not parallel (often the case in Blount's disease), the joint space contributes to the varus mechanical axis malalignment at the knee. Distal transfer of the proximal fibula is indicated to tauten the lateral collateral ligament of the knee.

H. Third, draw the mechanical axis of the femur from the center of the femoral head to the center of the knee and extend it distally.

Note: The mechanical axis of the femur is normal; the deformity is in the proximal tibial metaphysis and epiphysis.

The segment of the normal mechanical axis of the femur is extended inferior to the knee joint, representing the mechanical axis of the tibia superior to the apex of the deformity. The objective of surgery is to align the center of the ankle with this line.

I. Fourth, draw a line parallel to the medial or lateral cortex of the tibial shaft; extend it upward from the center of the ankle and perpendicular to the ankle joint orientation line.

The level of intersection of these two mechanical axis lines represents the apex of the deformity. The angle formed between the two mechanical axis lines is the magnitude of angular deformity—in this illustration it is 56 degrees.

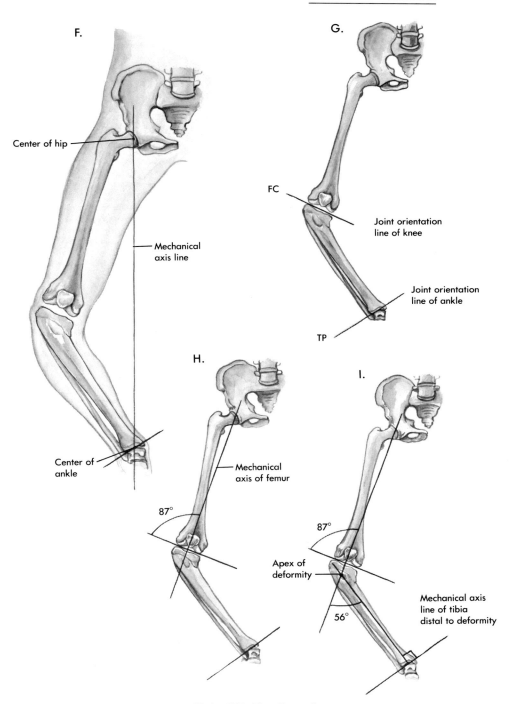

F.

Center of hip

Mechanical axis line

Center of ankle

G.

FC

Joint orientation line of knee

Joint orientation line of ankle

TP

H.

Mechanical axis of femur

87°

I.

87°

Apex of deformity

56°

Mechanical axis line of tibia distal to deformity

Plate 251. (Continued)

Varus Mechanical Axis Deviation Due to Lateral Knee Joint Laxity with Normal Femur and Normal Tibia

J. First, draw a longitudinal line from the center of the femoral head to the center of the ankle.

Note: The center of the knee lies lateral to the mechanical axis line.

K. Second, draw a transverse line across the subchondral bony plate of the medial and lateral femoral condyles (FC). Measure the lateral angle formed by mechanical axis of the femur and the joint orientation line of the distal femur. It measures 87 degrees, demonstrating that the mechanical axis of the femur is normal.

L. Third, draw a transverse line across the superior surface of the subchondral bony plate of the tibial plateau (TP). Draw a longitudinal line parallel to the medial cortex of the tibial diaphysis from the center of the ankle joint and perpendicular to the plafond of the distal tibia. Extend it proximal to intersect the tibial plateau joint line. The medial angle formed between the tibial plateau joint line and the mechanical axis of the tibia is 87 degrees, indicating that the mechanical axis of the tibia is normal.

M. Fourth, the femoral condyle joint line (FC) and the tibial plateau joint line (TP) are not parallel; they are open 7 degrees laterally, indicating that lateral ligamentous joint laxity is the cause of varus mechanical axis malalignment of the lower limb.

LATERAL JOINT LAXITY

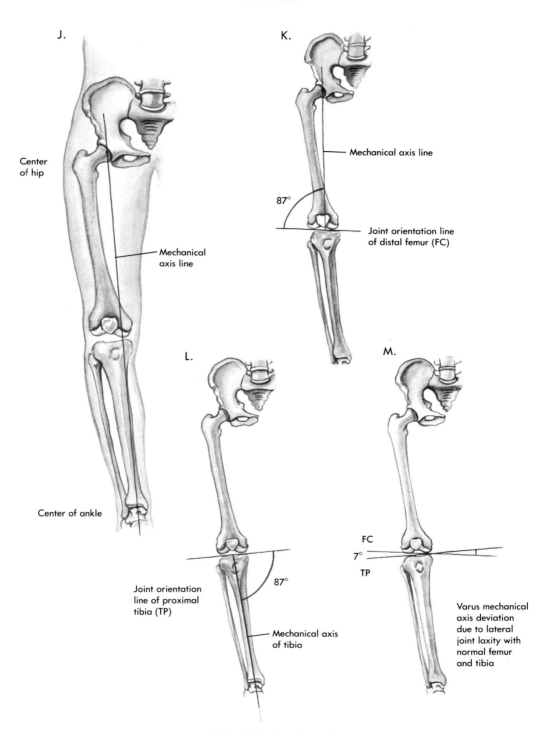

J.

Center
of hip

Mechanical
axis line

Center of ankle

K.

Mechanical axis line

87°

Joint orientation line
of distal femur (FC)

L.

Joint orientation
line of proximal
tibia (TP)

87°

Mechanical axis
of tibia

M.

FC
7°
TP

Varus mechanical
axis deviation
due to lateral
joint laxity with
normal femur
and tibia

Plate 251. (Continued)

Varus Mechanical Axis Deviation Due to Uniapical Varus Deformity of the Femoral Diaphysis with Normal Tibia

N. First, draw the mechanical axis line from the center of the hip to the center of the ankle.

O. Second, draw the *hip joint* orientation line from the tip of the greater trochanter to the center of the femoral head. Then draw the *knee joint* orientation line; draw a horizontal line across the subchondral bony plate of the lateral and medial condyles of the distal femur (line FC), and then draw a line across the superior bony surface of the tibial plateau (line TP). The lines FC and TP are parallel, indicating that the knee joint is normal and joint laxity is not present.

P. Third, draw the *ankle joint* orientation line, a horizontal line across the tibial plafond. Then, draw a line from the center of the ankle to the center of the knee. The medial angle between the mechanical axis of the tibia and the tibial plateau is 87 degrees, indicating that the tibia is normal. Extend the mechanical axis of the tibia proximally above the knee. This upward extended line represents the mechanical axis of the lower segment of the femur distal to the apex of the angular deformity.

FEMORAL DIAPHYSEAL DEVIATION

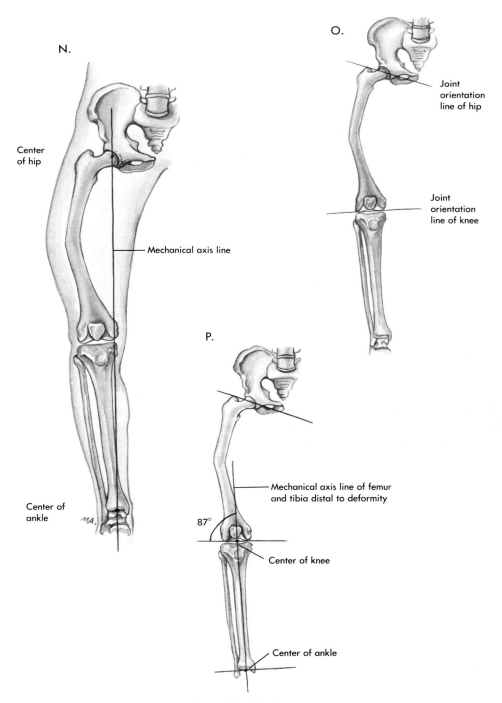

Plate 251. (Continued)

Q. Fourth, determine the mechanical axis of the proximal femur on the deformed side:

1. Draw the mechanical axis of the contralateral normal lower limb from the center of the femoral head to the center of the knee and to the center of the ankle.

2. Draw the hip joint orientation line of the opposite normal side from the tip of its greater trochanter to the center of the femoral head.

3. Measure the angle formed between the mechanical axis of the femur and the hip joint orientation line of the normal lower limb (LB). Compare it with that of the deformed lower limb (LA).

4. When the two angles are similar, use this angle to calculate the mechanical axis of the proximal femur on the deformed side. For example, when the angle between the hip joint orientation line and the mechanical axis of the femur is 90 degrees, draw a line on the deformed side from the center of the femoral head and extend it distally at a 90-degree angle to its hip joint orientation line. This extended line represents the mechanical axis of the proximal segment of the deformed femur.

5. The point of intersection of the mechanical axis of the proximal femur with that of the distal femur (a proximal extension of the mechanical axis of the normal tibia) is the apex of the deformity.

6. The angle subtended between the two lines (the degree of angulation) is 23 degrees here.

Alternate Method

R. An alternate method of determining mechanical axis of the proximal femur of the deformed side is by the use of the lateral cortex of the proximal femur of the normal side.

1. Draw a line along the lateral cortex of the femur.

2. Measure the angle subtended between the mechanical axis line and the lateral cortex line; it is 10 degrees here.

3. Draw the lateral cortex line on the proximal segment of the deformed femur.

4. Draw a line from the center of the femoral head, and extend it distally parallel to the lateral cortex line of the normal femur.

5. Draw a longitudinal line from the center of the femoral head; extend it distally at an angle identical to the angle formed by the lateral cortex line and mechanical axis line of the contralateral normal femur (10 degrees). This line represents the mechanical axis of the proximal segment of the malaligned femur.

6. The point of intersection of the mechanical axis lines of the proximal and distal segments of the deformed femur is the apex of the deformity; the angle subtended by these mechanical lines is the degree of angular deformity. This alternate method is used when the degree of coxa vara or valga is clinically insignificant and correction of the neck-shaft is not indicated. The proximal femoral lateral cortex method is based on the observation that the femoral diaphysis is not parallel to the anatomic axis of the femur and that the mechanical axis of the femur and anatomic axis of the femur subtend a constant angle of 5 to 7 degrees.

FEMORAL DIAPHYSEAL DEVIATION

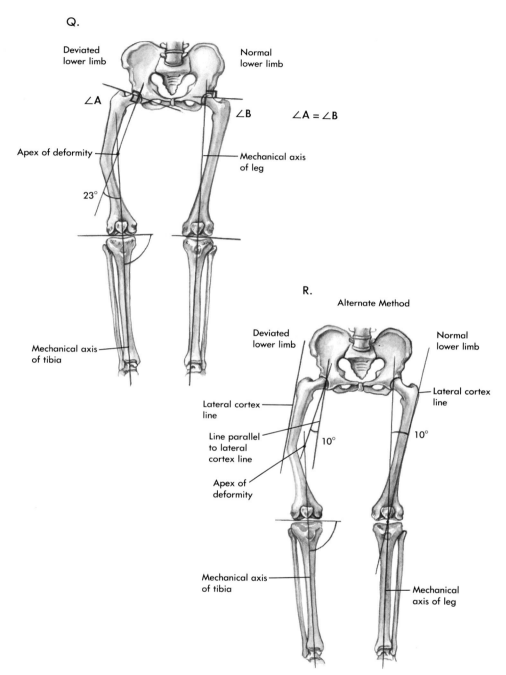

Q.

Deviated lower limb

Normal lower limb

∠A

∠B

∠A = ∠B

Apex of deformity

Mechanical axis of leg

23°

Mechanical axis of tibia

R.

Alternate Method

Deviated lower limb

Normal lower limb

Lateral cortex line

Lateral cortex line

Line parallel to lateral cortex line

10°

10°

Apex of deformity

Mechanical axis of tibia

Mechanical axis of leg

Plate 251. (Continued)

Juxta-articular Varus Angular Deformity of the Distal Femur with Normal Tibia

S. First, draw the mechanical axis of the lower limb from the center of the femoral head to the center of the ankle. Note the magnitude of varus malalignment.

T. Second, draw the joint orientation lines of the hip and knee.

U. Third, draw the mechanical axis line of the tibia from the center of the ankle to the center of the knee, and extend it proximally. The mechanical axis of the tibia is normal. The proximal (above-the-knee) extension of the mechanical axis line of the tibia represents the mechanical axis line of the femoral segment distal to the apex of deformity. The objective of surgical correction is to align the femur and to ensure that the lines drawn distally from the center of the femoral head come to lie on the mechanical axis line of the tibia.

FEMORAL JUXTA-ARTICULAR DEVIATION

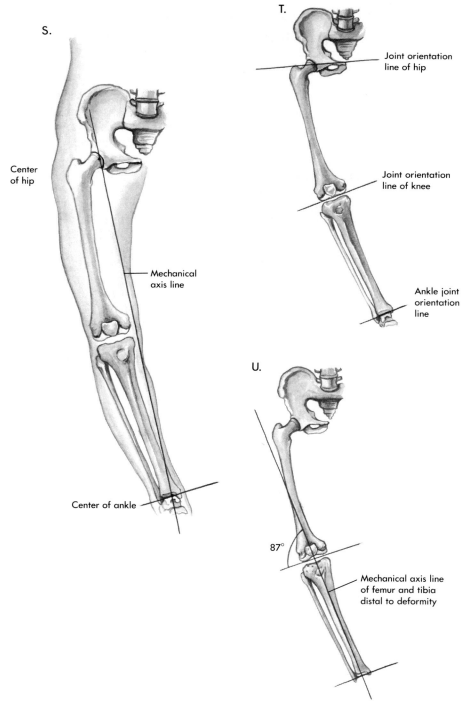

S.

Center
of hip

Mechanical
axis line

Center of ankle

T.

Joint orientation
line of hip

Joint orientation
line of knee

Ankle joint
orientation
line

U.

87°

Mechanical axis line
of femur and tibia
distal to deformity

Plate 251. (Continued)

V. Fourth, determine the mechanical axis of the proximal segment of the malaligned femur. Follow the same steps as outlined for preoperative planning of correction of diaphyseal angular deformity of the femur:

1. On the normal lower limb radiogram, draw the hip joint orientation line and the mechanical axis line of the femur and determine the angle subtended between these two lines ($\angle$B).

2. Measure the angle ($\angle$A) between the hip joint orientation line and the mechanical axis line of the malaligned lower limb. When these angles between the malaligned and normal limb ($\angle$A and $\angle$B) are similar, determine the mechanical axis of the proximal segment of the femur as follows:

3. Draw a line from the center of the femoral head of the malaligned limb and extend it distally at the angle ($\angle$A) to the hip joint orientation line. This line represents the mechanical axis of the proximal segment of the deformed femur.

4. The point of intersection of the mechanical axis of the proximal segment of the femur and that of the distal segment of the femur (i.e., proximal extension of the mechanical axis of the normal tibia) is the apex of the deformity and the angle formed between the two lines is the degree of angulation.

W. An alternate method is the use of the lateral cortex line. Follow the same steps as those outlined for correction of diaphyseal deformity of the femur.

FEMORAL JUXTA-ARTICULAR DEVIATION

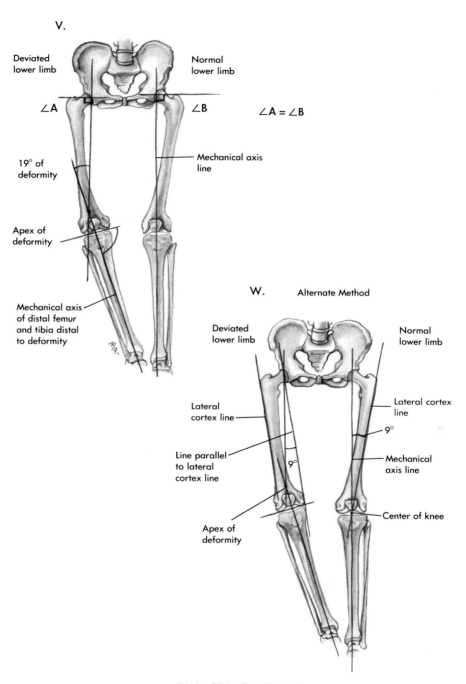

V.

Deviated lower limb

Normal lower limb

∠A   ∠B   ∠A = ∠B

Mechanical axis line

19° of deformity

Apex of deformity

Mechanical axis of distal femur and tibia distal to deformity

W.   Alternate Method

Deviated lower limb

Normal lower limb

Lateral cortex line

Lateral cortex line

9°

Line parallel to lateral cortex line

Mechanical axis line

9°

Center of knee

Apex of deformity

Plate 251. (Continued)

Varus Mechanical Axis Deviation of the Lower Limb Due to Varus Angular Deformity of Both Femur and Tibia

X. First, draw a line from the center of the femoral head to the center of the ankle.

Note: The center of the knee is located lateral to the mechanical axis of the lower limb.

Y. Second, draw the hip, knee, and ankle joint orientation lines.

Z1. Third, locate the center of the knee. Starting at that point, draw a longitudinal line at an 87-degree angle to the knee joint line (3 degrees of varus). Distal and proximal extensions of the line represent the mechanical axis of the proximal tibia and distal femur. This method of determining the mechanical axis is employed because both the femur and the tibia are deviated into varus deformity and normal mechanical axis of one long bone cannot be used as the mechanical axis of the other long bone.

Z2. Fourth, draw a mechanical axis line from the center of the femoral head to the center of the knee. The point at which the two lines intersect is the apex of the femoral deformity; the angle between the two lines is the magnitude of angular deformity (16 degrees here).

Draw a longitudinal line from the center of the ankle joint perpendicular to the tibial plafond, and extend it proximally parallel to the distal tibial diaphysis. The point at which this line intersects the mechanical axis line is the apex of tibial deformity and the angle between the two lines (14 degrees here) is the magnitude of varus deformity of the tibia. An opening-wedge or closing-wedge osteotomy at the apex of the angulation will correct the deformity.

In preoperative planning, correct the deformity of one long bone, then plan correction of the other long bone. For example, when the tibia is corrected first and normal mechanical axis of the tibia is achieved, plan correction of the femoral deformity by following the steps of preoperative planning of correction of femoral deformity with normal tibia and vice versa when the femoral deformity is corrected first.

Juxta-articular deformation about the hip and ankle present a complex problem. A translational deformity will result when simple closing-wedge or opening-wedge osteotomy is performed without translation. When supramalleolar tibial osteotomies or proximal femoral osteotomies (intertrochanteric or subtrochanteric) are performed, it is vital to combine angulation with translation because the level of osteotomy is not at the apex of the deformity.

FEMORAL/TIBIAL MECHANICAL DEVIATION

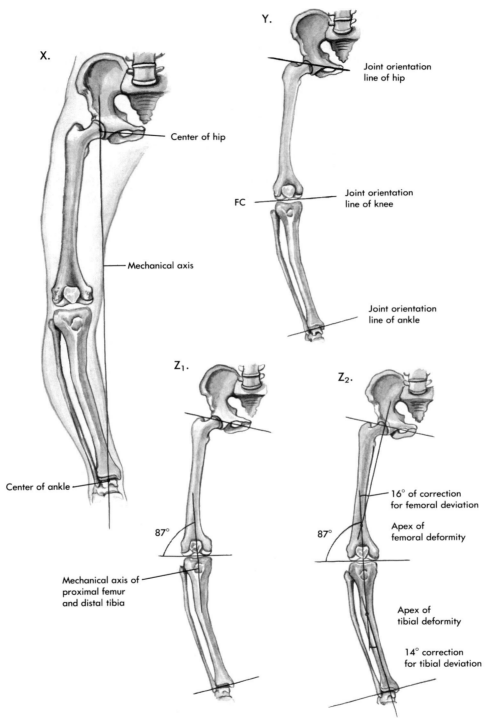

X.

Center of hip

Mechanical axis

Center of ankle

Y.

Joint orientation line of hip

FC   Joint orientation line of knee

Joint orientation line of ankle

Z₁.

87°

Mechanical axis of proximal femur and distal tibia

Z₂.

16° of correction for femoral deviation

Apex of femoral deformity

87°

Apex of tibial deformity

14° correction for tibial deviation

Plate 251. (Continued)

Deformity of the Ankle

AA. In the *frontal plane,* the tibial plafond may be tilted into valgus or varus, causing malalignment of the ankle joint orientation line. There is no deviation of the mechanical axis—longitudinal line drawn from the center of the femoral head to the centers of the knee and ankle. The apex of the deformity is the center point of the tibial plafond.

BB. The angular deformity (varus or valgus) is measured by the angle between a line drawn perpendicular to the tibial plafond and the mechanical axis.

CC. To provide space for internal fixation, perform a supramalleolar osteotomy to correct ankle valgus or varus. This causes a translation deformity and deviation of the mechanical axis.

DD. and **EE.** Therefore, correction of angulation should be combined with translation—*lateral* translation when correcting ankle *varus* and *medial* translation when correcting ankle *valgus.* I recommend the Wiltse technique as described in Plate 168.

TIBIAL PLAFOND

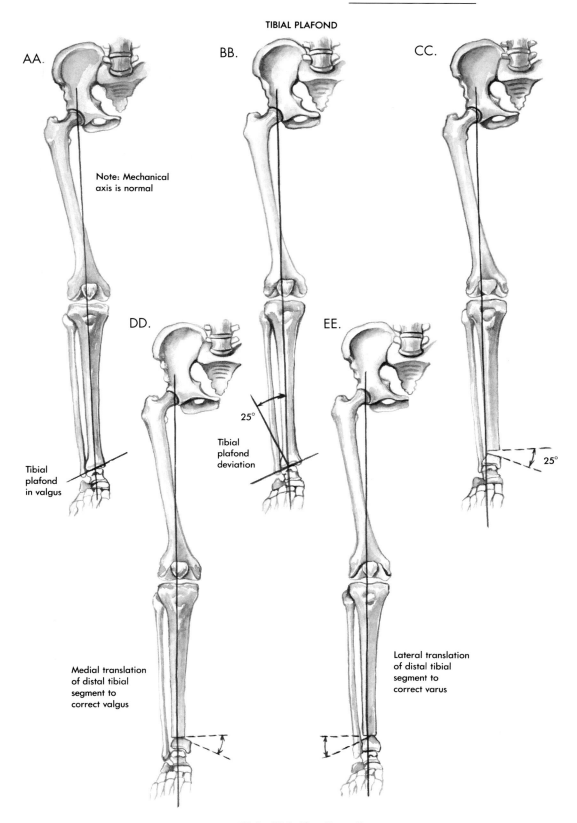

AA.

Note: Mechanical axis is normal

BB.

CC.

DD.

25°

Tibial plafond deviation

EE.

25°

Tibial plafond in valgus

Medial translation of distal tibial segment to correct valgus

Lateral translation of distal tibial segment to correct varus

Plate 251. (Continued)

Hip Deformity in the Frontal Plane

Coxa Vara

FF. The mechanical axis is normal; i.e., the line drawn from the center of the femoral head to the center of the knee and to the center of the ankle is colinear. The knee and ankle joint orientation lines are normal, whereas the hip joint orientation line is malaligned. The angle formed between the mechanical axis and the hip joint orientation line is greater than 90 degrees (in this illustration, 120 degrees), indicating a coxa vara deformity.

Measure the degree of varus angulation by drawing a line perpendicular (90 degrees) to the hip joint orientation line. Begin at the center of the femoral head, and extend it distally. The angle formed between this perpendicular line and the mechanical axis is the degree of varus angulation (30 degrees).

GG. When the coxa vara is corrected by simple lateral closing-wedge or medial opening-wedge osteotomy at the intertrochanteric or subtrochanteric level, the mechanical axis is deviated laterally.

HH. Therefore, both angulation and *lateral* translation of the distal segment are required to restore normal alignment of the mechanical axis.

Coxa Valga

II.–KK. Measure the degree of angular deformity as in coxa vara.

Correction of valgus deformity by simple medial closing-wedge or lateral opening-up wedge osteotomy at the intertrochanteric or subtrochanteric level results in medial mechanical axis deviation; therefore, correction of coxa valga requires angulation and *medial* translation of the distal segment to restore mechanical axis to normal.

REFERENCES

Paley, D., and Tetsworth, K: Mechanical axis deviation of the lower limbs. Clin. Orthop., 280:65–71, 1992.

JUXTA-ARTICULAR HIP DEFORMITY

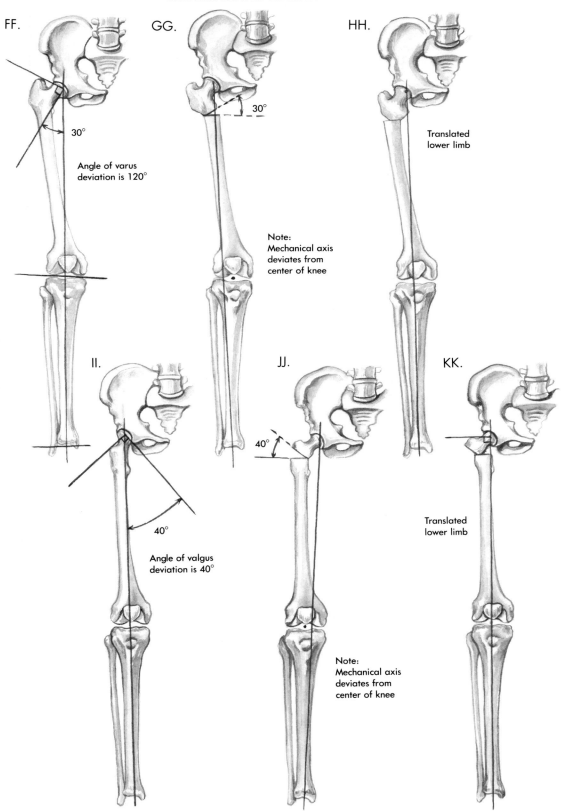

FF.

30°

Angle of varus
deviation is 120°

GG.

30°

Note:
Mechanical axis
deviates from
center of knee

HH.

Translated
lower limb

II.

40°

Angle of valgus
deviation is 40°

JJ.

40°

Note:
Mechanical axis
deviates from
center of knee

KK.

Translated
lower limb

Plate 251. (Continued)

PLATE 252 | Uniapical Valgus Deformity of the Diaphysis of the Tibia and Fibula Corrected by Ilizarov Technique

Indications. Valgus deformity of the tibial shaft and fibula as seen in malunion or fibrous non-union.

Preoperative Measures. Presurgical planning as outlined in Plate 251.

Special Apparatus. Complete set of Ilizarov instruments.

Blood for Transfusion. No.

Radiographic Control. Image intensifier.

Patient Position. Supine.

Operative Technique. Assemble the proximal pair and distal pair of rings according to measurements on the patient's leg and on radiograms.

Insertion of Transverse Wires

A. Insert the wires under image intensifier radiographic control.

First, from the lateral side, insert the proximal transverse olive wire parallel to the knee joint.

Second, insert the distal transverse olive wire from the lateral side parallel to the ankle joint. The olives on the proximal and distal transverse wire are on the concave side of the angular valgus deformity and act as antifulcrum or distraction point wires.

B. Near the apex of the deformity, from the medial side, insert a transverse olive wire proximal to the apex of the deformity and parallel to the knee joint. Then insert another transverse olive wire from the medial side distal to the apex of the deformity and parallel to the ankle joint. These two transverse wires have their olives on the convex side of the valgus deformity; they are called *fulcrum wires*.

Placement of Preconstructed Two-Ring Frame on the Proximal Pair of Transverse Wires

C. Progress from proximal to distal. Remove one of the central bolts from the superior ring and also from the inferior ring. Open the two connected rings as a clasp, and place it around the tibia and between the wires.

Insert the central bolts, and close the rings. Temporarily fix the transverse wire to the rings. An assistant holds the rings two fingerbreadths from the leg. The rings should be perpendicular to the tibia. The anterior cortex of the tibia should be parallel to the anterior and posterior rods. The bolts are retightened, and the wires are tensioned on the proximal two rings.

A.

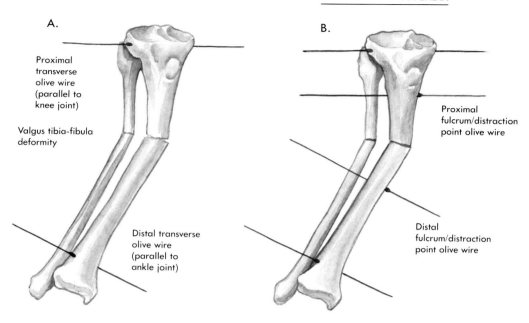

Proximal transverse olive wire (parallel to knee joint)

Valgus tibia-fibula deformity

Distal transverse olive wire (parallel to ankle joint)

B.

Proximal fulcrum/distraction point olive wire

Distal fulcrum/distraction point olive wire

C.   Placement of proximal ring block

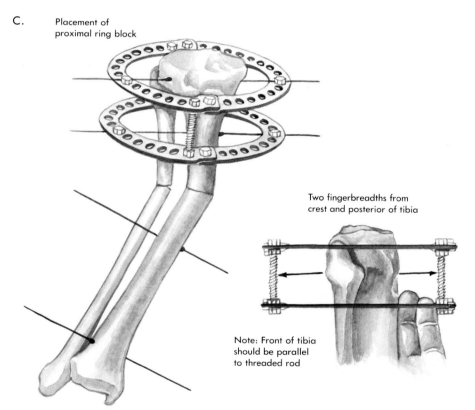

Two fingerbreadths from crest and posterior of tibia

Note: Front of tibia should be parallel to threaded rod

Plate 252. **A.–L.,** Uniapical valgus deformity of the diaphysis of the tibia and fibula corrected by Ilizarov technique.

Hinge Reconstruction and Positioning

D. The following parameters are critical in hinge reconstruction and positioning:

1. The point of rotation axis of the hinge should be on the horizontal level with the apex of the deformity.

2. Two hinges provide greater stability in correction of simple angular deformity in the frontal plane—in this plate, tibia valga. One hinge is placed anteriorly, the other hinge posteriorly.

3. The threaded rod of the anterior hinge should be parallel to the anterior convex surface of the tibia. The threaded rod of the posterior hinge should be parallel to the threaded rod of the anterior hinge. Orient the two hinges on the same plane and along the same plane of the deformity.

4. Hinge position and movement of the axis of rotation of the hinges affect movement of the bone fragments. When the hinge is placed on the convex side of the deformity, it causes distraction of the fragments. When the hinge is placed on the concave side, it compresses the fragments. In this plate, the hinges are positioned on the convex cortex of the deformity—an opening-wedge hinge.

The hinges are attached to the middle rings, near the apex of the deformity. In this plate, two female half-hinges are connected to the threaded rods, which in turn are connected to the rings. Other types of hinges that may be assembled in the Ilizarov technique are one male half-hinge (attached to the ring) and one female hinge, two supports or two posts to two plates connected to each other, or one support and one post connected to each other. No matter what type of assembly is utilized, the connecting bolt is the axis of rotation. Fixation of the bolt should be secure but not too tight, as it will prevent rotation and movement of the hinge. Ordinarily, the bolt is fixed either by two thin half-nuts tightened to each other or by lock nuts with nylon inserts.

First, attach the threaded rod of the proximal female half-hinge to the proximal middle ring next to the apex of the deformity.

Note: The threaded rod is of appropriate length so that the hinge overlies the apex of the deformity.

The threaded rod is parallel to the convex surface of the tibia proximal to the apex of the deformity. The hinge is positioned on the medial border of the cortex of the convex side of the deformity so that the correction obtained is an opening-wedge type.

Next, place the posterior hinge; it should be parallel to the anterior hinge, with its rotation axis on the horizontal level of the apex of the deformity.

E. Attach the anterior and posterior distal female half-hinge to the proximal female half-hinges. The connecting rod of the distal female half-hinge should be parallel to the medial convex border of the distal tibia, distal to the apex of the deformity.

D.   Hinge construction

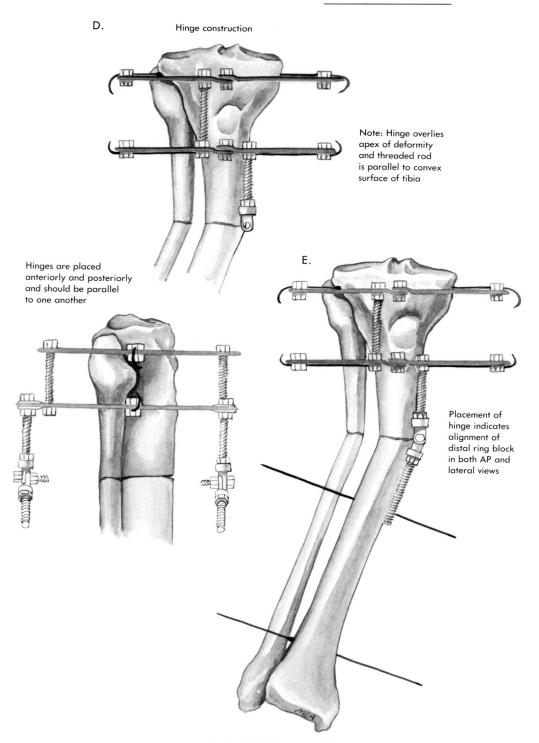

Note: Hinge overlies
apex of deformity
and threaded rod
is parallel to convex
surface of tibia

Hinges are placed
anteriorly and posteriorly
and should be parallel
to one another

E.

Placement of
hinge indicates
alignment of
distal ring block
in both AP and
lateral views

Plate 252. (Continued)

F. and **G.** Insert the distal pair of preconstructed rings by removing the central bolt and opening the rings like a half-shell. Place the rings around the lower leg, and close them by tightening the central bolts.

Insert the threads of the anterior and posterior distal female half-hinges to the corresponding holes of the lower middle rings near the apex of the deformity, similar to the proximal block of rings. Double-check and ensure that the rings are positioned correctly. The apparatus should completely mimic the deformity. The proximal pair of rings should be perpendicular to the axis of the proximal segment of the tibia, and the distal pair of rings is perpendicular to the axis of the segment of the tibia distal to the apex of the deformity. The angle between the rings near the apex of the deformity should be equal to the degree of angular deformity of the tibia in the frontal plane.

Insert the bolts for the wires and tension the four transverse wires. (Next, insert smooth wires in the proximal and distal middle rings at an angle to the transverse wires and tension them.)

Insert two fibular wires: One proximal wire is inserted from the head of the fibula into the tibia; attach it by bolts to the most proximal ring. The second wire is inserted laterally from the shaft of the fibula into the tibia and attached to the most distal ring. Tension all of the wires.

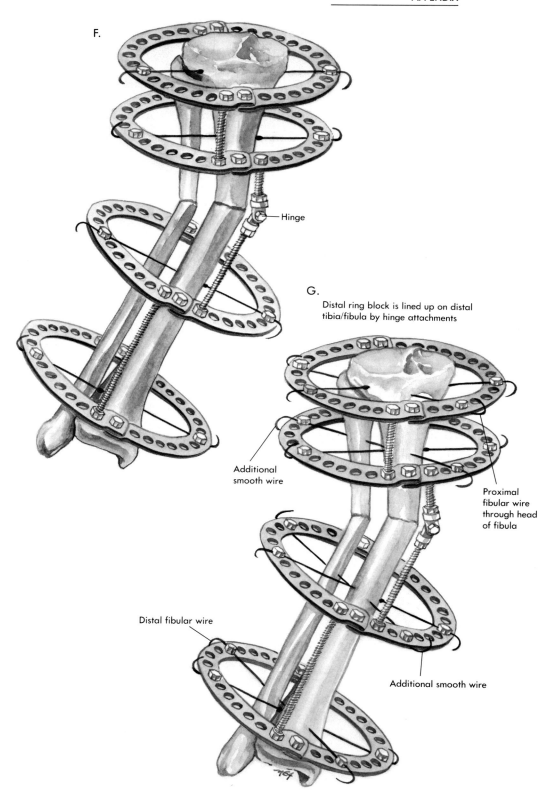

F.

Hinge

G.

Distal ring block is lined up on distal
tibia/fibula by hinge attachments

Additional
smooth wire

Proximal
fibular wire
through head
of fibula

Distal fibular wire

Additional smooth wire

Plate 252. (Continued)

Positioning and Attachment of Distraction Rods

H. The distraction rods are usually graduated telescoping rods; they are placed on the concavity of the deformity opposite the hinges, which are placed on the convexity of the curve. The distraction rods are connected to the most proximal and most distal rings with twisted plates and one-hole posts. The two nuts are on the inside. With distraction, the hinges rotate to accommodate changes in position of deformity.

The rate of correction with hinges is slower than the speed of distraction because the distraction graduated telescoping rod is situated at a distance from the axis of rotation of the hinges. The rate of correction of angular deformity is determined by the rule of triangles—a 3:1 factor; i.e., 3 mm. of distraction achieves 1 mm. of angular correction. Soft-tissue contracture on the concave side of the deformity should be considered because it will further slow the rate of angular correction.

I. When the deformity is corrected, the distraction rods become parallel to the shaft of the tibia. The hinges are straight, and the proximal and distal pair of rings are parallel to each other.

Opening-Wedge Hinge

As stated, the hinge is positioned on the concave side of the angular deformity. The exact placement of the axis of rotation varies, depending on the bone structure at the site of the deformity, the magnitude of opening wedge desired, and the degree of distraction-compression forces necessary to achieve union with simultaneous correction of deformity.

When the axis of rotation is in the center of the bony contour, the opening wedge on the concave side and the compression forces on the convex side will be small; this is indicated when the bone structure is normal, such as in an osteotomy of normal bone. When the axis of rotation of the hinges shifts more toward the convex side of the angular deformity, the opening wedge at the concave side of the deformity will be large whereas the opening on the convex side will be small; this type of positioning of hinge axis is indicated in hypertrophic non-union with sclerosis at bone ends. When the axis of rotation of the hinge shifts more on the concave side of the deformity, the opening of the wedge becomes smaller on the concave side and the compressive forces are greater on the convex side.

Hinge positions can vary, depending on the type of deformity correction required.

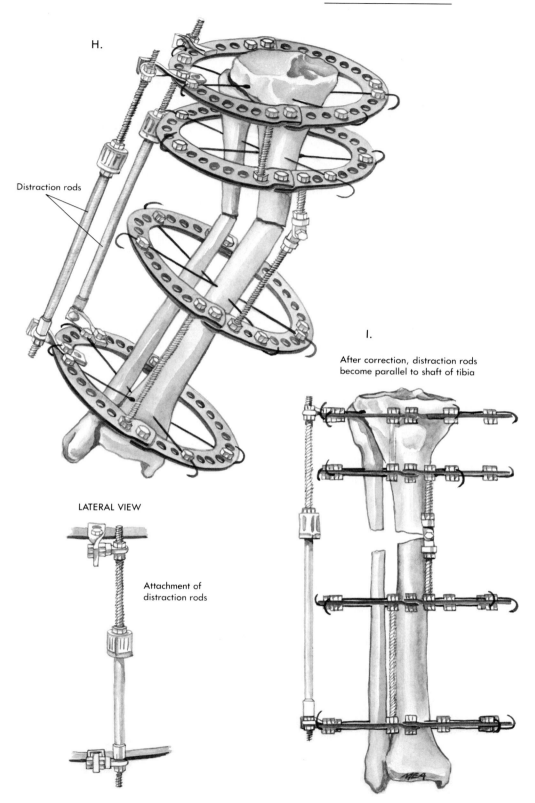

H.

Distraction rods

I.

After correction, distraction rods
become parallel to shaft of tibia

LATERAL VIEW

Attachment of
distraction rods

Plate 252. (Continued)

Distraction Hinge

J. When the axis of rotation of the hinge is positioned beyond the convex side of angulation, a wide opening is provided on both the concave and convex sides by distraction and straightening of the deformity. The farther away the hinge is from the bone, the greater the opening. The magnitude of distraction is limited by the distance of the hinge from the bone. The use of the distraction hinge is indicated when limb lengthening is required with correction of angular deformity.

Compression Hinge

K. The axis of rotation of the compression hinge is at the non-unicn site. With distraction and straightening, the bone ends are compressed.

Translation Hinge

L. A translation hinge is indicated when correction of both angular and translational deformity is desired. The axis of rotation of the hinges is positioned outside the level of the apex of the deformity. When the distal fragment of the tibia is displaced medially, the threaded rod of the upper female half-hinge is connected to two holes from the central bolt of the upper ring and the threaded rod of the lower female half-hinge is connected to one hole away from the central bolt of the lower ring. Distraction and straightening of the angular deformity translate the distal fragment toward the convexity and anatomically align the upper and lower bone fragments.

If the distal fragment is displaced lateral to the proximal fragment, the proximal connection of the rod of the hinge is one hole away from the central bolt of the upper ring and the distal connection of the rod of the hinge is two holes away from the central bolt of the lower ring.

Postoperative Care. Pin site care is provided as described in basic Ilizarov technique. Physical therapy in the form of passive range of motion exercises of the ankle and knee are performed several times a day. Partial weight bearing is allowed with three-point crutch support. Periodic radiograms (every two to three weeks) are made to determine the degree of correction and the status of bone healing.

When the osteosynthesis of the non-union or osteotomy site is adequate, the frame is dynamized for two to three weeks and the fixator is then removed. Depending on the individual case, a period of external support in the form of an orthosis—knee-ankle-foot (KAFO) or ankle-foot (AFO)—may be necessary.

J.   Distraction hinge

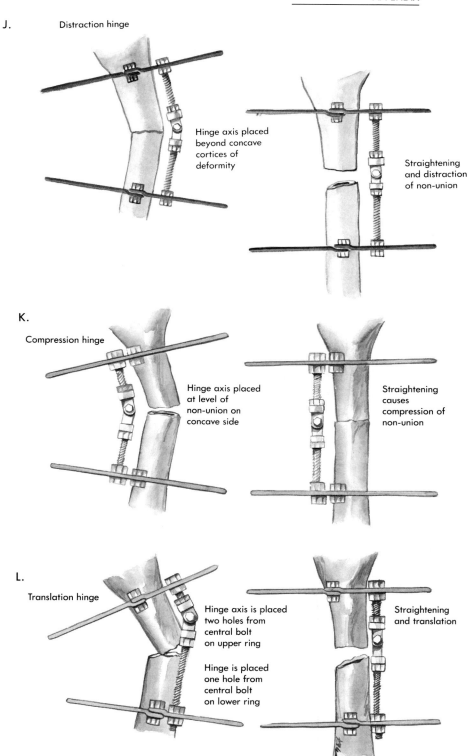

Hinge axis placed beyond concave cortices of deformity

Straightening and distraction of non-union

K.

Compression hinge

Hinge axis placed at level of non-union on concave side

Straightening causes compression of non-union

L.

Translation hinge

Hinge axis is placed two holes from central bolt on upper ring

Hinge is placed one hole from central bolt on lower ring

Straightening and translation

Plate 252. (Continued)

PLATE 253 — Treatment of Pseudarthrosis of the Tibia with Correction of Anterior Angulation and Lengthening with Ilizarov Technique

Indications. Pseudarthrosis of the tibia and fibula with anterior angulation of the tibia. (When limb lengths are equal, the steps **J.** and **K.** are deleted.)

Blood for Transfusion. No.

Radiographic Control. Image intensifier.

Special Instrumentation. Complete Ilizarov set.

Patient Position. Supine.

Operative Technique

Preconstruction of the Apparatus. If feasible, it is desirable to make a plastic model of the deformed leg and construct the apparatus by measurements made clinically on the patient's leg and on radiograms. In the growing skeleton, do not disturb the distal and proximal growth plates of the tibia and fibula.

    A. and **B.** The apparatus consists of a long Ilizarov plate of appropriate length that is placed directly anterior to the convex tibia. Two full rings, one proximal and one distal, are connected with regular nuts to the long plate with three-hole and four-hole posts. The posts are attached to the hole in the rings immediately next to the central bolt connecting the two half-rings. The proximal and distal full rings should be exactly perpendicular to the respective segments of the tibial shaft. The level of the rings should be 2 to 3 cm. away from the respective growth plates of the tibia.

    Be sure that the proximal ring allows adequate knee flexion (about 90 degrees). In the heavy child or in the adult, it is desirable to use a five-eighths (⅝) ring and full ring proximally for secure fixation. Connect the proximal full ring and ⅝ ring in the usual fashion.

    In the middle of the leg are two half-rings—one superior and the other inferior to the site of pseudarthrosis. The level of the half-rings should be 2 to 3 cm. away from the site of union; insert the pins through good bone stock.

    The half-rings are placed and centered immediately anterior to the tibia. The middle two half-rings should be parallel to each other. They are connected with four threaded rods of appropriate length. The rods are attached to the half-rings with regular nuts—one rod at each end of the half-ring and the central two rods evenly dispersed. The middle two half-rings are connected by nylon nuts to the long plate by the female hinge and post. Connection by nylon nuts allows superior and inferior angulation of the middle half-rings without varus or valgus deviation.

Insertion of Wires. With the patient under general anesthesia and with a pneumatic tourniquet on the proximal thigh, the lower limb is prepared and draped sterile in the usual fashion. The limb is inserted through the apparatus. The level of the proximal and distal full rings and middle two half-rings is double-checked and appropriate adjustments are made. Avoid injury to the proximal and distal tibial physis. The long plate and hinge should be directly anterior to the anterior convexity of the tibia. Under image intensification radiography, double-check the proposed level of insertion of the wires. There should be good bone stock for the middle segment wires.

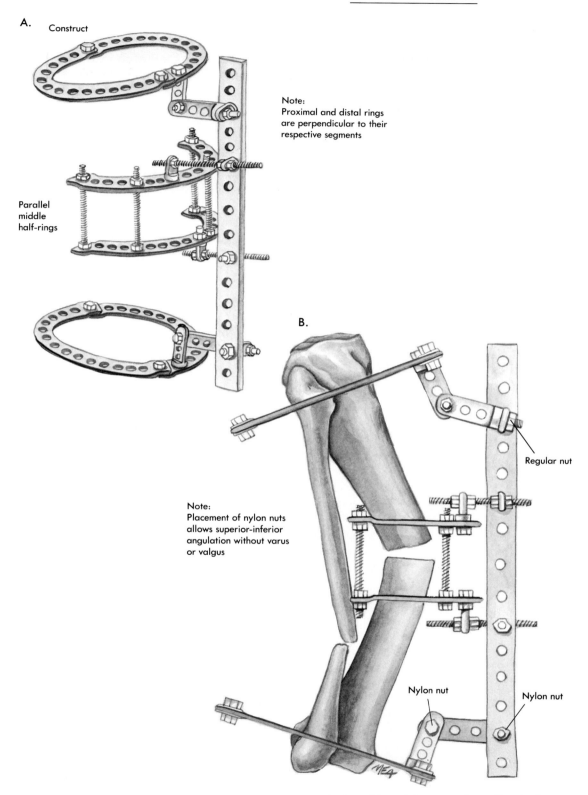

A. Construct

Note:
Proximal and distal rings are perpendicular to their respective segments

Parallel middle half-rings

B.

Regular nut

Note:
Placement of nylon nuts allows superior-inferior angulation without varus or valgus

Nylon nut   Nylon nut

Plate 253. A.–K., Treatment of pseudarthrosis of the tibia with correction of anterior angulation and lengthening with Ilizarov technique.

C. and **D.** First, insert the proximal transverse wire and then the distal transverse wire, according to basic Ilizarov technique as described in Plate 250.

E. Insert the proximal fibular and distal fibular wires. After double-checking the position of the middle half-rings, connect and tension the proximal and distal transverse and fibular wires.

C. Application of transverse wires
    (proximally)

D.

    Application of transverse wires
    (distally)

E.

    Fibular wires

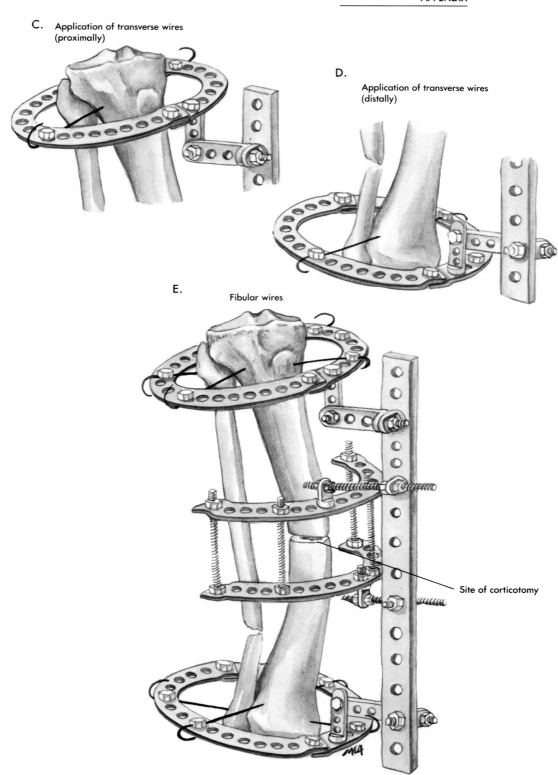

Site of corticotomy

Plate 253. (Continued)

Insertion of Middle Segment Wires and Attachment of Distraction Rod

F. Insert one Ilizarov wire in the proximal segment of the tibia and another Ilizarov wire in the distal segment of the tibia, 2 to 3 cm. away from the pseudarthrosis site. Attach and tension the middle segment wires.

Connect the distraction graduated rod to posts at the center of the proximal full ring and the distal full ring. The distraction rod should be straight posterior to the anteriorly angulated tibia and opposite the long plate.

Gradually, the tibial segments are distracted and the anterior convexity is straightened.

G.–I. After correcting anterior angulation, insert half-pins in the anterior aspect of the lower part of the proximal segment and the upper part of the distal segment. Connect the half-pins to the respective half-rings by Rancho cubes. With the graduated telescoping rod, the tibial bone segments are compressed.

F.

Distraction rod

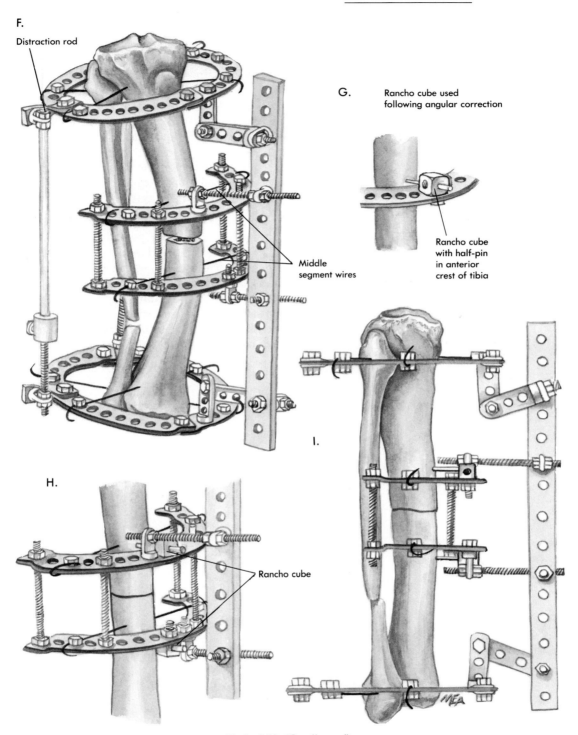

G.   Rancho cube used
following angular correction

Rancho cube
with half-pin
in anterior
crest of tibia

Middle
segment wires

I.

H.

Rancho cube

Plate 253. (Continued)

J. and K. When the tibia is short and lengthening is indicated, the distal full ring is fixed rigidly by regular nuts to the lower end of the long plate by a twisted plate. The proximal full ring is loosely secured to the long plate by a sliding buckle. The proximal ring is connected to the distal ring by two graduated telescoping rods—one inserted anterolaterally and the other anteromedially—parallel to each other. Leave the posterior distraction-compression rod as it is, or replace it by two graduated telescoping rods—one placed posteromedially and the other posterolaterally. The posterior and anterior graduated telescoping rods should be parallel to each other.

The rods are loosened. Prepare a corticotomy of the proximal tibial metaphysis and fibular shaft (see the steps described Plate 250, p. 1450). The rods are reconnected and lengthening of the tibia is carried out as described in Plate 158 (p. 896).

Postoperative Care. See Plate 158. After a latency period of three to five days, begin lengthening by distraction. The rate of distraction is 1 mm. per day, achieved in incremental gains of 1.25 mm. each turn, four times per day. When the desired length is obtained, the apparatus is securely fixed for immobilization. The pseudarthrosis site is compressed. When there is adequate healing of the elongated segment and the pseudarthrosis, the apparatus is dynamized (see Plate 158) and removed in a few weeks. It is vital that the tibia be supported in a knee-ankle-foot orthosis (KAFO) with an anterior shell.

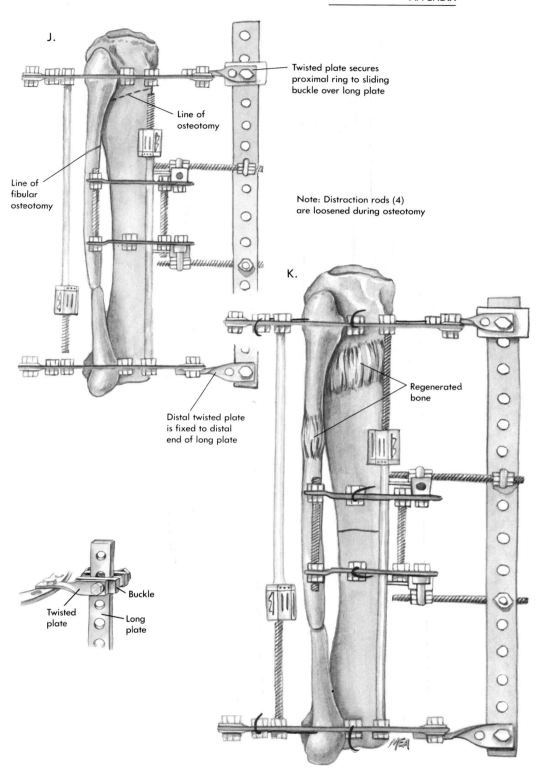

J.

Twisted plate secures
proximal ring to sliding
buckle over long plate

Line of
osteotomy

Line of
fibular
osteotomy

Note: Distraction rods (4)
are loosened during osteotomy

K.

Regenerated
bone

Distal twisted plate
is fixed to distal
end of long plate

Buckle

Twisted
plate

Long
plate

Plate 253. (Continued)

PLATE 254 **Tibial Lengthening with Foot Construct Using Ilizarov Technique**

Indications. Limb length disparity of the tibia of greater than 5 cm. with instability of the ankle due to longitudinal deficiency of the fibula or other causes with or without foot deformity.

Requisites

1. The knee and ankle joint should be stable.
2. Circulation should be normal.
3. There should be no skin or soft-tissue problems.
4. Bone structures should be normal.
5. The patient should be psychosocially stable.
6. The patient should be cooperative and cognizant of the postoperative program.

Blood for Transfusion. No.

Radiographic Control. Image intensifier.

Patient Position. Supine.

Preassembly

A. The frame is assembled prior to surgery to save time on the operating table (see Plate 158, p. 896). The proximal block of rings consists of a five-eighths (⅝) upper ring open posteriorly, so that it does not restrict knee flexion, and a lower full ring. The two rings are connected by hexagonal screws, as described in Plate 158. The distal block of rings consists of a proximal full ring connected by offset posts to a half-ring closed posteriorly. The proximal and distal blocks are connected with anterior and posterior telescoping threaded rods. For details as to the level of the rings and the technique of connection of the rings with the rods, refer to Plate 158.

Operative Technique

B. With the patient under general anesthesia and supine on the operating table, the frame is placed on the leg by inserting the foot through the rings. The levels of the rings are double-checked clinically and verified by radiography.

A.

Construct

B.

Placement on leg

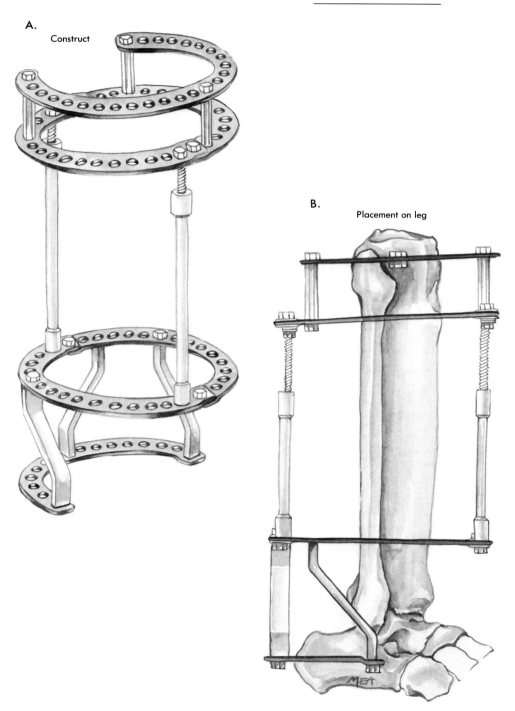

Plate 254. A.–N., Tibial lengthening with foot construct using Ilizarov technique.

C. Insert the *proximal* transverse reference wire in the frontal plane. This 1.8-mm. olive wire should be at an inclination of 7 degrees to the knee joint. It is inserted from the lateral side and should exit more proximally on the medial than on the lateral side. Its plane is similar to the inclination of the proximal block of rings.

Insert the *distal* transverse reference wire, a 1.8-mm. smooth wire, from the lateral side in the frontal plane just proximal to the ankle joint and parallel to the tibial plafond. Extend the frame so that it fills the space between the two wires. The proximal block should be flush with the proximal reference wire, and the distal block should be flush with the distal reference wire.

D. Next, insert the fibular wires: the first one in the most proximal ring through the head of the fibula, the second one through the proximal fibula from the lateral side in the distal ring of the proximal block, and the third one through the distal diaphyseal-metaphyseal region of the fibula and tibia through the proximal full ring of the distal block. The wires are tensioned, as described in Plate 250.

Next, insert a medial face wire in the distal ring of the proximal block. It is perpendicular to the fibular wires (see Plate 158).

C.

Proximal transverse
reference wire

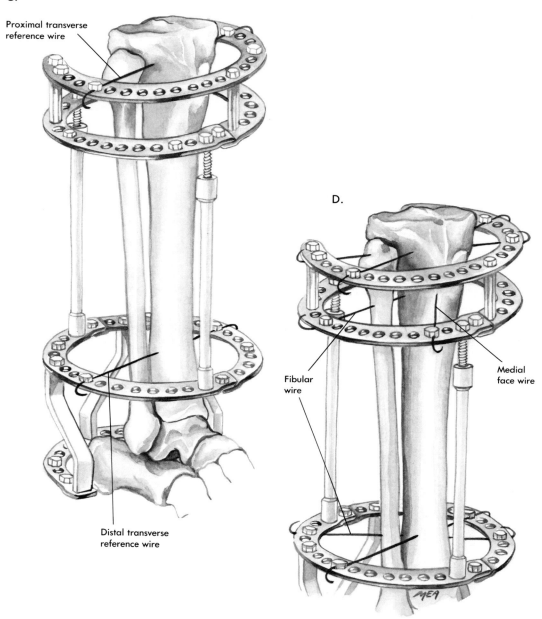

Distal transverse
reference wire

D.

Fibular
wire

Medial
face wire

Plate 254. (Continued)

E. and **F.** Center the distal half-ring in the coronal axis. It should correspond in size to the distal full ring. Connect the half-ring to the distal full ring by three offset posts (one at each end and one posteriorly in the center of the half-ring) or by two threaded rods inserted at each end of the half-ring. The half-ring must be lined up with the side of the calcaneus.

Insert two olive wires, one from the lateral side of the calcaneus and one from the medial side. The wires should pass through the posterior part of the calcaneus and should be slightly proximal to the body of the os calcis. This measure provides enough bone structure so that the wires will not cut out through the calcaneus from the pull of the Achilles tendon. With the foot in neutral dorsiflexion at the ankle joint, tension the calcaneal wires.

G. Determine the lines of the corticotomies of the tibia and fibula on the radiogram as shown.

E.   Calcaneal wires

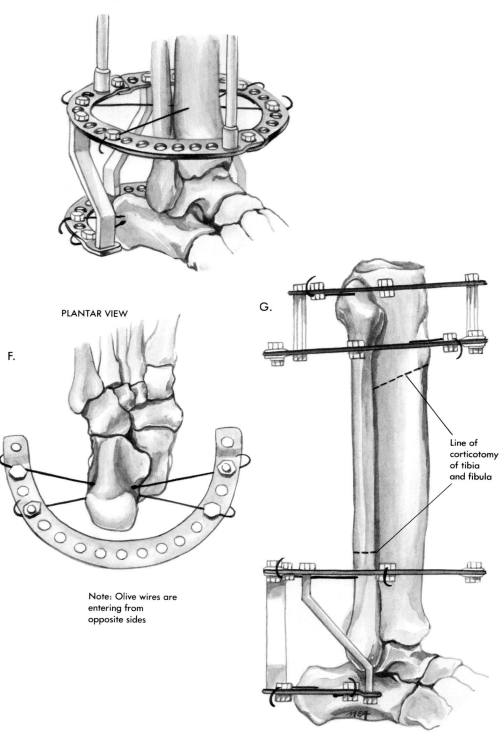

PLANTAR VIEW

F.

G.

Line of
corticotomy
of tibia
and fibula

Note: Olive wires are
entering from
opposite sides

Plate 254. (Continued)

H.–J. If the fibula is present, first perform a corticotomy of the fibula at the juncture of its medial and distal thirds through a 2-cm. lateral longitudinal incision. Next, perform a tibial corticotomy through a 1-cm. anterior incision over the anterior crest of the tibia immediately distal to the second proximal ring.

Note: The direction of the corticotomy is posteromedial.

Section the anterior cortex of the tibia with a sharp osteotome with the protection of subperiosteally inserted Chandler retractors. Divide the medial and lateral cortices of the tibia with a 5-mm. sharp osteotome. The proximal and distal blocks of rings are disconnected and the posterior cortex is sectioned by twisting the osteotome. Perform osteoclasis by lateral rotation of the distal segment of the tibia. Then reconnect the graduated telescoping rods between the proximal and distal blocks of rings. Verify the completeness of corticotomy by image intensifier radiography. Place a clicker on the rods for distraction and compression. Be sure there are 5 degrees of varus and 7 degrees of recurvatum between the proximal and distal blocks. The foot construct prevents ankle valgus and equinus.

K. Five to 7 days after corticotomy, the tibia is elongated. The elongation technique and postoperative care are described in Plate 158.

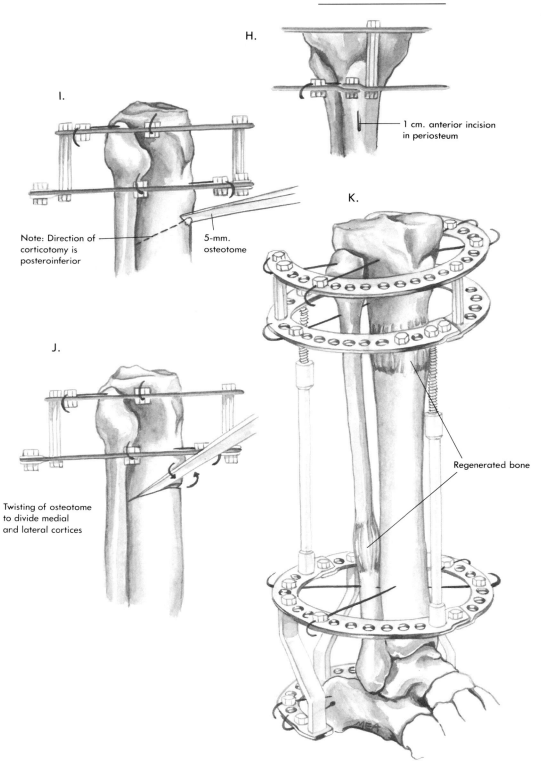

H.

1 cm. anterior incision
in periosteum

I.

Note: Direction of
corticotomy is
posteroinferior

5-mm.
osteotome

J.

Twisting of osteotome
to divide medial
and lateral cortices

K.

Regenerated bone

Plate 254. (Continued)

L.–N. When there is a foot deformity, insert a transverse wire through the anterior calcaneus, another wire through the talus, and a third wire across the distal end of the metatarsals. The metatarsal and anterior calcaneal wires are attached to half-rings and tensioned in the usual fashion. Attach the transverse wire through the anterior part of the talus (if used) to the one-hole posts, which are attached to the proximal half-ring on the dorsum of the foot. The offset posts are connected to the full ring on the distal block by conical washers.

The proximal half-ring on the foot is connected to the full ring of the distal block by a hinge with its apex over the axis of the ankle joint. The half-rings on the dorsum of the foot are connected to the posterior half-ring of the distal block by graduated distraction rods with clickers. This system allows correction of the varus-valgus deformities of the foot, equinus of the forefoot, and equinus of the ankle.

Postoperative Care. See Plates 158 (p. 896) and 250 (p. 1450).

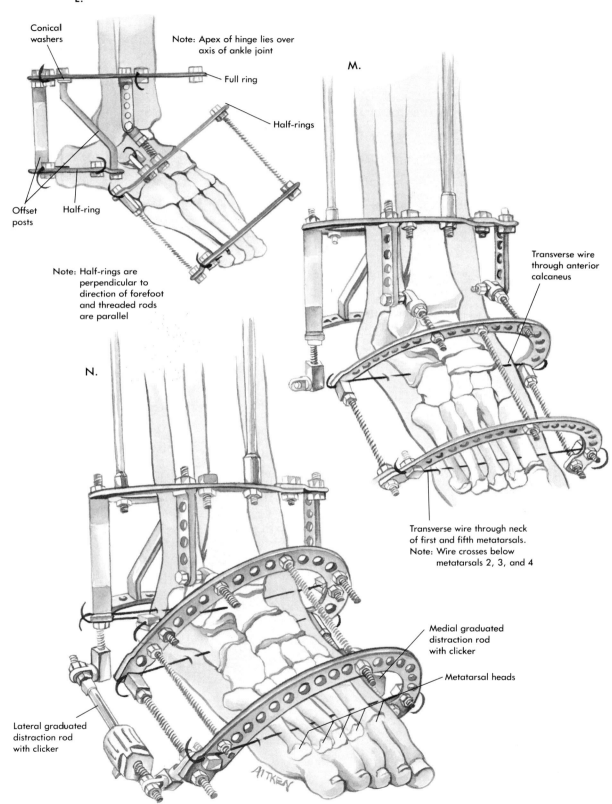

L.

Conical washers

Note: Apex of hinge lies over axis of ankle joint

Full ring

Half-rings

Half-ring

Offset posts

Note: Half-rings are perpendicular to direction of forefoot and threaded rods are parallel

M.

Transverse wire through anterior calcaneus

Transverse wire through neck of first and fifth metatarsals.
Note: Wire crosses below metatarsals 2, 3, and 4

N.

Medial graduated distraction rod with clicker

Metatarsal heads

Lateral graduated distraction rod with clicker

AITKEN

Plate 254. (Continued)

PLATE 255 ### Correction of Complex Deformity of Femoral Diaphysis (Varus, Antetorsion, and Translation) with Lengthening of the Short Femur

Indications. Varus and severe antetorsion deformity of femoral shaft with shortening caused by malunion or developmental bone dysplasia.

Blood for Transfusion. Yes.

Radiographic Control. Image intensifier.

Special Instrumentation. Complete Ilizarov set.

Patient Position. Supine.

Operative Technique. The sequence of correction of deformities is as follows:

1. Varus.
2. Elongation of the short femur.
3. Correction of femoral antetorsion.
4. Correction of translational deformity, which in this case is created by the derotation.

Preconstruction of the Apparatus. The completed apparatus consists of the following:

1. A proximal arc connected to the femur with two half-pins.
2. A full ring connected to the proximal segment of the femur with two crossed olive wires.
3. A full ring connected to the upper part of the distal segment of the femur with two crossed olive wires.
4. A distal five-eighths (⅝) ring connected to the lower part of the distal femoral shaft with one smooth wire and an olive wire. Each ring level has two wires or pins; a translation device is added later on.

A. and **B.** Connect the distal block of two rings—a distal ⅝ ring open posteriorly for knee flexion and a full ring—in the standard fashion.

Note: Two of the threaded rods are attached to the ends of the ⅝ ring and to the corresponding holes of the full ring. The middle rod is connected proximally to the hole of the full ring medial and next to the central bolt and distally attached to the ⅝ ring two holes medial to its central hole.

Use hinges for connecting the distal block of rings to the proximal block of rings; the hinges are required for correction of the varus deformity. Construct one ring by connecting two half-rings in the standard fashion. Choose a pair of threaded rods of appropriate length and hinge assembly consisting of hinge bolts and nylon nuts. Connect the full ring of the proximal block to the distal block by attaching the rods at the first hole adjacent to the central bolt both anteriorly and posteriorly. Connect the hinge assembly to the lower full ring at the first hole adjacent to the central bolt both anteriorly and posteriorly.

It is critical that the two full rings be of the same size. Flex and extend the two full rings several times, and tighten the connections with the two full rings in the flexed position; this measure ensures that the two rings do not jam when the hinges rotate into flexion.

Next, assemble an arc of appropriate size with two oblique supports connected to the end holes of the arc. Choose two 40-mm. sockets that are connected to the proximal full ring. In the preconstruction of the arc to the proximal full ring, the degree of antetorsional deformity should be taken into consideration by connecting the socket to the appropriate holes of the proximal full ring. The anterior socket is connected to a more lateral hole on the full ring, and the posterior socket is connected to a more medial hole on the full ring.

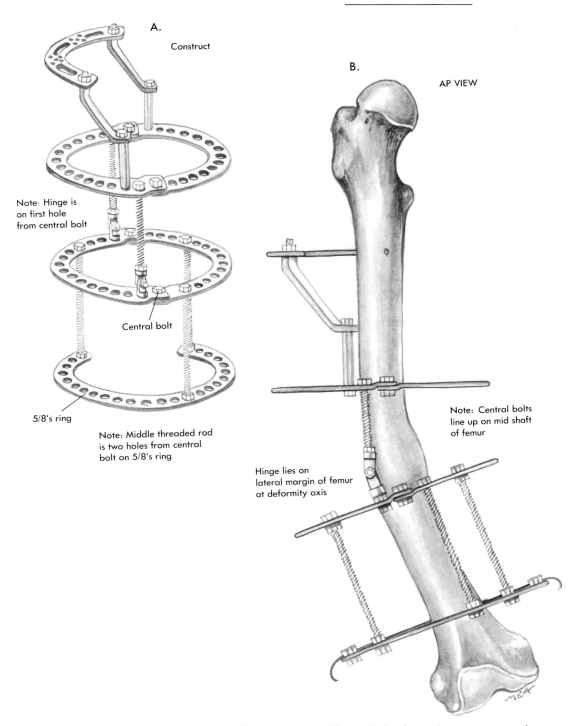

A. Construct

Note: Hinge is on first hole from central bolt

5/8's ring

Central bolt

Note: Middle threaded rod is two holes from central bolt on 5/8's ring

B. AP VIEW

Note: Central bolts line up on mid shaft of femur

Hinge lies on lateral margin of femur at deformity axis

Plate 255. A.–N., Correction of complex deformity of femoral diaphysis (varus, antetorsion, and translation) with lengthening of the short femur.

C. Prepare the entire lower limb, hip, and lower abdomen sterile, and drape in the usual orthopedic fashion. The sterilized, previously preconstructed frame is slipped upward over the patient's foot and leg.

Insert a 1.8-mm. olive wire through the distal femur perpendicular to the distal femoral shaft. *All of the wire must be inserted perpendicular to the femoral shaft for correction of the midshaft angular deformity.*

An alternate method of wire insertion is parallel to the joint orientation lines of the knee and hip, as described for realignment of the mechanical axis (see Plate 251). When the deformity is midshaft and severe, the method of insertion of the wires perpendicular to the femoral shaft is relatively simple.

Center the distal ⅝ ring of the preconstructed frame over the distal reference wire. Be sure that there is ample room for the soft tissues and that the knee flexes adequately through the posterior opening of the ⅝ ring. Next, pivot the apparatus and align it in the lateral view so that the rods are parallel to the femoral shaft.

D. With the apparatus properly aligned, insert one half of a pin through the posterior end of the arc perpendicular to the femoral shaft. The apparatus should be level with the anterior aspect of the femur in the lateral projection, the distal block of rings perpendicular to the distal segment of the femoral shaft, and the proximal block of rings perpendicular to the proximal segment of the femoral shaft.

Check the length of the apparatus, and shorten or lengthen the connecting rods as necessary. The hinges should be level with the apex of the deformity in order to avoid translation at the osteotomy site. The upper and lower parts of the hinge should align with each segment of the femoral deformity; i.e., the threaded rod of the hinge should line up with the proximal part of the femoral shaft above the apex of the deformity and the lower part of the hinge should align with the distal segment of the femoral shaft below the apex of the deformity.

Fulcrum Wire Insertion and Fixation

E. and **F.** The fulcrum wires are inserted *obliquely* from the *lateral* side, with the olives on the lateral side acting as counterpoints for correction of the angular deformity. The oblique 45-degree angle direction of insertion of the olive-fulcrum wires from the lateral side avoids entrapment of the fascia lata and restriction of knee motion and posteriorly it avoids the hamstrings.

Before inserting the wire, pull the skin and soft tissues toward the osteotomy site where the lengthening will occur. The knee is in flexion when the wire traverses the anterior aspect. When the wire exits the posterior surface of the femur, it is tapped through the soft tissues with the knee in extension. That is, when the wire is drilled through the anteromedial aspect of the thigh (at a 45-degree oblique angle), the knee is in flexion to avoid the fascia lata and the quadriceps muscle fibers at increased length. When the wire traverses the postero-medial compartment, the knee is in full extension to avoid the hamstrings. When the wire is about to puncture the skin, pull the soft tissues and skin toward the osteotomy site. When the olive-fulcrum wire is inserted on the distal middle ring, pull the skin up proximally. When the wire is inserted through the proximal middle ring, pull the skin down distally.

1. Insert the olive wire for fixation to the distal middle ring.
2. Insert the olive wire for fixation to the proximal middle ring.
3. Insert the olive-fulcrum wire for fixation to the distal ⅝ ring.
4. Insert a half-pin proximally for fixation to the arc as far anteriorly as possible.

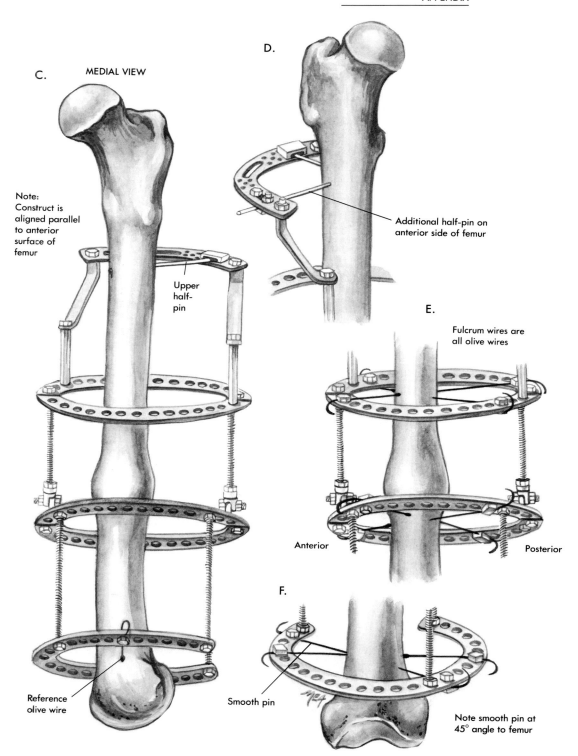

C. MEDIAL VIEW

D.

Note:
Construct is
aligned parallel
to anterior
surface of
femur

Upper
half-
pin

Additional half-pin on
anterior side of femur

E.

Fulcrum wires are
all olive wires

Anterior   Posterior

Reference
olive wire

F.

Smooth pin

Note smooth pin at
45° angle to femur

Plate 255. (Continued)

Positioning and Fixation of the Distraction Rod

G. Apply the distraction rod to the two full middle rings with two-hole twisted plates and a one-hole post or hinge. Insert the threaded rod through the hole of the posts. Tighten the base of the hinge or post with nylon insert nuts, which will allow pivot motion, change in angle, and self-adjustment between the distraction rod and twisted plates as the angle between the rings changes with straightening of the angular deformity.

Corticotomy

H. From the upper middle ring, remove the rods connecting the hinges, leaving the hinges locked in place, and disconnect the distraction rod by removing the nuts on it.

Perform a corticotomy through a lateral approach at the apex of the deformity following the standard Ilizarov technique. The hinges should be in line with the level of corticotomy at the apex of the deformity.

Correction of Varus Angulation

I. Reconnect the threaded rods, and reattach the distraction rod on the concavity of the deformity.

Distraction begins the second to the fourth day, and the varus deformity is gradually corrected hinging at the apex. When the hinge is positioned at the convex cortex of the apex of the deformity, distraction or opening-wedge type of correction of the angular deformity is achieved. With straightening, the rings become parallel to each other.

G.   Two-hole plate and
      distraction rod

MEDIAL VIEW

H.

Distraction rod
removed

I.   Varus correction

Connecting
rods to hinges
are removed

Line of
corticotomy

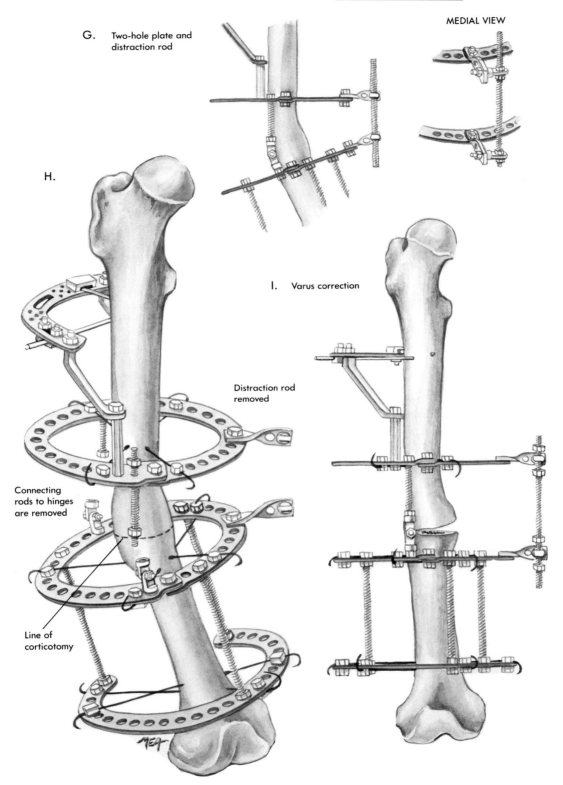

Plate 255. (Continued)

Elongation of the Short Femur by Use of the Distraction Hinge

J. and **K.** When moderate elongation with correction of varus angulation is desired, the hinges are positioned at a certain distance lateral to the convex cortex at the apex of the deformity. With distraction, the angular deformity is corrected and the femur is elongated.

J.

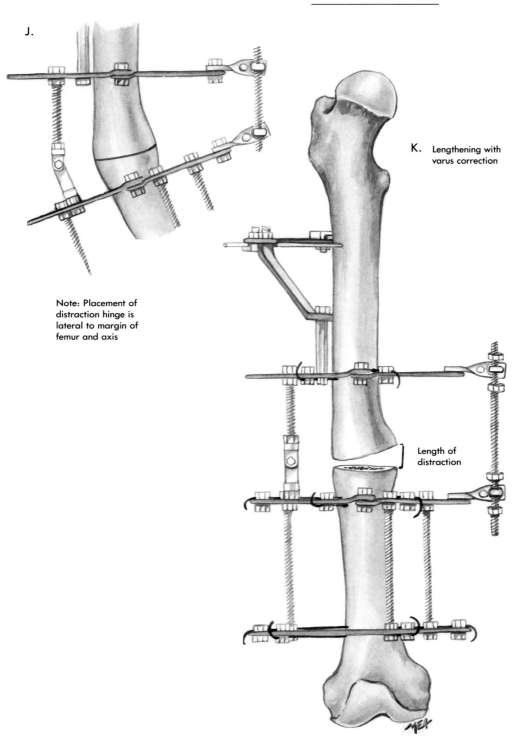

K.   Lengthening with
     varus correction

Note: Placement of
distraction hinge is
lateral to margin of
femur and axis

Length of
distraction

Plate 255. (Continued)

Correction of Antetorsion

L. Derotation is performed after distraction in order to prevent disruption and compression of the blood vessels in the newly formed bone regenerate. Connect the rotational devices to the two rings immediately above and below the apex of the deformity. A total of four rotational devices are required; they are spread evenly among the rings. Position the horizontal rods at a level with the apex of the deformity (which is now corrected) and in the center of the regenerate bone of the elongated segment.

The rotational device is constructed as follows:

Insert a long threaded rod from the superior ring down, and apply a bushing (a short cylinder with a *smooth* aperture and two *threaded* holes perpendicular to and midway between the smooth holes). Insert the threaded rod through the threaded holes of the bushing, which is locked to the threaded rod on either side by one nut. Add one more nut on the threaded rod distal to the bushing, and choose a buckle without its plate. Insert the lower end of the threaded rod through the threaded hole in the buckle, and thread it only *partially*. The buckle should lie smoothly against the ring so that it can easily slide on the ring. When the threaded rod is threaded all the way through the hole of the buckle and the ring, the buckle will not slide. Tighten the nut against the buckle using a wrench.

Then take a three-hole or four-hole post, and place it away from the threaded rod in the direction of derotation. Connect the post to the ring, and pass it through the top hole of the post; extend it into the bushing, and thread it into the hole of the bushing. Do not overthread it, or it will impact. Then tighten all the nuts around the bushing. The post and the threaded rod are tightened securely, but the nut holding the post to the ring (a nylon insert nut) should not be too tight in order to allow rotation of the post as derotation is carried out. Next, construct the remaining three rotation connection devices as described above.

When the distal fragment is rotated medially, there is *medial* translation of the distal fragment; when it is laterally rotated (as shown in this illustration) to correct antetorsion, there is *lateral* translation of the distal fragment. The translation of the distal fragment on derotation is caused by the eccentric location of the femur in the ring.

L.

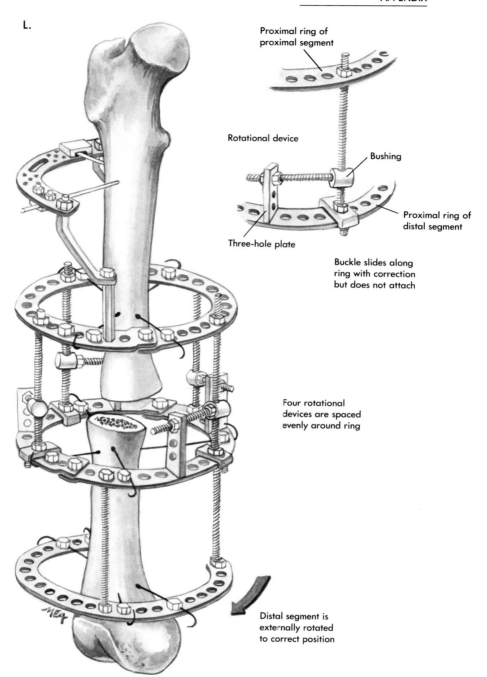

Proximal ring of
proximal segment

Rotational device

Bushing

Three-hole plate

Proximal ring of
distal segment

Buckle slides along
ring with correction
but does not attach

Four rotational
devices are spaced
evenly around ring

Distal segment is
externally rotated
to correct position

Plate 255. (Continued)

Correction of Translational Deformity

M. Apply the translational apparatus. It consists of a 17-hole plate on the lateral aspect of the femur, which is anchored to the upper arc ring with a twisted plate. At the lower end, the plate is attached to the distal ⅝ ring with a threaded rod and a female poster hinge.

In the front and back of the femur, construct a rail device, which consists of a horizontal threaded rod in the direction of the translational deformity. Insert a bushing on the horizontal threaded rod. In the anterior aspect of the femur, connect the horizontal threaded rod to the proximal full ring next to the osteotomy by vertical rods. Tighten all of the nuts.

As the bushing moves ("rails") along the horizontal rod, it carries along the upper ring. Construct a similar rail device, and posteriorly connect it to the distal full ring next to the osteotomy. The horizontal rail rods should be parallel to each other.

N. Correct the translational deformity by lateral translation of the proximal segment.

Postoperative Care. When the regenerate bone in the elongated segment is healed, the fixator is dynamized for two to three weeks (see Plate 158, p. 896). The external support, in the form of a hip-knee-ankle-foot orthosis (HKAFO), is often indicated to prevent stress fracture. The orthosis is worn for two to four months after removal of the fixator.

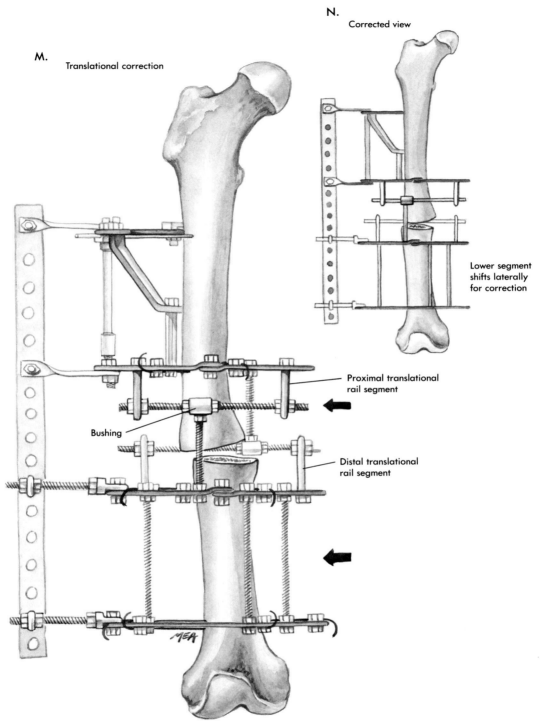

N.
Corrected view

M.
Translational correction

Lower segment
shifts laterally
for correction

Proximal translational
rail segment

Bushing

Distal translational
rail segment

Plate 255. (Continued)

PLATE 256

Treatment of Pseudarthrosis (Non-union) by Bone Transport Using Ilizarov Technique

Indications. Segmental bone loss with non-union and congenital pseudarthrosis of the tibia with marked shortening of the leg.

1. Reconstruction of non-unions, such as in congenital pseudarthrosis of the tibia.

2. Major post-traumatic defects in long bones as a complication of severe limb injuries in which contaminated, devascularized segments of cortical bone have been excised or lost.

3. Chronic osteomyelitis, in which infected necrotic bone is removed to enhance healing. Ordinarily, for defects greater than 2.5 to 3 cm., bone transport is required.

4. Tumor resection.

Blood for Transfusion. Yes.

Radiographic Control. Yes.

Special Apparatus. Complete Ilizarov set.

Patient Position. Supine.

Operative Technique

Preconstruction of the Apparatus

A. and **B.** The apparatus is constructed before surgery according to measurements on the patient's leg and radiograms. In difficult cases, make a plastic model of the leg and preconstruct the apparatus on the model. Preoperative planning is vital.

The apparatus consists of these components:

1. The *proximal ring block* comprises a proximal ⅝ ring (to allow knee flexion) and a full ring. The two are connected by three 40-mm. hexagonal sockets attached to the rings by short bolts on either side. The middle hexagonal socket is placed directly in the middle, whereas the other two sockets are placed at the ends of the ⅝ ring.

2. The *distal ring block* consists of two full rings connected by one 40-mm. hexagonal socket placed anteriorly and another 40-mm. hexagonal socket placed posteriorly on equivalent holes on either side of the ring.

3. The *middle transport segment* consists of a single transport ring with two long threaded rods appropriate to the length of the patient's tibia and a 20-mm. socket at one of its ends locked with a nut.

Connect the *distal block* to the middle block with threaded rods anteriorly and posteriorly. All of the fixation rods and sockets connecting the rings together are anterior and posterior. The threaded rods are attached to the ring one hole away from the central bolt connecting the two half-rings together, and the hexagonal sockets are one hole away from the central bolt on the other side.

Connect the *proximal block* of rings to the middle transport rings by bolts fixed to the socket; the connection is one hole away from the central bolt.

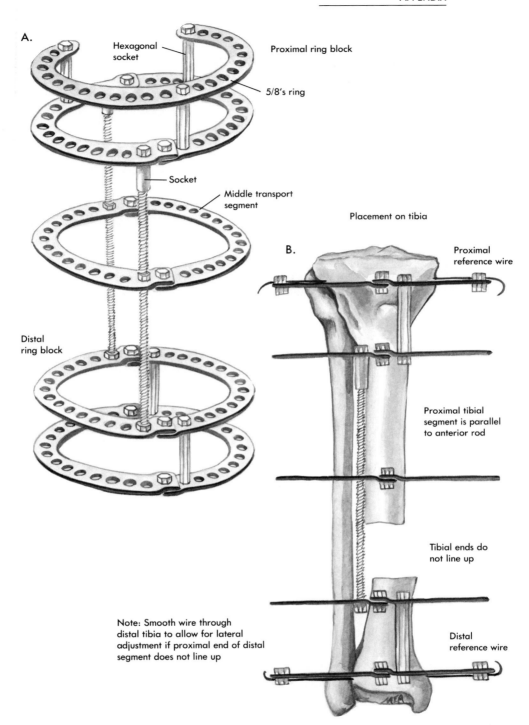

A.

Hexagonal
socket

Proximal ring block

5/8's ring

Socket

Middle transport
segment

Placement on tibia

B.

Proximal
reference wire

Proximal tibial
segment is parallel
to anterior rod

Distal
ring block

Tibial ends do
not line up

Note: Smooth wire through
distal tibia to allow for lateral
adjustment if proximal end of distal
segment does not line up

Distal
reference wire

Plate 256. **A.–L.,** Treatment of pseudarthosis (non-union) by bone transport using Ilizarov technique.

C. On the lateral view of the completed apparatus on the leg, the fixation rods and sockets are directly anterior and posterior to the tibia. The anterior rod is parallel to the anterior crest of the tibia, and there are two fingerbreadths of space between the skin and the rings.

Reference Wires

D. First, insert the most proximal wire; it is an olive wire drilled from the lateral side parallel to the knee joint and perpendicular to the proximal tibial segment.

Second, apply the apparatus on the patient's leg and insert the most distal wire. It is a smooth 1.8-mm. wire parallel to the ankle joint. Adjust the frame so that the proximal block of rings and the distal block of rings are parallel to each; this is made simple by having the most distal wire smooth. It allows mediolateral translation of the distal segment of the tibia. The central bolts connecting the half-rings are aligned along the crest of the tibia proximally and distally. Be sure that the anterior threaded rod connecting the rings is parallel to the crest of the tibia both in the anterior and lateral projections.

Next, insert two more wires, one for the second ring proximally and the other for the second ring from the bottom. These are olive wires directed in the frontal plane and inserted from the medial side. Be sure that there is no sag of the most distal ring. The tibial segments should be anatomically aligned. The rings are parallel to each other, and the anterior rod is parallel to the crest of the tibia.

C.

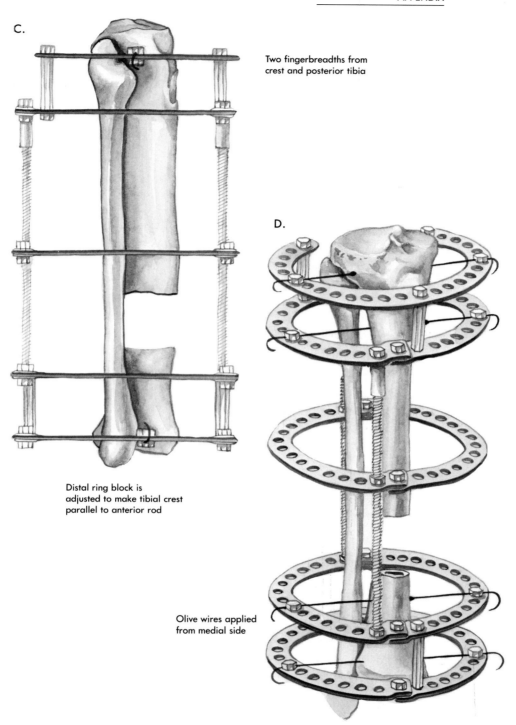

Two fingerbreadths from
crest and posterior tibia

D.

Distal ring block is
adjusted to make tibial crest
parallel to anterior rod

Olive wires applied
from medial side

Plate 256. (Continued)

Proximal Segment Fixation

E. First, insert a wire from the lateral side into the fibular head. Direct it obliquely across the tibia to exit inferiorly toward the second ring to which it is fixed. This wire is a cross between the two rings, providing greater stability of fixation.

Caution! Avoid injury to the common peroneal nerve.

An alternative (not illustrated) is to direct the wire horizontally from the fibular head across the tibia to be fixed to the ⅝ ring.

Second, insert a wire for the second ring from the top parallel to the medial cortex of the tibia parallel to the medial face of the tibia. The fibular wire and the medial tibial face wire for the second ring are about at right angles to each other, providing maximal stability of fixation.

Wire Fixation of the Distal Block of Rings

F. First, insert an olive wire parallel to the medial face of the tibia, between the tendons of the anterior tibial and extensor hallucis longus and exiting posteromedially.

Second, insert a wire through the fibula and direct it to exit anteromedially through the tibia. These two wires should be perpendicular to each other to provide maximal stability of fixation.

Wire Fixation of the Transport Ring

G. Position the ring in the correct location. It should be 4 to 5 cm. proximal to the lower end of the proximal fragment, and there should be enough length of bone between the distal ring and the transport ring to allow compression.

Insert these wires through the transport ring. All the wires are smooth and are 1.5 mm., not 1.8 mm., the size that was used for fixation of the proximal and distal pair of rings. Insert the wires on the transport ring in cruciate fashion.

Insert the first wire on the medial surface of the tibia. The second wire is inserted just anterior to the fibula and directed to exit on the medial side of the tibia. The third wire is a drop wire, attached to posts and suspended superior to the ring. Tension the drop wire to only 80 or 90 kg. The rest of the wires are tightened and tensioned to 130 kg.

E.   Proximal segment fixation

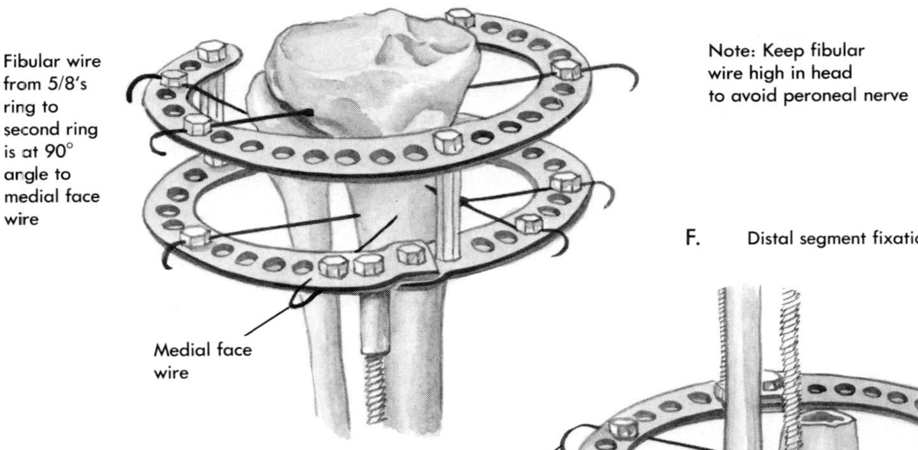

Fibular wire
from 5/8's
ring to
second ring
is at 90°
angle to
medial face
wire

Note: Keep fibular
wire high in head
to avoid peroneal nerve

F.   Distal segment fixation

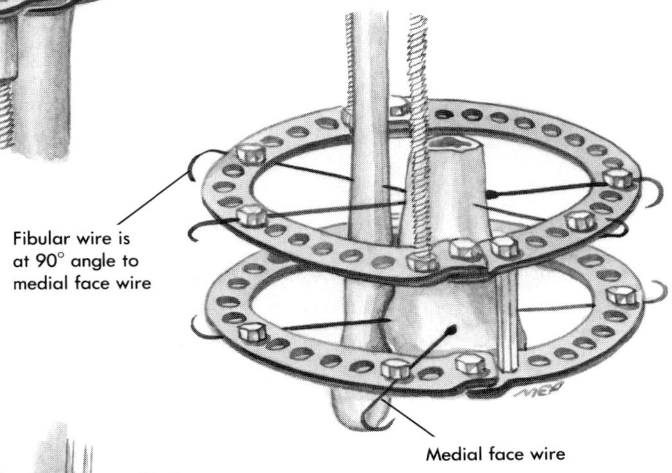

Medial face
wire

Fibular wire is
at 90° angle to
medial face wire

Medial face wire

G.   Transport ring fixation

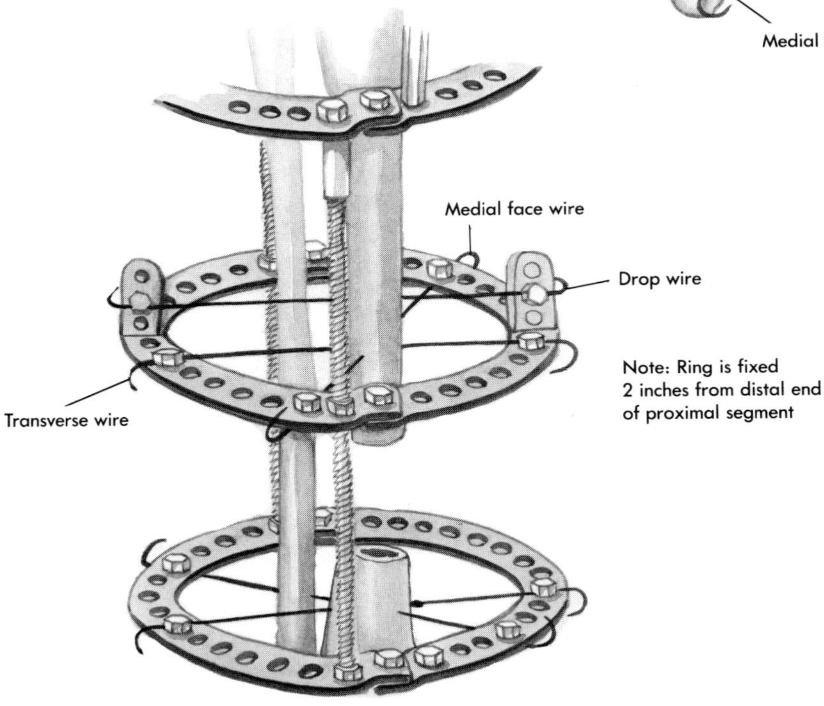

Medial face wire

Drop wire

Note: Ring is fixed
2 inches from distal end
of proximal segment

Transverse wire

Plate 256. (Continued)

Preparation for Corticotomy

H. Insert additional threaded rods medially and laterally between the transport ring and the second ring from below the distal block of rings. The rods are inserted through the same numbered holes and tightened with bolts. This connection converts the transport ring and the distal pair of rings into one solid block.

Next, disconnect the distal block of three rings from the proximal block of rings by removing the short post connected to the socket. Back up the socket out of the way to allow room for exposure of the anteromedial surface of the proximal tibia for corticotomy and rotational osteoclasis.

Prior to corticotomy, check the stability of fixation of the proximal block of rings. Wiggle the proximal block ("toggle test"). If the fixation is stable and rigid on flexion-extension and varus-valgus stress, the proximal block of rings and the upper segment of the tibia move in one piece. *It is essential that there be no motion between the two, as the rest of the apparatus levers on the proximal fixation after corticotomy.*

Corticotomy

I. See the Ilizarov technique (Plate 250, p. 1450). Make a 1-cm.-long longitudinal incision over the anterior crest of the tibia. The periosteum is incised and elevated medially and laterally. Insert a 1-cm.-wide sharp osteotome, and divide the anterior cortex of the tibia. Then insert a 5-mm.-wide sharp osteotome under the protection of the periosteum; section the medial cortex and, similarly, the lateral cortex of the tibia.

Take a wrench, and turn the 5-mm. osteotome 90 degrees. First spread apart the divided posteromedial and, following similar technique, the posterolateral cortices of the tibia. This maneuver, mimicking a laminar spread, cracks open the posterior wall of the cortex. Perform a rotational osteoclasis; twist the distal block *laterally.*

Under image intensifier radiography, confirm the completeness of corticotomy. An alternate method of sectioning of the posterior cortex is to use a Gigli saw.

H.   Preparation for corticotomy

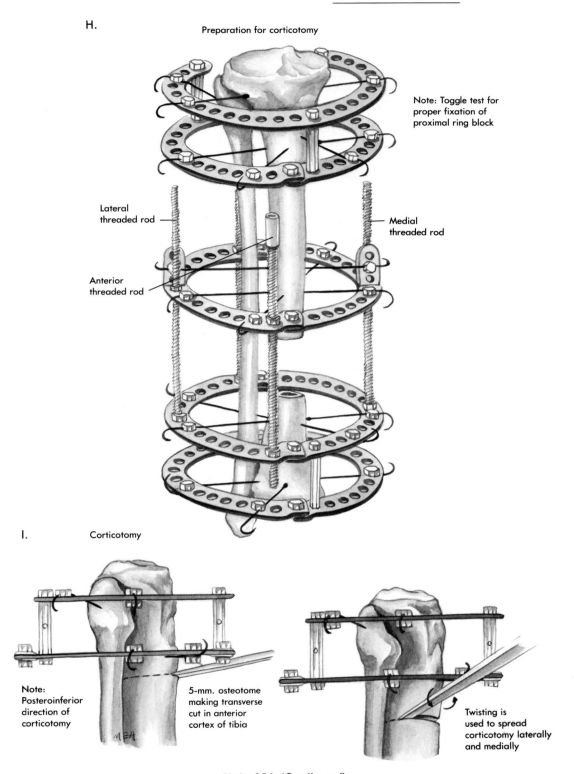

Note: Toggle test for
proper fixation of
proximal ring block

Lateral
threaded rod

Medial
threaded rod

Anterior
threaded rod

I.   Corticotomy

Note:
Posteroinferior
direction of
corticotomy

5-mm. osteotome
making transverse
cut in anterior
cortex of tibia

Twisting is
used to spread
corticotomy laterally
and medially

Plate 256. (Continued)

Reconstruction of the Apparatus in Preparation for Transport

J. Reposition the upper bone segments to their pre-corticotomy position, and reattach the transport ring (with the distal pair of rings) to the proximal pair of rings by connecting the socket to the hole to which it was fixed originally. Connect the medial, lateral, and posterior threaded rods to their original holes. Be sure that rotational alignment of the tibial segments is anatomic and that the entire bone transport apparatus is rigidly fixed.

Transport and Compression at the Docking Site

K. The middle bone segment is transported distally following the technique described in tibial lengthening. It is best to use graduated telescoping rods.

When contact is made between the middle and distal tibial bone segments, continue to advance the transport segment ring and apply compression at the non-union site. When adequate compression is applied, the wires will become bowed and the transport ring will be slightly more advanced than its wires.

Stabilization of the Proximal Block Ring Fixation by Insertion of a Half-Pin Anteriorly

L. This is often indicated when there is a major segmental loss of the tibia.

Insert one half-pin anteriorly, and fix it by combining a buckle and a two-hole post.

Postoperative Care. When the non-union site and regenerated bone between the proximal and middle tibial segments is adequately healed, the fixation is decompressed for two to three weeks and then removed (see Plate 158, p. 896). Modifications are made as required by the soft-tissue pathology. External support to the leg in the form of a knee-ankle-foot orthosis (KAFO) or ankle-foot orthosis (AFO) is utilized for three to six months.

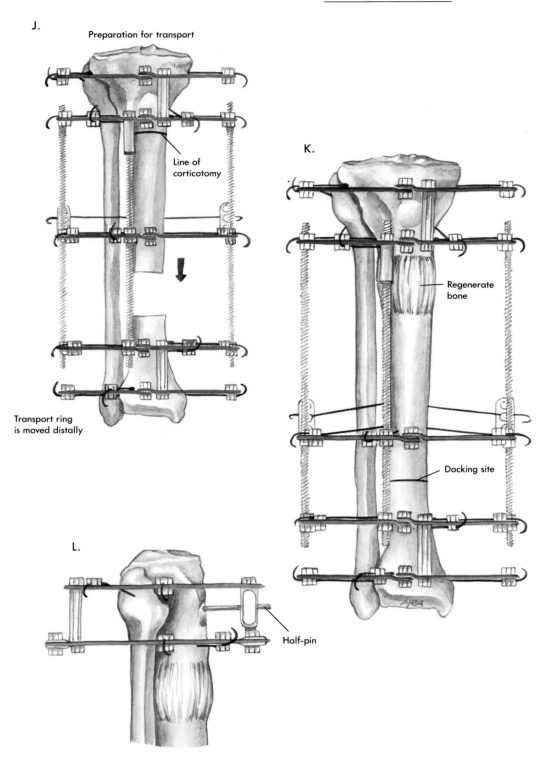

J.

Preparation for transport

Line of corticotomy

Transport ring is moved distally

K.

Regenerate bone

Docking site

L.

Half-pin

Plate 256. (Continued)

Index

Note: Page numbers in *italics* refer to illustrations; page numbers in **boldface** refer to surgical plates. Roman numerals refer to the principles of practice preceding Chapter 1.

I

ISBN 0-7216-5449-5